Reproductive BIOLOGY

Reproductive
BIOLOGY

GAYATRI PRAKASH

Alpha Science International Ltd.
Oxford, U.K.

Gayatri Prakash
Department of Zoology
Daulat Ram College
Delhi University
Delhi 110 007, India

Alpha Science International Ltd.
7200 The Quorum, Oxford Business Park North
Garsington Road, Oxford OX4 2JZ, U.K.

www.alphasci.com

ISBN 978-1-84265-416-3

Printed in India

Preface

This book on reproductive biology and human welfare represents a complete textbook in the field of reproduction based on more than three decade of teaching undergraduate students of Zoology, Biology, Physiology, Medicine, and Veterinary Sciences at the University of Delhi as well as to provide a source of basic information for postgraduate students and research workers. The book has been designed in such a way as to cover the entire syllabus of various universities.

The book consists of Twenty Nine Chapters in all. The first twenty-seven chapters divided into Four Parts cover various aspects of reproduction and the remaining chapters give the acronyms and the glossary.

The first part deals with various aspects of endocrinology such as its basic concepts, hormones, hypothalamus and pituitary, pituitary hormones, steroids, prostaglandin, and mechanism of hormone action.

The second part deals with the biology of reproduction. It covers development and differentiation of genital system, biology of sex, germ cells and gamete formation, puberty, adolescence and menopause. This part gives detailed account of male reproductive system and physiology of the epididymis and accessory glands of reproduction, and also of female reproductive system along with its physiological aspects which include reproductive cycles, ovulation, fertilization, implantation, pregnancy, parturition and lactation.

Part three of this book is on reproductive health and human welfare. It deals with infertility, assisted reproductive technologies, contraception and abortion and demographic terminologies used in family planning in addition to certain important topics such as AIDS and Cancer, which have been included keeping in view the general interest in these topics in the present day world.

The fourth part on animal husbandry covers techniques of improving reproductive efficiency in farm animals and effects of nutrition on reproduction and poultry.

Acknowledgements

I am very grateful to my students who provided me the motivation to write this book. I owe my sincere thanks to my husband, Dr. Jai Prakash and our children, Dr. Amol Prakash and Mrs. Ela Goyal for the continued help and encouragement at every stage during the preparation of the manuscript. Their untiring efforts had enabled me to complete this vast project. I thank all the publishers who allowed me to use the photographs.

Contents

Part IV: Animal Husbandry

Part I

Introduction to Endocrinology

- Basic Concepts of Endocrinology
- Hormones
- The Hypothalamus
- The Pituitary
- Sex Steroids
- Prostaglandins
- Hormone Action

Chapter 1

Basic Concepts of Endocrinology

1.1 The Endocrine and Nervous Systems

There are two linking systems in vertebrate's body which co-ordinate functions of all the organs of the biological systems. These are the **endocrine** and the **nervous systems**. Both of these are the major means by which the body communicates information between different cells and tissues, and the transmitted information results in the regulation of numerous body functions. The nervous system coordinates the activities of the body through **nerve impulses** and **neurotransmitters** while the endocrine system does so through the mediator molecules called **hormones**. Hormones are chemical messengers that are released from cells into the blood stream to exert their action some distance away on the target cells. These blood-borne messengers of the endocrine system (the hormones) can be distinguished from the neurotransmitters, which are the chemical messengers released from neurons into a synapse between the nerve and its effecter cell, such as muscle cells, secretory cells or other neurons (Figure 1.1). However, the endocrine system does not act alone-it interacts with the nervous system to coordinate and integrate the activities of body cells. The regulatory controls in terms of mediator molecules, speed, duration of action etc. used by these two systems are very different. Table1.1 compares the characteristics of these two systems.

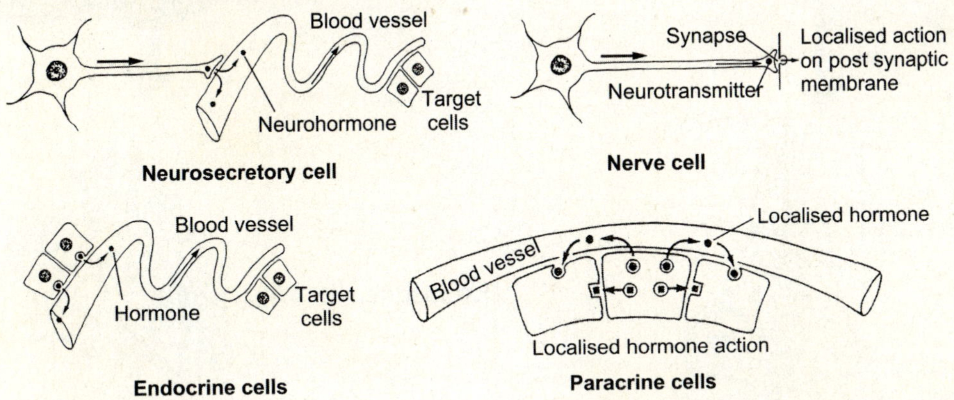

Figure 1.1: Types of chemical communication between cells.

The nervous system regulates the activity of muscles and glands via electrochemical impulses delivered by neurons and these organs respond within milliseconds. On the other hand, the endocrine system influences the metabolic activities of cells by means of hormones, and the tissues or organ responses to hormones typically occur after a lag period of seconds or even days. But once initiated, these responses tend to be much more prolonged than those induced by the nervous system. It must be mentioned here that a type of localized chemical communication between cells occurs in some tissues through the chemical messenger, which is not transported any distance in blood but acts in a highly circumscribed area. These secretory cells are not true endocrine cells and are termed **paracrine cells** (Figure 1.1). Further, as a result of histochemical studies pioneered in the 1940s, it emerged that certain nerve cells are neurosecretory, that is, they release chemical agents called neurohormones into the blood. However, distinction between neurotransmitter, neurohormones, and hormone may not always be obvious on the basis of chemical identity alone, and the same substance may possess different functions in different body tissues.

Table 1.1: Characteristics of the nervous and endocrine systems

System Characteristic	Nervous System	Endocrine System
Mediator molecules	Neurotransmitters released in response to nerve impulses	Hormones delivered by blood to tissues throughout the body
Cells affected	Muscle cells, gland cells, other Neurons	Virtually all body cells
Time of onset of action	Typically within milliseconds	Varies from seconds to days
Duration of action	Generally brief	Generally longer

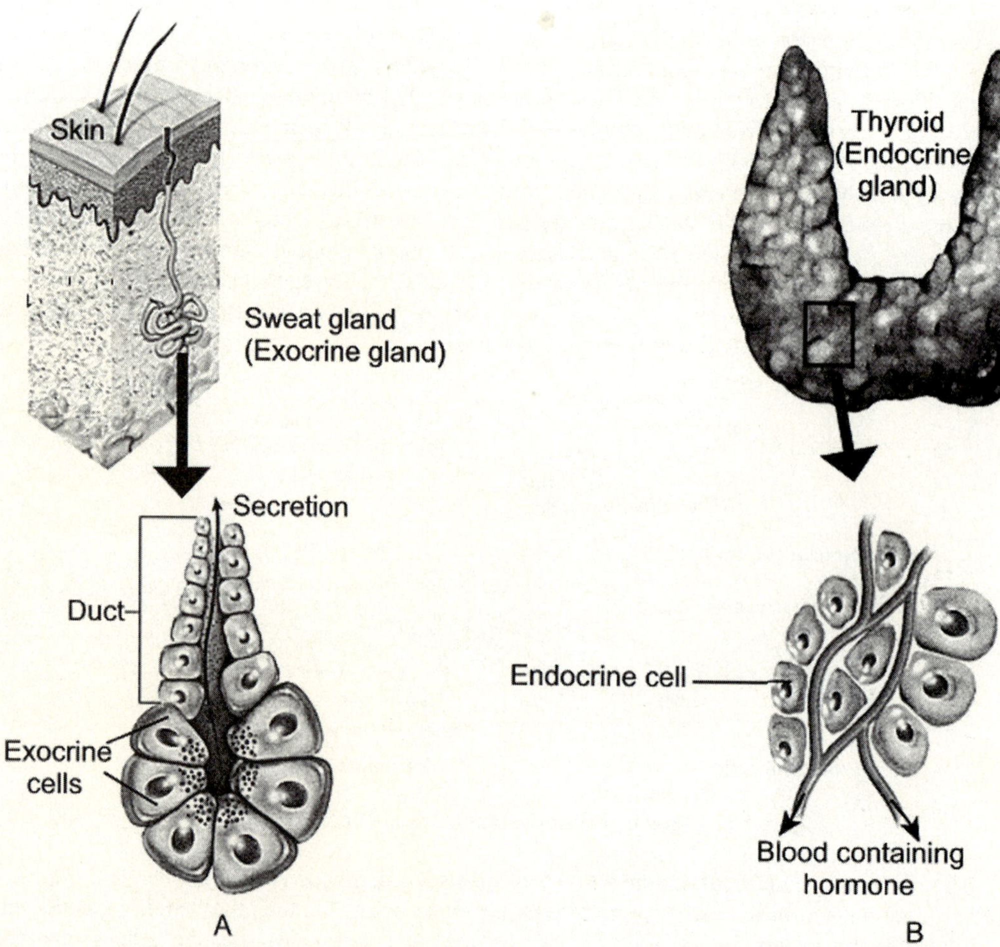

Figure 1.2: Exocrine (A) and endocrine (B) glands.

The endocrine system includes a number of glands that secrete hormones into body fluids (internal environment). The scientific study of the structure and function of endocrine glands is called **endocrinology** (endo = with in; *-crin* = to secrete; *-ology* = study of) and Thomas Addison is the father of endocrinology.

1.2 Exocrine and Endocrine glands

The glands of the vertebrates fall into two distinct categories: i) **exocrine glands**, and ii) **endocrine glands** (Figure 1.2). Exocrine (*exo* = outside, *-crine*=to secrete) glands have ducts and secrete their non-hormonal products via ducts into lumen of an organ, into body cavities, or to the outer surface of the body, e.g. digestive glands, mucous glands, sebaceous and sudoriferous glands (Figure 1.2 A). In contrast, endocrine (*endo* = within; *-crine* = to secrete) glands release their products called hormones into the surrounding tissue fluid rather than into ducts and therefore, are also called as **ductless glands** (Figure 1.2 B). Endocrine glands typically have a rich vascular and lymphatic drainage for secreting their hormones. Further, most hormone-producing cells are arranged in cords and branching networks in a manner that maximizes the contact between them and the surrounding capillaries.

1.3 Glands of Endocrine System

The endocrine glands are scattered throughout the body (Figure 1.3). **Glands of endocrine system** whose functions are solely endocrine in nature are **pituitary (hypophysis)**, **thyroid**, **parathyroid**, **adrenal**, **pineal**, and **thymus** glands. In addition, several organs of the body contain discrete areas of endocrine tissue and produce hormones and also exocrine products and therefore, are not exclusively endocrine glands. These include **pancreas** and **gonads** (the **ovaries** and **testes**). These are also major endocrine glands. The **hypothalamus** also falls into this category. Along with its neural functions, it produces and releases hormones and is therefore, considered a **neuroendocrine organ.** Compared to other organs of the body, the organs of endocrine system are small. In addition, the anatomical continuity typical of most organ systems of the body does not exist between the endocrine glands. Instead, they are widely scattered in the body. Location of the major endocrine glands of the body is shown in Figure 1.3, and the hormones produced by them are shown in Table 1.2. Details of the major endocrine glands in mammals, human in particular is described below:

Hypothalamus: Hypothalamus is a region of the diencephalon (a part of brain) that includes many nuclei. It derives its name due to its position below the thalamus. It caps the top of the brain stem and forms the inferolateral walls of the third ventricle. Merging into the midbrain inferiorly, hypothalamus extends from the optic chiasma to the posterior margin of the mammillary bodies. Between the optic chiasma and mammillary bodies exists the **infundibulum**, a stalk of the hypothalamic tissue that connects the **pituitary gland** to the base of the hypothalamus. Nerve fibers connect the hypothalamus to the cerebral cortex, thalamus, and parts of the brain stem so that it can receive impulses from them and send impulses to them. The hypothalamus helps to maintain homeostasis by regulating a variety of brain functions such as body temperature, appetite, thirst, sexual behavior, body rhythms, defensive reactions, and also by linking the nervous and endocrine systems. The hypothalamus contains two types of neurosecretory cells that propagate action potentials, and release hormones. These are regulated by inputs of both hormonal and central nervous systems. **Hypophysiotropic neurons** secrete releasing and inhibiting hormones into the median eminence and regulate the hormonal output of the anterior pituitary. **Neurohypophyseal neurons** traverse the hypothalamic-pituitary stalk and synthesize two hormones called vasopressin and oxytocin and export them to the posterior pituitary for storage and later release.

Pituitary Gland (Hypophysis): Bean shaped pituitary gland is securely sealed in the cavity called **sella turcica** of the sphenoid bone (cavity of the third ventricle). The tiny pituitary gland secretes at least nine major hormones, which are mentioned below. Its funnel shaped stalk, **infundibulum**, connects it superiorly to the hypothalamus. In humans, the pituitary gland has two major lobes an **anterior** and a **posterior**. A third region called **pars intermedia** or **intermediate lobe** atrophies during fetal development and ceases to exist as a separate lobe in adults. However, some of its cells migrate into adjacent parts of the anterior pituitary gland where they persist.

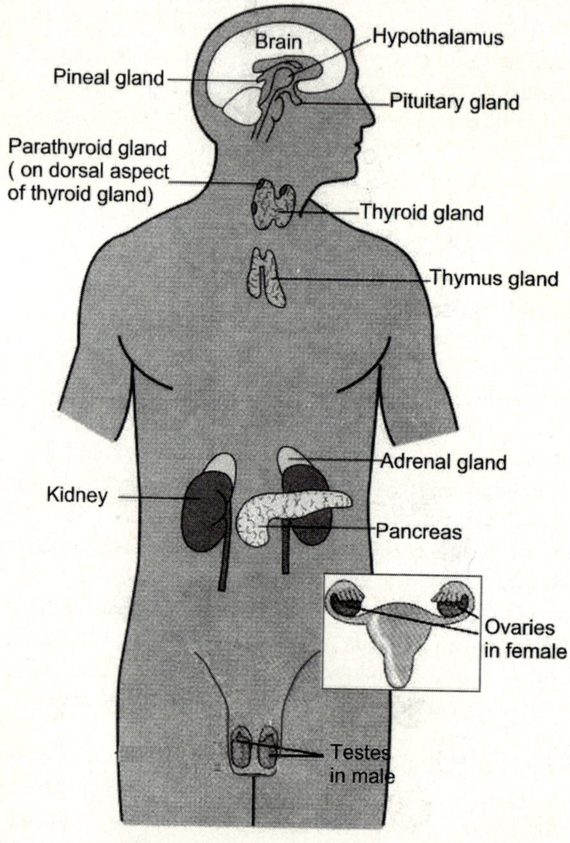

Figure 1.3: Locations of major endocrine glands in Human.

The **anterior lobe or adenohypophysis** is composed of glandular tissue. It manufactures and releases six hormones. These are **Growth hormone (GH), Thyroid-stimulating hormone (TSH), Adrenocorticotropic hormone (ACTH), Follicle stimulating hormone (FSH), Luteinizing hormone (LH)** and **Prolactin (PRL)**. Four of these (TSH, ACTH, FSH, and LH) are **trophic (tropic) hormones** or **tropins**, since these regulate the functions of other endocrine glands. The **posterior lobe** is composed of neural tissue and together with infundibulum make up the region called the **neurohypophysis.** The axon terminals in the posterior pituitary gland are associated with specialized neuroglia called **pituicytes**. Posterior pituitary releases two neurohormones, **oxytocin** and **anti-diuretic hormone** (ADH) or **vasopressin**, which it receives ready-made from the hypothalamus via **hypothalamohypophyseal tract**. Thus posterior lobe of the pituitary is in reality a hormone storage area and not a true endocrine gland in the precise sense. During fetal development, a narrow region appears between the anterior and posterior lobes of the pituitary gland called the **intermediate lobe** or **pars intermedia**. This region produces **melanocyte-stimulating hormone (MSH)**.

Thyroid Gland: The butterfly-shaped thyroid gland is composed of two lobes. It is located just inferior to the larynx in the neck region (Figure 1.3). Its right and left lateral **lobes** lie on either side of the trachea. A mass of tissue called **isthmus** lying anterior to trachea connects the two lobes of the thyroid gland. This gland is made up of **thyroid follicles** filled with a secretory substance called **colloid**. The wall of each follicle consists of follicular cells and the secretions of these thyroid cells are stored within this colloid. Thyroid gland secretes two hormones, namely, **thyroxine** or **tetraiodothyronine (T_4)** and **triiodothyronine (T_3)**. Thyroid hormones affect the general metabolism of the body.

Table 1.2: Hormones produced by major endocrine glands and their abbreviations

Gland		Hormone (Abbreviation)
Hypothalamus		Corticotropin-releasing hormone (CRH)
		Gonadotropin- releasing hormone (GnRH)
		Growth hormone release-inhibiting hormone (GIH)
		Growth hormone-releasing hormone (GHRH) / Somatostatin (SS)
		Prolactin release-inhibiting hormone (PIH)
		Prolactin-releasing hormone (PRH)
		Thyrotropin-releasing hormone (TRH)
Pituitary	Anterior	Growth hormone (GH) / Somatotropin (STH)
		Follicle-Stimulating hormone (FSH) / Follitropin
		Luteinizing hormone (LH) / Interstitial cell stimulating hormone (ICSH) / Lutropin
		Corticotropin / Adrenocorticotropic hormone (ACTH)
		Thyroid- Stimulating hormone (TSH) / Thyrotropin
		Prolactin (PRL)
	Intermediate	Melanocyte-stimulating hormone (MSH)
	Posterior	Antidiuretic hormone (ADH) / Vasopressin
		Oxytocin (OT)
Thyroid		Thyroxin (T_4)
		Triiodothyronine (T_3)
Parathyroid		Parathyroid Hormone (PTH) / Parathormone
Adrenal	Cortex	Mineralocorticoid (Aldosterone)
		Glucocorticoid (Cortisol)
		Gonadocorticoid-androgen
	Medulla	Epinephrine (EPI) / Adrenalin
		Norepinephrine (NE) / Noradrenalin
Pancreas		Glucagon
		Insulin
		Somatostatin (SS)
Testes		Testosterone (T)
Ovaries		Estrogen (E)
		Progesterone (P)

Parathyroid Glands: Sandstrom described parathyroid glands first in 1880. These are small, round masses of tissue, usually one superior and one inferior and are attached to each lateral lobe of the thyroid gland. They secrete **parathyroid hormone (PTH)** also known as **parathormone**. Parathyroid hormone acts on bones and kidneys and regulates the blood calcium level.

Adrenal Glands: The adrenals are flattened pyramid shaped, paired glands lying superior to each kidney, and therefore, also known as **suprarenal glands**. During embryonic development, the adrenal glands differentiate into two structurally and functionally distinct regions. The large peripherally located region called **adrenal cortex** develops from the mesoderm and the small centrally located region called **adrenal medulla** develops from the ectoderm. The adrenal cortex produces **steroid hormones** such as **mineralocorticoid (aldosterone), glucocorticoid (cortisol)** and **gonadocorticoids (weak androgens)**. The adrenal medulla produces two **catecholamines** and these are **epinephrine (adrenaline)** and **norepinephrine (nor adrenaline)**. Catecholamines are any catechol-derived compound (such as adrenaline or dopamine), which exerts an action similar to that of sympathetic nervous system. Hormones of adrenal glands exert variety of effects in the body. Aldosterone maintains the electrolyte balance of different ions in the blood. It increases absorption of sodium and chloride ions and secretion of potassium and hydrogen ions. Cortisol has metabolic function, anti-inflammatory function, anti-allergic effect and other systemic effects. Catecholamines show effects on heart, blood pressure and peripheral circulation. Both adrenaline and nor adrenaline cause an increase in free fatty acid (FFA) content in blood and basal metabolic rate (BMR). They increase blood pressure and blood sugar concentration.

Pancreas: The pancreas is located within the curve of the duodenum. It is a compound gland and therefore, functions both as an endocrine gland and also as an exocrine gland. The exocrine part consists of lobules or acini and produce digestive enzymes. Scattered among these exocrine acini are tiny clusters of endocrine tissue called **pancreatic islets or islets of Langerhans.** Among pancreatic islet, **alpha** or **A cell** secretes hormone **glucagon, beta** or **B cells** secrete hormone **insulin**, and **delta** or D cells secrete hormone **somatostatin**. Glucagon hormone raises blood glucose level while insulin hormone lowers blood glucose level. Thus, interplay of these two hormones maintains the blood sugar levels to normalcy. On the other hand, somatostatin inhibits the secretion of glucagon, insulin, growth hormone, thyroid stimulating hormone (TSH) and also has effects on gut and central nervous system (CNS).

Gonads: Gonads represent a pair of **testes *in* males** and a pair of **ovaries** in **females**. The **testes** are oval structures lying inside the scrotum. They produce male hormone called **testosterone**. The **ovaries** are also paired oval structures but located in the pelvic cavity. They produce female sex hormones called **estrogens** and **progesterone**. The male and female sex hormones promote the growth, development and maintenance of gonads and accessory glands of reproduction. They also regulate the development of secondary sex characteristics in male and female respectively.

Pineal Gland: It is a small endocrine gland attached to the roof of the third ventricle of the brain at the midline. Pineal gland is also called as **epiphysis**. Histologically, it consists of thin walled parenchymatous cells. It contains high concentration of serotonin (5 hydroxytryptamine) and an enzyme called hydroxy-indole-o-methyl transferase (HIOMT), which converts serotonin to melatonin. The pineal gland therefore, secretes **melatonin**, an amine hormone derived from serotonin. The function of pineal gland in adult humans is yet unknown as it atrophies at the age of seven years. It may function as a neuroendocrine transducer, mediating the effects of light on gonads.

Thymus Gland: In mammals' thymus gland is located in the mediastinum just in front of the heart in the thorax region between the lungs. It is large and conspicuous in infants and young children but diminishes in size with age. Thymus gland weighs about 10-12 gm at birth, about 20-30 gms in adolescence, and only 3-6 gm in old age. Thymus is endodermal in origin and is composed largely of adipose and fibrous connective tissues and lymphocytes. Thymus is essentially a lymphoid organ. The major hormonal product of the thymus epithelial cells is a family of peptide hormones, including

thymopoietins (thymin) and **thymosins**. These are essential for the normal development of T lymphocytes or T cells and the immune response.

Endocrine glands and the hormones help to regulate metabolic processes in the body. They control the rates of certain chemical reactions, aid in transporting substances through membranes, and help to regulate water balance, electrolyte balance, and blood pressure etc. in the body. They also play vital roles in development, growth and reproduction.

Endocrine glands are derived from all three embryonic germ layers. While the mesoderm-derived endocrine glands produce steroid hormones, all others produce amines or amino acid and protein hormones.

Endocrine glands function smoothly throughout life until old age. However, aging may bring about changes in the rates of hormone secretion, their breakdown and excretion, or in the sensitivity of target cell receptors to their respective hormones.

Various other tissues and organs in the mammalian body also produce hormones. For example, pockets of hormone-producing cells are found in the walls of stomach, small intestine (duodenum), kidneys, heart, liver, skin and placenta. Placenta is a temporary endocrine organ formed during pregnancy. Details of such hormones are given in Table 1.3 along with their effects on the human body.

Table 1.3: Hormones produced by organs other than major endocrine glands and their effects on Human

Source and Chemical composition	Hormone	Target organ	Effect
Stomach (Peptide)	Gastrin	Stomach	Stimulates glands to release hydrochloric acid (HCl)
	Serotonin	Stomach	Causes contraction of stomach muscles
Duodenum (Peptide)	Intestinal gastrin	Stomach	Inhibits HCl secretion and gastrointestinal tract mobility
	Secretin	Pancreas	Stimulates release of bicarbonate-rich juice
		Liver	Increases release of bile
		Stomach	Inhibits secretory activity
	Cholecystokinin (CCK)	Pancreas	Stimulates release of enzyme-rich juice
		Gall bladder	Stimulates expulsion of stored bile
		Sphincter of Oddi	Causes sphincter to relax, allowing bile and pancreatic juice to enter duodenum
Kidney (Glycoprotein)	Erythropoietin (EPO)	Bone marrow	Stimulates production of red blood cells
Skin-epidermal cells (Steroid)	Cholecalciferol (provitamin D_3)	Intestine	Stimulates active transport of dietary calcium across intestinal cell membrane
Heart-atria (Peptide)	Atrial natriuretic peptide (ANP)	Kidney	Inhibits sodium ion resorption and renin release
		Adrenal cortex	Inhibits secretion of aldosterone, decreases blood pressure

1.4 Hypophysiotropic Hormones, Tropic Hormones and Target Glands

In the endocrine system, while a single gland has its own independent functions, the interdependence of various glands is of equal importance. The release of hormones by one gland may be dependent on the release of a hormone from another gland. For example, pituitary gland affects the hormonal activity of adrenal cortex, thyroid, and gonads etc. The pituitary hormones that have this control over other endocrine glands are called **tropic hormones**, while the glands influenced by the pituitary secretions are called the **target glands**. The pituitary gland in turn is controlled by the humoral factors released by the hypothalamus, called **hypophysiotropic factors**. These factors are inhibitory or stimulatory to pituitary secretions and therefore, are known as inhibiting releasing hormone/factor and stimulatory releasing hormone/factor respectively.

1.5 Endocrine Gland Stimuli

The endocrine glands are stimulated to manufacture and release their hormones by three major types of stimuli. These are i) humoral, ii) neural, and iii) hormonal. Endocrine gland stimuli are shown in Figure 1.4

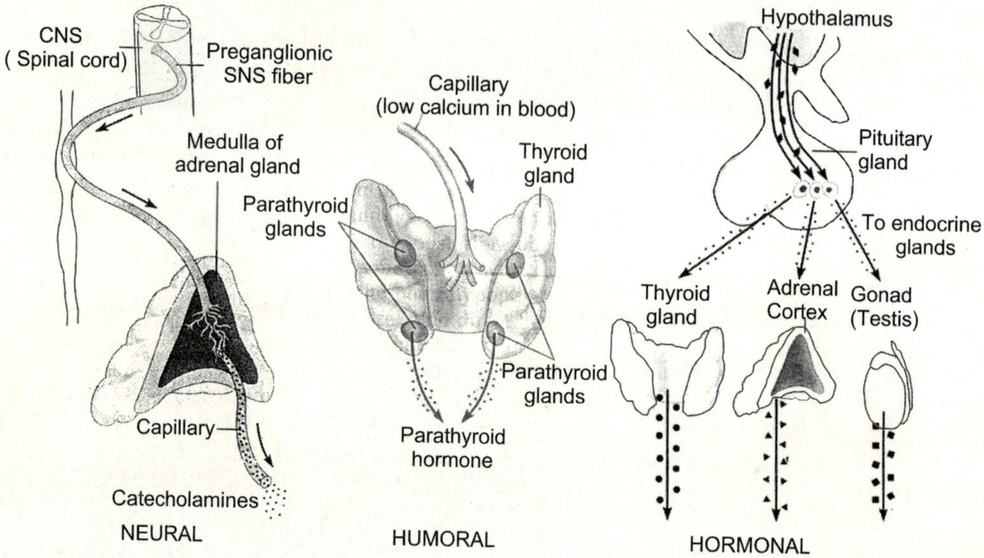

Figure 1.4: Three major types of endocrine gland stimuli-Neural, Humoral and Hormonal.

Neural Stimuli: In a few cases, nerve fibers stimulate hormone release. The example is sympathetic nervous system (SNS) stimulation of the adrenal medulla to release catecholamines (epinephrine and norepinephrine) during periods of stress. Also, oxytocin and anti-diuretic hormone are released from the posterior pituitary in response to nerve impulses from hypothalamic neurons.

Humoral Stimuli: Some endocrine glands secrete their hormones in direct response to changing concentration of certain ions and nutrients in blood. These stimuli are called humoral stimuli to distinguish them from hormonal stimuli, which are also blood borne chemicals. The term humoral dates back to the ancient use of the word humor, as it refers to various body fluids (blood, bile, and others). This is the simplest of the endocrine control systems. For example, cells of the parathyroid glands directly monitor the concentration of calcium ions in blood and when they detect a decline from normal Ca++ values, they secrete parathyroid hormone (PTH). Since PTH acts by several routes to reverse that decline, blood Ca++ levels soon rise, ending the initiative for PTH release. Other hormones released in response to humoral stimuli include insulin, produced by the pancreas, and aldosterone, one of the adrenal cortex hormones.

Hormonal Stimuli: Many endocrine glands release their hormones in response to hormones produced by other endocrine organs. For example, releasing and inhibiting hormones produced by the hypothalamus regulates release of most of the anterior pituitary hormones. And further, many anterior pituitary hormones in turn stimulate other endocrine glands to release their hormones into the blood.

As the hormones produced by the final target gland increase in the blood, they inhibit the release of anterior pituitary hormones and thus their own release (feedback inhibition). The hormonal mechanism promotes rhythmic hormone release, with the rising and falling levels of hormone in blood in a specific pattern.

While these three stimuli mechanisms typify most systems that control hormone release, yet they are by no means all-inclusive or mutually exclusive, and some endocrine glands respond to multiple stimuli. Both "turn on" factors (humoral, hormonal and neural stimuli) and "turn off" factors (feedback inhibition) may be modified or modulated by the nervous system. The nervous system can, in certain cases, override normal endocrine controls as needed to maintain homeostasis. For example, blood sugar levels are normally kept within a range of 90-110 mg glucose per 100 ml of blood by the action of insulin and several other hormones. However, when the body is under severe stress, blood sugar levels rise much higher because the hypothalamus and sympathetic nervous system centers are strongly activated. This ensures that body cells will have sufficient fuel for the more vigorous activity required of them during such periods.

Summary

The nervous and endocrine systems are the major controlling systems of the body. The nervous system exerts rapid controls via nerve impulses while endocrine system's effects are mediated by hormones and are more prolonged.

Glands in the body may be exocrine or endocrine.

The endocrine system consists of endocrine glands and several organs containing endocrine tissue. The endocrine glands are small and widely separated in the body.

Endocrine glands are ductless, and well vascularised. They release their products called hormones directly into the blood or lymph.

Major endocrine glands are pituitary, thyroid, parathyroid, adrenal, pineal, thymus, pancreas and gonads. The hypothalamus is a neuroendocrine organ.

Endocrine glands via hormones regulate many processes in the body such as reproduction, growth and development, maintenance of electrolyte, water and nutrient balance, mobilization of body defenses to stressors, and regulation of cellular metabolism.

Endocrine glands are derived from all three germ layers. Those derived from mesoderm produce steroidal hormones, while others produce the amino acid-based hormones.

The hypothalamus lies below the thalamus and extends from the optic chiasma to the posterior margin of the mammillary bodies. A stalk of the hypothalamic tissue connects the pituitary gland to the base of the hypothalamus.

Pituitary gland consists of a hormone-producing glandular portion (anterior pituitary) and a neural portion (posterior pituitary). Pituitary-hypothalamic relationship exists through hypophyseal portal system.

The thyroid gland is located in the anterior throat. Thyroid follicles store thyroglobulin, a colloid from which thyroid hormone is derived. Thyroid hormone includes thyroxine and triiodothyronine.

The parathyroid glands are located on the dorsal aspect of the thyroid gland. They secrete parathyroid hormone.

The paired adrenal (suprarenal) glands sit atop the kidneys. The adrenal gland has two functional portions, outer cortex and inner medulla. The cortex secretes mineralocorticoids (primarily aldosterone), glucocorticoids (primarily cortisol) and gonadocorticoids (mainly androgens). Adrenal medulla produces catecholamines, epinephrine and norepinephrine.

The pancreas located in the abdomen close to the stomach is both an exocrine and an endocrine gland. The endocrine portion (pancreatic islets) secretes insulin and glucagon.

The male gonads, testes are located in the scrotum. These secrete testosterone.

The female gonads, ovaries are located in the pelvic cavity. These release two hormones, estrogen and progesterone.

The pineal gland is located in the diencephalone. It produces hormone melatonin.

The Thymus gland lies posterior to the sternum and between the lungs. Its size diminishes with age. Its hormones, thymosins and thymopoietins, are important to the normal development of the immune response.

Besides major endocrine organs, various other tissues and organs also produce hormones

In the endocrine system, a single gland has its own independent functions, but of equal importance is the interdependence of various glands.

Endocrine glands operate smoothly throughout life until old age.

Endocrine glands are activated to release their hormones by humoral, neural, or hormonal stimuli. Nervous system, acting through hypothalamic controls, can in certain cases override or modulate hormonal effects.

Questions

1. Enumerate the characteristics of endocrine and nervous systems.
2. Contrast the control of homeostasis by the nervous and endocrine systems.
3. Distinguish between exocrine and endocrine glands.
4. List the major endocrine organs and give their location in the body.
5. Besides the major endocrine organs, what are the other hormone-producing cells clusters?
6. Explain how the nervous system controls hormonal secretion.
7. How endocrine glands are stimulated to release their hormones? Discuss all the phenomena in brief.
8. List the hormones secreted by cells in tissues and organs other than endocrine glands and give their functions.
9. What is the name of the endocrine portion of the pancreas?
10. Where is the pineal gland located? What is the function of the pineal gland?
11. The major stimulus for release of parathyroid hormone is a) hormonal, **b) humoral**, c) neural.

Chapter 2

Hormones

William M. Bayliss and his brother-in-law Ernest H. Starling, both of London University College in 1903 used the term 'hormone' for the first time while referring to a gastrointestinal tract hormone, secretin. Subsequently, a number of other hormones were discovered based on the principle that a chemical is responsible for many biological phenomena. These substances were then called as 'Chemical messengers'.

Hormone *(hormon* = to excite or get moving) is a chemical substance secreted by the glands of the endocrine system into blood stream and is virtually carried to all cells throughout the body. Hormones have powerful effects even in very low concentration and as a rule, affect only a few types of cells, called **target cells**.

2.1 Characteristics of hormones

The endocrine glands secrete hormones into the interstitial fluid surrounding the secretory cells. The secretion then diffuses into capillaries and is carried away by the blood to distant target organ or cell to exert its action. The concentration of a circulating hormone in blood at any time reflects its rate of release, and the speed of its inactivation and removal from the body. Enzymes within their target cells rapidly degrade some hormones, but most are removed from the blood by kidney and liver enzyme systems, and their breakdown products are excreted from the body in urine or, to a lesser extent, in feces. As a result, the persistence of a hormone in the blood, referred to as its **half-life**, is usually brief-from a fraction of a minute to 30 minutes.

The time required for hormone effects to occur varies greatly. Some hormones provoke target organ responses almost immediately, while others, particularly the steroid hormones, require from hours to days before their effects are seen. Additionally, some hormones such as testosterone secreted by the testes, are secreted in a relatively inactive (*prohormone*) form and must be activated in the target cells. The duration of action of hormone is limited. Depending on hormone it ranges from 20 minutes to several hours. Effects may disappear rapidly as the hormone levels in blood drop, or these may persist for hours even after very low levels of hormone in blood have been reached. Because of these many variations, hormonal blood levels must be precisely and individually controlled to meet the continuously changing needs of the body.

2.2 Hormonal Regulation

The concept of regulatory mechanisms initially arose from the work of Claude Bernard, a French Physician who by 1859 had suggested the importance of maintaining the constancy of the "*milieu interieur*" (or internal environment). He pointed out that it is through the *milieu interieur* that foods, wastes and gases are exchanged and chemical messengers are distributed.

The development of control system theory in the 1940s provided a framework to describe physiological and biochemical regulatory mechanisms. The function of a hormone is to regulate the metabolic activity of its specific target cells. To perform this function, an endocrine gland requires constant and rapid information on the state of the system, which it is regulating. Two major categories of control systems exist, and these are '**open loop**' and '**closed loop**'. In the open loop control system input is not affected by the output, while in the closed loop a part of the output is fed back and participates as an input to the system. Most physiological homeostatic mechanisms are closed loop systems operating via the principle of negative feedback. An American Physiologist, Walter B. Cannon coined the term 'homeostasis' (*homoios* = same, *stasis* = state) in 1932. Homeostasis is the tendency to maintain uniformity in the internal environment of the organism and to maintain the normal composition of the body fluids. Hormones play an important and decisive role in homeostatic regulation of internal environment in an organism's body.

2.3 Feedback Mechanisms

The synthesis and release of most hormones is regulated by some type of **negative and positive feedback system** (Figure 2.1) and as a result, blood levels of many hormones vary only within a narrow "desirable" range (Figure 2.2). Release of a hormone from the parent gland, is controlled by its levels in the blood. In general, each gland has a tendency to over-secrete, but once its physiological effect is achieved, information is transmitted back to the gland to check further secretions. This is called negative feedback. Once the secretion of a hormone is reduced below optimum levels, positive feedback system operates to stimulate the involved gland to increase its secretion. In such a feedback system, an endocrine gland or the system controlling it is sensitive to the concentration of a substance the gland secretes or to the concentration of a product from a process it controls. For example, increase in the levels of a target-gland hormone in blood signals the hypothalamus-pituitary axis to decrease output of the stimulating hormone (a negative effect), which in turn decreases the secretory activity of the target-gland (Figure 2.3). Hypothalamic control of the peripheral endocrine glands may utilize as many as three types of hormones, with multiple negative feedback controls as indicated by negative signs in Figure 2.3. A positive effect on the secretory activity of the gland occurs with a decrease in the levels of its hormone in blood. For example, the function of the thyrotropic hormone from the pituitary is to stimulate the thyroid gland to produce more thyroxin. When the thyroid produces a sufficient amount, the blood level of thyroxin rises, and as the blood circulates back to the hypothalamus and pituitary, the pituitary reduces its output of the stimulating hormone-thyrotropin. This in turn results in decreased production of thyroxin. Vice versa occurs with low levels of thyroxin in blood. Such negative and positive feedback systems, work to keep the hormones concentrations relatively stable.

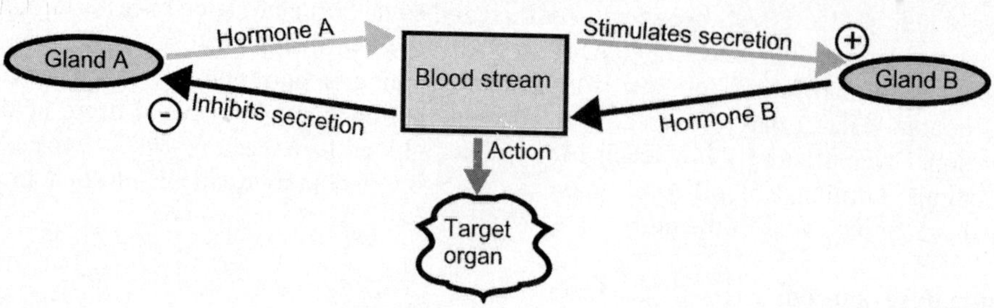

Figure 2.1: Hormone regulation through negative (-) and positive (+) feedback systems, hormone A stimulates secretion of gland B, hormone B has action on target cells and also inhibits secretion of gland A.

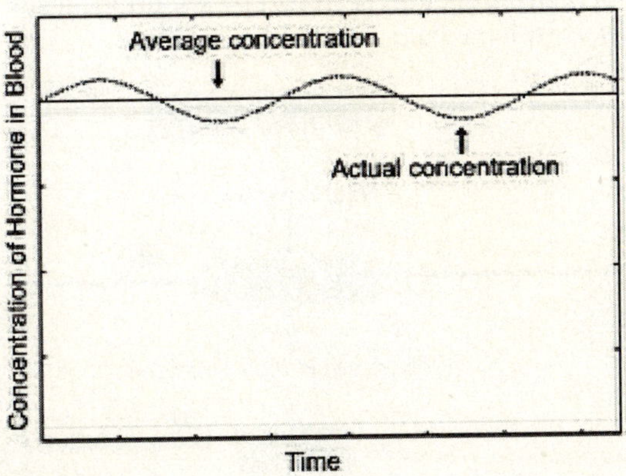

Figure 2.2: Fluctuations in hormone concentration.

Long and Short-Loop Feedback Mechanisms: Three mechanisms of feedback control of hypophysiotropin and hypophyseal hormone secretion are recognized. Hormones from peripheral target tissue may feed back through **a long-loop system** to act at the level of the pituitary gland, at the level of the hypothalamus, or even at the higher brain centers. In contrast, **a short-loop system** involves circulation of hypophyseal hormones by retrograde portal system blood flow to affect secretion of hypothalamic hypophysiotropic hormone. Also, the secreted hypophyseal hormones may feed back on their cells of origin to inhibit their own secretion. This is referred **as autofeedback inhibition or autoinhibition** (Figure 2.4).

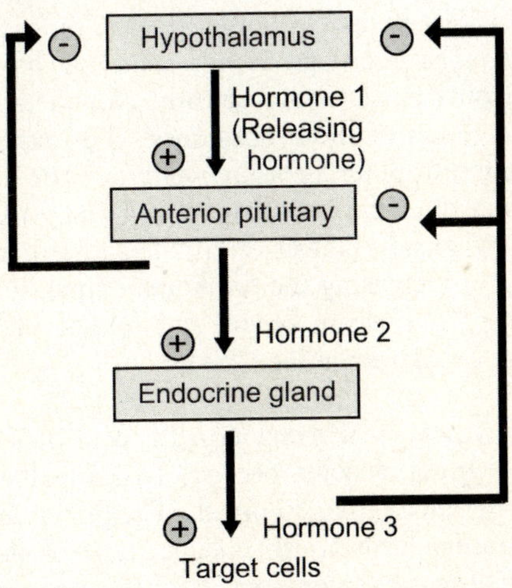

Figure 2.3: Hypothalamic control mechanism of peripheral endocrine glands.

Thus, a hormone secreted by a target gland can have both a direct feedback on the adenohypophyseal hormone and an indirect feedback on the release of the hypothalamic hormone. This involvement of the hypothalamus is particularly important in the control of hormones secreted by the adrenal cortex and gonads (Figure 2.4). There is some evidence for the existence of a short feedback loop in the control of pituitary function whereby a pituitary hormone has a negative feedback action on the secretion of a hypothalamic releasing or release-inhibiting factor. Prolactin is one hormone, which is thought to regulate its own secretion by a short feedback mechanism. However, the general circulation could just as well mediate a short-loop feedback.

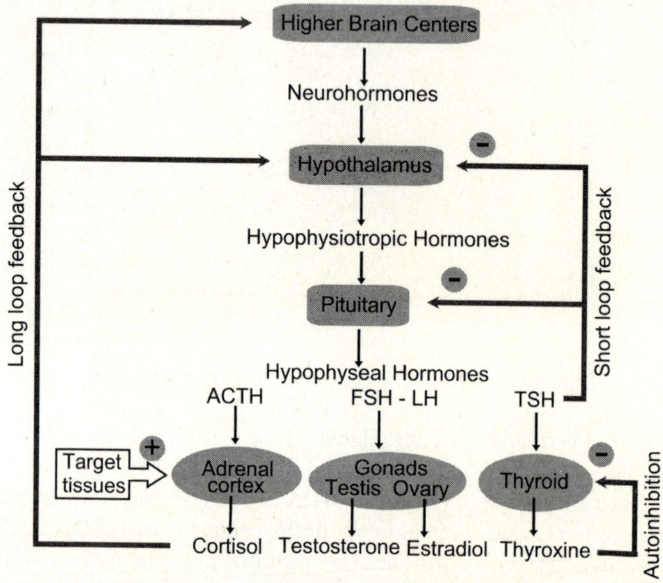

Figure 2.4: Feedback mechanisms in hormones secretion-autoregulation, short-loop and long-loop.

Although some of the pituitary hormones such as prolactin, melanotropin, and neurohypophyseal hormones stimulate peripheral target tissues, these target tissues themselves do not secrete hormones and therefore, their secretion is not controlled by long-loop hormonal feedback mechanisms. The reflex mechanisms and other sensory stimuli reaching the hypothalamus from sensory receptors control the secretion of these hormones. For example, suckling of breast by the infant leads to secretion of oxytocin from the neurohypophysis. The hormones from the pancreas and parathyroid are not under the control of the hypothalamus-pituitary axis, and in these, it is the blood level of certain substance that the gland controls, and not the hormone itself. The substance is the stimulating factor for decreasing or increasing the hormonal output. For example insulin release from the pancreas depends on levels of glucose in blood, and release of parathormone (PTH) from the parathyroid depends on the levels of calcium in the blood

There is at least one example in the endocrine system of a positive feedback mechanism. These are extremely rare in biological systems because basically they are unstable and lead to an 'explosive' situation when no other factors are involved. The principle of positive feedback is that an increase in a hormone concentration leads to an enhancement of its effect by stimulating further release. This situation occurs prior to ovulation when estrogens are secreted in increasing amounts by the developing ovarian follicle (s). Normally these steroids have a negative feedback action on pituitary gonadotropin secretion but when they reach a critical plasma concentration, they stimulate the release of gonadotropins from the pituitary. This results in a surge of luteinizing hormone (LH) and follicle stimulating hormone (FSH) secretion. This surge acts on the ovary to cause follicular rupture and release of the ovum (see chapter 16). The reason why this positive feedback does not become uncontrollable is that by some unknown mechanism the feedback effect of estrogen reverts to a negative feedback action thereby stabilizing the system.

The endocrine system is not dependent solely on circulatory communication, since the nervous system has a stimulating effect on the release of hormones from the posterior pituitary, adrenal medulla, and the pineal. As such, the posterior pituitary and the adrenal medulla are of neural origin, and thus a part of the autonomic nervous system, and if these glands are destroyed, their function is taken over to some extent by the nervous system.

2.4 Circulation of Hormones

Hormones circulate in the blood either in a free form or in a form bound to protein. Free hormones are generally considered as the active fraction that is directly available to target tissue. Protein-bound hormones represent the hormone reserve in the plasma. Protein binding may act to prevent excretion of this hormone reserve through the kidney glomerulus. Also, in this protein-bound form, hormones may be able to cross certain plasma membranes to be more available to a specific tissue.

2.5 Types of Hormones

Hormones may be classified in a number of ways. This can be on the basis of how far they act from their site of production, their solubility characteristics, with the kind of molecule a hormone is made of or its mechanism of action on the basis of location of receptors.

Principally hormones are classified into two groups on the basis of how far from their site of production they act. These are- i) **Circulating (general) hormones** also called **endocrine hormones** and ii) **Local hormones**. Circulating hormones are those that pass into blood and act on distant target cells, for example, the adrenocorticotropic hormone (ACTH) from the anterior pituitary gland stimulate the adrenal cortex. These hormones stay in the blood and exert their effects for a few minutes or for a few hours, and then get inactivated by the liver and excreted by the kidneys. Local hormones are those that act locally without first entering the blood stream and usually are inactivated quickly. These hormones have specific local effects, for example, secretin released by the duodenal wall act directly on the pancreas, or cholecystokinin released from the small intestine causes the gall bladder to contract, or nitric oxide (NO) hormone released by endothelial cells lining the blood vessels, causes relaxation of nearby vascular smooth muscle fibers resulting in vasodilation and increase in blood flow in that region. The eicosanoids (prostaglandin and leukotriene) are important local hormones, and they may act as circulating hormones as well. Figure 2.5 compares the sites of action of circulating and local hormones. Among local hormones, those act on neighboring cells, are called **paracrines** (*para* = beside or near, *crin* = to secrete), and those that act on the same cell which secrete them, are termed **autocrines** (*auto* = self, *crin* = to secrete).

2.6 Chemical Classes of Hormones

Chemically, hormones can be divided into two broad classes:

- **Lipid soluble hormones** such as steroids, thyroid hormones and nitric oxide (NO).
- **Water soluble hormones** such as peptides, proteins, glycoproteins, amines and eicosanoids (prostaglandin and leukotriene).

Water-soluble hormone molecules mostly circulate in a "free" form in blood whereas, lipid-soluble hormone molecules circulate in the form bound to **transport proteins** (Table 2.1). However, 0.1-10 % of the molecules of a lipid-soluble hormone are not bound to a transport protein and remain free. This 'free fraction' diffuses out of capillaries, binds to receptors, and triggers responses. As free hormone molecules leave the blood and bind to their receptors, transport proteins release new ones to replenish the free fraction.

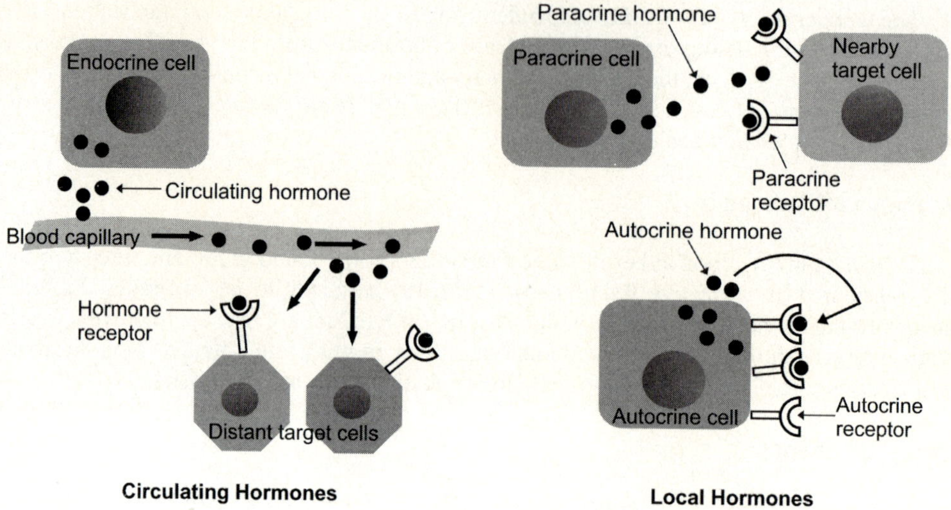

Figure 2.5: Sites of action of circulating and local hormones.

Table 2.1: General features of hormone classes

Character	Group I	Group II
Types	Steroids, iodothyronine, calcitriol, gas nitric oxide	Polypeptides, proteins, glycoproteins, amines (catecholamines), eicosanoids
Solubility	Lipophilic	Hydrophilic
Transport Proteins	Yes	No
Plasma half-life	Long (hours to days)	Short (minutes)
Receptor	Intracellular	Plasma Membrane
Mediator	Receptor-hormone complex	cAMP, cGMP, Ca++, metabolites of complex phosphoinositols, kinase cascades

Based on their chemical structures, hormones may also be classified into:

- **Peptide and protein hormones** such as all hypothalamic releasing and inhibiting hormones, pituitary hormones, insulin, glucagon, parathyroid hormone, etc.
- **Steroid hormones** such as sex steroids, corticosteroids, aldosterone, and calcitriol.
- **Thyroid hormones such** as triiodothyronine (T_3) and thyroxin (T_4).
- **Biogenic amines** which include the **catecholamines** such as epinephrine norepinephrine and dopamine, and the **indolamines**, which include histamine, melatonin and serotonin.
- **Gas (NO) Nitric oxide.**
- **Eicosanoids**, which include prostaglandins and leukotrienes.

Table 2.2 lists some examples of lipid-soluble and water-soluble hormones along with the type of compound they are made of and their sites of production. Hormones exhibit a variety of structures ranging from that of simple amino acid derivative to steroid like structures and huge glycoproteins. Chemically, most hormones are either **steroids** that are synthesized from cholesterol (see Chapter 5) or they are **amines**, **peptides**, **proteins**, or **glycoproteins** that are synthesized from amino acids. Vitamin D is a modified steroid and can be converted into a hormone (calcitriol).

Some neurons produce hormones called **amines** (as they retain an amino group $-NH_3^+$) that are synthesized by decarboxylating and modifying certain amino acids. The **catecholamines** (epinephrine, norepinephrine and dopamine) and **thyroid hormones** (triiodothyronine and thyroxine) are synthesized by modifying amino acid **tyrosine**. **Mast cells** (one of the cells in connective tissue present alongside the blood vessels) and **platelets** synthesize **histamine** from **histidine**. On the other hand, **melatonin** and **serotonin** are derived from amino acid **tryptophan**.

Table 2.2: Chemical classes of hormones

Class	Compound	Sites of Production	Example
Lipid – Soluble	Steroids	Ovary	Estrogen, Progesterone
		Testes	Testosterone
		Adrenal Cortex	Aldosterone, Cortisol
		Kidneys	Calcitriol
	Amino Acids	Thyroid Gland	Triiodothyronine (I_3), Thyroxin (I_4)
		Endothelial Cells lining blood vessels	Nitric Oxide (NO)
Water - Soluble	Amines	Adrenal Medulla	Epinephrine and Nor Epinephrine
		Pineal Gland	Melatonin
		Mast Cells in Connective Tissue	Histamine
		Platelets in Blood	Serotonin
	Peptides and Proteins	Hypothalamic Neurosecretory Cells	All Hypothalamic Releasing and Inhibiting Hormones
		Posterior Pituitary Hormones	ADH, OT
		Anterior Pituitary Hormones	PTH, GH, PRL, ACTH
		Pancreas	Insulin, Glucagon, SS
		Parathyroid	Parathyroid Hormone/Parathormone
	Glycoproteins	Anterior Pituitary Hormones	FSH, LH, TSH
	Lipids (20-carbon fatty acids)	All cells except red blood cells	Eicosanoids- Prostaglandins and leukotriene

The **peptide** and **protein** hormones are synthesized on rough endoplasmic reticulum. The peptide hormones are short chains of amino acids, while protein hormones are composed of long chains of amino acids. These include hormones produced in the hypothalamus, anterior pituitary gland, parathyroid gland and pancreas, and the ones associated with posterior pituitary gland. The small size peptide hormones range from a tripeptide like thyroid stimulating hormone (TRH) to octapeptides like vasopressin and oxytocin to decapeptides like gonadotropin releasing hormone (GnRH) to polypeptides like melanocyte stimulating hormone (MSH), adrenocorticotropic hormone (ACTH), insulin, glucagon, prolactin, etc. Some of the protein hormones produced by the anterior pituitary gland, such as thyroid stimulating hormone (TSH), follicle-stimulating hormone (FSH) and lureinizing hormone (LH) have attached carbohydrate groups and thus are **glycoprotein hormones**.

A group of chemical mediators are known as **eicosanoid hormones**. These are derived from a 20-carbon fatty acid, the **arachidonic acid** and include prostaglandins and leukotrienes and are described in detail in chapter 6. Prostaglandins occur in a wide variety of cells, such as those of liver, heart, lungs, kidneys, thymus gland, pancreas, brain, and reproductive organs.

Summary

Hormone is a chemical substance secreted by the glands of the endocrine system into blood stream. It is carried to all cells throughout the body.

Hormones affect only a few types of cells, called target cells. They exert powerful effects even in very low concentrations. They have a brief half-life.

Some type of negative feedback system regulates the synthesis and release of the hormones. Therefore, as a result, blood levels of many hormones vary only within a narrow desirable range.

The feedback loops concerned with the control of adenohypophyseal hormones involve hormones secreted by their target glands whereas those regulating posterior pituitary hormones involve neural feedback control. In both cases, the important feature of the regulation of hypophyseal hormone release is the ability of other brain regions to override or finely adjust those feedback mechanisms, which operate principally at the level of the hypothalamus.

Hormones can be of circulating and local type depending on how far from their site of production they act. Local hormones can be paracrine or autocrine in nature.

Hormones circulate in the blood in a free form and also in a form that is bound to proteins.

Hormones may be water or lipid soluble.

Chemically, most hormones are either steroids that are synthesized from cholesterol or they are amines, peptides, proteins, or glycoproteins that are synthesized from amino acids.

Steroid hormones include sex hormones, such as estrogen, progesterone, and testosterone, and the ones secreted by the adrenal cortex include aldosterone and cortisol.

Some neurons and adrenal medulla produce amines such as epinephrine and nor-epinephrine, derived from amino acids.

The peptide hormones are short chains of amino acids, produced in the hypothalamus.

Protein hormones are long chains of amino acids secreted by parathyroid gland and anterior pituitary gland.

Some of the anterior pituitary gland hormones, such as TSH, LH and FSH are glycoproteins, which consist of a protein joined to a carbohydrate.

Questions

1. Define hormone and target cell.
2. Distinguish between circulating and local hormones.
3. Describe how hormones interact with target-cell receptors.
4. Compare the two chemical classes of hormones based on their solubility.
5. Distinguish between down and up-regulation of a hormone.
6. Identify the chemical classes of hormones. Give an example of each.
7. How are hormones transported in the blood?
8. Describe the three types of signals that can control hormone secretion.
9. What is a feedback system and why is it important?
10. How do negative and positive feedback systems differ from one another?
11. Explain how hormone release is regulated.
12. Describe the effect of aging on endocrine system functioning.
13. How does the negative feedback system of the parathyroid glands differ from that of the thyroid gland?

Chapter 3

The Hypothalamus

For many years, the **pituitary gland**, also known, as **hypophysis** was famous as **"master" gland** because its hormones control the activity levels of other endocrine glands. Then it was discovered that the pituitary gland itself has a "**super master**"- the **hypothalamus**.

The neuroendocrine research has shown that a minute region of the mammalian forebrain, called the hypothalamus, is an important region of neurohormone production and that the pituitary gland, situated directly beneath it acts as the principal target organ or mediator for the action of these neurohormones. The important role of the hypothalamus in control of endocrine processes via the pituitary was first recognized around the middle of nineteenth century. Thereafter, over next two decades, more critical experiments involving hypophysectomy, pituitary grafts, and sections of the portal vessels made it clear that blood-borne factors from the median eminence and the hypothalamus were necessary for the synthesis and secretion of the pituitary peptide hormones.

In the 1950s, the demonstration of blood flow from hypothalamus to pituitary provided a framework for the concept of a neuro-humoral control of anterior pituitary function. Ironically, recent evidences indicate an upward flow in some vessels (retrograde flow) although flow towards the pituitary predominates.

Geoffrey Harris provided enough data suggesting that the release of pituitary hormones is controlled by humoral factors of hypothalamic origin. For their contribution to the isolation and determination of the structures of hypothalamic regulatory peptides, Roger C.L. Guillemin and Andrew V. Schally received a Noble prize in 1978 in physiology/medicine. Many other scientists provided important discoveries that contributed to the determination of the structures and roles of hypothalamic peptide hormones.

The human fetal anterior pituitary analogue is recognizable as early as at 4-5 weeks of gestation, and by 8th week, the median eminence of tuber cinereum and the primordial pituitary can easily be recognized. During this period gonadotropin-releasing hormone (GnRH) can also be detected immuno-cytochemically in the fetal hypothalamus while gonadotropins become detectable a couple of weeks later. Further development and differentiation leads to the formation of a mature hypothalamic-pituitary unit at 20 weeks.

The hypothalamus and pituitary gland form a joint unit, which exerts control over the functioning of several other endocrine glands. This unit constitutes a paradigm of brain-endocrine interactions, study of which is known as **neuroendocrinology**. Neuroendocrinology is defined as the study of the physiological processes involved in integrating neural and endocrine functions.

3.1 Relationship of Brain with Hypothalamus and Pituitary

The **forebrain** or **prosencephalon** of vertebrates can be divided into two parts. These are the anterior **telencephalon** or **cerebral hemispheres** and the posterior **diencephalon**. The lateral walls of the diencephalon are further subdivided into four horizontal zones. These are the **epithalamus**, the **dorsal thalamus**, the **ventral thalamus** and the **hypothalamus** (Figure 3.1). The central lumen of the diencephalon is the **third ventricle**, which possesses lateral extensions into parts of the hypothalamus. The structure that forms part of the floor of the third ventricle of the brain, and extends downward to connect the hypothalamus with the hypophysis (pituitary gland) is called the **infundibulum**. This connecting region is also known as the **infundibular stalk** (Figure 3.1).

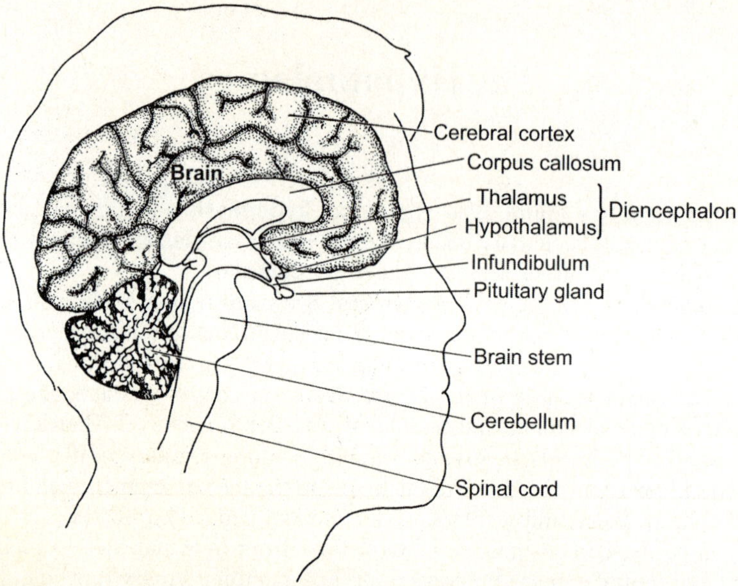

Figure 3.1: Locations of brain, hypothalamus and pituitary gland in Human.

Within the brain, the neurosecretory cells are usually grouped together into discrete areas or nuclei, and those controlling pituitary activity are located in the hypothalamus (Figure 3.2). The structure of hypothalamic nuclei and the cells within them show a high degree of uniformity throughout the vertebrates. Multipolar cell bodies known as **perikarya** are characteristic of the hypothalamic nuclei of adult mammals. The hypothalamus is responsible for integration of a whole range of inputs from other brain centers and for the control of visceral functions, in many cases via its effects on the secretions of the pituitary gland.

3.2 Structure of Hypothalamus

The hypothalamus is the basal part of the diencephalon, and as its name suggests, lies below the thalamus (Figure 3.1). It forms the walls and lower part of the third ventricle, which is one of the chambers of the brain filled with cerebrospinal fluid.

The hypothalamus is bound rostrally (towards the nose) by the optic chiasma, caudally by the mamillary bodies, laterally by the optic tracts of the eyes, and dorso-laterally by the brain region called the thalamus. A part of the third ventricle floor that extends downward toward the infundibulum is the **tuber cinereum**. Its lower part is richly supplied with blood vessels and is known as the **median eminence** (Figure 3.2). The vascular link between the median eminence and the pituitary gland is known as the **hypophyseal portal system**.

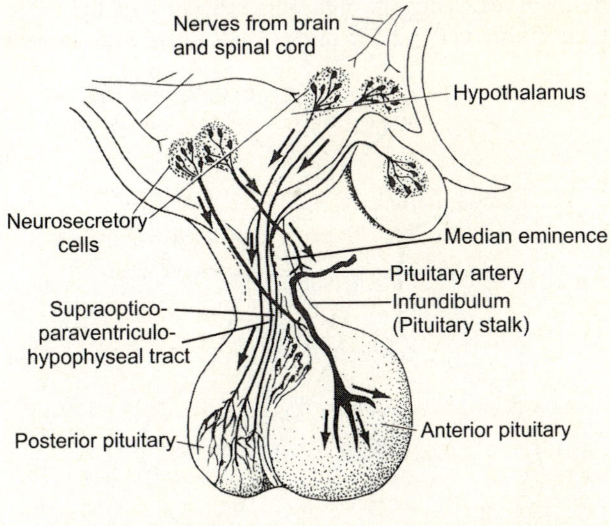

Figure 3.2: Hypothalamus in relation to pituitary.

Within the hypothalamus, symmetrically placed clusters of neurons are present around the third ventricle. These are known as the **hypothalamic nuclei**. Those nuclei concerned with pituitary regulation tend to a medial distribution, whilst those of the lateral hypothalamus are involved in other functions such as regulation of food intake etc. There are species differences in the presence and distribution of the hypothalamic nuclei and also in the arrangement of the hypothalamic-hypophyseal tissues. The two bilaterally placed-paired nuclei in the hypothalamus are the **supraoptic nuclei (SON)** and the **paraventricular nuclei (PVN)**. The axons from these cell bodies extend into the median eminence and then into the neurohypophysis and constitute the **supraoptico-paraventriculo-hypophyseal tract** (Figure 3.2).

The hypothalamus is connected to the pituitary gland by both nerve fibers and blood vessels, through which it regulates its activity. Hypothalamus is the major integrating link between the nervous and endocrine systems. It constantly receives information about the internal environment from neural connections and cerebrospinal fluid. This is made possible by its location near both the thalamus and the third ventricle. Cells in the hypothalamus synthesize at least nine different hormones known as the releasing and inhibiting factors, and the pituitary secretes seven more called the tropic hormones and these hormones together play important roles in the regulation of virtually all aspects of functions and physiological processes in the body.

3.3 Structure of Pituitary Gland

The pituitary gland (also called **hypophysis**) is an unpaired organ, weighing nearly 600 mg in adult man. It is a pea-shaped structure measuring about 1-1.5 cm in diameter. It hangs from the base of the brain by a delicate stalk called **infundibulum** and is lodged in a depression of the sphenoid bone called **sella turcica,** just at the back of the optic chiasma.

Hypophysis or Pituitary gland consists of three parts. Morphologically these vary in size and relationship in different species. These are- i) a hormone-producing glandular portion called **adenohypophysis** or **pars anterior** or **anterior lobe** with **pars distalis** and **pars tuberalis**, ii) a neural portion called **neurohypophysis** or **pars nervosa** or **posterior lobe**, which is an extension of the hypothalamus, and iii) a third region called the **pars intermedia** or **intermediate lobe** (Figure 3.3 and Table 3.1). Pars intermedia atrophies during fetal development and ceases to exist as a separate lobe in adults. However, some of its cells migrate into adjacent parts of the anterior pituitary gland and persists there. Pars intermedia are not found in birds, whale, elephants, Armadillo and adult humans.

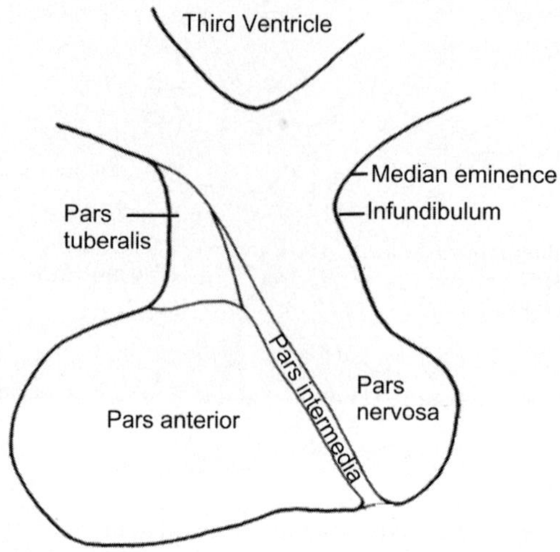

Figure 3.3: Major subdivisions of the pituitary gland.

Table 3.1:Derivation of hypophysis and its components

Derivation	Divisions	Components	Lobes of Pituitary
Oral ectoderm	Adenohypophysis	Pars tuberalis	Anterior lobe
		Pars anterior- Pars distalis	
		Pars intermedia	Posterior lobe
Neural ectoderm	Neurohypophysis	Pars nervosa (neural lobe)	
		Infundibulum (neural stalk), median eminence	Infundibulum

3.4 Origin of Pituitary Gland

The pituitary gland is ectodermal in origin but contrasting histology of its two lobes reflects the dual origin of this tiny gland (Figure 3.4). The **posterior lobe** is an evagination of the diencephalon (part of the brain) and is derived from a down growth of hypothalamic (nervous) tissue. It maintains its neural connection with the hypothalamus via a nerve bundle called the **hypothalamic hypophyseal tract** (Figure 3.2), which runs through the infundibulum. This tract arises from neurons in the **supraoptic** and **paraventricular** nuclei of the hypothalamus. These neurosecretory cells synthesize two **neurohormones, oxytocin** and **antidiuretic hormone**, which are transported along the length to their axon terminal in the posterior pituitary. **Oxytocin** is made by the **paraventricular neurons** and **antidiuretic hormone (ADH),** also called **vasopressin** is synthesized by the **supraoptic neurons**. When these hypothalamic neurons fire, they release the stored hormones into a capillary bed in the posterior pituitary for distribution throughout body. In contrast, the **anterior lobe** of the pituitary gland originates from a superior out pocketing of the oral mucosa or buccal cavity (*Rathke's pouch*) and is also formed from the epithelial tissue (Figure 3.4). After touching the posterior lobe, the adenohypophysis loses its connection with the oral mucosa and adheres to the neurohypophysis to form the composite organ. The **pars intermedia** differentiate from the wall of Rathke's pouch and in some species forms a cup around the neural lobe. The remainder of the pouch thickens and becomes **pars**

distalis. Pars distalis is glandular with sinusoidal tissue and developing blood vessel. Paired lateral extensions differentiate from the pars distalis (analogue) or eventually fuse to produce a mini plate of tissue, called the **pars tuberalis**. It grows around the infundibulum stalk and spreads below the hypothalamus as a non-secreting tissue. Figure 3.4 describes the development of the pituitary gland and Figure 3.5 diagrammatically represents the division, components and parts of the pituitary gland.

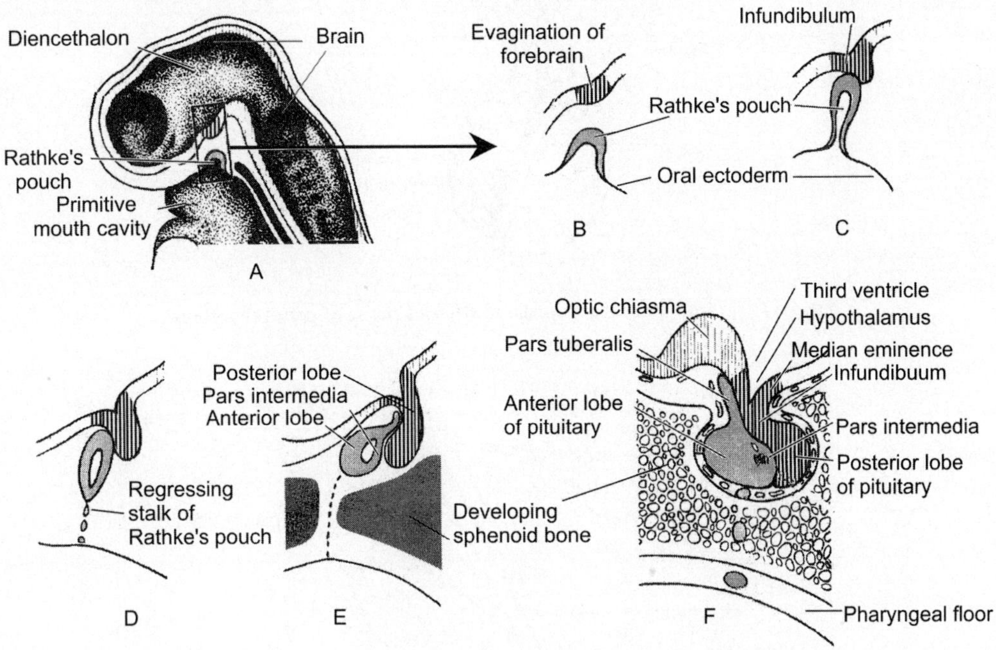

Figure 3.4: Development of the pituitary gland.

3.5 Vascular Supply to the pituitary gland

The vessels supplying blood to the anterior pituitary were first studied in detail in the 1930s and 1940s when it was demonstrated for the first time that the blood flowed downwards in the hypophyseal portal vessels (previous view was of blood flow towards the brain). The blood vessels were first described by histological methods and subsequently more sophisticated techniques enabled direct observation on blood flow in several species.

The vascularization of the mammalian pituitary is highly complex compared to that in lower vertebrates. However, it is similar in most mammals. The arterial supply to the adenohypophysis, particularly to the pars distalis, is independent to that of the neurohypophysis and the whole organ is drained by means of short veins. The arterial supply to the pituitary is from branches of the **internal carotid arteries**. The **blood supply** to the **posterior pituitary gland** comes from both the **superior** and **inferior hypophyseal arteries** (Figure 3.6). The **superior hypophyseal artery** supplies the **upper part of the neurohypophysis**, the **median eminence** and the **infundibular stem**, whereas the **inferior hypophyseal artery** chiefly supplies the **lower part of the neurohypophysis** (Figure 3.6). There is usually no direct arterial supply to the pars distalis, or to the largely avascular pars intermedia. Blood drains into the pars distalis from the median eminence via several long portal vessels, and also from the capillary bed of the neural lobe via a few short portal vessels. The **trabecular artery** connects the superior and inferior arteries (Figure 3.6). Venous blood from all parts of the pituitary is drained into the systemic circulation via the intracranial venous sinuses.

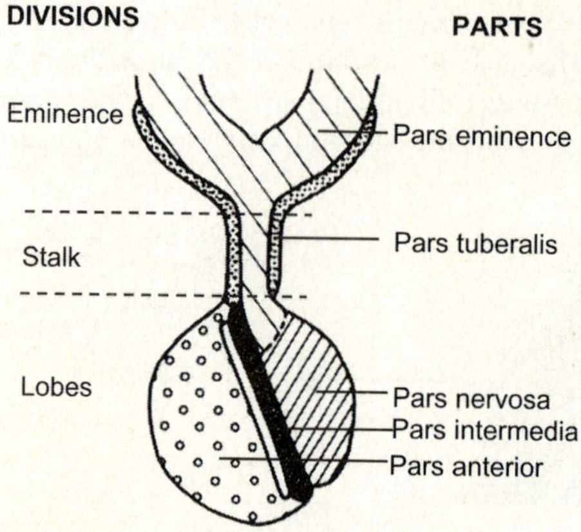

Figure 3.5: Diagrammatic representation of parts of pituitary gland.

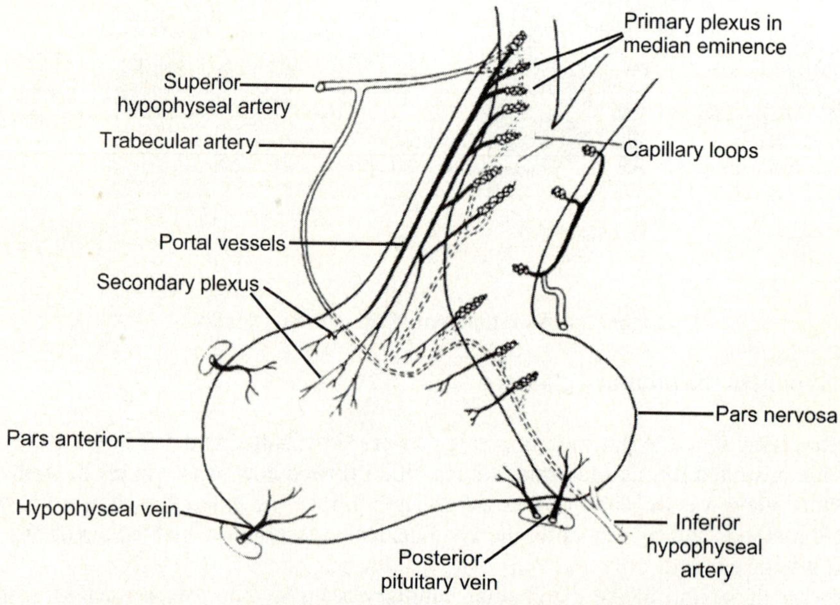

Figure 3.6: Major blood vessels of pituitary gland (Human).

The **superior hypophyseal arteries,** the branches of the **internal carotid arteries** supply blood to the anterior pituitary. These arteries supply the **primary capillary plexuses** of the **hypothalamo-hypophyseal portal vessels**, which travel down the pituitary stalk. Specifically, the primary capillary plexus in the infundibulum communicates inferiorly via the small **hypophyseal portal veins** with a **secondary capillary plexus** in the adenohypophysis. The primary and secondary capillary plexuses and the intervening hypophyseal portal veins make up the **hypophyseal portal system**. The hormones secreted by anterior pituitary gland cells pass into the **anterior hypophyseal veins** via the secondary plexus of the hypophyseal portal system for distribution to the target tissues located throughout the body.

3.6 Anatomic Connections between Hypothalamus and Pituitary

Adenohypophysis and neurohypophysis are connected to the hypothalamus through **vascular** and **neural connections** respectively (Figure 3.7 A and B).

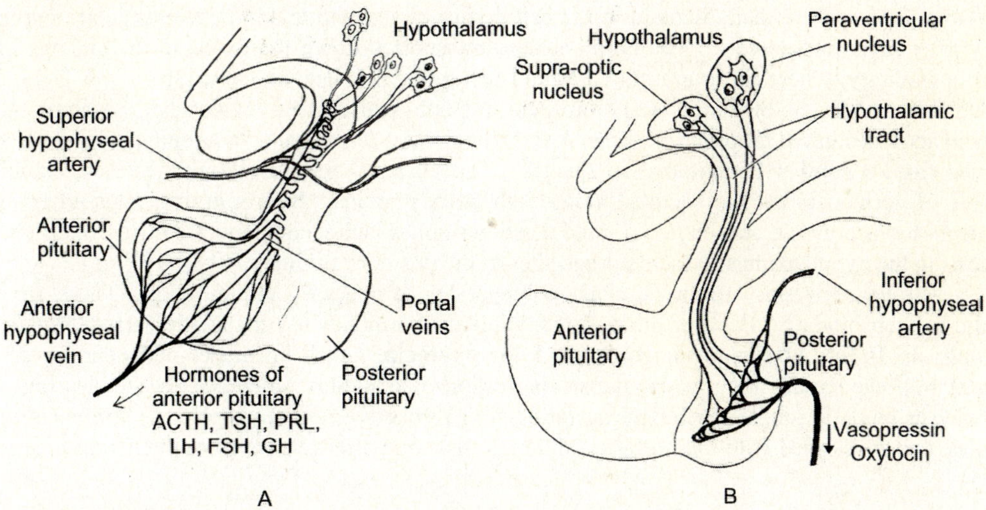

Figure 3.7: Anatomic connections between hypothalamus and pituitary, A -vascular and B- neural.

In vertebrates, except teleosts, the vascular link between the floor of the brain and pituitary is particularly important because it carries various factors from the central nervous system that controls the cell activity of the adenohypophysis. This vascular connection is via a system of portal vessels within the median eminence, so that virtually all blood reaching the adenohypophysis passes through this specialized area. Within the adenohypophysis, vascular channels are extensive, and almost all cells contact a capillary or sinusoid, essential for the transport of secreted peptide hormones and for receiving nutrients and controlling signals from the hypothalamus.

The capillaries in the anterior pituitary form sinusoids similar to those seen in the liver, thus providing close contact between the blood and the glandular cells. Via this **portal system**, **releasing** and **inhibiting hormones** secreted by neurons in the ventral hypothalamus circulate directly to the adenohypophysis, where they regulate the secretory activity of its hormone-producing cells (Figure 3.7 A). All of these hypothalamic regulatory hormones are amino acid-based, but these vary widely in size from amines to polypeptides. This direct route of blood supply permits hypothalamic hormones to act quickly on anterior pituitary gland cells, before the hormones are diluted or destroyed in the systemic circulation.

Since embryologically, the posterior pituitary arises as an evagination of the floor of the third ventricle, it essentially retains its neural character and receives an abundant supply of nerve fibers called the hypothalamo-hypophyseal tract from the supraoptic and paraventricular nuclei (Figure 3.7 B). In contrast, the anterior and intermediate lobes of the pituitary arise in the embryo from Rathke's pouch, which is an evagination from the roof of the pharynx. Therefore, though sympathetic and parasympathetic nerve fibers reach the anterior lobe, but very few nerve fibers pass to it from hypothalamus.

3.7 Functions of Hypothalamus

Hypothalamus has the following functions:

Origin and control of posterior pituitary hormones: The hormones Vasopressin (also known as ADH) and Oxytocin are manufactured in the cell bodies of supraoptic and paraventricular neurons of the hypothalamus respectively. The hormones are transported down the axons to the endings in the posterior pituitary, where these are stored bound to a protein called **neurophysin**. Van Dyke *et al* isolated this protein (30,000 mol. wt.) from neurohypophyseal extracts, which had vasopressor and oxytocin activities in the ratio of 1:1. Later Van Dyke protein was named "neurophysin" and has been obtained from a number of mammalian species. The posterior pituitary hormones thus, exhibit an example of hormones that are secreted along with other proteins. Neurophysins, released from the precursors to vasopressin and oxytocin, bind these hormones and accompany them from their sites of synthesis in the hypothalamus to their storage sites in the posterior pituitary.

The neurophysins are single chain polypeptides of about 95 amino acids. These are very specific in their binding. Each of the posterior pituitary hormones has a specific carrier protein, the **neurophysin II for ADH** and **neurophysin I for oxytocin**. Both hormones and neurophysin are released into the circulation by exocytosis in response to action potentials in the neurons. The neurophysin binds in single stochiometric ratios with respective neurohypophyseal hormones in the granules, and is released with the hormone although their role after release from the neural lobe is not known.

Control of Anterior Pituitary Secretions: The hypothalamus plays an important stimulatory role in regulating the secretion of adrenocorticotropic hormone (ACTH), thyroid stimulating hormone (TSH), growth hormone (STH), follicle stimulating hormone (FSH) and luteinizing hormone (LH). It also regulates secretion of prolactin, but its effect is predominantly inhibitory rather than stimulatory. The area from which the hypothalamic releasing and inhibitory hormones are secreted is the median eminence of the hypothalamus. This region contains many nerve endings in close proximity to the capillary loops from which the portal vessels originate. The hormones are secreted from these endings.

Role of the Hypothalamus in Regulating Pituitary Hormones: The hypothalamus regulates the secretions from the pituitary gland by producing and secreting hormones called hypothalamic releasing factors (RFs) and inhibitory factors (IFs). A releasing factor from the hypothalamus triggers the anterior pituitary to secrete a tropic hormone that stimulates a target gland or tissue. In similar fashion, inhibitory factor from the hypothalamus triggers the anterior pituitary to inhibit the secretion of a tropic hormone and in turn a target gland. In regulating the pituitary, the hypothalamus responds to messages it receives from both the circulatory and the nervous systems. There are nine important factors or hormones (six RFs and three IFs) that control the secretion of adenohypophysis. Table 3.2 summarizes the elements in the hypothalamic-pituitary-target axis: the releasing and inhibitory factors from the hypothalamus, the tropic hormones released by the anterior pituitary, and the target glands or tissue stimulated by the tropic hormones. The secretion of thyroid stimulating hormone (TSH) is controlled by thyrotropin releasing hormone (TRH), that of adrenocorticotropic hormone (ACTH) by corticotropin releasing hormone/factor (CRH/F), and of both gonadotropins, LH and FSH by gonadotropin releasing hormone (GnRH), also termed as luteinizing hormone releasing hormone (LHRH). However, secretion of growth hormone (GH) and prolactin (PRL) appear to be regulated by a dual control mechanism from hypothalamus i.e. by both releasing and release-inhibiting factors. Somatostatin inhibits the release of GH, although the predominant hypothalamic influence on GH release in basal condition is predominantly inhibitory in nature.

Table 3.2 Hypothalamus - pituitary - target gland

Hormones From Hypothalamus	Hormones From Pituitary Gland	Target Organs
Thyrotropin-releasing hormone (TRH)	Thyroid stimulating Hormone (TSH) or Thyrotropin	Thyroid
Prolactin-releasing hormone (PRH)	Prolactin (PRL)	Mammary Gland
Prolactin release-inhibiting hormone (PIH)		
Corticotropin-releasing hormone (CRH)	Adrenocorticotropic hormone (ACTH) or Corticotropin	Adrenal Cortex
Gonadotropin-releasing hormone (GnRH)	Luteinizing hormone (LH) or Interstitial Cell Stimulating Hormone (ICSH)	Gonads (Testis and Ovary)
	Follicle Stimulating Hormone (FSH)	
Growth Hormone releasing hormone (GHRH) or Somatocrinin	Growth Hormone (GH) or Somatotropin	Bone, Muscle, Adipose tissue, Liver
Growth hormone-inhibiting hormone (GHIH) or Somatostatin (SS)		
Melanocyte-releasing hormone (MRH)	Melanocyte-stimulating Hormone (MSH) or Intermedin	Skin Pigmentation
Melanocyte-inhibiting hormone (MIH)		

3.8 Neurosecretory cells and Neurohormones of Hypothalamus:

The predominant neurosecretory cells in the hypothalamus are those, which largely terminate in the neurohypophysis and release hormones into general circulation. Other groups of neurosecretory cells in the hypothalamus are the ones, which mostly terminate in the median eminence (the tubero-infundibular system), and release their products into the hypophyseal portal vessels. These hypothalamic neurosecretory cells are also peptidergic neurons and their secretory products are peptides. Since the neurosecretory cells need to manufacture large amounts of neurohormones in their cell bodies, their neurosecretory peptidergic neurons are morphologically characterized for this purpose. These cells therefore, have predominant protein synthetic apparatus that is common with other active peptide hormone-secretory cells, and abundant rough endoplasmic reticulum (RER), Golgi apparatus, and membrane bound granules (Figure 3.8). Generally, the neurosecretory peptide is synthesized in the cell body as an inactive larger precursor polypeptide by the usual process of ribosomal protein synthesis on the RER. This material is then packaged into granules in the Golgi complex together with specific peptidase enzymes, and then the granules are transported from cell body to nerve terminal down the axon by means of an active axonal transport process. During transportation and subsequent storage of the granules, the active hormone or secretory product is processed from the precursor by the action of the co-packaged peptidase enzymes. Neurosecretory cells release their active hormones by mechanisms identical with those widely described for neurotransmitter release.

3.9 Neurohumoral Control Mechanisms

The demonstration of blood flow from the hypothalamus to pituitary provided a framework for the concept of a neurohumoral control of anterior pituitary function. The neural control of endocrine function is exerted in a number of ways (Figure 3.9). This can occur either through hypothalamic neurosecretory neurons releasing a hormone into the blood (Figure 3.9 A, B) or by a neuron directly innervating a secretory cell (Figure 3.9 C,D). The neurons of the tubero-infundibular system release their peptides into the hypophyseal portal blood vessels in which they are carried down to the anterior pituitary and stimulate or inhibit the release of various adenohypophyseal hormones (3.9 A). The neurohypophyseal neurons release the two peptide hormones, oxytocin and vasopressin from the posterior pituitary into the general circulation (3.9 B). The release of the intermediate lobe hormone

(MSH, and others) is controlled by hypothalamic neurons, which directly innervate the intermediate secretory cells (3.9 C). The secretion of catecholamines (adrenaline and nor adrenaline) from the chromaffin cells of the adrenal medulla in the periphery is controlled by acetylcholine (Ach) released from preganglionic sympathetic neurons (3.9 D). The chromaffin cells are modified postganglionic neurons and may be considered as neurosecretory cells, in the sense that they release hormone directly into general circulation.

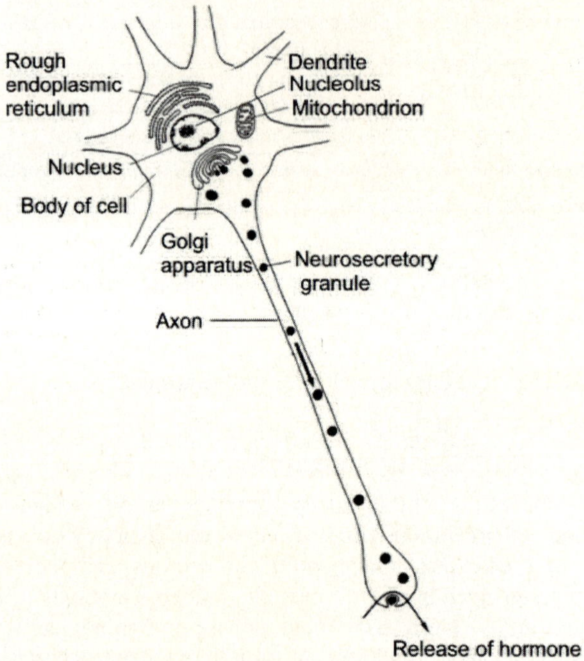

Figure 3.8: Components of neurosecretory cell.

The neurosecretory neurons of the neurohypophyseal and tubero-infundibular system convert neural signals into endocrine signals and can be classified as the transducer cells. Their inputs are electrical, and outputs hormonal. Thus, their secretory activity depend on any input that may alter their electrical excitability, thereby generating nerve impulses or action potentials to result in secretion. Inputs to neuroendocrine transducer cells can be both, neuronal via neurotransmitters from other neurons that impinge on the hypothalamic neurosecretory neurons and also via the feedback action of peripheral hormones. For example, ovulation, the process of release of mature ova from the ovary, is stimulated by a surge of LH released from the pituitary gland in response to an increased secretion of gonadotropin releasing hormone (Gn-RH or LH-RH) from specific hypothalamic neuroendocrine cells. The LH surge is not only dependent on the feedback action of hormones secreted by the ovary, but also on the neural signals (neurotransmitters) from the brain. In this way, factors such as stress, depression, duration of daylight and tactile stimulation associated with copulation can, in particular circumstances, affect both the occurrence and timing of ovulation. Thus, integration of a broad spectrum of information operates through the final common pathway of the neuroendocrine cells. This enables an extremely "fine tuning" of a particular endocrine system. Another example of neuroendocrine transducer cells is the one that occur in the pineal gland.

Apart from aminergic innervations of the pars intermedia, neurosecretory peptidergic neurons from paraventricular nucleus in the hypothalamus directly innervate the intermediate lobe. Two hypothalamic factors seem to be involved in this peptidergic control, one which stimulates melanocyte stimulating hormone releasing factor (MSH-RF), and the other which inhibits (melanocyte stimulating hormone inhibiting factor -MSH-IF) the release of α-MSH from the pars intermedia (Figure 3.10). The hypothalamic inhibitory control of α-MSH secretion involves a complex but direct neural mechanism, which contrasts the neurohumoral control system of the anterior pituitary. Dopamine inhibits the secretion of all intermediate lobe peptides from its cells. In addition, adrenaline, nor adrenaline, γ-amino butyric acid and 5-hydroxytryptamine also modify the release of α-MSH from neurointermediate lobe cells. These transmitters may be involved in the neural control of the neurointermediate lobe (Figure 3.10).

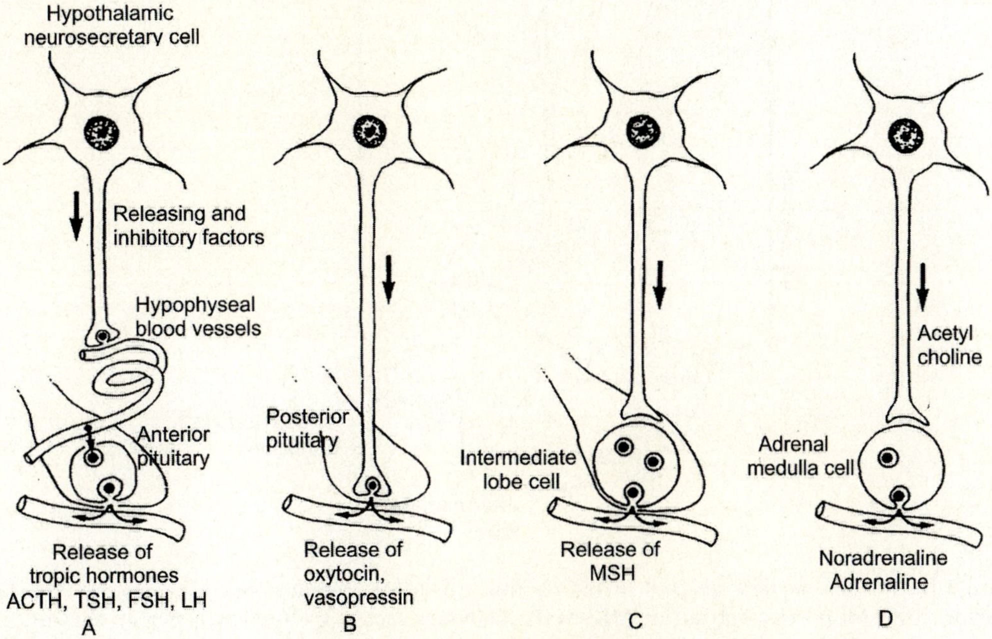

Figure 3.9: Neural control of endocrine functions.

3.10 Neurotransmitters and Neuropeptides

In addition to the specific peptide-releasing hormones, it is now known that the neurons in the brain, including the hypothalamus, produce other substances that modify the secretion of one or more pituitary hormones, either directly or indirectly by varying the release of releasing hormones. These substances can be classified as neurotransmitters and neuropeptides.

Neurotransmitters: Neurotransmitters are small chemical mediators involved in the transfer of information from one neuron to the next via synapses. The classical neurotransmitters are amines or amino acids (adrenaline, nor adrenaline, serotonin or 5-hydroxytrytamine, dopamine, acetylcholine, and γ-amino butyric acid) whose structural formulae are given in Figure 3.11. Evidences indicates involvement of dopamine and acetylcholine in release of oxytocin and vasopressin; acetyl choline, dopamine, γ-amino butyric acid, nor adrenaline and 5-hydroxytryptamine in gonadotropin release; dopamine and 5-hydroxytryptamine and possibly also acetyl choline and noradrenaline in prolactin (PRL) release; nor adrenaline, dopamine and 5-hydroxytryptamine in growth hormone release; nor adrenaline and 5-hydroxytryptamine in TSH release; and 5-hydroxytryptamine, and possibly nor adrenaline and acetylcholine in ACTH release.

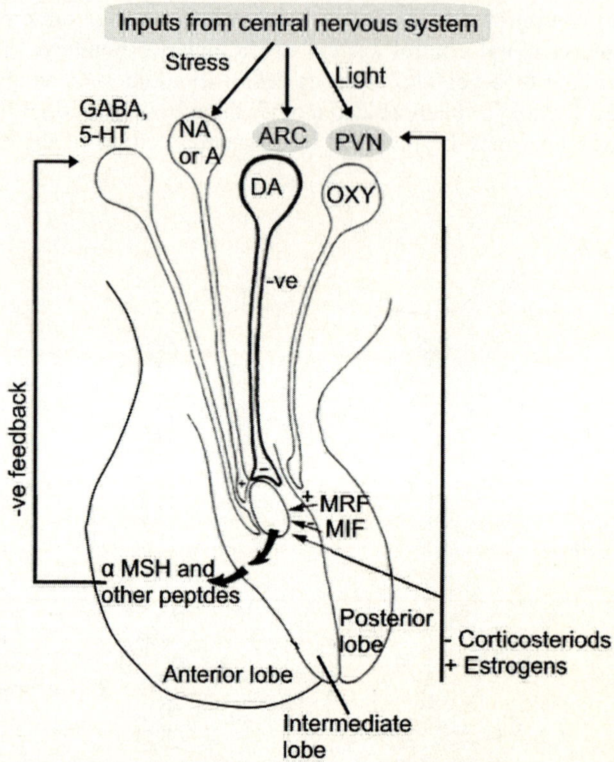

Figure 3.10: Possible factors involved in the control of α-MSH secretion, MSH-melanocyte stimulating hormone, MRF-MSH releasing factor, MIF-MSH inhibitory factor, PVN-paraventricular nucleus, ARC-arcuate nucleus, OXY-oxytocin, DA-dopamine, A-adrenaline, NA-nor adrenaline, GABA-γ amino butyric acid, and 5 HT-5-hydroxytryptamine.

Neuropeptides: Several neuropeptides have been detected in the portal blood and have been found to have effects on the secretion of particular pituitary hormones. The effects may be similar to those of the neurotransmitters, that is modifying the activity of hypothalamic neurons producing releasing hormones, or at the pituitary cell level working as "**neuromodulators**". A neuromodulator is a substance that is released in the vicinity of the synapse and augments or blocks the release of the neurotransmitter. Some of these include **substance P** (an 11-amino acid polypeptide of tachykinin family, distributed throughout the body in tissues of neural crest origin), neurotensin (a 13-amino acid polypeptide found extensively in nerve cells in the CNS), **bombesin** (a peptide found in frog and shares biologic activity with mammalian gastrin-releasing peptide-GRP), **proopiomelanocortins** (a large precursor molecule from which ACTH is processed), and the **gastrointestinal peptides**.

3.11 Mechanism of Action of Hypothalamic Hormones on Pituitary Cells

The hypothalamic hormones, both releasing and inhibiting factors, exert their effects on pituitary cells through binding to specific receptors on the cell membrane. Each receptor is usually highly specific for a particular factor (**secretagogue**). For some factors, such as LH-RH, TRH, pituitary cells appear to possess two types of receptors, a low-affinity, high-capacity type and a high-affinity, low capacity type. In some cells, two or more substances may have additive or opposing effects on hormone secretions that results in either blockade of a single receptor or form separate and independent binding at different receptors. Also, the number and concentration of receptors vary under the influence of local and systemic "modulating" factors such as neurotransmitters, steroids, hormonal feedback, so that the response of the cell to its primary secretagogue is regulated by the availability of its receptors.

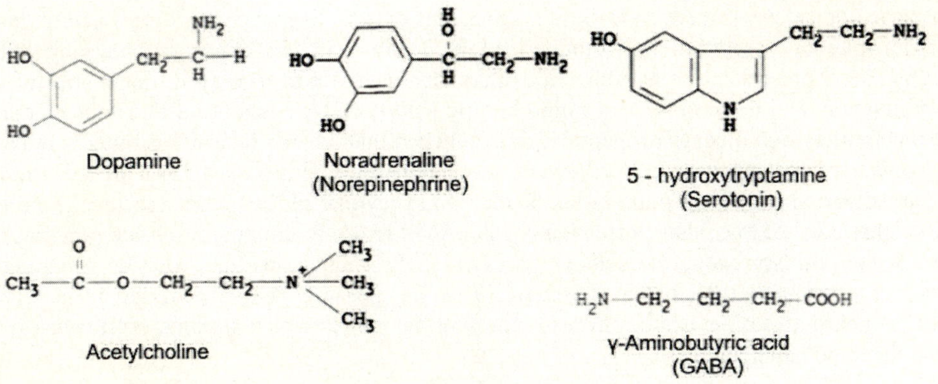

Figure 3.11: Structure of principal nonpeptidergic neurotransmitters.

The exact intracellular pathway leading to increased or decreased hormone secretion following secretagogue binding to a pituitary cell is still not clear. Two mechanisms have been implicated involving either the adenyl cyclase enzyme system or changes in intracellular cAMP concentration, or changes in intracellular calcium ion concentration due to influx or mobilization of intracellular stores or both. However, the process of exocytosis in all cells is known to be calcium dependent. Figure 3.12 shows the possible pathway. Changes in secretion by the cell may be effected by action at three points in the intracellular secretory pathway. These are synthesis of new hormone by the rough endoplasmic reticulum, release of hormone from granules at the cell membrane, and degradation of old hormone by lysosomes. In some cases the processes of synthesis and release appear to be activated independently. For example, LH-RH stimulation of LH secretion from the mammalian gonadotroph is not accompanied by *de novo* protein synthesis unless the cell has received a prior exposure or 'priming' to LH-RH.

In addition to the established hypophysiotropic hormones, the hypothalamus contains numerous other biologically active peptides with known structure and action on the anterior pituitary, but their possible physiological function as hypophysiotropic hormones or regulators of other hormones is not clearly understood. Further, a number of biogenic amine neurotransmitters present in the hypothalamus converge on the median eminence and indirectly or directly influence the secretion of the anterior pituitary hormones. This implies a second, "higher" level of control over the production of the hypothalamic hormones. This may be by inhibitory or stimulatory input from other extra hypothalamic areas of the brain, directly or indirectly from the special sense organs (vision, smell, hearing), exteroreceptors (temperature, pain, reproductive stimuli), chemoreceptors, stress, or inbuilt rhythms. Alternatively, control may be resulted through changes in the levels of hormones, ions and other substances in the blood supply to the hypothalamus and in the cerebrospinal fluid.

A major aminergic pathway, which terminates in the median eminence, is the intra-hypothalamic dopamine pathway. The neurons have both a neurosecretory function in that they can release dopamine into the hypophyseal portal capillaries, and may also modulate the release of other hypothalamic hormones as demonstrated by the existence of axo-axonic connections with peptidergic nerve terminals in the median eminence, and also by pharmacological studies. Table 3.3 gives the possible roles of brain neurotransmitters in the regulation of anterior pituitary secretion. There may be four possible mechanisms by which neurotransmitter modulation of pituitary secretion might operate (Figure 3.13). These are i) action via one or several neurons in a neural pathway converging on the neurosecretory neuron ii) direct synapse on the soma or dendrite of the neurosecretory neuron, iii) axo-axonic synapse on the nerve endings of the neurosecretory neuron, and iv) neurotransmitter neurons secrete directly into portal vessels and neurotransmitter acts directly at pituitary level. Physiological and pharmacological evidence for all these mechanisms exists. Responses of theses neurotransmitters on anterior pituitary secretion are summarized in Table 3.3. Evidence is emerging that other neurotransmitters present in the hypothalamus may also have a part to play in the control of anterior pituitary function, and these include γ-amino butyric acid (GABA-amino acid transmitter), adrenaline (amine transmitter), and other neuropeptide. It is believed that when a neurotransmitter is released at a synapse on a hypothalamic neuron, it causes an action potential. This passes down the axon and results in the depolarization and calcium ion influx, leading to exocytosis of the neuro secretory granules at the ending (Figure 3.8). It may also cause changes in cAMP levels in the neuron by the same mechanism as seen for the pituitary endocrine cells (Figure 3.12). Prostaglandins have also been implied in the regulation of hypophysiotropic hormone release. This may possibly be by modifying or modulating the effect of the neurotransmitters, and may also represent the way in which steroids exert their controlling effects at the hypothalamic level.

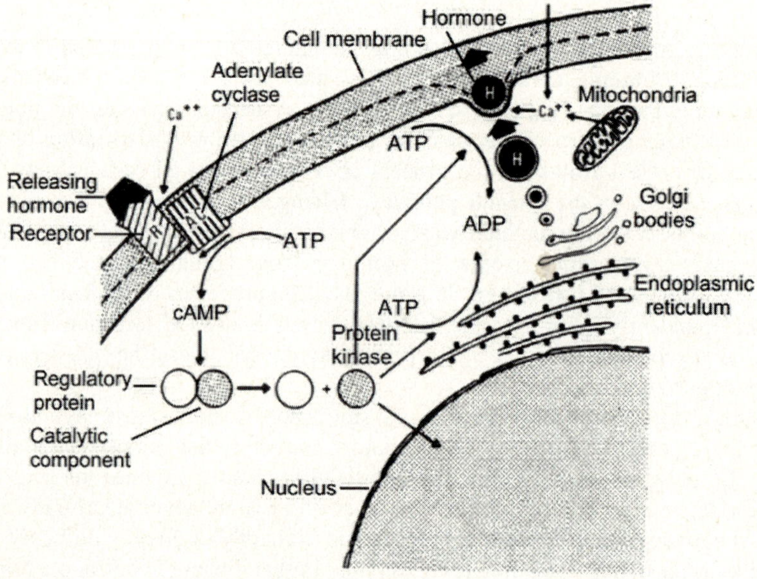

Figure 3.12: Intracellular pathway and biochemical events following stimulation of hormone release, ADP-Adenosine Diphosphate, ATP-Adenosine Triphosphate.

3.12 Peptides and Sexual Behavior

The hypothalamic gonadotropin-releasing hormone (GnRH), which induces the secretion of LH and FSH from the anterior pituitary, are considered as a likely mediator of sexual behavior since peripherally injected GnRH potentiates mating behavior (lordosis) in estrogen primed ovariectomized rats which have been adrenalectomized or hypophysectomized, indicating a control action independent of gonads, adrenals, or pituitary gland. Similar results have been observed in the mating behavior of male rats as well as an acceleration of ejaculation. The GnRH induced copulatory behavior is dependent on the presence of testosterone in the male and estrogen in the female. TRH is known to inhibit mating behavior. Both the GnRH and TRH-sensitive sites for these behavioral effects are confined to the medial pre-optic area, the arcuate ventromedial nuclei in the hypothalamus and the central grey in the mid-brain, an area of the brain from which descending axons originate and which are responsible for eliciting the lordosis response. In the female rats, GnRH is particularly active in the mid-brain central grey. It has been suggested that the ventromedial nucleus exerts an estrogen dependant tonic bias on the mesencephalic central gray and those GnRH neurons, also present in the ventromedial nucleus, may project to the same area. Thus, in female rodents, GnRH may act to synchronize the timing of ovulation with sexual receptivity thereby maximizing the chances of fertilization. Since GnRH is known to facilitate mating behavior in rats, it may be used to treat human disorders leading to sexual dysfunction and impotence.

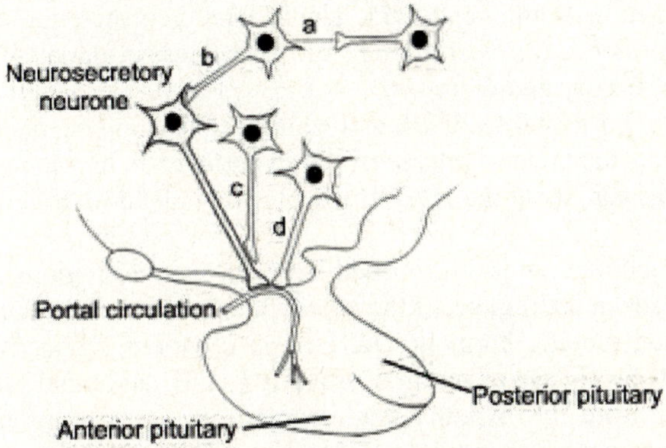

Figure 3.13: Four possible mechanisms by which neuro-transmitters modulate function of anterior pituitary -a) action via one or several neurons in a neural pathway converging on neurosecretory neuron, b) direct synapse on the soma or dendrite of neurosecretory neuron, c) axo-axonic synapse on nerve endings of neurosecretory neuron, and d) neurotransmitter neuron secretes directly into portal vessels and neurotransmitter acts directly at pituitary level.

Table3.3: Brain neurotransmitters in regulation of anterior pituitary secretion

Neuro-transmitters	**Corticotropin (ACTH)**	**Gonadotropins (LH/FSH)**	**Growth Hormone (GH)**	**Prolactin (PRL)**	**Thyrotropin (TSH)**
Acetylcholine	++	+	0	-	?
Γ-Amino butyric acid (GABA)	-	+	+	-	-
Dopamine	-	+ -	+ -	- -	+ -
Histamine	+ -	+ -	?	+ -	+ -
Nor adrenaline	- -	+	+ +	+ -	+ ?
Serotonin	+ -	- +	+ +	+ +	+ -

+ = Stimulation, - = Inhibition, 0 = No apparent regulation, ? = Unknown regulation

Summary

The hypothalamus and pituitary gland form a joint unit, which exerts control over the functions of several endocrine glands.

The hypothalamus lies at the base of the brain, and is a composite of nerve tissue. It controls the functions of pituitary, and is the "top boss" of endocrine activity.

Specific interactions between the hypothalamus, pituitary, and target endocrine glands form a series of closed-loop regulatory units that are the core of the endocrine system.

The hypothalamus is connected to the pituitary by both nerve fibers and blood vessels, through which it regulates the hormonal activity. It regulates the hormonal output of the anterior pituitary via releasing and inhibiting hormones and synthesizes two hormones that it exports to the posterior pituitary for storage and later release.

Hypothalamic hormones are small peptides which cause i) acute release or inhibition of the anterior pituitary hormone, ii) an increase in the synthesis of the pituitary hormone.

With the exception of growth hormone (GH) and prolactin (PRL), all the anterior pituitary hormones regulate the function of other endocrine glands, and their secretion rates are controlled by the feedback action of the hormones released by their target endocrine gland coupled with the integrated information from various sensory neural inputs.

The integration of hormonal feedback and neural information occurs chiefly at the level of the hypothalamus and regulates the rates of release of the hypothalamic hormones. However, feedback of some circulating hormones can act at the level of the pituitary gland to affect its responsiveness to the hypothalamic hormones.

Very different functional units are formed between specific regions of the hypothalamus and the posterior pituitary. Cells in the regions of the supraoptic and paraventricular nuclei synthesize large molecules that contain anti-diuretic hormone (ADH) and oxytocin, respectively. The hormones are released from these depots by change of serum osmolarity (ADH) and nipple stimulation (oxytocin).

A release factor from the hypothalamus triggers the anterior pituitary to secrete a tropic hormone that stimulates a target gland or tissue.

Questions

1. Explain why the hypothalamus is an endocrine gland.
2. How the hypothalamo-hypophyseal tract and the hypophyseal portal veins are functionally similar and structurally different?
3. How do hypothalamic releasing and inhibitory hormones influence the secretions of the anterior pituitary gland?
4. Describe the structure and importance of hypothalamo-hypophyseal tract.
5. Describe the structural and functional relationships between the hypothalamus and the pituitary gland.
6. The pituitary is often referred to as the master endocrine gland, but it too has a "master". What controls the release of pituitary hormones?

Chapter 4

The Pituitary

The pituitary gland is the hub around which a majority of the activities of the endocrine system revolve. It affects most of the functions of the body. To understand how the pituitary gland controls the activities of other glands, it is essential to study the structural and functional anatomy of this important gland.

4.1 Structure of Pituitary Gland

The pituitary is a compound gland located in the concavity of the sphenoid bone, sella turcica. It is encapsulated by the dura mater. Pituitary gland is one of the best-protected and most inaccessible organs of the body. Structurally and physiologically, the **pituitary** or **hypophysis** is divided into two parts: the **anterior pituitary** (**adenohypophysis**), comprising nearly 75 percent of the gland (mainly as **pars distalis**), and the **posterior pituitary** (**neurohypophysis**) comprising nearly the remaining 25 percent. Between these two parts is a small strip of tissue called the **pars intermedia** (Figure 4.1), which is a very small vestigial structure in man but is much larger and more functional in some lower animals. **Pars tuberalis** is a thin sheath of non-glandular cells surrounding the infundibular peduncle or stalk of the pituitary and is a part of the adenohypophysis. The anterior pituitary originates from the pharyngeal epithelium (roof of the mouth), while the posterior pituitary originates from the neural tissue (an outgrowth of the hypothalamus). Details of components of pituitary gland and their derivation are given in chapter 3. Because of the dual origin of this tiny gland, anatomical differences exist between the two lobes of the pituitary gland.

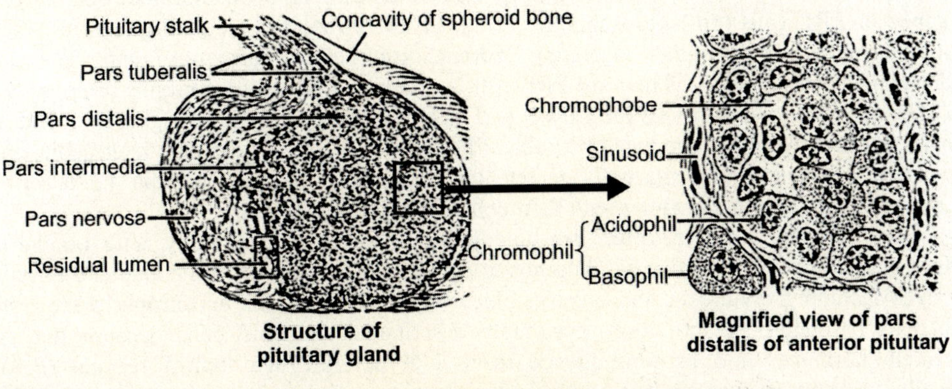

Figure 4.1: Structure of the pituitary gland and magnified view of pars distalis to show two types of chromophils (acidophil and basophil) and undifferentiated chromophobes.

4.2 Microscopic Structure of Anterior Pituitary

Anatomically, anterior pituitary consists of two parts, the pars tuberalis and pars distalis. The pars tuberalis is a thin epithelial plate of cells, which is formed by the fusion of two outgrowths from the embryonic pars distalis and in adults, it may surround the infundibular stalk and extend some distance below the tuber cinereum. The pars distalis is the main component of the anterior pituitary. It contains an irregular mass of epithelial cells separated by sinusoids and supported by a loose framework of connective tissue. The cells of pars distalis (**adenohypophyseal cells**) are glandular in nature containing certain characteristic granules. They are known as **chromophils.** On the basis of selective staining techniques, two major classes of these gland cells can easily be identified. These cells take either acid stain (40%) or basic stain (10%) or do not take any stain (50%), and hence, accordingly they are designated as **acidophil**, **basophils**, and **chromophobe** cells, respectively (Figure 4.1). Chromophobes are the biggest of the three and are named so because they do not stain as readily as the other two types. These cells are assumed to be the progenitors and thus represent undifferentiated acidophils and basophils and are not associated with the secretion of any hormone. On the other hand, acidophils are smaller than the basophils and the components of the stain react with particular cells according to the nature of the stored hormone, for example acidophils take up acidic dyes and basophils take up basic dyes. Staining properties of anterior pituitary or adenohypophyseal cells are shown in Table 4.1. Some of the acidic stains are orange G, eosin, acid fuchsin, alizarin blue etc, while basic stains are periodic acid –Schiff (PAS), aldehyde -fuchsin etc. The term amphilic (amphophil cell) is used to describe the nature of the cytoplasmic granules of thyrotrophic cells, since these PAS positive granules, by varying the fixatives and stains, can be made to appear either basophilic or acidophilic.

Table 4.1: Staining properties of adenohypophyseal cells

Cell Type	Staining Property
Adrenocorticotrophs, ε cells	Acidophilic, erthrosinophilic, alizarin blue+ (Aliz B+)
Gonadotrophs, β and γ cells	Basophilic, PAS+
Lactotrophs/PRL cells, η cells	Acidophilic, erthrosinophilic
Somatotrophs, α cells	Acidophilic, orangeophilic (OG+)
Thyrotrophs, δ cells	Amphilic, PAS+, aldehyde fuchsin+ (AF+)

Immunocytochemical and electron microscopic techniques now permit classification of cells by their specific secretory products, such as **somatotrophs** (growth hormone-secreting cells), **lactotrophs** or **PRL cells** (prolactin-secreting cells), **thyrotrophs** (cells secreting thyroid stimulating hormone), **corticotrophs** (cells secreting adrenocorticotropic hormone), and **gonadotroph** (gonadotropin secreting cells). The term PRL cell is preferred because lactotrophs refers only to the action of prolactin hormone (PRL) on growth and differentiation of mammary glands, found only in mammals. Further, ACTH is produced by cells of both the pars distalis and pars intermedia, although only cells of the pars distalis normally secrete the complete molecule. Table 4.2 describes the hormones of the pituitary gland along with their cellular source and actions.

Somatotrophs and lactotrophs are acidophilic, staining preferentially with orange G and erythrosin or azocarmine respectively. Adrenocorticotrophs are also acidophilic and tend to stain with acidic dyes including erythrosin and alizarin blue. Gonadotrophs and thyrotrophs were originally described as basophils, but are more accurately described as mucoid cells because they secrete glycoprotein hormones and in consequence react with periodic acid Schiff reagent (PAS) that specifically identifies polysaccharide-containing molecules. Thyrotrophs also react with aldehyde fuchsin that stains acid mucopolysaccharide. However, various cell types do not always give exactly the same reaction in different animal species.

Table 4.2: Hormones of the pituitary gland

Part of Pituitary Gland	Hormone	Chemical Structure	Secreted by (Cell Type) Target Tissue	Principal Action and Effects Hypo secretion ↓ Hyper secretion ↑
Anterior Pituitary (Pars Distalis)	Thyroid stimulating Hormone (TSH) or Thyrotropin	Glyco-protein	Basophil (Thyrotrophs) Thyroid	Stimulate the thyroid gland to form and release thyroid hormones; ↓Cretinism in children; Myxedema in adults ↑ Graves' disease, exophthalmos
	Prolactin (PRL) or Lactogenic hormone or luteotrophin	Poly-peptide	Acidophil (Lactotroph or Mammotroph) Mammary Epithelium	Proliferation of mammary gland and initiation of milk secretion ↓Poor milk production in nursing women ↑Galactorrhea; cessation of menses in females; impotence in males
	Adrenocortico-tropic hormone (ACTH) or corticotropin	Poly-peptide (39 amino acids)	Basophil (Corticotrophs) Adrenal Cortex	Stimulates secretion of adrenal cortex; promotes release of glucocorticoids and androgens, (to a lesser extent mineralocorticoid) ↓ Rare ↑ Cushing's disease
	Luteinizing hormone (LH) or Interstitial Cell Stimulating Hormone (ICSH)	Glyco-protein	Basophil (LH-gonadotroph) Testis-Leydig cells; Ovary-Interstitial and follicular cells; Corpus luteum	On Gonads (Testis and Ovary) In males, stimulates Leydig cells to promote secretion of androgens; In females, triggers ovulation and stimulates ovarian production of estrogen and progesterone; ↓Failure of sexual maturation ↑No important effects
	Follicle Stimulating Hormone (FSH)	Glyco-protein	Basophil (FSH-gonadotroph) Testis-Sertoli Cells; Ovary-Granular cells	On Gonads (Testis and Ovary) Testes-promotes spermatogenesis Ovary-causes growth and maturation of ovarian follicles; estrogen production; ↓ and ↑- same as LH
	Growth Hormone (GH) / Somatotropin (STH)	Poly-peptide (191 amino acids)	Acidophil (Somatotrophs) Liver, muscle, adipose, bone, cartilage, etc.	Stimulates somatic growth; mobilizes fats; target organs- bone, muscle, adipose tissue, liver, etc.; ↓ Pituitary dwarfism in children ↑ Gigantism in children, acromegaly in adults
Pars Inter-media	Melanocyte-stimulating Hormone (MSH) or Intermedin	Peptide	Basophil (Corticotrophs) Skin	Promotes skin pigmentation, results in dispersion of pigment granules in the melanophores, thus causing darkening of skin
Posterior Pituitary or Neurohy-pophysis	Antidiuretic hormone (ADH) or Vasopressin	Peptide	Neurons in supraoptic nucleus of hypothalamus Kidneys	Promotes reabsorption of water by kidney tubules; elevates BP; ↓ Diabetes insipidus ↑ Syndrome of inappropriate ADH secretion (SIADH)
	Oxytocin	Peptide	Neurons in paraventricular nucleus of hypothalamus Uterus, Breast	Stimulates uterine contraction; initiates labor; affects sperm transport in female tract; initiates milk ejection

4.3 Ultra structure of Adenohypophyseal Cell

The pituitary cells or the peptide-hormone-secreting cells have the typical organization of glandular epithelial cells (Figure 4.2). Peptide synthesis is very energy demanding; therefore, these cells have numerous mitochondria. The basic components of these cells are cytoplasmic organelles concerned with peptide synthesis, including rough endoplasmic reticulum (RER), mitochondria, hormone storage granules, and smooth endoplasmic reticulum forming the Golgi complex. They store their product in secretory granules. The process of peptide synthesis occurs in the RER. Messenger RNA (mRNA), encoded by nuclear DNA, passes to ribosome attached to RER membranes. By sequential processing of transfer RNAs (tRNA) with their attached amino acids, the specific peptide chain is assembled. A specific signal sequence causes the membrane of the RER to recognize the beginning of the peptide molecule and attach to it, thus enabling the growing peptide to pass into the lumen of the RER cisternae. The signal sequence is cleaved and a particular peptide of the adenohypophysis passes along the RER lumen until a specialized area of membrane, without attached ribosome, is reached. This is the Golgi complex and it is here that peptides are parceled. Finally, by a pinching-off process at the membrane of the innermost cisternae of the Golgi stack, they are released into the cytoplasm as membrane-bound granules, and are stored until the hormone is released by exocytosis. This process involves fusion of the granule membrane with the cell membrane so that the granule contents are released into the extra cellular space and ultimately into the lumen of the capillary.

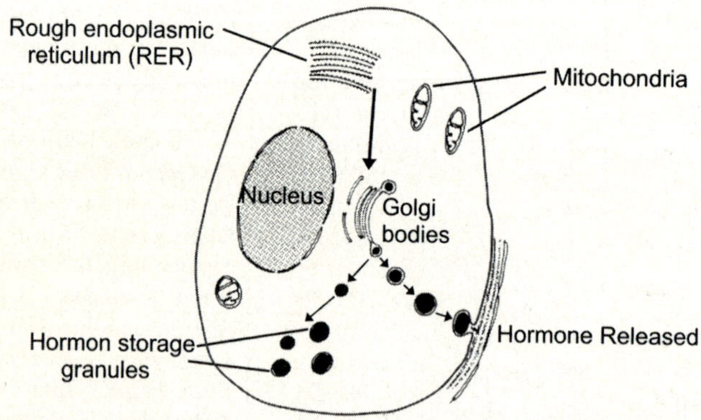

Figure 4.2: Structure of peptide-hormone-secreting cell showing intracellular secretory pathway, amino acids assembled into peptides in RER pass to the Golgi bodies to be parceled into membrane-bound granules for release or storage.

4.4 Hormones of Anterior Lobe of Pituitary Gland

The anterior pituitary gland acts like a composite of independent glands, since it secretes seven major hormones. Each of these hormones is produced by a specific group of cells (Table 4.2). There are five types of cell in mammalian pars distalis, and a single MSH-secreting cell in the pars intermedia secreting seven hormones since both gonadotropins (FSH and LH) are secreted by the same cell. These hormones are thyroid stimulating hormone (TSH), follicle stimulating hormone (FSH), luteinizing hormone (LH), adrenocorticotropic hormone (ACTH), growth hormone (GH, also called somatotropic hormone or STH), prolactin (LTH), and melanocyte tropic hormone (MTH). Four of these hormones, ACTH, TSH, FSH and LH induce cellular growth and increased secretions in **specific target glands** and therefore, are designated as **tropic hormones**, meaning "turning toward" in Greek. The remaining three anterior pituitary hormones, LTH, GH (STH), and MSH have direct metabolic effects on target tissue. However, α-MSH, β-MSH, and, β-lipotropin (LPH) are produced by cells of the pars intermedia. β-lipotropin is a lipotropic peptide, named for its action on adipose tissue and possibly functions as anti-pain (analgesic) hormone. Figure 4.3 indicates how the anterior pituitary hormones exert their control on the target organs.

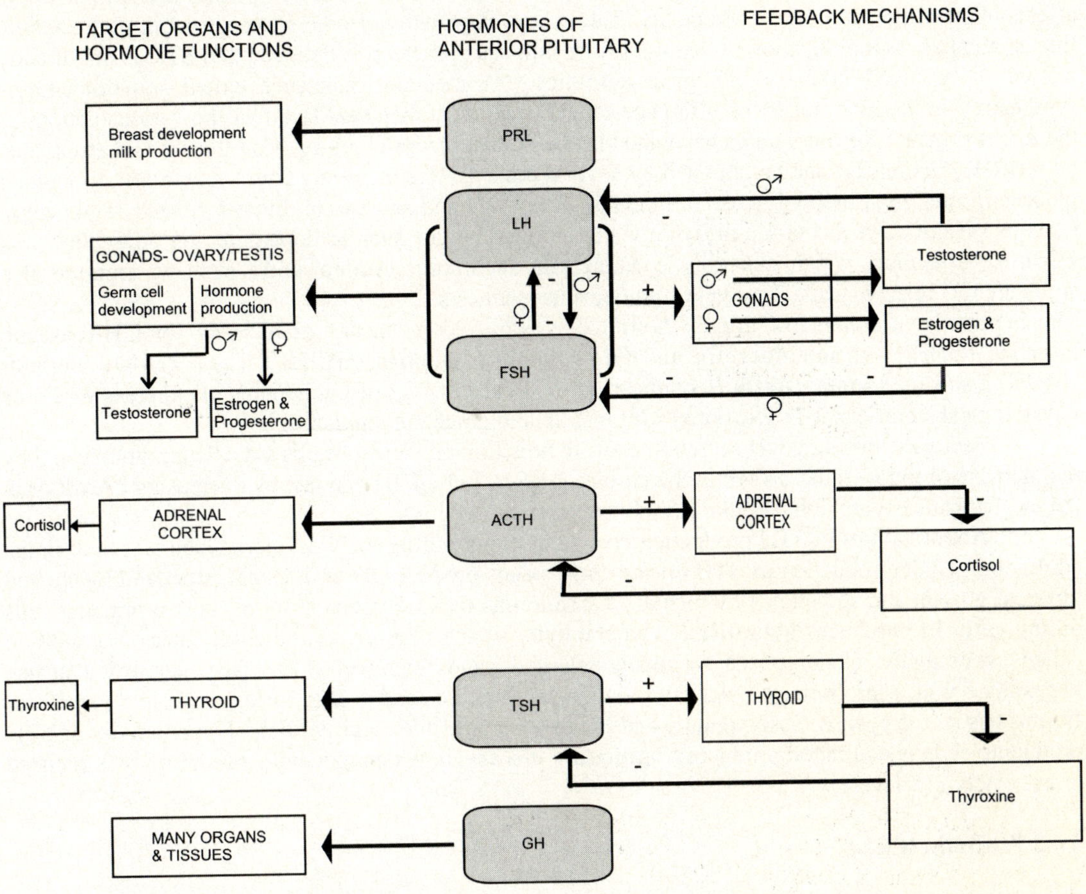

Figure 4.3: Target organs and functions controlled by the hormones of anterior pituitary; + = Stimulation and - = Inhibition.

4.4.1 Growth Hormone (GH)

Growth hormone is also called as **Somatotropin (STH)**. It is a peptide containing 191 amino acids in a single chain with two intra-molecular disulfide bridges. Acidophilic cells (somatotrophs) of the adenohypophysis produce it and its molecular weight in man is 22,000 Dalton. Somatotrophs normally contain spherical secretory granules. These are the most numerous cell types in non-pregnant animals and also are more numerous in males than females.

Growth hormone is released episodically from the pituitary. It is not a tropic hormone, as it does not exert its effect on a specific target gland. The effects of growth hormone are particularly striking in bones, muscles, kidneys, adipose tissue, and liver. One of the important functions of STH is growth and differentiation of epiphyseal cartilage during preadolescent period and ossification of chondrocytes at maturity. It causes the growth of all tissues of the body that are capable of growing. It promotes both, the growth and mitotic activity of the cells resulting in the development of increased number of cells. It also increases the rate of protein synthesis in all cells of body by increasing the amino acid transport through the cell membrane. Another important function of STH is initiation of gluconeogenesis. Decreased peripheral utilization of glucose, hyperglycemia and increased oxygen consumption are characteristic effects of excess growth hormone. These responses are similar to the effects of starvation and are diabetogenic. The excess of growth hormone has a strong lipolytic action, that is, it enhances mobilization of depot fat from adipose tissues. It is believed that STH is not directly related or involved in these biological activities. A mediator substance called somatomedin is synthesized in the liver under the influence of STH, which is then said to effect the various actions in the target organs. Recent studies have shown that somatomedin C inhibit secretion of GH stimulated by GHRH. GH release can be obtained by several other factors including stress, starvation, low blood glucose in rats, high blood glucose in humans, anesthesia and short-term direct feedback. The central nervous system plays a coordinating role via neurotransmitters, such as dopamine, nor adrenaline, and 5-hydroxytrptamine, which generally enhance GH secretion. Amino acids, such as arginine also stimulate GH release, while thyroxine stimulates its synthesis.

The hypothalamic control of growth hormone is achieved by means of STH-RH or GH-releasing hormone (GHRH) or **somatocrinin** and GH-inhibitory hormone (GHIH). The STH-RH inhibitor (GHIH) also called **somatostatin** is synthesized in D cells of islet of Langerhans in pancreas where its physiological significance is associated with insulin and glucagon regulation.

Factors controlling GH secretion exert their action on somatotrophs via calcium uptake and by the increase of intracellular cAMP in the case of GHRH, but GHIH may act by decreasing cAMP or in the mechanisms beyond intracellular cAMP conversion.

Abnormalities in STH production can occur either during early developmental stages or in the adulthood. Underproduction of STH during early stages produces **dwarfism**, characterized by stunted physical growth and sometimes by mental retardation as well. Hyperactivity of STH producing cells during early life produces **gigantism.** Hyperactivity of the pituitary in the adult causes a condition called **acromegaly**, characterized by much enlarged hands and feet. The face acquires a coarse appearance with a protruding lower jaw, and widely spaced teeth. Due to the excessive growth of fibrous tissue, the eyelids, nose, tongue, and the lips become thick and swollen. Hyperactivity of STH producing cells in adulthood produces **Simmond's disease**, in which metabolic rate of body is reduced to extremely low levels.

4.4.2 Prolactin (PRL)

Prolactin (PRL) is also called as **Lactogenic hormone** or **mammotropic hormone (MH)** or **luteotropic hormone (LTH)**. It is a protein hormone, chemically similar to GH and is secreted by acidophil. Lactotrophs or PRL-cells are larger than somatotrophs with more irregularly shaped pleomorphic secretory granules. They are distributed uniformly in the pars distalis, and increase in size and number during pregnancy and lactation. Prolactin cells are unique among pituitary pars distalis in being principally under tonic inhibitory control from hypothalamus, and generally exhibit autonomous secretion.

Human PRL is a single –chain polypeptide with a molecular weight of about 22,500daltons. PRL is continuously inhibited by a hypothalamic inhibitory hormone (PIH), and therefore, is stimulated by abolishing the release of PIH in the hypothalamus. In mammals, the hypothalamic inhibitory factor is considered to be dopamine. Other factors that may be concerned with control of PRL secretion include vasoactive intestinal peptide (VIP), thyrotropin releasing hormone (TRH), steroid hormones and neurotransmitters (Figure 4.4). A potent stimulant for PRL release, peculiar to mammals, is suckling of the mammary gland.

PRL is highest at term (that is end of pregnancy), and it drops rapidly immediately after labor to a basal level during the first few days of delivery. Every time, when there is stimulation of the nipples during suckling, there are bursts of release of PRL, giving rise to high plasma concentrations. Therefore, existence of PRL-releasing hormone (PRH) has also been postulated to explain this phenomenon. And when the mother stops breast-feeding, PRL level gradually decreases and eventually stops. Hypothalamic TRH stimulates PRL secretion in addition to that of TSH. Muscular exercise, sleep, emotional and physical stress are some other stimuli which seem to work through hypothalamus on PRL. Further, PRL has a short-loop negative feedback inhibitory effect on the hypothalamus to stop its own release.

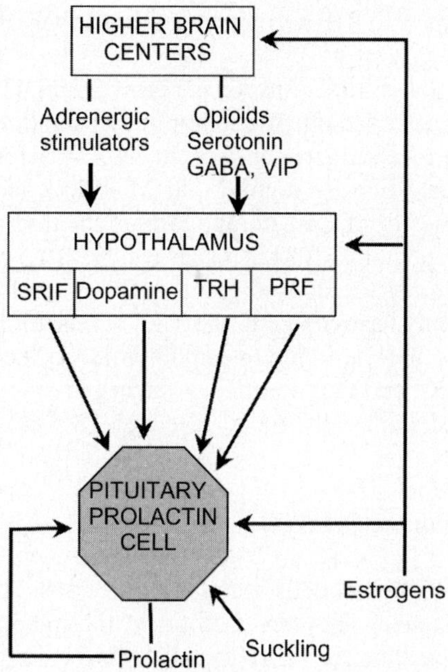

Figure 4.4: Factors controlling the secretion of prolactin, GABA-γ-amino butyric acid, VIP- Vasoactive intestinal peptide, SRIF-Somatostatin, TRH-Thyrotropin-releasing hormone and PRF-Prolactin-releasing factor.

Prolactin is involved in i) growth and development, ii) osmoregulation (both of these are primitive actions), and iii) reproduction. The most familiar role of PRL in reproduction is stimulation of mammary gland growth and milk production. PRL increases mitosis of mammary epithelial cells during development. It acts on the breast to produce milk. The continued secretion of prolactin during pregnancy causes growth of the mammary glands but due to inhibitory effect of the large amounts of estrogen and progesterone secreted by the placenta, production of milk does not occur at that time. After delivery, this inhibition is removed, and PRL initiates and maintains milk production. PRL release during breast-feeding exerts negative effect on the ovaries and suppresses the menstrual cycle by decreasing the sensitivity of the ovaries to gonadotropins. In mammals, PRL can be luteolytic and luteotropic. High circulating levels of PRL in primates cause amenorrhea, due in part to action on the ovary, but PRL also interferes with pituitary gonadotropin production, particularly episodic LH secretion, which would normally initiate and maintain the corpus luteum. In males PRL acts on the testes and accessory sex glands, causing increase in the weight of seminal vesicles.

The wide range of PRL actions in vertebrate physiology suggest that the molecule is very ancient and has played a vital part in vertebrate survival and evolutionary radiation.

4.4.3 Thyroid Stimulating Hormone (TSH)

Thyroid Stimulating Hormone (TSH) or **Thyrotropin** is a glycoprotein secreted by basophilic cells (thyrotrophs) with molecular weight 28,000 Daltons. TSH has two subunits, one (α) that is common to LH, FSH, and human placental lactogen (HPL), and the other (β) that expresses TSH hormone bioactivity. TSH is released from pituitary gland under the influence of thyroid releasing factor/hormone (TRH), secreted from hypothalamus. Hormones of the thyroid gland, thyroxine (T4) and tri-iodothyronine (T_3) in turn control the levels of TRH. These hormones decrease the responsiveness of the thyrotrophs to TRH by reducing the number of TRH-binding sites on the cell membrane.

As the name implies, TSH is important for the growth and development of the thyroid gland. It stimulates the secretion of thyroxin and other iodothyronine from thyroid gland. The actions of TSH are mediated by cyclic AMP via receptor sites on thyroid cells. TSH accelerates the process of iodine trapping and therefore its concentration by thyroid gland. It also activates the proteolytic enzymes, which release the thyroid hormones from their storage form in the thyroglobulin molecules.

Primary pituitary deficiency of TSH or its exces is rare. Thyroid disease, however, is common and this is usually due to diseases of the thyroid gland itself. Therefore, high or low TSH is usually secondary to thyroid disease. In hyperthyroidism, the TSH levels are found to be low due to negative feedback effect of the excess T_3 and T_4, while in hypothyroidism the levels of TSH are high due to diminished thyroid hormone levels, and thus absence of the negative feedback. However, in the case of endemic goiter, due to iodine deficiency, the blood levels of TSH are found elevated, resulting in the enlargement of the thyroid gland.

4.4.4 Adreno-corticotropic Hormone (ACTH)

Adrenocorticotrophs are small polyhedral cells with long processes. These make up about 4 % of the total cell population of pars distalis. They are distributed throughout the pars distalis except for a narrow region besides the pars distalis. ACTH (also called **Corticotropin**) molecule has only recently been characterized. It is a single chain polypeptide, containing 49 amino acids of which only 23 amino acids constitute the active core. Its secretion is under the control of hypothalamus through corticotropin-releasing hormone (CRH). This hormone is under the control of circulating adrenal glucocorticoid hormones through a negative feedback mechanism. The primary action of ACTH is to stimulate adrenal cortex or internal cells to secrete glucocorticoids, mainly cortisol and corticosterone, which exercise feedback inhibition on release of ACTH by pituitary corticotrophs. The adrenal steroids in the circulation act directly on both corticotrophs and hypothalamic nuclei.

In mammals, basal secretion of ACTH is episodic, with bursts of hormone released every 1-3 hour. These occur rhythmically and in relation to dark or light and activity cycles, so that the highest circulating levels of ACTH and glucocorticoids occur just before start of activity, i.e. waking time and reach their lowest just before cessation of activity, i.e. sleeping time. ACTH is rapidly released in response to physical or emotional stress and hypoglycemia. This response to stress is a part of the general preparation to counteract injury, infections and various other stressful conditions.

ACTH is necessary for the healthy growth and repair of the adrenal cortex and for maintaining healthy vascularity of the gland. In cases of ACTH deficiency, the adrenal cortex atrophies and its blood vessels disappear while its excess causes hypertrophy of the adrenal cortex. ACTH stimulates the synthesis of cortisol and 17-keto-steroids by the adrenal cortex. It has little or no effect on the aldosterone secretion. It acts on adenyl cyclase and a protein kinase to increase the lipid content of the adrenal cortex. Free cholesterol is also increased. ACTH has a melanocyte-stimulating action causing pigmentation of the skin in conditions where high ACTH levels are found. ACTH decreases the ascorbic acid content of the adrenal cortex. It stimulates insulin secretion and also mobilization of free fatty acids (FFAs) from adipose tissue. The levels of ACTH are elevated in Addison's disease due to destruction of the adrenal cortex, and absence of inhibitory feedback effect of the glucocorticoids.

4.4.5 Gonadotropic Hormones

The gonadotropic hormones **are follicle stimulating hormone (FSH)** and **luteinizing hormone (LH)** or **interstitial cell stimulating hormone ICSH)**, which control both male and female gonadal functions. The same cell (gonadotrophs) secretes both FSH and LH. Gonadotrophs are scattered throughout the pars distalis, but tend to be more numerous in the cephalic region near the infundibular attachment. Secretion of gonadotropins by the pituitary is controlled by a hypothalamic releasing hormone, GnRH, or LH-RH. In mammals, the basal levels of LH and FSH secretion necessary for gonadal integrity are maintained by a succession of episodic discharges, regulated by negative feedback of the gonadal steroids.

Both FSH and LH are double-chain glycoproteins with molecular weights in order of 30,000-35,000 Dalton. The molecules are composed of two subunits, α and β, each containing a carbohydrate moiety. The smaller unit (α –subunit contains 96 amino acids) is common to all the pituitary glycoprotein hormones-LH, FSH and also TSH. The β-subunit (about 120 amino acids) confers biological specificity on the hormone. Both subunits are required for hormonal activity. Carbohydrates of gonadotropins are a variable proportion of the total molecular weight, most frequently between 10 and 15 %. They include hexose, hexosamine, and sialic acid, which is only a small part of the total carbohydrate in LH but a significantly higher proportion in FSH. Carbohydrate is attached to both peptide subunits and presence of carbohydrate is important for biological activity of the molecule.

The secretion of FSH and LH is controlled by hypothalamus as well as by the hormones of the gonads. The rate of secretion of gonadotropin hormones is controlled by gonadotropin releasing hormone (GnRH), a peptide of the hypothalamus. GnRH (LH-RH) was the second hypothalamic hypophysiotropic hormone to be isolated and characterized and its structure was first published in 1971. GnRH is released from hypothalamic nerve terminals into the hypophyseal portal vessels and transported to the anterior pituitary where it stimulates the synthesis and release of LH and FSH. There has been debate as to whether, the hypothalamus secretes two releasing factors-**luteinizing hormone releasing hormone (LHRH)** for the secretion of luteinizing hormones, and **follicle-stimulating hormone releasing hormone (FSH-RH)** for follicle stimulating hormone or only one as GnRH. The biological responses induced by the action of GnRH on pituitary are an increased release and synthesis of both LH and FSH. GnRH is secreted in a pulsatile fashion, as are the gonadotropins, and the rate and amplitude of such pulses appear to be of paramount importance in determining the magnitude of response of the pituitary. The receptors for the gonadotropins as for all glycoprotein hormones are proteins located on the plasma membrane of target cells. They have a high affinity for their respective hormones, with dissociation constants in the order of 10^{-10M}. Both FSH and LH act on their gonadal target cells by stimulating adenylate cyclase, which causes an increase in the intracellular concentration of cAMP (see Chapter 7).

The hormones of the gonads, **androgens** and **estrogens**, have been found to act directly on hypothalamus and inhibit the release of releasing hormones. In the males, LH is also called as ICSH as it stimulates interstitial or Leydig cells to promote testosterone production in the testes to maintain spermatogenesis and development of accessory sex organs. In the females, LH stimulates the synthesis of female sex hormones. The final maturation of ovarian follicles and ovulation is under the influence of LH. A modified follicular structure, corpus luteum is formed. LH also maintains the corpus luteum during the secretory phase of the menstrual cycle. Binding studies of FSH in the gonad have indicated that FSH receptors are located on only one cell type in either the testis or ovary-namely, the Sertoli cells or the granular cells respectively. FSH functions to maintain the spermatogenic epithelium in the male and promotes the early growth of ovarian follicles in the female. In the female, estrogen is produced under FSH influence, in the growing Graafian follicle. In addition, it also stimulates protein synthesis and mitotic activity of the granulosa cells. In the male, under the influence of FSH, the Sertoli cells of germinal epithelium in testis produce a glycoprotein called ABP (androgen binding protein), which is responsible for transport of androgens in the tubules of epididymis where functional maturation of spermatozoa occurs. In the testis, the Sertoli cells play an important role in spermatogenesis providing nutrients for the developing sperm and forming a unique blood-testis barrier, which serves to protect the maturing sperm. Sertoli cells are also believed to produce another protein, called inhibin that normally appears in seminal plasma. Inhibin inhibits FSH production.

4.5 Microscopic Structure and Hormones of Intermediate Lobe of Pituitary

Intermediate lobe of pituitary has polygonal cells (**basophil-corticotrophs**) that can be stained with basic dyes. It has vesicles, lined with low columnar epithelial cells, with or without basophilic granules in their cytoplasm. Their lumens are filled with colloid. Follicles lined with basophilic cells are often present and some of the cells contain secretory granules. This lobe secretes only one hormone known as **melanocyte stimulating hormone (MSH)** or **melanotropin** or **intermedin**. However, a peptide hormone secreted by the adenohypophysis is called **corticomelanolipotropins**, which include **α-** and **β-melanotropin (MSH), adrenocorticotropin (ACTH),** and **β-lipotropin (LPH)**. Cells of pars intermedia produce α-MSH, β-MSH, and β-LPH by cleavage of a large molecule, **proopiocortin**. MSH is a polypeptide and structurally similar to ACTH molecule.

MSH increases melanin biosynthesis by acting on melanocytes present in the dermis and epidermis of the skin. It promotes dispersion of the melanin pigment in entire cells making them dark in appearance. MSH is thus involved in color adaptation in lower vertebrates. In mammals, MSH is a vestigial hormone and therefore, its role in man is not clear. It may influence deposition of pigment in nipples, areolae and other parts of skin in pregnant women and participate in darkening the areas already pigmented.

The release of MSH, both in mammals as well as lower vertebrates, is under hypothalamic inhibitory control. This control, unlike that of pars distalis is mediated directly by neurons, which terminate in the vicinity of the hormone-secreting cells and appears to involve both catecholamines and peptidergic substances (see Chapter 3). Both, MSH release-inhibiting factor (MIF) and MSH releasing factor (MRF), derived from oxytocin have been characterized but their physiological significance remains to be demonstrated.

Another intermediate lobe hormone called **Corticotropin-like intermediate lobe peptide (CLIP)** has been described but the control of its secretion etc. requires further study.

4.6 Microscopic Structure and Hormones of Posterior Lobe of Pituitary

The posterior pituitary gland is recognized by the presence of nerve fibers and is composed of glial cells of nervous system called **pituicytes**. However, pituicytes act simply as terminal nerve endings that originate in the supraoptic and paraventricular nucleus of the hypothalamus and thus do not secrete hormones. Thus, posterior pituitary gland is responsible for the storage of hormones synthesized in these nuclei of the hypothalamus. **Antidiuretic hormone (ADH)**, also known as **vasopressin**, is produced in the supraoptic nuclei of the hypothalamus while hormone **oxytocin** is produced in the paraventricular nuclei of the hypothalamus. These hormones travel down the nerve fibers and remain as storage granules in the nerve endings with in the neurohypophysis until they are released by specific stimuli.

4.6.1 Antidiuretic Hormone (ADH)

ADH also called, **Vasopressin** or **Pitressin** is a nanopeptide. Its principal action is to increase water reabsorption in the collecting ducts of the kidney, and hence named anti-diuretic. The name vasopressin has also been given to ADH because of the powerful vasoconstrictor effect of this hormone. Two main stimuli are known to result in its secretion. One is an increase in the osmotic pressure of the extra cellular fluid (ECF). This occurs in the state of dehydration, due to either excessive water loss or water deprivation. High osmotic pressure stimulates osmoreceptors in the anterior hypothalamus. These receptors are located near the supraoptic nucleus and the impulses generated in them stimulate the release of ADH. The second stimulus to result the release of ADH is a fall in blood volume. This may occur in conditions leading to dehydration or after blood loss. Hemorrhage causes a fall in the blood pressure and one of the earliest responses to hemorrhage is ADH release. The response to volume receptor stimulation is more powerful than that due to osmo-receptors. Both mechanisms tend to release ADH, which in turn causes the kidney tubules to reabsorb water. The volume of urine is consequently greatly decreased and water is retained in the body so as to correct the volume and osmolarity of the extra cellular fluid.

Emotional stress, physical trauma, pain, and certain drugs such as barbiturates, nicotine, morphine etc also release ADH. Alcohol inhibits the secretion of ADH.

4.6.2 Oxytocin

Oxytocin (also called **Pitocin**)is also a nanopeptide hormone and chemically similar to ADH. It causes ejection of milk from the lactating breasts and contractions of the uterus during labor. Oxytocin is released in response to two types of secretory stimuli- i) by stimulation of the nipples of the lactating mother or suckling of the offspring to result in ejection of milk and therefore, facilitates breast-feeding, and ii) distension of the uterus and stretching of the cervix also stimulates release of oxytocin which in turn facilitates contraction of the uterine muscles leading to gradual expulsion of the fetal head through the birth canal. Also, stimulation of vagina and the genital organs during coitus causes release of oxytocin, resulting in repeated contractions of the uterus and fallopian tubes. Fear and use of alcohol inhibits oxytocin release while pain, anxiety may release oxytocin. These 'reflex' pathways therefore, have a neural (afferent) input with a hormonal (efferent) output. The stimuli that release oxytocin work at the level of hypothalamic nuclei and impulses from the paraventricular nuclei travel in the hypothalamo-hypophyseal tracts to release the stored hormone from the nerve endings in the neurohypophysis directly in the bloodstream.

Oxytocin is secreted in male of mammals but its physiological actions and control mechanisms are not understood.

4.7 Feedback Mechanisms in the Control of Pituitary Function

Feedback mechanisms are of great importance in regulating the levels of pituitary secretion. They are best exemplified by the pituitary-target gland model (Figure 4.6), which shows that the pituitary, under the influence of a hypothalamic factor, secretes a tropic hormone that stimulates a target gland to release its hormone, known **as long-loop feedback** (see also Chapter 2). There is also evidence that some pituitary hormones can exert positive or negative regulation of their own secretion by **short-loop feedback** (Figure 4.5). It is also possible that some hypothalamic hormones might control their own release by **ultra-short-loop feedback** via either a vascular route or a system of axosomatic synapse.

Feedback effects of gonadal steroids in the control of gonadotropin secretion: One of the major mechanisms controlling the secretion of gonadotropin is the feedback effect of the steroids both at the brain and the pituitary gland. In the adult male, the rate of gonadotropin secretion does not show cyclical changes and remain relatively constant due to the negative feedback effects of testosterone. However, the mature female shows a cyclical rhythm of gonadotropin release and estrogens have been shown to exert both positive and negative feedback effects. The positive feedback action occurs at midcycle, when estrogen levels are high due to increased secretion from the mature follicle(s). These relatively high levels of estrogen stimulate what is known as the pre-ovulatory LH surge (positive feedback) and this surge is responsible for rupture of the mature follicle and release of the ovum (ovulation). The hormonal events, which occur during the estrous or menstrual cycle, are dealt in chapter 15.

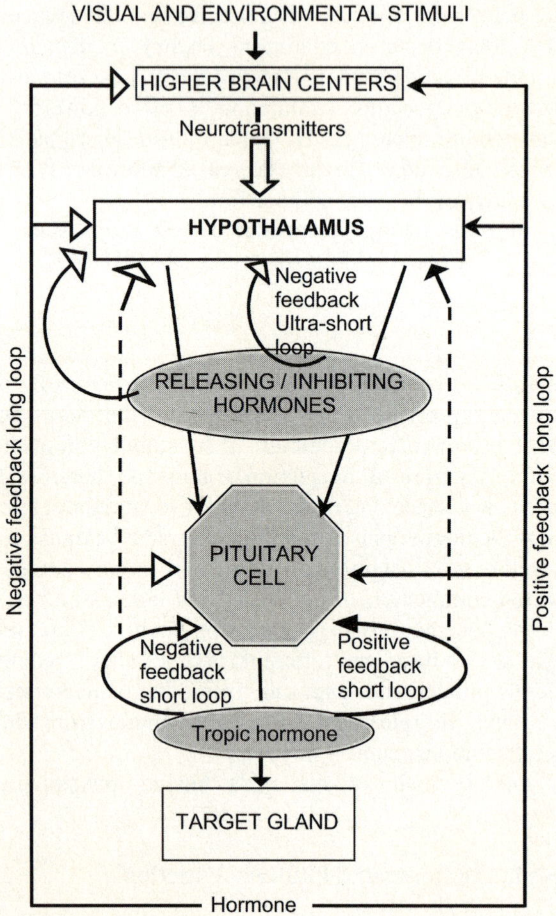

Figure 4.5: Pituitary-target gland model to show feedback pathways controlling secretion of pituitary hormones.

Generally at the pituitary level, high concentration of estrogens are known to increase the amount of LH secreted in response to GnRH, as occurs prior to ovulation whereas, testosterone inhibits GnRH effects on pituitary LH release. Progesterone appears to have a biphasic effect, initially promoting GnRH responsiveness followed by an inhibitory effect. In contrast, all three steroids have an exclusively stimulating action on the release of FSH in response to GnRH (Figure 4.6). Apart from steroid modulation of the GnRH response in the anterior pituitary, there is also substantial evidence showing that gonadal steroids can act at the level of the hypothalamus to alter rate of GnRH secretion in both sexes. In the female, the pre-ovulatory surge of LH is associated with an increased concentration of GnRH in hypophyseal portal blood (thought to result from an increased frequency and/or amplitude of the pulsatile GnRH secretion). In the rat gonadectomy results in a rise of both GnRH and gonadotropin secretion due to the loss of negative feedback of steroids.

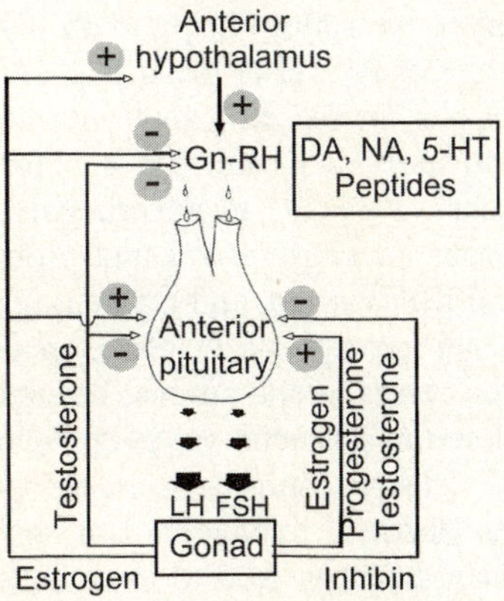

Figure 4.6: Feedback effects of sex steroids on the hypothalamus and anterior pituitary. DA-dopamine, NA-noradrnaline, 5-HT-5-hydroxytryptamine, GnRH-Gonadotropin releasing hormone, LH-Luteinizing hormone, FSH-Follicle stimulating hormone.

It is clear that mechanisms, which trigger the pre-ovulatory surge of LH, are complex and appear to involve steroid modulation of pituitary responses to GnRH and stimulation of GnRH release by an action on the hypothalamus. It seems that the increase in pituitary responses observed prior to and during the LH surge occurs in two phases. The first occurs gradually due to the elevated levels of estrogen and the second phase occurs rapidly and abruptly (10 fold), just prior to ovulation, perhaps largely due to the self-priming capacity of GnRH. Progesterone can also augment the effects of estradiol but, because of the timing of the progesterone surge in many species, it is not certain whether this plays a major role in stimulating ovulation. Pituitary seems to be the major site of steroid feedback.

4.8 Hypophysectomy

Removal of pituitary gland or hypophysis is termed as hypophysectomy. In young animal, it results in cessation of growth, retention of juvenile hair-coat and other immature features. In adults, it results in atrophy of adrenal cortex, and thyroid. The testes and ovaries become non-functional with no germ cells and gonadal hormones to maintain functional status of accessory sex organs. Metabolism of carbohydrates, lipids, and proteins gets disturbed with reduction in blood glucose, decrease in glycogen in liver and muscle. Metabolization of fat and nitrogen loss from body gets retarded. Color adaptation in fish, amphibians and reptiles is lost.

4.9 Abnormalities of Pituitary Function

Several clinical syndromes are known to be associated with disorders of pituitary especially with its hyper or hypo functions. However, disorders of pituitary function are not as common as other endocrine disease like diabetes mellitus and mostly develop from the development of a tumor, e.g. an adenoma. Pituitary dysfunction can also result from disorders of the hypothalamus, again via a tumor, e.g. a craniopharyngioma. Other causes of pituitary dysfunction are trauma after injury, vascular disorders, such as a pituitary infarct (pituitary apoplexy), subarachnoid hemorrhage, or very rarely inflammatory problems resulting from infectious diseases such as encephalitis or meningitis. Sheehan's syndrome occurs in mothers with post-partum hemorrhage and necrosis of the anterior pituitary resulting in congenital disorder with GnRH deficiency.

Hyperpituitarism: Over activity (hyper secretion) of pituitary is hyperpituitarism. This may result in increased secretion of growth hormone or ACTH or prolactin. If it is hyperactive during childhood or adolescence before closure of epiphysis, increased growth hormone results in gigantism (precocious growth), or mentally subnormal and individuals die by or before the age of 20yrs. If pituitary is hyperactive after the epiphysis closure, it results in **acromegaly**, in which bone gets thickened and deformed, drastic facial changes occur causing growth and protrusion of jaw, enlargement of nose, growth and enlargement of hands and feet, viscera, and thickening of the skin. Increased ACTH causes formation of adrenal tumor or adrenal hyperplasia resulting in **Cushing's disease** due to prolonged excessive production of cortisol. The contra lateral adrenal becomes atrophic due to negative feedback and therefore, low ACTH. Raised serum prolactin (**hyperprolactinemia**) may occur during normal pregnancy and lactation, stress sleep, drugs use, as well as hypothalamic disorders. Hyperprolactinemia can lead to galactorrhea, hypogonadism, amenorrhea, and infertility in women. This condition is less common in man, but may lead to impotence, ejaculatory failure or galactorrhea due to reduced actions of gonadotropins on the gonads in the presence of high prolactin and inhibition of the positive feedback of estrogens, which trigger the LH surge. Hyperprolactinemia caused by pituitary or hypothalamic disease may be treated with a long-acting dopamine receptor agonist drug, Bromocriptine (α-bromo- α ergocrytine). Vasopressin excess is called **syndrome of inappropriate ADH (SIADH)**, and is fairly common in clinical medicine. It tends to complicate many diseases of chest and brain. SIADH results when a reduction in plasma osmolarity does not reduce vasopressin secretion and this may cause **hyponatremia** (low plasma sodium concentration) due to excess water reabsorption. Oxytocin excess or deficiency is not associated with any disease. SIADH does not require any treatment other than water deprivation.

Hypopituitarism: Under activity or low activity of pituitary is hypopituitarism. A single adenohypophyseal hormone deficiency is rare, but condition of inappropriate growth hormone and gonadotropin occur most frequently. The gonadotropins are usually affected first. Evidence of TSH and ACTH involvement appears later. In children, the predominant feature is failure to grow. Underproduction of STH results in dwarfism with permanent retarded sexual development, i.e. sexually immature condition. Due to lack of TSH or symptoms of hypothyroidism, pituitary myxedema is resulted showing reduced BMR, low heart beat, puffy skin and edematous tissues. Hypo secretion of adrenals due to low ACTH causes Addison's disease with low BP, loss of appetite and muscular weakness.

Panhypopituitarism is a term given to a generalized hypo function of pituitary. In this condition, most, if not all of the pituitary hormones are involved. It causes **Sheehan's syndrome** and **Simmond's disease** resulting in genital atrophy, gradual regression of secondary sex characteristics, loss of body hair, reduced BMR, subnormal body temperature, low heart rate and arterial pressure, disturbed carbohydrate metabolism resulting in hypoglycemia. These individuals live only for 6-12 months.

Deficiency of the neurohypophyseal hormone, vasopressin, also occurs rarely resulting in diabetes insipidus. The condition is characterized by the lack of antidiuretic activity, which result in frequent micturition (urination) and insatiable thirst. A synthetic long-acting analogue of vasopressin, known as desmopressin (DDAVP) has greater antidiuretic potency than vasopressor activity and therefore, desmopressin is administered through intranasal mode to treat patients of diabetes insipidus.

Summary

The pituitary gland is located at the base of the brain in the sella turcica of the sphenoid bone and attached to the hypothalamus by the pituitary stalk or infundibulum.

The pituitary gland consists of two distinct portions, an anterior lobe or adenohypophysis, and a posterior lobe or neurohypophysis.

During fetal development, a narrow third region appears between the anterior and posterior lobes of the pituitary gland called the intermediate lobe or pars intermedia. This region produces melanocyte stimulating hormone (MSH), which regulates the formation of melanin pigment in the skin.

Within the epithelial tissue of the anterior pituitary, five types of secretory cells can be recognized. They are somatotrophs, which secrete growth hormone (GH), thyrotrophs that secrete thyroid-stimulating hormone (TSH), corticotrophs that secrete adrenocorticotropic hormone (ACTH), gonadotrophs that secrete follicle stimulating hormone (FSH) and luteinizing hormone (LH), and mammatrophs that secrete prolactin (PRL).

Secretion of the anterior pituitary hormones is regulated by the releasing and release-inhibitory factors secreted by the hypothalamus.

Four of the anterior pituitary hormones induce cellular growth and increased secretion in specific target glands and therefore, are designated as tropic hormones. These are ACTH, TSH, FSH and LH. The remaining, i.e. LTH, GH or STH, and MSH have direct metabolic effects on target tissue.

The gonadal steroids secreted by the gonads exert feedback effect on the gonadotropin secretion from the anterior pituitary.

The posterior lobe of the pituitary gland largely consists of neuroglial cells and nerve fibers that originate in the hypothalamus. The two hormones of the posterior pituitary are secreted by special neurons called neurosecretory cells located in the hypothalamus. These two hormones are anti-diuretic hormone (ADH) and oxytocin (OT). These are stored in posterior pituitary and are released from there when required.

Surgical removal of pituitary is called hypophysectomy. Under activity and over activity of the pituitary gland is called hypopituitarism and hyperpituitarism respectively. These conditions lead to various abnormalities such as acromegaly, Cushing's disease, hyperprolactinemia etc. Panhypopituitarism term is given to a generalized hypofunction of pituitary.

Questions

1. Describe the location, histology, hormones and functions of anterior and posterior pituitary.
2. In what respect is the pituitary gland actually two glands.
3. Describe the development of pituitary gland.
4. List and describe the chief effects of adenohpophyseal hormones.
5. Discuss the structure of the neurohypophysis and describe the effects of the two hormones it releases.
6. Where is the pituitary gland located? Give a list of hormones that the anterior and posterior lobes of the pituitary gland secrete.
7. What effects does oxytocin produce in females?
8. Describe the functions of FSH and LH in a male and in a female.
9. What is a gonadotropin? Give its functions.
10. Summarize the functions of prolactin.
11. Compare the cellular structures of the anterior and posterior lobes of the pituitary.
12. The posterior pituitary is not really an endocrine gland. What is it and why?

Chapter 5

Sex Steroids

The term steroid has been derived from *stereos* meaning 'solid'. Steroid is the generic name for the compounds comprising the **sterols, bile acids** and **steroid hormones**. These are a class of biological compounds often found in association with fat and represent a group of **derived lipids** as they are derived from simple and compound lipids. The steroids synthesized in the sex organs, such as testes, ovaries are called **sex steroids**, and more commonly, as **sex hormones**.

5.1 Steroids

All steroids are derivatives of a fused and fully saturated ring system known as **cyclopentanoperhydrophenanthrene** or **sterane** (Figure 5.1). This ring system consists of three cyclohexane rings, A, B and C fused in nonlinear or phenanthrene manner to which a cyclopentane ring D is attached. The carbon atoms in the parent substance, cyclopentanoperhydrophenanthrene are conventionally numbered and the letters are assigned to the rings as shown in Figure 5.2. The six-member (hexagonal) rings in steroids are as in hexane and not as in benzene. This means that the valences of carbon atoms are fully satisfied by hydrogen bonds and if double bonds are present, they are shown as such. Most steroids made by living organisms have one or more double bonds, methyl groups (C 18 and 19) attached at position C 13 and C 10 respectively, and alcoholic and/or ketonic groups. Several types have side chains attached to C 17. The methyl groups C 18 and C 19 are known as the angular methyl groups (Figure 5.2). One exception to this generalization is found in the natural estrogens, the female sex hormones where ring A is aromatic (that is, ring A has three, alternate double bonds). Vitamin D and related calciferols are with one open ring, and are called secosteroids. The common steroids present in animals and humans are cholesterol, bile acids, as well as steroid hormones (Table 5.1).

Each of the three-cyclohexane rings in cyclopentanoperhydrophenanthrene nucleus is capable of existing in 3-dimentional corrugation or conformation in two forms. These are either of a '**chair**' or of a **'boat'** ('**bed**') type (Figure 5.3). The 'chair' form is rigid and resists distortion and when it is changed to the 'boat' form, some angular deformity invariably takes place. All the rings are in 'chair' form in the naturally occurring steroids. In addition, with respect to each other, the rings can be either *–cis* or *–trans*. The junction between the rings A and B (A/B) may be either *–cis* or *–trans* but between the rings B/C and C/D are always in *–trans* configuration with certain exceptions. When the hydrogen atom on C 5 is on the same side of the plane of molecule as the methyl group on C 10, then rings A and B are *–cis* to each other and the molecule belongs to **normal configuration**. On the other hand, if the hydrogen atom on C 5 is on the opposite side of the plane of molecule in comparison to the methyl group on C 10, the rings A and B are *–trans* to each other and the molecule is of **allo configuration**. Estrogens do not show such isomerism since in them, ring A is aromatic. In the structural representation of steroids, substituents that are above the plane of ring are β-oriented and are shown by solid lines. In addition, those, which are below the plane of the ring, are α-oriented and are represented by broken lines. For example, methyl groups at C 10 and C 13, the hydroxyl group on C 3 and the side chain at C 17 are all β-oriented in cholesterol molecule (Figures 5.2 and 5.3). In contrast, hydroxyl groups at 3, 7 and 12 positions in cholic acid are all α-oriented.

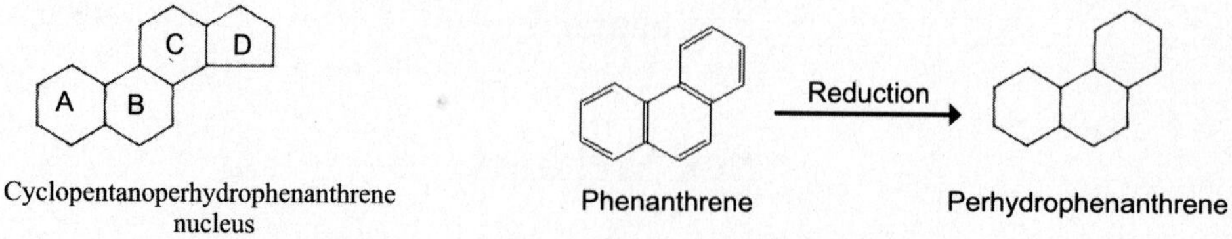

Figure 5.1: Cyclopentanoperhydrophenanthrene (Sterane).

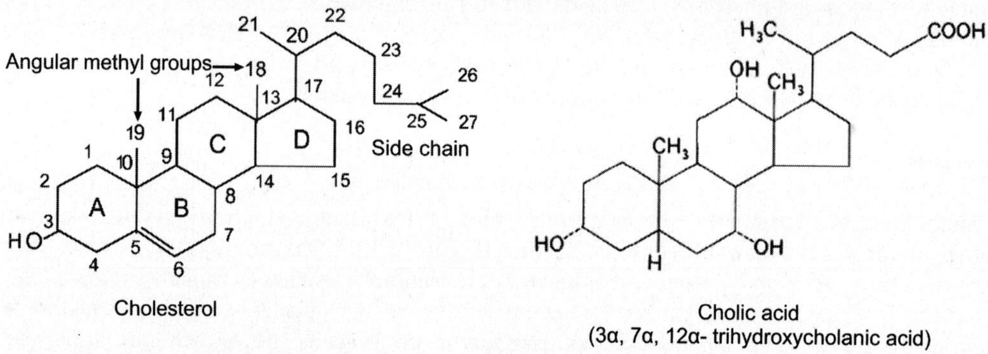

Figure 5.2: Structure of cholesterol and cholic acid.

5.2 Structure of Cholesterol

Cholesterol (cholest-5-en-3β-ol) is the best-known steroid (a sterol found in all eukaryote cells) having the parent nucleus, cyclopentanoperhydrophenanthrene (Figure 5.2). Corrugation of rings A, B, and C are of the '**chair**' and not the '**bed**' or '**boat**' type (Figure 5.3). It has a hydroxyl group at C 3, an unsaturated bond between C 5 and C 6, two methyl groups at C 10 and C 13, and 8 carbon side-chain attached to C 17 (Figure 5.2). Cholestane is a 27-carbon saturated steroid used as the "parent" structure for nomenclature of cholesterol (Figure 5.2), calciferols, bile acids and steroid hormones.

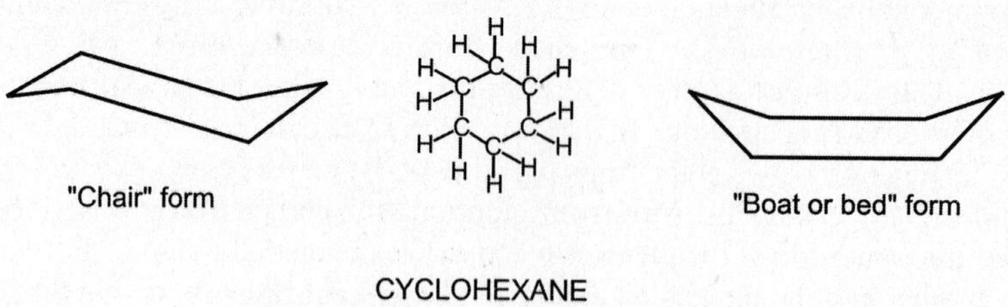

Figure 5.3: Isomerism of cyclohexane.

Modifications of the parent structure arise largely by the introduction of: i) unsaturation. e.g. double bonds between carbon atoms (-HC=CH-), as at C-5 and C-6 in cholesterol, ii) hydroxyl substituents, e.g. as at C-3 in cholesterol, and iii) carbonyl groups, e.g. oxidation of the secondary alcohol group of cholesterol to yield cholesten-3-one (Table 5.2). The position of these modifications is always indicated by the appropriate carbon number and the introduction of unsaturation change the vowel in the stem name (as shown in steroid hormones in Table 5.3)). Prefixes and suffixes are used to indicate the presence of substituents such as hydroxyl, carbonyl etc. Any number of prefixes is permitted but only one suffix may be used. The common substituents with their respective prefix and suffix forms are given in Table 5.2 and examples in Table 5.3.

Table 5.1: Some common steroids, their occurrence and biological roles

Steroid Group		Representative	Occurrence	Biological Role
Sterols	C_{30}	Lanosterol	Wool fat	Biosynthesis of cholesterol
	C_{28}	Ergosterol	Yeast	Provitamin D
	C_{27}	Cholesterol	Animal fat	Structural component of cells and precursor for other steroids
	C_{27}	7-dehydro cholesterol	Skin	Provitamin D
Bile acids	C_{24}	Cholic acid	Intestine and gall bladder	Absorption of fats
Hormone	C_{21}	Progesterone	Corpus luteum	Female hormone
	C_{21}	Dehydrocorticosterone	Adrenal cortex	Hormone in males and females
	C_{21}	Cortisol	Adrenal cortex	Hormone in males and females
	C_{19}	Testosterone	Testes	Male hormone
	C_{18}	Estradiol	Ovaries	Female hormone

Table 5.2: The common substituents with their respective prefix and suffix forms

Substituent Group		Prefix	Suffix
Group	Formula		
Acetate	$-OCOCH_3$	Acetoxy-	-yl acetate
Aldehyde	CHO	–	–al
Carbonyl	C=O	Oxo–	–one
Carboxylic acid	COOH	Carboxy–	–oic acid
Double bond	–C=C–	Δ– *	–ene
Hydroxyl	–OH	Hydroxy–	–ol
Triple bond	–C≡C–	–	–yne

❖ Not used in systematic nomenclature.

With the firm establishment of the structure of cholesterol, intensive studies were made to discover and isolate other steroid compounds from endocrine glands. Doisy and Butenand isolated estrone and Marrian isolated pregnanediol in 1929 from the urine of pregnant women. Little later, Marrian (1930) isolated estradiol from the urine of women showing advanced stage of pregnancy, while Butenandt isolated and characterized androsterone (1931) and dehydroepiandrosterone (1934) from the urine of males. However, estradiol and testosterone were obtained first time from the endocrine tissues in 1935: estradiol from sow's ovaries by Doisy and testosterone from bull's testes by Lacqueur. In 1934, four groups of scientists (Butenandt, Slotta, Allen and Wintersteiner, and Hartmann) simultaneously isolated progesterone.

As long as the number of steroids isolated remained small, each was referred by its 'trivial name', such as testosterone, estradiol, progesterone etc. However, when the list of naturally occurring steroid compounds became too long, introduction of systemic nomenclature became essential. Table 5.3 gives 'trivial' and 'systematic' names of most commonly known gonadal steroids and cholesterol.

Table 5.3: Trivial and systematic names of gonadal steroids

Trivial name	Systematic name
Cholesterol	Cholest–5–en–3β–ol
Estrone	3–hydroxy–estra–1,3,5 (10) –triene–17–one
Estradiol–17β	Estra–1,3,5 (10) –triene–3,17β–diol
Estradiol–17α	Estra–1,3,5 (10) –triene–3,17α–diol
Estriol	Estra–1,3,5 (10) –triene–3,16α, 17β–triol
Androsterone	3α–hydroxy–5α–androstan–17–one
Androstenedione	Androst–4–ene–3,17–dione
Testosterone	17β–hydroxy androst–4–en–3–one
Progesterone	Pregn–4–ene–3,20–dione
Pregnenolone	3β–hydroxy pregn–5–en–20–one
Pregnanediol	5β–pregnane–3α, 20α–diol
Pregnanetriol	5β–pregnane–3α, 17,20α–triol

5.3 Synthesis of Cholesterol

Cholesterol is the primary precursor of steroid hormones and bile acids. Therefore, it is important to understand the biosynthesis of cholesterol before dealing with the sex steroids.

Cholesterol is the most known molecule because of the correlation between its high levels in blood and incidence of cardiovascular diseases in humans. It is an important component of cell membranes and of plasma lipoproteins. It is especially abundant in nerve tissues and in gallstones. Egyptians and Greeks named it as cholesterol (*chole*-bile, *steroids*-solid) as it was found in bile stone (gallstone). However, cholesterol is not found in plant fat. Adolph Windaus received Nobel Prize in chemistry in 1928 for determining the structure of cholesterol.

Large part of the cholesterol is synthesized in the body and only small amount is provided by the average diet. It is synthesized from **acetyl coenzyme A (acetyl-CoA)** in many tissues of the body involving participation of both cytosolic and membrane-bound enzymes (Figure 5.4). Liver is the principal organ for its synthesis. Other tissues, which can also synthesize cholesterol, include adrenal cortex, intestine, skin, kidney, ovary and testis. Some cholesterol is obtained from food packaged into chylomicrons in the small intestine, and delivered to the blood stream via large lymphatic vessels. Hepatocytes take up cholesterol from chylomicrons and from other lipoprotein particles, and package it along with synthesized molecules, into low-density lipoprotein particles (LDLs), which are released to the bloodstream. Although circulating LDLs are major sources of cholesterol for most cell types, the sterol is also synthesized locally for internal use, especially when LDL levels are low.

Biosynthesis of cholesterol may be divided into five stages: i) formation of six carbon compound, mevalonate from three molecules of acetyl CoA, ii) isoprenoid units are formed from mevalonate by loss of CO_2, iii) condensation of six molecules of isoprenoid units through a series of phosphorylated intermediates into C-30 hydrocarbon, the squalene, iv) oxidation of squalene to 2,3-oxido-squalene followed by cyclization to give the tetra cyclic C-30 parent steroid, the lanosterol, and finally, v) modification of lanosterol by a number of oxidation and reduction steps, which result in the removal of three methyl groups and rearrangement of double bond to produce the C-27 product, the cholesterol (Figure 5.4).

In steroidogenic tissues, it is probable that the bulk of the steroids produced are derived primarily from acetate with cholesterol as an intermediate product. However, direct synthesis of steroids from cholesterol also occurs. Thus, both de novo biosynthetic and plasma cholesterol taken up by the tissue can serve as precursors to steroids and steroid hormones. All the important steroids are produced from cholesterol during steroid hormone biogenesis by desmolase or lyase enzymes, which break C-C bonds in vicinity of usually a tertiary carbon atom. Most important metabolic products formed from cholesterol in mammals are- i) the **C_{18}, C_{19}** and **C_{21} steroid hormones** derived by removal of the sterol side chain, ii) the fecal neutral sterols such as 5α-cholestan-3β-ol and 5β-cholestan-3β-ol; iii) the C_{24} bile acids obtained by removal of the terminal isopropyl group of the side chain, and iv) Vitamin D. A series of hydroxylases, oxido-reductases etc. carry out all the stereo specific transformations to give rise to a spectrum of steroid hormones. Quantitatively, the amount of cholesterol metabolized to steroid hormones may not be very large relative to the production of the other metabolites but is of vital physiological importance. The rate-limiting step in the synthesis of gonadal hormones from cholesterol is its delivery to the inner membrane of the mitochondria by the transport protein called steroidogenic acute regulatory protein (STAR).

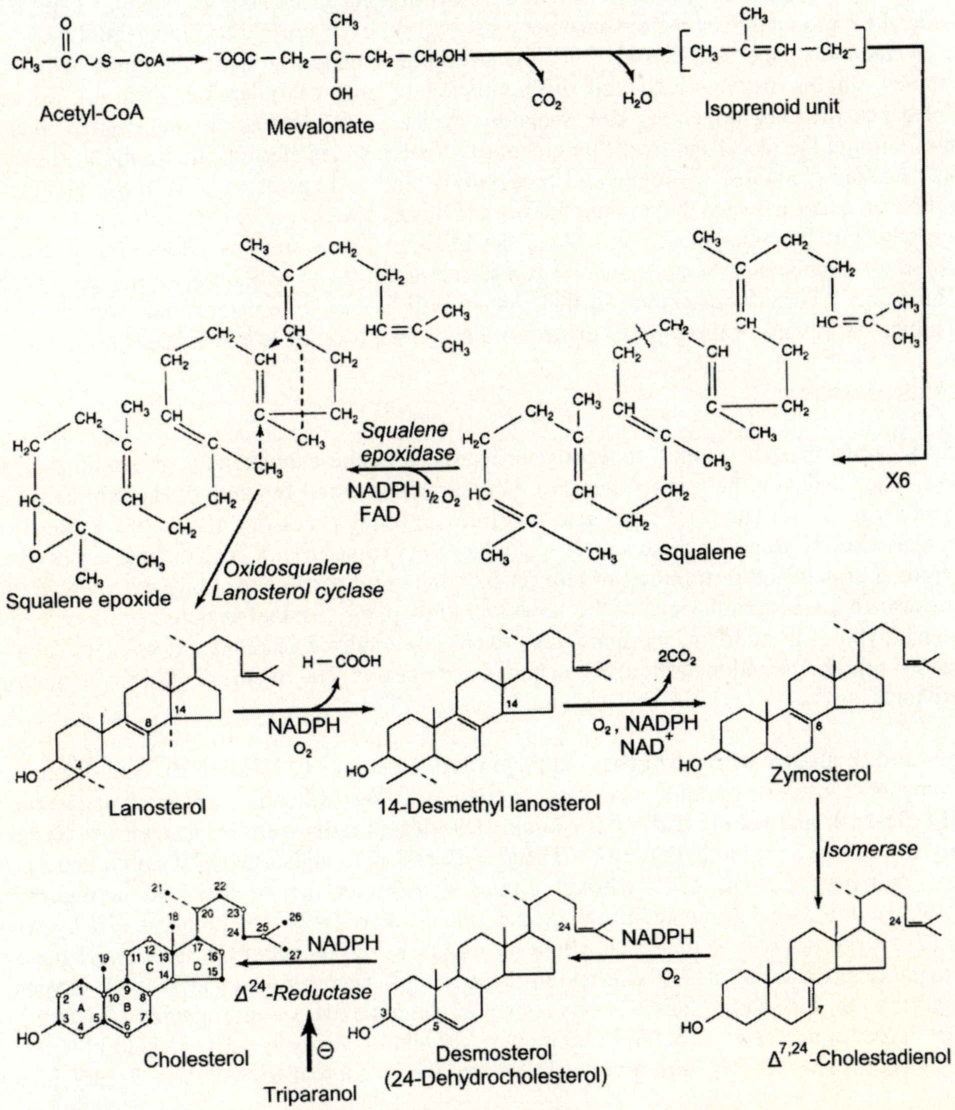

Figure 5.4: Biosynthesis of cholesterol.

5.4 Sex Steroids

The sex steroids are **gonadal hormones (sex hormones)** that are synthesized from cholesterol in the gonads. They are produced by testes, ovary and corpus luteum and in small quantities by the placenta and adrenal cortex. Naturally occurring sex steroids are a class of chemically related compounds and their basic structure is similar to that of cholesterol consisting of 4 fused rings, the cyclopentanoperhydrophenanthrene nucleus (called more simply as the **steroid nucleus**). There are three types of gonadal hormones: i) **Androgens** or **male hormones**, ii) **Estrogens** or **female hormones**, and iii) **Progestational hormones** or **gestogens**.

Sex hormone target tissues are widely distributed throughout the body. They include the gonads, the reproductive tracts, the accessory sex organs, liver, muscle and the central nervous system. The interaction of the sex steroids with their receptors induces a wide spectrum of tissue-specific responses ranging from growth and differentiation to enzyme induction, anabolic responses, and maintenance of spermatogenesis and ovulatory cycles. Sex steroids are transported to their target tissues through the blood and over 90 percent of circulating sex steroids are bound to specific plasma proteins called globulins. Estrogen and testosterone bind to a specific sex hormone binding globulin. Equilibrium exists between the amount of free and bound circulating sex steroids but it is only the free form, which is biologically active. Thus, the binding of sex steroids allows for a large potential 'reserve' of circulating free hormone. It is also important for protection against rapid metabolism of the hormone. Further description in this chapter will be on the structure, biosynthesis, metabolism, and biological actions of the gonadal or sex hormones, that is on male and female hormones.

5.5 Male Hormones

Androgens are male hormones concerned primarily with the characteristic masculinizing effects in males. They maintain the spermatogenesis, normal structure and function of the seminal vesicles and prostate, with the formation of citric acid and fructose in the accessory glands of reproduction. These hormones also influence development of secondary sex characteristics such as hoarseness of voice and differential growth and distribution of hair on face and other parts of the body in males. Furthermore, they cause an increase in the size of the testes, scrotum, penis, seminal vesicles, prostate, vas deferens, and epididymis. In addition, the androgens exert a generalized anabolic effect in the body causing increased protein formation particularly in bones and muscles, and retention of nitrogen, potassium and phosphorus.

Types and Structure of Androgens: Androgens are a class of **C 19 steroids** with distinct structural and functional features. Naturally occurring androgens are **testosterone, 5α–dihydrotestosterone (5α–DHT), 5α-androstanediol, androstenedione, dehydroepiandrosterone**, and **androsterone** (Figure 5.5). All of these have methyl group (–CH_3) at C 10 and C 13 and contain 19 carbon atoms. The most potent androgens possess 17β–hydroxyl groups with either the 4–en–3–oxo configuration as in testosterone or a 3–oxo group and a saturated A ring as in 5α–DHT. Oxidation of 17β–hydroxyl group to a 17–oxo group as in 4–androstenedione results in a loss of about 80 % of androgenic potency. Furthermore, presence of a 17α–hydroxyl group as in epi– testosterone or lack of 17–oxygen function altogether as in 4,16–androstadien–3–one results in complete loss of androgenicity. In addition, 3-oxo groups is also a necessary structural requirement for androgenicity because reduction to a compound like 5α–androstane–3β, 17β–diol gives only 60% of the potency of testosterone (Figure 5.6 and Table 5.4).

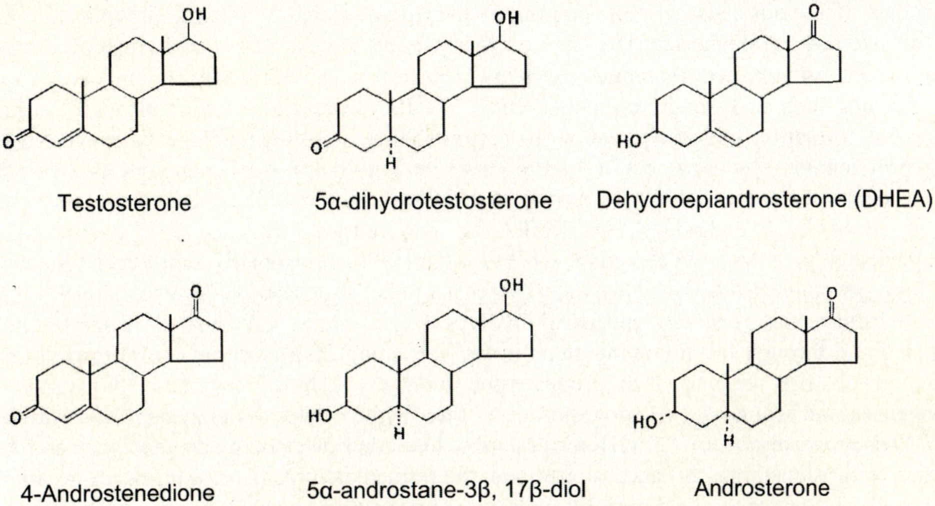

Figure 5.5: Structure of some naturally occurring androgens.

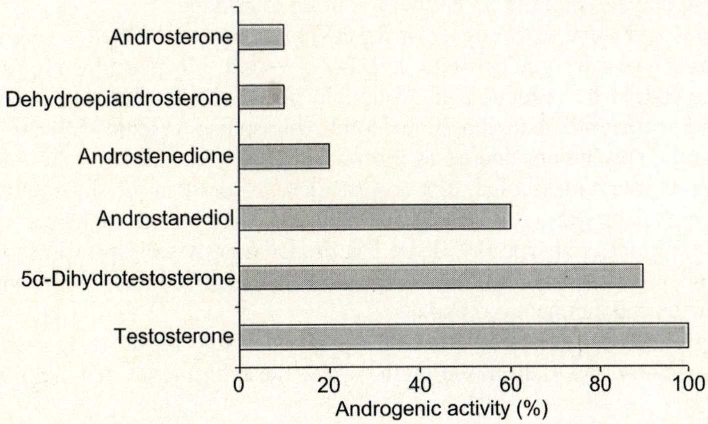

Figure 5.6: Androgenic activity (relative to testosterone) of some C-19 steroids.

Table 5.4: Percentage of relative potency of natural androgen

Androgen	Relative potency (%)
Testosterone	100
5α-dihydrotestosterone	90
Androstanediol	60
Androstanedione	20
Dehydro-epiandrosterone	10
Androsterone	10

Biosynthesis of androgens: Bulk of androgen production occurs mainly by the Leydig cells of the interstitial tissue of testes. It is also produced in adrenal cortex and in minute quantities in the ovary and placenta. Androgens are synthesized (**androgenesis**) from acetate and cholesterol through the following steps: i) cholesterol, C-27 compound is converted to pregnenolone (C-21 compound) in the mitochondria of Leydig cells, ii) pregnenolone is then translocated to smooth endoplasmic reticulum where testosterone is synthesized by any of the two pathways: Δ5 or **dehydroepiandrosterone pathway,** and Δ4 or **progesterone pathway** (Figure 5.7). **Δ5 pathway** involves 5-ene-3β-hydroxysteroids such as 17-hydroxypregnenolone and dehydroepiandrosterone through the following steps for the formation of testosterone from pregnenolone. i) Pregnenolone is converted to 17α–hydroxy pregnenolone by enzyme 17α–hydroxylase, ii) 17α–hydroxy pregnenolone is then converted to dehydroepiandrosterone (DHEA) with the help of enzyme lyase by cleaving the side chain and converting it to C-19 compound, iii) DHEA is then reduced by enzyme 17β–hydroxy steroid dehydrogenase to give Δ5-androstenediol, which on reduction and isomerization forms testosterone, or DHEA may get converted by enzymes dehydrogenase plus isomerase to androstenedione, which then reduces to form testosterone. **Δ4 pathway** involves 4-en-3-oxosteroids such as progesterone and 4-androstenedione through the following steps in the formation of testosterone from pregnenolone. i) Pregnenolone is first converted to progesterone with the help of enzymes 3β–hydroxy steroid dehydrogenase and isomerase, ii) progesterone is then hydroxylated by enzyme 17α–hydroxylase to form 17–OH–progesterone, iii) 17–OH–progesterone loses its side chain by enzyme lyase to form C-19 compound, androstenedione, iv) androstenedione, the immediate precursor of testosterone, finally gets reduced at C-17 position by enzyme 17β–hydroxy steroid dehydrogenase to give rise to testosterone. Various workers have worked to determine the relative importance of the two pathways in androgen biosynthesis. It has been found that in rat testes and mouse testes, the Δ4 pathway takes preference while in man, rabbit, dog and pig, the Δ5 pathway is more important.

In the testes and some extra-testicular tissues, testosterone itself exerts its action, but in few others such as seminal vesicles and prostate, it gets converted into more 'active' and 'potent' form, dihydrotestosterone (DHT) by reduction of Δ5-double bond with the help of enzyme reductase and NADPH, reduced nicotinamide-adenine dinucleotide phosphate (Figure 5.8) to exert its effects. Therefore, testosterone may be considered as a prohormone for seminal vesicles and prostate as it is converted into a more potent metabolite, dihydrotestosterone, and that too outside the testes. In these tissues, nearly 0.4-mg testosterone is reduced to dihydrotestosterone daily. There are two forms of 5 α-reductase. These are type I and type II. Type I is predominantly expressed in liver while type II is expressed in reproductive tissues and peripheral target organs. Mutations of type II enzyme are associated with male pseudohermaphroditism.

A small percentage of testosterone is also converted into estradiol by aromatization (Figure 5.9), and this is especially important in the brain, where these hormones may help in determining the five sexual behavior.

Numerous studies have shown that both the Δ5, and Δ4 pathways for androgen synthesis also occur in the adrenal cortex and ovaries. Further, circulating dehydroepiandrosterone sulphate (DHEA-SO4) from the adrenal cortex can be converted in the testes by enzyme sulfatase to 'free DHEA' that may provide an additional source of testosterone precursor.

The importance of **16-androstenes**, which are major metabolites in boar testis is now becoming better understood. Some 16-androstenes have been found in men and women, and are probably important in human social interactions. It has been shown that the odors of both 5α–androstenone and 5α–androst-16-en-3α–ol cause sows in estrus to adapt the mating behavior and wait for the boar to mount them. A non-estrus sow will not respond in this way. Infect, 5α–androstenone is now marketed in aerosol-spray form and is also used extensively in the pig-breeding industry to determine the time of estrus.

Androgen Levels: The Leydig cells of testis begin to proliferate at about eighth week of fetal life and the fetal testis starts secreting androgen probably by the ninth week. There is a relative deficiency of 3β–OH-dehydrogenase activity in the adrenal cortex during the fetal life. Therefore, a large amount of dehydroepiandrosterone is secreted by the fetal adrenal cortex. Consequently, much of it is converted to 16α –OH-dehydroepiandrosterone sulphate in the fetal liver. This compound is then transported to the placenta to serve as the major precursor for estriol synthesis (see Chapter 18).

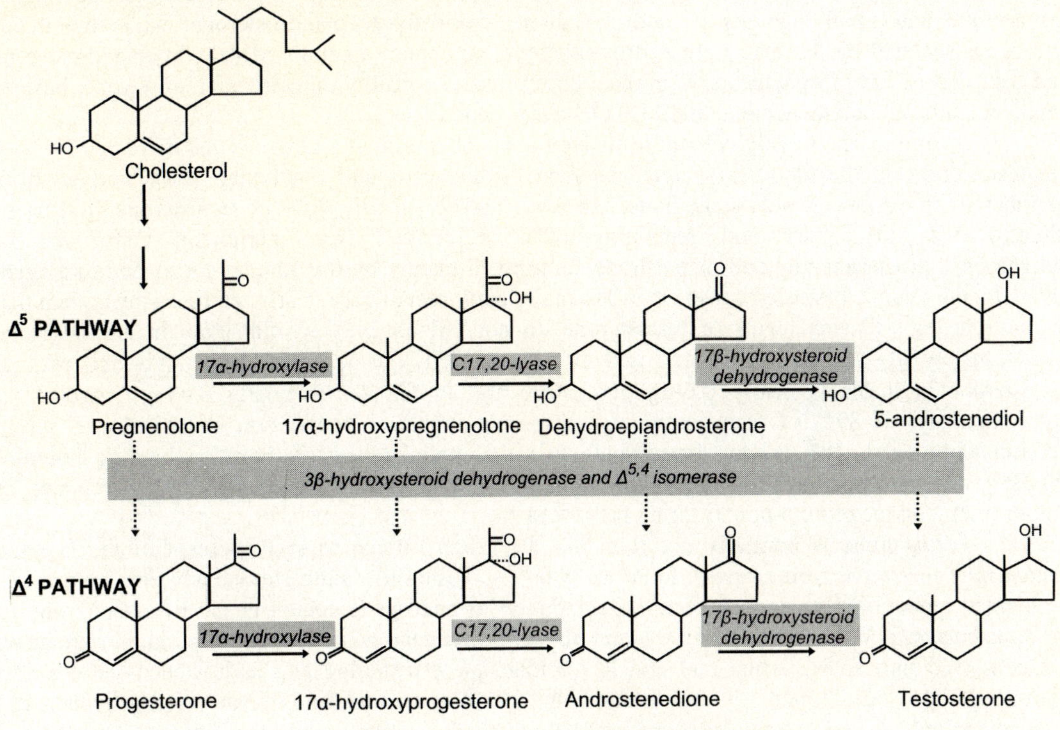

Figure 5.7: Biosynthesis of androgens.

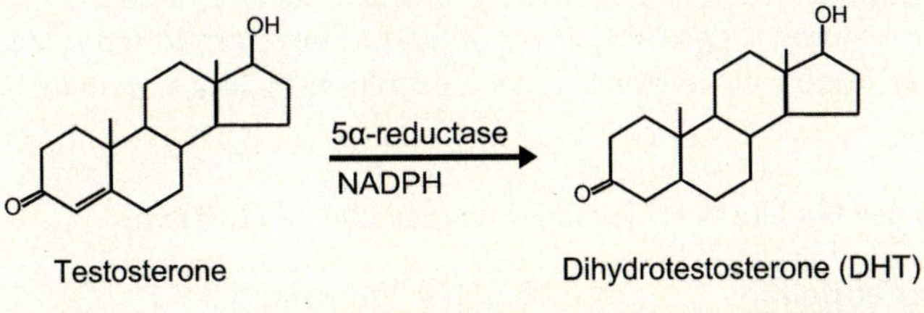

Figure 5.8: Formation of DHT from testosterone with the help of enzyme 5α-reductase.

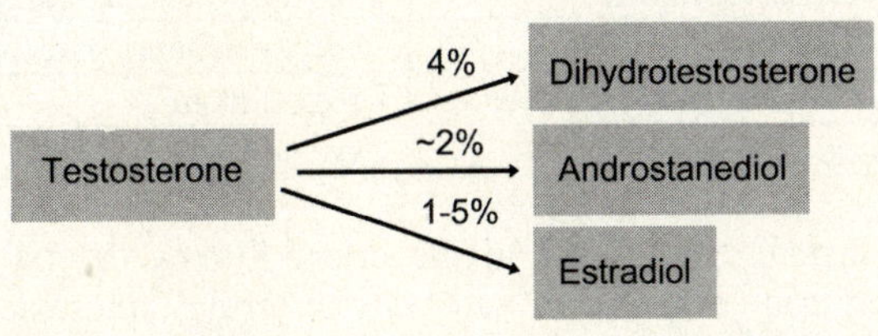

Figure 5.9: Production of other hormones from testosterone.

Plasma level of testosterone is elevated in both sexes in the immediate neonatal period but there is no significant sex difference in the secretion of testosterone at this time. Plasma testosterone levels fall quickly after birth to values that are at or below the normal female range and remain at this level until puberty. As puberty approaches, there is a gradual increase in the plasma levels of luteinizing hormone (LH) and testosterone in the male. In the adult, the testis secretes mainly testosterone and small amounts of androstendione and dehydroepiandrosterone, while the major androgens secreted by the ovary are androstenedione, and small amounts of dehydroepiandrosterone and testosterone. On the other hand, adrenal cortex secretes mainly dehydroepiandrosterone, besides small amounts of androstenedione and 11β–OH-androstenedione.

In adult males, Leydig cells of testis are the major source of androgens and more than 95% of the testosterone in the blood is secreted as such by the testis and remaining 5% is derived from peripheral conversion of androstenedione. In adult females, nearly 40% of testosterone is secreted directly from the ovary and remaining 60% is derived from peripheral conversion of dehydroepiandrosterone and androstenedione contributed mainly by the adrenal cortex and to a small extent by the ovary. Testosterone levels in plasma of adult females are nearly ten times lower than that in adult males. Plasma levels of testosterone do not fall abruptly in old age. In normal male, approximately 4 –12 mg testosterone and 10-15 mg DHEA is secreted daily. Plasma level of testosterone in males is nearly 0.6-μg percentage and in females is nearly o.o3 μg percentage. Approximately, 87-89% of testosterone is transported in blood bound non specifically to serum albumin while nearly 10% is bound specifically to a β–globulin, called 'sex hormone binding globulin' (SHBG) or 'testosterone-estrogen binding globulin' (TEBG). The remaining 1-3% circulates in equilibrium with the protein-bound form (Table 5.5).

Testosterone is normally not found in the urine. Fifteen to sixty percent of the injected testosterone recovered from urine is found as two '17-oxosteroid', androsterone and etiocholanolone with small amounts of epiandrosterone. Degradation of androgens occurs in the liver along any of these pathways: i) With the help of 5α – and 5β-steroid reductases, testosterone and androstenedione are converted into androsterone and etiocholanolone, ii) testosterone and androstenedione are first converted into 5α – and 5β-androstanediols which on oxidation forms androsterone and etiocholanolone, iii) or testosterone and androstenedione are converted into estrone and estradiol respectively. These metabolites are conjugated with sulphuric or glucuronic acid in liver and excreted as water-soluble conjugates. A portion of the conjugates and/or metabolites is either excreted in the bile or subsequently reabsorbed to undergo 'enterohepatic circulation' or return to the systemic blood stream with possible excretion in urine. In humans, biliary excretion is less important in case of androgens than of estrogens.

Table 5.5: Hormone binding to sex hormone binding globulin (SHBG)

Steroid Bound	Steroid Not Bound
Testosterone	17α-Testosterone
Dihydrotestosterone	Conjugated androgens
17β-Estradiol	Dehydroisoandrosterone
Other 17β-hydroxysteroids	Progesterone
Estrone	Cortisol

Testosterone is normally not found in the urine. Fifteen to sixty percent of the injected testosterone recovered from urine is found as two '17-oxosteroid', androsterone and etiocholanolone with small amounts of epiandrosterone. Degradation of androgens occurs in the liver along any of these pathways: i) With the help of 5α – and 5β-steroid reductases, testosterone and androstenedione are converted into androsterone and etiocholanolone, ii) testosterone and androstenedione are first converted into 5α – and 5β-androstanediols which on oxidation forms androsterone and etiocholanolone, iii) or testosterone and androstenedione are converted into estrone and estradiol respectively. These metabolites are conjugated with sulphuric or glucuronic acid in liver and excreted as water-soluble conjugates. A portion of the conjugates and/or metabolites is either excreted in the bile or subsequently reabsorbed to undergo 'enterohepatic circulation' or return to the systemic blood stream with possible excretion in urine. In humans, biliary excretion is less important in case of androgens than of estrogens.

Regulation of androgen secretion: Secretion of testosterone by the interstitial cells of Leydig in the testis is regulated by luteinizing hormone (LH) or interstitial cell stimulating hormone (ICSH) of the anterior pituitary (Chapter 4). A high level of testosterone in blood exerts a "feed-back" inhibition of LH secretion, and low level is associated with a compensatory rise in the secretion of LH (Chapter 2). Hypothalamic LH-releasing hormone (LH-RH) regulates the secretion of LH from the pituitary since the receptor sites of the neuro-endocrine feedback are in the hypothalamus, and is susceptible to influences that may stimulate or inhibit the formation or secretion of LH-RH (Chapter 3).

Administration of human chorionic gonadotropin (hCG), which has LH-like activity, to normal males produces a quick rise in plasma testosterone while to normal females it increases the urinary excretion of dehydroepiandrosterone. This is because androgen secretion from the ovary is also under the control of pituitary LH. Evidences indicate that maternal hCG stimulates androgen secretion from human fetal testis. In both men and women, adrenocorticotrophic hormone (ACTH) stimulates the production of dehydroepiandrosterone and androstenedione from the adrenal cortex. Further, administration of gluco-corticoids suppresses the production of dehydroepiandrosterone and androstenedione. The primary action of both the gonadotropins as well as ACTH appears to be the conversion of cholesterol into 20α-OH-cholesterol and subsequent cleavage of the side chain. Stimulation of steroid hormone production by the tropic hormone may be mediated by the cyclic nucleotide 3',5'-AMP. It is assumed that the tropic hormone activates adenyl cyclase in the membrane of the cell, where transformation of ATP to 3', 5'-ATP presumably occurs. This in turn causes increased biosynthesis of total steroidal products of the testis.

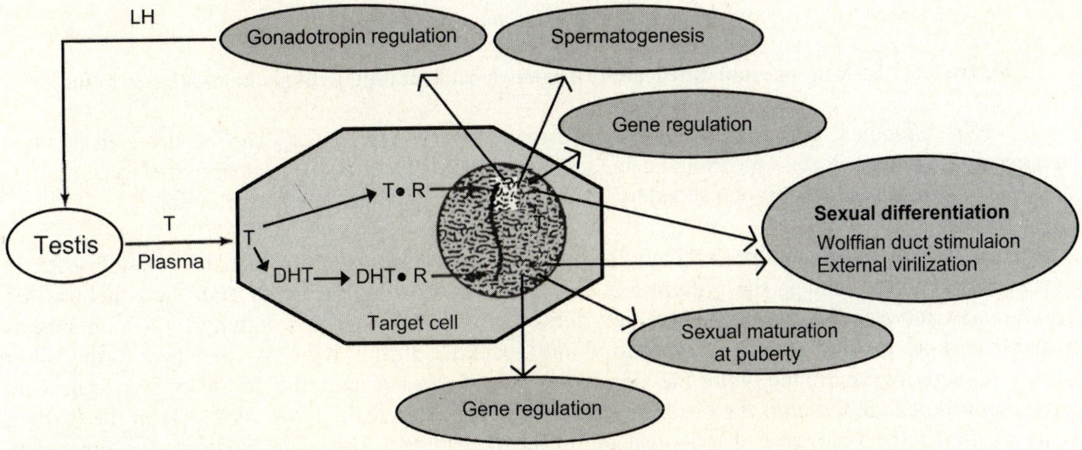

Figure 5.10: Mechanism of action of androgens, T-Testosterone, DHT-Dihydrotestosterone, LH-luteinizing hormone, R-Androgen receptor.

Biological effect of androgen: The androgens have widespread effects on the body (Figure 5.10). The action of an androgen secreted by an endocrine gland on a particular target tissue depends on a number of factors. Generally, free testosterone enters the target cells by simple diffusion or facilitated diffusion. Weaker androgens may be converted to testosterone either in peripheral tissue or in the target tissue, and the proportion of testosterone in the plasma, which is able to reach the target tissue, depends on the concentration of SHBG in plasma. In the cytoplasm of some tissues, conversion of testosterone to its 'active' form, dihydrotestosterone (DHT) is necessary before exerting its action on the target cell (Figure 5.10). For example, in the ventral prostate, action of testosterone is exclusively through conversion to the 5α –reduced metabolite (Figure 5.11). External genitalia and genital skin are other target organs, which have high 5α-reductase activity. Targets for testosterone include embryonic Wolffian structures, spermatogonia, bone, muscles, kidney, and brain. There are specific 'androgen receptors' present in the cytosol and the hormone is tightly bound to the receptor to form 'hormone-receptor complex', which in turn binds to 'hormone-responsive element' (HRE) present with specific nuclear genes (Chapter 7). This induces the effects of hormone in terms of transcription of those genes, which lead to increased synthesis of respective proteins to produce cellular effects.

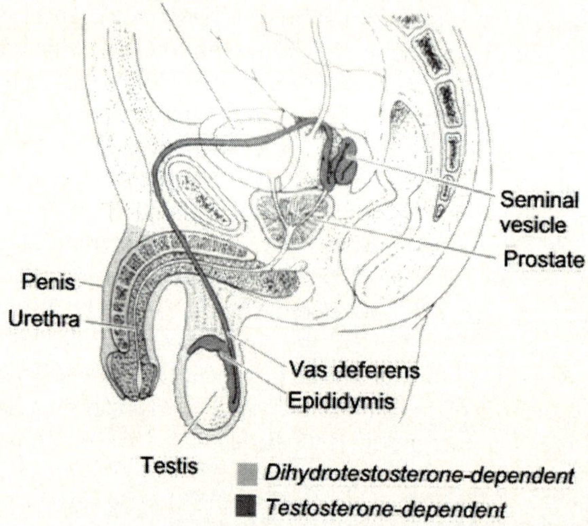

Figure 5.11: Testosterone and dihydrotestosterone-dependent regions of genital system in Man.

The biological effects of androgens are many and diverse. They can be grouped in three categories- i) actions on sex organs and accessory glands of reproduction, ii) anabolic effects, and iii) action on non-sexual organs or on secondary sex characteristics including male behavior.

Action on reproductive system: Fetal androgens first appear around eighth week of intrauterine life in human male embryo, and in the presence of functional testes, fetal testicular androgens help in the development and stabilization of male genital ducts and glands. After this activity by 4-5th month of pregnancy, testes go through a quiescent period until just after birth. There may then be a further short period of activity associated with the descent of the testes. Again, the testes remain quiescent throughout the childhood until the onset of puberty. The testis, which grows very little in the first ten years of life, is the first organ to manifest the onset of puberty. The rising testosterone along with follicle stimulating hormone (FSH) from pituitary brings about maturation of the seminiferous tubules and active spermatogenesis begins around the age of 11 years. Accompanying growth of the testes, increase in the sizes of the scrotum and penis occurs and these become pigmented. Simultaneously growth and secretory activity of secondary sex organs, such as epididymis, vas deferens, seminal vesicles, prostates are also stimulated by androgen and these become fully mature. Androgens promote protein synthesis in male accessory glands. They result in fructose production by seminal vesicles and utilization of this sugar by the seminal plasma for enhancing the activity of both aldose reductase as well as keto reductase. At puberty, ejaculation of semen starts. At this time, secondary sex characteristics also appear in males, such as change in voice, appearance of hair on face and body, and increase in muscles etc. in the body.

Anabolic effects: Anabolic effects include increase in muscle protein, bone matrix, and skeletal length. This rapid growth of bone and muscle tissue gives rise to the well-known increase in height and weight in boys at puberty. Stimulation of protein anabolism by androgen results in an increased urinary creatinine and a decrease in urinary nitrogen without an increase in blood urea. Androgens are also known to cause an increase in the activity of numerous enzymes, such as amino acid oxidase and arginase, which are involved in nitrogen metabolism. Androgens also act at the mitochondrial level to increase the respiratory rate. Further, it shows a "renotropic" action, that is, causes a rather selective increase in size and weight of the kidneys. In addition, androgen reduces the excretion of citrates in the urine by increasing its reabsorption by renal tubular epithelium. It may also cause an increase in the red blood cell and hemoglobin content of blood.

Action on secondary sex characteristics and behavior: Under the influence of androgen, growth of pubic, axillary and facial hair is stimulated at puberty. Secretion from sebaceous glands of skin and axillary glands enhances with androgen stimulation leading to an increased sebum production. Oiliness increases, and this results in acne formation in some individuals. Skin pigmentation and tanning effect of ultraviolet light on skin is intensified by androgen. In addition to effects on skin, thickening and enlargement of vocal cords and enlargement of larynx occurs, leading to deepening of the voice. Androgen plays an important role in the development of male psychosexual behavior. It results in the development of a more aggressive attitude, an attraction towards girls and stimulates libido and sexual potency.

Hormonal Defects: Lack of testosterone synthesis is called **hypogonadism. Primary hypogonadism** is due to processes, which cause failure of the testicular growth and functions, and **secondary hypogonadism** is due to defective gonadotropins secretion. The secondary sex characteristics fail to develop if lack of testosterone synthesis occurs before puberty. At least five distinct genetic defects in testosterone biosynthesis in the Leydig cell have been found. Enzyme deficiencies in Leydig cell affect side-chain cleavage, 17 α-hydroxylase, conversion of C_{21} to C_{19}, reduction of 17-ketone, and oxidation of A ring to Δ^4-3-ketosteroid. At the target cell level, a 5α-reductase deficiency, receptor disorders or receptor-positive resistance may affect the action of testosterone or dihydrotestosterone (Figure 5.12). Genetic males, who completely lack functioning receptors, have testes and produce testosterone but have complete feminization of the external genitalia, and such a condition is called as **testicular feminization syndrome**.

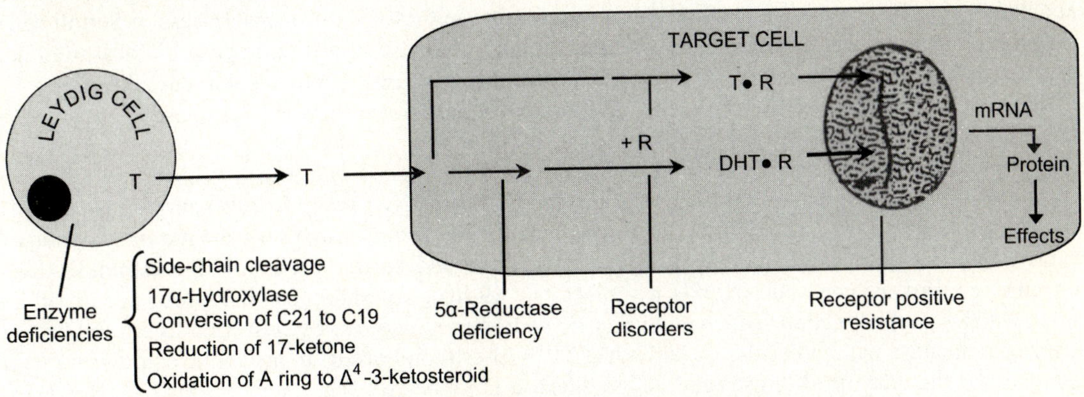

Figure 5.12: Defects in testosterone biosynthesis.

5.6 Female Hormones

Ovary secretes mainly two hormones called female sex hormones. These are i) **estrogens** or **follicular hormones**, and ii) **progesterone**. Biosynthesis and metabolism of ovarian hormones are similar to those of male hormones.

Estrogens: The naturally occurring estrogens are all steroid hormones capable of producing certain biological effects in females. Estrogens induce the growth and functions of female sex organs and are responsible for the development of secondary sex characteristics of females. They also influence the gonadotropin secretion by the pituitary. The secondary sex characteristics (also called extra genital characters) of females are development and growth of the mammary glands and duct system, typical female body shape, texture of skin and differential growth of hair on the body.

Types and structure of estrogens: Three types of estrogens exist in human females. These are **Estradiol**, **Estrone**, and **Estriol** (Figure 5.13). 17β-Estradiol is the principal and most active estrogenic hormone in circulation. Activity of estrone depends upon its metabolic conversion to estradiol. Estriol is a weak estrogen and gains importance during pregnancy. It is the principal estrogen found in the urine of pregnant women and in the placenta.

All naturally occurring estrogens are **C-18** compounds with **aromatic** character or three double bonds in ring A. The methyl ($-CH_3$) group is absent at C 10, and OH group at C 3 possesses the properties of a phenolic (–OH) group or weak acid. Estrogens are produced in the ovary by the theca and granulosa cells of developing Graafian follicles and in corpus luteum, in the adrenal cortex, placenta, and in small amounts in testes.

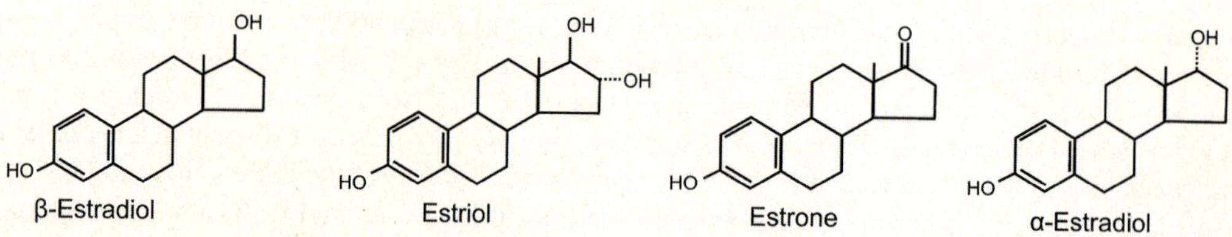

Figure 5.13: Types of estrogens.

Biosynthesis of Estrogens: Estrogen biosynthesis in the ovary is very complicated due to constantly changing population of cells in the ovary with the processes of follicular development, ovulation, corpus luteum formation and its regression with each menstrual cycle. Androgens such as testosterone and androstenedione are the immediate precursors for the synthesis of estrogens. In case of Sertoli cells and granulosa cells, enzyme aromatase becomes important as it converts androgens like testosterone, androstenedione into 17β-estradiol. In human, estrogens may arise from five sources: i) ovaries, ii) adrenal cortex, iii) testes, iv) fetoplacental unit, and v) other tissues, such as liver, muscle and adipose tissue.

Biosynthesis of estrogens from androgens requires mainly two steps i) conversion of C 19 compound to C 18 compound by removing angular methyl ($-CH_3$) group from position C 10, and ii) aromatization of ring A (Figure 5.14). A microsomal enzyme, aromatase brings about aromatization of ring A by three successive hydroxylation of testosterone and converts it into 17β - estradiol. The enzyme requires oxygen and NADPH as cofactors. 19-hydroxy androgens have been identified as intermediates in the reaction sequence. Similarly, androstenedione can be converted to estrone by the enzyme aromatase with molecular O_2 and NADPH. 17β-estradiol occurs in metabolic equilibrium with estrone and the enzyme, 17β-estradiol dehydrogenase is involved in the inter-conversion. However, both 17β-estradiol and estrone can also be produced in extra-gonadal tissues such as liver, muscle, adipose tissue etc. from testosterone, androstenedione and DHEA. These estrogens are also interconvertible in liver, placenta, etc. with the help of enzyme 17β-estradiol dehydrogenase.

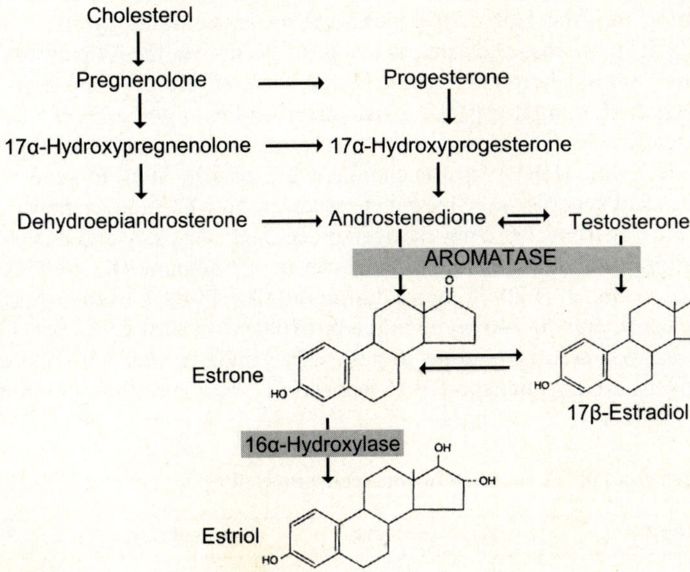

Figure 5.14: Biosynthesis of estrogens.

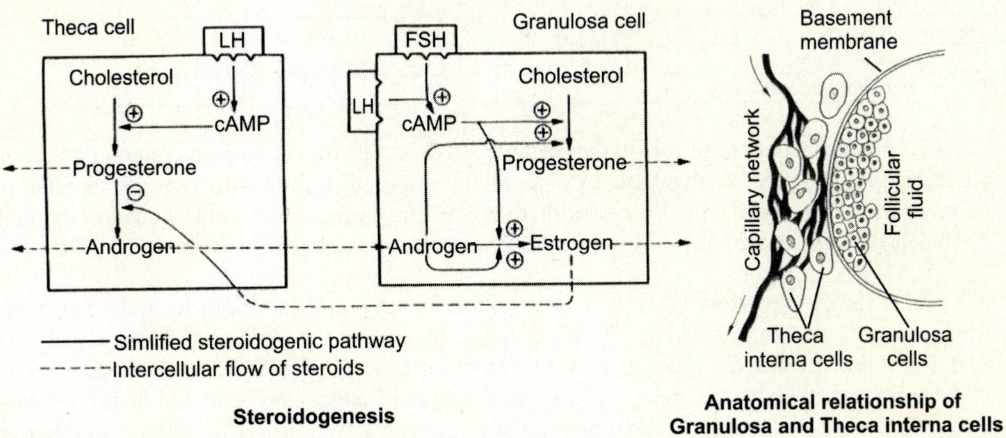

Figure 5.15: Steroidogenesis and structures showing anatomical relationship in ovarian follicle.

Estrogens are mainly formed in the ovarian follicles. Both, the granulosa and theca cells are required for estrogen formation. The structural relationship between the theca interna cells and the granulosa cells of the follicle (Figure 5.15) indicates that the theca cells, which have a rich blood supply are in association with a vascular granulosa cells. The steroid synthesized by theca cells can readily pass into circulation while any steroid formed in granulosa cells would have to cross to the theca interna in order to enter the circulation. It appears that the steroids secreted by the granulosa cells may be altered by the theca cells before these reach the circulation and conversely, steroid produced in the theca interna may be altered by the granulosa cells before they reach the follicular fluid. However, both the granulosa and the theca cells appear to have all the enzymes necessary for the biosynthesis of estrogens and each cell type individually is less efficient in synthesizing estrogens than a combination of the two cell types. Further studies suggest that in the theca cells, where main estrogen production in the ovary occurs during the first half of the menstrual cycle, hormone synthesis occurs by the $\Delta 5$ pathway. However, in the granulosa cells steroid synthesis occurs via the $\Delta 4$ pathway.

Like any other steroid hormone, estrogens are secreted directly into blood and through its circulation, these reach their 'target organs'. After entering the target cells, the hormone binds to a specific receptor present in the cytosol and form " receptor-steroid complex", which in turn binds to 'hormone-responsive-element' (HRE) in association with specific nuclear genes. This gene then translocates the synthesis of specific proteins and enzymes to show hormone action.

In adult females, nearly 0.1-0.2 mg estrogen is secreted every day and this amount increases to nearly 0.5 mg/day during ovulation (Table 5.6). However, the amount of estrogens in plasma varies according to menstrual cycle. It is 20-70 pg/ml during the first 10 days of the cycle, 50-290 pg/ml in the next 8 days of the cycle, and 70-140 pg/ml in the last 10 days of the cycle. Specific carrier protein, a β-globulin known as "sex-steroid binding protein"(SBT) mainly transports estrogens by binding tightly to them. Estrogens are also transported in free form (1-3%) and through binding less tightly to serum albumin.

Table 5.6: Production rates of sex steroids/day during menstrual cycle

Sex steroids	Early follicular	Pre-ovulatory	Mid-luteal
Estradiol (μg)	36	380	250
Estrone (μg)	50	350	250
Progesterone (mg)	1	4	25
17-OH Progesterone (mg)	0.5	4	4
Testosterone (μg)	144	171	126
Androstenedione(mg)	2.6	4.7	3.4
Dehydroepiandrosterone (mg)	7	7	7

Liver plays an important role in the metabolism of estrogens. It converts them into their more soluble form, by conjugation with sulfate or glucuronide, which then returns to systemic circulation for excretion in the urine. Estrogens are reabsorbed in the blood stream in 'enterohepatic circulation". Liver efficiently picks up estrogens from the systemic circulation and secretes them in the bile.

Biological effects of estrogens: Estrogens are responsible for the development and growth of the female sex organs and duct system. They promote the growth of the uterus, cervix, vagina and fallopian tubes and prepare the reproductive tract to receive the fertilized ovum. Estrogens primarily act on the surface epithelium and glands in the endometrium of uterus and results in its proliferation. It influences the tonicity of the uterine musculature and stimulates contractions. Estrogens primarily act during the proliferative phase of menstrual cycle. Increased contractility of the myometrium helps the sperms deposited in the vagina to move quickly towards the outer end of the fallopian tube for fertilization to occur in short time. Estrogen increases the content of RNA, protein, lipids, glycogen and sialic acid in the uterus. In the cervix, estrogen results in a marked increase in cellular proliferation and secretions of cervical glands. Estrogens cause enlargement of breast due to growth of stromal tissue, proliferation of ducts and deposition of fat in the breast, pigmentation of areola and growth of nipple. Estrogen favors retention and elevation of calcium and phosphorus in the body, and in turn calcification and ossification of bones and thus, prevents osteoporosis. They also have a cholesterol lowering effect and reduce plasma cholesterol level.

Synthetic Estrogens: Besides naturally occurring estrogens, estrogenic activity is also exhibited by certain derivatives of phenanthrene and dibenzanthracene. These are commonly referred to as synthetic estrogens and are synthesized commercially for therapeutic purposes. One of the first developed synthetic estrogens was **diethylstilbestrol (DES)**. Other examples of synthetic estrogens are **17α-ethinyl estradiol** and **mestranol**, which are used in oral contraceptives (Figure 5.16). Numerous compounds with anti-estrogenic activity have also been synthesized, and have several clinical applications. The most familiar example of this category is **Clomiphene** (Figure 5.17), which was originally designed as an antifertility drug but is used now for the opposite effect in the treatment of certain types of infertility. Clomid or Clomiphene citrate has a particular affinity for the estrogen receptor in the hypothalamus, and it competes with estradiol for hypothalamic receptor sites. Thus, GnRH release is not restrained and increased amounts of FSH and LH are released. In response to clomiphene, multiple follicles often mature simultaneously. The other common estrogen antagonists are Nafoxidine, a non-steroidal compound, and Tamoxifen, which combine with the estrogen receptor to form very stable complexes with chromatin, thus inhibiting the action of estradiol for prolonged periods. These antagonists are used in the treatment of estrogen receptor-dependent breast cancer. A new class of compounds known as selective estrogen receptor modulators (SERMs) exerts estrogen agonist activity in some target cells and as an antagonist in others. These are useful in the treatment of osteoporosis as they mimic the anabolic action of estrogens in bone without affecting reproductive tissues.

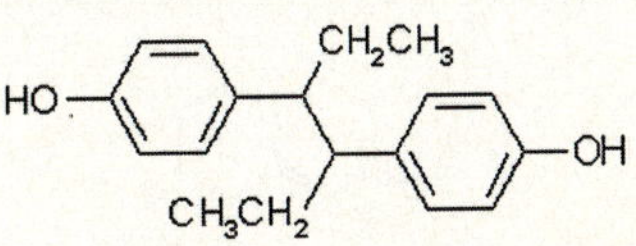

Diethylstilbestrol (DES)

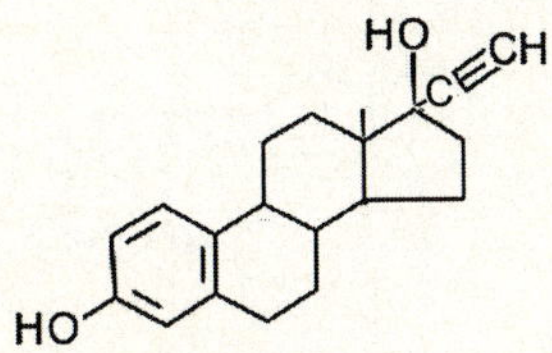

17α-Ethinyl estradiol

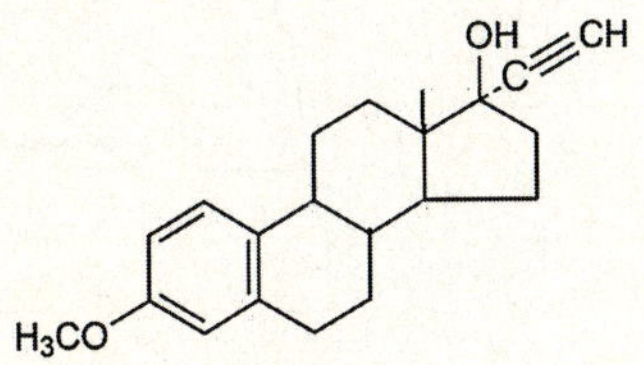

Mestranol

Figure 5.16: Synthetic estrogens.

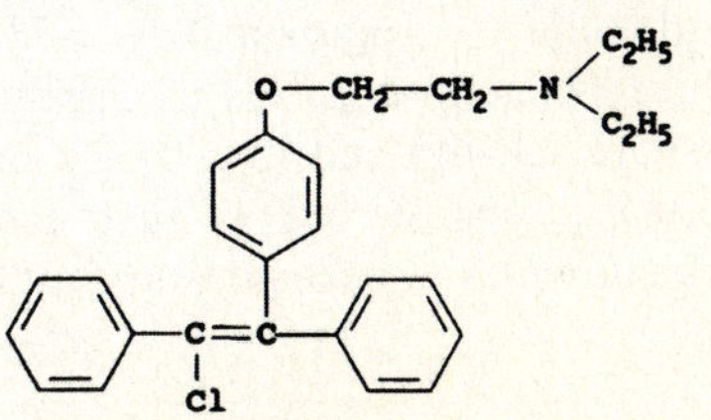

Clomiphene

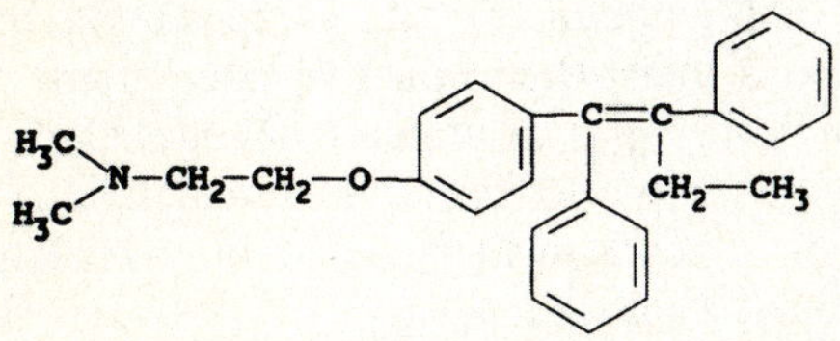

Tamoxifen

Figure 5.17: Anti-estrogens.

Progesterone (Progestational or Luteal hormones): Progesterone (the hormone of corpus luteum) is the other major ovarian hormone. It is secreted mainly by the corpus luteum during the period of its functional activity, and by the placenta during the later part of pregnancy. It is also formed in the adrenal cortex and testes as a precursor of both C 21 and C 19 steroid hormones. Progesterone prepares the uterus to receive embryo, and maintains it during pregnancy. It stimulates growth of mammary glands, but suppresses milk secretion.

Types and structure of progesterone: Progesterone is a **C 21** steroid hormone. It has methyl (–CH_3) group at positions C 10, and C 13 (Figure 5.18). It is a derivative of pregnane and is chemically designated as '4-pregnane-3, 20-dione. Progesterone has 100% relative potency, while 17α-hydroxyprogeserone has 40-70 % and 20α-hydroxyprogeserone has only 5 % relative potency.

Biosynthesis of progesterone: Like other steroids, progesterone is also synthesized from acetate via cholesterol and pregnenolone is the immediate precursor (Figure 5.18). Theca cells provide pregnenolone to the granulosa cells, which convert it to progesterone. Progesterone is an important intermediate for all steroid hormones in all tissues. 17α-hydroxyprogesterone is secreted along with estrogens from the ovarian follicle and its secretion parallels that of 17β-estradiol. Because the liver actively metabolizes progesterone to several compounds, progesterone is ineffective when given orally. Sodium-pregnanediol-20-glucuronide is the major progestin metabolite found in human urine.

Progesterone levels in blood is very low during the follicular phase but becomes evident on the day of ovulation or a day or two earlier and remains at high levels in the latter half of the menstrual cycle. This is to prepare the estrogen-primed endometrium of the uterus for the implantation of the fertilized ovum. It is secreted at the rate of nearly 2mg/day during follicular phase, which increases to nearly 25 mg/day in luteal phase. During early pregnancy, progesterone is produced by the corpus luteum of pregnancy but later mainly the syncytial cells of placenta produce it.

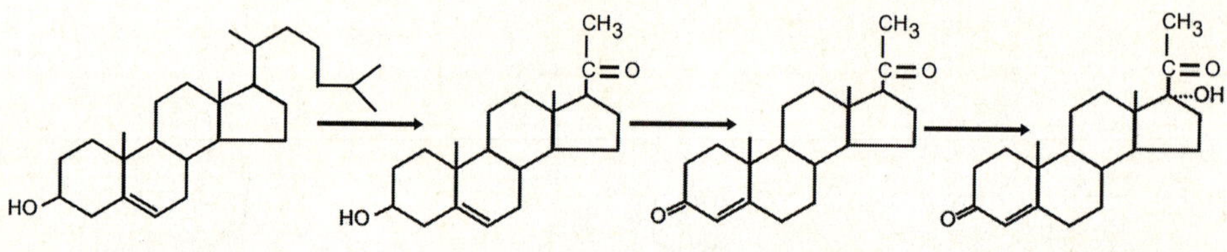

Figure 5.18: Structure and biosynthesis of progesterone.

In contrast to androgens and/or estrogens, nearly 40% of progesterone is tightly bound to and carried by a β-globulin, called "corticosteroid binding globulin". Approximately 1-5% of total progesterone is transported in active "free" form while the remaining is carried as tightly bound to albumin and other plasma proteins. Progesterone has a short half-life and liver is the main organ involved in its removal from the circulation. In the liver, progesterone is first converted to pregnanediol, which is then converted into its sulfates or glucuronides to become water-soluble and is finally excreted via urine.

Biological effects of progesterone: Like estrogens, progesterone also shows genital and extra-genital functions. Progesterone produces characteristic changes in the estrogen-primed endometrium. It brings about extensive development of endometrium, preparing the uterus for implantation of the embryo. It inhibits the myometrium contraction in the uterus. It results in the thickening of endocervical plug of mucus, thus reducing the chances of sperms passing through the cervical canal. Progesterone stimulates the mammary glands and in conjunction with estrogen, causes development of alveolar system of breast. Extra-genital effects of progesterone include effects on central nervous system to prevent ovulation. It is thermogenic and causes rise in basal temperature due to increase in basal metabolic rate.

For its action, progesterone combines with its receptors in the cytosol to form a receptor-hormone-complex, then moves to specific portion of specific DNA and is attached to it. This results in transcription of mRNA to synthesize new proteins including enzymes, which produce the biological effects of progesterone.

Synthetic Progestins: Substances that mimic the action of progesterone are sometimes called progestational agents, progestins, or gestagens. These are used along with synthetic estrogens as oral contraceptives (Chapter 23). Some synthetic progestins, which are in clinical use, are shown in Figure 5.19. It has been difficult to synthesize compounds that have only progestin activity but no estrogenic or androgenic action. The 17α-alkyl-substituted 19-nortestosterone derivative (e.g. norethindrone) have progestational activity but a minimal androgenic effect in most women and is used in oral contraceptives. Some of the commercially used **progestins** are Norethisterone (Lynestrenol, Norethynodrel, Ethynodiol diacetate), Norgestrel, Medroxyprogesterone acetate (Provera), and Chlormadinone acetate.

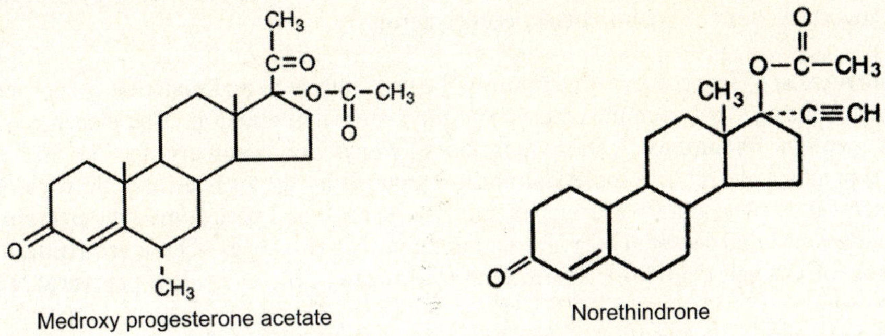

Figure 5.19: Synthetic progestins.

Hormonal Defects: Primary hypogonadism is caused due to the processes that directly involve the ovaries and cause ovarian hormonal deficiency such as decreased ovulation, decreased hormone production, or both. **Secondary hypogonadism** is caused due to loss of pituitary gonadotropin function. **Gonadal dysgenesis** or **Turner's syndrome** is a genetic disorder with XO karyotype, female internal and external genitalia, several developmental abnormalities, and delayed puberty. **Polycystic ovary syndrome (Stein-Leventhal syndrome)** is the overproduction of androgens causing hirsutism (excess hair growth, usually with male-type distribution in girls or women), obesity, irregular menses, and impaired fertility.

Besides these gonadal steroids (androgens, estrogens and progesterone), there are a few more hormones, which are secreted by the gonads or the associated structures. However, these hormones are polypeptides and not steroids, but are associated with reproduction, and fall in the category of gonadal hormones. Therefore, these hormones are also described in this chapter.

Relaxin: Relaxin hormone is secreted by corpus luteum in women and prostate gland in men. In women, it is produced during pregnancy, principally by corpus luteum and by placenta. In non-pregnant women, relaxin is found in the corpus luteum and endometrium only during the secretory phase and not during the proliferative phase of the menstrual cycle. In most mammals, maternal blood levels of relaxin rise soon after conception and therefore, its role in implantation have been suggested. In some, there is a much greater rise in relaxin levels several days before parturition, followed by an abrupt fall shortly before the onset of labor. This is believed to facilitate myometrial contraction. In others, high levels persist to the time of birth, and in these relaxin may contribute to fetal membrane rupture.

Relaxin is concerned mainly with the relaxation of pubic symphysis and other pelvic joints. Thus, it facilitates delivery by softening and dilating the uterine cervix joint. Relaxin helps to maintain pregnancy by inhibiting myometrial contractions. It is also implicated as a stimulant of uterine and vaginal growth, uterine vascularization and of mammary gland growth and maturation. In men, relaxin is found in semen, and probably help to maintain sperm motility thus aiding in sperm penetration for fertilization. High affinity binding sites have been identified in many brain regions, including the olfactory system, neocortex, hypothalamus and medulla oblongata. The hormone may gain access to neuron via circumventricular organs. It inhibits oxytocin and vasopressin release. Relaxin is used to treat dysmenorrhea and in some cases to arrest premature labor.

Relaxin is a polypeptide hormone. There is only one relaxin gene in most species. However, in human there are two genes on chromosome 9 that code for two structurally different polypeptides, both of which have relaxin activity. Only one of these genes is active in the ovary and prostate. Relaxin is made up of two polypeptide chains, A and B with 22 and 26 amino acids respectively. Two S-S bonds link these two chains and one intra-chain S-S bond is present in chain A. Relaxin is inactivated on breaking/reduction of S-S bond. Relaxin production is stimulated by progesterone and related adrenocortical steroids such as deoxy corticosterone.

Placental hormones: Placenta is an organ jointly formed from fetal and maternal tissues and provides the nutritional connection between the embryo and the maternal circulation. The placenta secretes both **steroid** and **protein hormones**. These hormones, which are necessary for the maintenance of pregnancy, supplement or replace those hormones produced by the ovaries and pituitary. The steroid hormones secreted by placenta are estrogens (chiefly as estriol) and progestins. The **protein** or peptide hormones synthesized and secreted by placenta are mainly of two types. These are **Human chorionic gonadotropin** (**hCG**), and **Chorionic somatomammotropin** (**CS**), also called **placental lactogen**.

Steroids: The placenta is like an 'incomplete endocrine gland as it is deficient in many of the essential enzymes necessary for complete synthesis of steroid hormones from acetate. Both, the maternal and fetal liver and adrenal glands supply preformed precursors to the placenta, which transforms them into hormones that are more active. The placenta converts cholesterol or pregnenolone from maternal blood to progesterone, which is secreted in large amounts by the placenta, as it is important in maintaining pregnancy in many species. Progesterone reduces the excitability and contractility of uterine muscle and helps to prevent premature expulsion of the fetus from the uterus. In human female, corpus luteum is the major source of progesterone during 6-8 weeks of pregnancy, following which placenta takes over and in the third trimester, placenta produces 30-40 times more progesterone than that by the corpus luteum.

Throughout pregnancy, plasma concentrations of all estrogens gradually increase but estriol is produced in the largest amount. Progesterone formed is also secreted from the placenta into the fetus via the umbilical vein and is converted by the fetal adrenal to adrenocortical steroids and variety of C 19 steroids, such as dehydroepiandrosterone (DHEA). An additional hydroxyl group is added to DHEA by the fetal liver and the 16-hydroxylated compound is then passed back to the placenta, where it is converted into estriol (Figure 5.20). The human placenta is incapable of converting DHEA directly to estriol as it lacks the 16-hydroxylase enzyme. The human placenta also synthesizes and secretes small quantities of estradiol-17 β and estrone from other C 19 precursors such as androstenedione. Placental estrogens, like ovarian estrogens promote the growth and development of the breast and the uterine muscle in pregnancy. It also induces widespread changes in maternal metabolism in terms of alterations in carbohydrate metabolism, protein synthesis and thyroid and adrenal function.

The human placenta also secretes large quantities of at least two protein hormones, hCG and CS. The placenta of other mammals, such as rat and sheep, also produce protein hormones, which are luteotropic (that is they maintain the life of the corpus luteum). The serum of pregnant mares contains high concentrations of a gonadotropic substance known as **pregnant mare's serum gonadotropin**

(**PMSG**), secreted by the endometrial cups of the pregnant uterus. PMSG shows follicle-stimulating hormone (FSH) like activity.

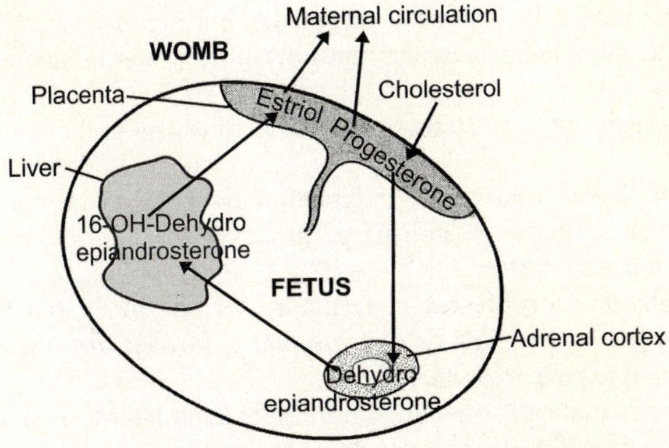

Figure 5.20: The Human feto-placental unit showing dependence of fetal structures on maternal compartment for the synthesis of steroids.

Human chorionic gonadotropin hormone (hCG): It is a glycoprotein consisting of two subunits α and β. α –chain is made up of 92 amino acids and is identical to human FSH, LH, and TSH while β-chain has 145 amino acids. hCG is formed by the syncytiotrophoblast of chorionic villi within 12-14 days of fertilization. It can be detected in blood after six days of conception. Presence of hCG in urine of women is a laboratory test for pregnancy. HCG exerts luteotrophic effect, that is, it results in the enlargement of corpus luteum as well as stimulates and maintains its secretion in first trimester. hCG has LH like activity and so stimulates the growth of interstitial cells of embryonic testes to produce testosterone.

Human Chorionic somatomammotropin (hCS) or Human Placental lactogen (HPL): This hormone was earlier called as chorionic growth hormone-prolactin (CGP) and human placental lactogen (hPL), but is now called human chorionic somatomammotropin (hCS). It is a peptide hormone with a structure very similar to that of human growth hormone. It is secreted by of placenta from about second week of pregnancy, rises slowly to reach a peak by 36 weeks of pregnancy. Chorionic somatomammotropin exerts both somatotrophic and luteotrophic effects. It exerts most of the actions of growth hormone and functions as a 'maternal growth hormone of pregnancy' promoting growth of maternal tissues. It stimulates the enlargement, growth and secretion of corpus luteum and helps to maintain a secretory corpus luteum. It stimulates alveolar growth of mammary glands and lactation. It also shows anti-insulin effect and thus decreases glucose utilization by mother but diverts glucose to the fetus.

Summary

Cholesterol is the precursor of all steroids in the body, such as, corticosteroids, sex hormones, bile acids, and vitamin D. It is synthesized entirely from acetyl-CoA in the body.

Excess cholesterol is excreted from the liver in the bile as cholesterol or as bile salts. A large proportion of bile salts is absorbed into portal circulation and returned to liver as part of enterohepatic circulation.

The first step in the biosynthesis of steroid hormones from cholesterol is its conversion to pregnenolone. This conversion is identical in adrenal, ovary, and testes. However, in gonads luteinizing hormone (LH) and in adrenals adrenocorticotropic hormone (ACTH) promotes this reaction.

The rate-limiting step in the synthesis of gonadal hormones from cholesterol is its delivery to the inner membrane of the mitochondria by the transport protein, steroidogenic acute regulatory protein (STAR).

Testicular androgens are C 19 steroids and are synthesized in the interstitial tissue of the testes by the Leydig cells.

Biosynthesis of testosterone from pregnenolone occur by any of the two pathways: i) dehydroepiandrosterone or Δ^5 pathway, and ii) progesterone or Δ^4 pathway. The Δ^5 pathway appears to be preferred in human testes.

A number of steroids are present in testicular venous blood but testosterone is the major steroid secreted by the adult testes. Dihydrotestosterone is formed from testosterone by reduction of the A ring with the help of enzyme 5α-reductase.

LH or ICSH (interstitial cell stimulating hormone) stimulates testicular steroidogenesis.

Androgens are responsible for the development and maintenance of the accessory glands of reproduction and secondary sex characteristics in males.

The ovary secretes two hormones, estrogen and progesterone. The follicular tissue forms the estrogen while the progesterone is formed by the corpus luteum.

The estrogens are C-18 steroids and differ from androgens in lacking the methyl group at position C-10 and their ring A is aromatic. Also, androgens are precursors for the synthesis of estrogens.

Estrogens are responsible for the growth of the uterus, vagina, pelvis, breasts, and pubic and axillary hair. They influence the menstrual cycle and secretion of the gonadotropic hormones from the anterior pituitary.

Progesterone is also synthesized from cholesterol. It is also formed in the adrenal cortex as a precursor of both C-19 and C-21 corticosteroids.

Progesterone causes development of the endometrium of the uterus, preparing it for the implantation of the fertilized ovum. It suppresses estrus, ovulation and production of LH from anterior pituitary. It is the hormone of pregnancy, and thus maintains it.

Placental hormones maintain pregnancy. The glycoprotein hormone, hCG supports the corpus luteum until the placenta produces sufficient progesterone to support the pregnancy.

Questions

1. What are steroids? Give examples of sex steroids.
2. Describe synthesis of male hormones.
3. What are female hormones? Describe their synthesis.
4. Enumerate the biological effects of male hormones.
5. Describe the biological effects of female hormones.
6. Discuss the physiological effects of estrogens and progesterone
7. What are synthetic estrogens and progestins? Give examples along with structural formulae of three each.
8. Describe placental hormones.

Chapter 6

Prostaglandins

In addition to hormones, there are number of compounds in the body which have been found to possess hormonal properties. These hormones are not transported between tissues in the blood, but act locally on the tissue in which they are produced, and hence called as **tissue hormones.** Tissue hormones fall in the category of **local hormones (paracrine)** and are effective at low concentrations. Examples of such hormones are**, pineal hormone (melatonin), renal hormones (erythropoietin and renin)**, and **eicosanoids.**

6.1 Eicosanoids

Eicosanoid hormones or simply eicosanoids (*eikosan-* = twenty, *-oid* = resembling) are fatty acid derivatives possessing potent hormone-like properties. These are important local hormones, and may also act as circulating hormone. The eicosanoids are synthesized from 20-carbon polyenoic (polyenes are compounds with many conjugated double bonds) fatty acids commonly called eicosanoic acids from which they take their general name eicosanoid meaning twenty. Eicosanoids are derived from the essential fatty acids, **linoleate** and **α-linolenate**, or directly from **arachidonate** and **eicosapentaenoate** present in the diet. Arachidonic acid is one of the phospholipids normally present in cell membranes. It is released from membrane bound phospholipids by the activity of phospholipase A_2.

There are three classes or groups of eicosanoid. The number of double bonds in the side chains characterizes these classes of eicosanoids. One eicosanoid class is represented by **prostaglandins (PGs)**, second by **prostacyclin (PGIs)** and **thromboxanes (TXs)**, and the **leukotrienes (LTs)** and **lipoxins (LXs)** represent the third class of eicosanoid derivatives. Prostaglandins (PGs), prostacyclin (PGIs) and thromboxanes (TXs) together comprise the **prostanoids**. Many classify prostaglandins and prostacyclins together as prostaglandins and thus consider three groups of eicosanoids as PG, TX and LT. Physiologically, eicosanoids function through G-protein linked receptors to elicit their biochemical effects (see chapter 7).

6.2 Prostaglandins

Prostaglandins are most important eicosanoids that are released from nearly all cell membranes. Although these biologically active lipids are present in very small quantities in cells and tissues yet they are very potent. Prostaglandins are not stored in cells, but are synthesized just before they are released, as they have a short half-life of 5 minutes or less. This property makes them act as local hormones, either within the cells in which they are formed or on the organ in which they are released. Both, the liver and lungs rapidly metabolize prostaglandins, in the body. Therefore, prostaglandins have a high turnover rate. And the short half-life ensures their transient and limited response at the intermediate site of production. Prostaglandins can act as mediators of hormone action and influence either protein synthesis or other precursors within the cell. Therefore, their knowledge becomes an important part in the study of hormones or endocrinology.

In 1930, Kurzrok and Lieb observed for the first time that the human semen when placed in the uterus is able to bring about strong muscular contraction or relaxation. This was later attributed to the presence of a number of structurally –related compounds in the semen, collectively termed as prostaglandins. However, name prostaglandin (PG) was given to this lipid-soluble acidic substance by Von Euler, a Swedish Nobel Prize Winner in Chemistry in 1935 as these were observed in the secretion of prostate gland. Now prostaglandins have been found to occur in a wide variety of mammalian tissues including brain, spinal cord, thymus, liver, lungs, kidneys, pancreas, uterus, menstrual fluid and placenta, yet semen remains one of the richest sources of prostaglandins.

Chemical Structure and Synthesis of Prostaglandins and other eicosanoids: Chemically, prostaglandins are variants of a basic 20-carbon carboxylic fatty acid- prostanoic acid (Figure 6.1). They differ from all other hormones in being fatty acids i.e. incorporating COOH group in their molecule. These are synthesized from polyunsaturated C-20 cyclic fatty acid called arachidonic acid that contains a 5-carbon ring called cyclopentane ring. The carbon atoms 8 to 12 in its molecule are involved in the formation of this ring (Figure 6.1). Arachidonic acid (arachidonate) is usually derived from the membrane phospholipid as a result of phospholipase A_2 activity (Figure 6.2).

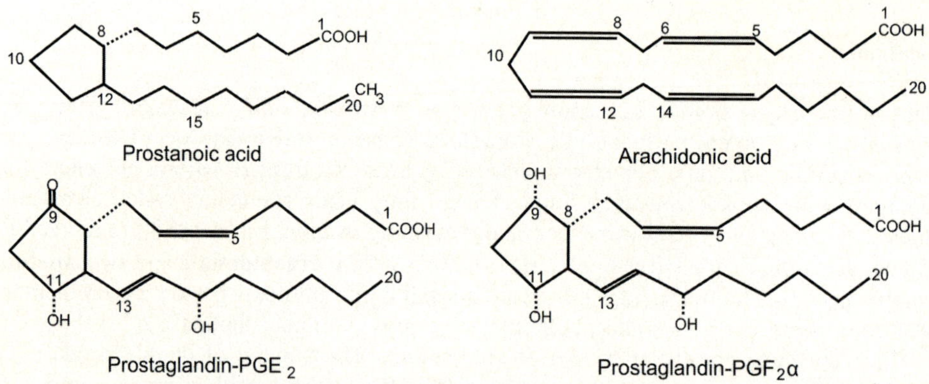

Figure 6.1: Prostanoic acid, arachidonic acid and two common prostaglandins.

However, the synthetic pathways of prostanoids and leukotrienes are divergent. These two pathways are known as the **cyclo-oxygenase** and **lipoxygenase pathways** respectively (Figure 6.2). The synthesis of prostanoid occurs via cyclooxygenase pathway and requires the consumption of two molecules of oxygen and two molecules of reduced glutathione and is catalyzed by prostaglandin synthetase complex. On the other hand, the lipoxygenase pathway in response to both immunologic and nonimmunologic stimuli forms leukotrienes. Figure 6.3 gives an outline of the synthesis of prostanoids that is of prostaglandins, prostacyclins and thromboxanes and the ring structures of these compounds are given in Figure 6.4. Variations in the position of double bonds and in the ketone and hydroxyl groups give rise to 9 groups of prostaglandins designated as PGA, PGB, PGC, PGD, PGE, PGF, PGG, PGH, and PGI. Originally, two groups of prostaglandins were recognized. These were PGE and PGF. Prostaglandin E (PGE) is ether soluble, and hence designated as E (from ether) with a keto group at C_9. On the other hand, prostaglandin F (PGF) is phosphate buffer soluble, and therefore, is designated as F (from *fosfat* in Swedish) with a hydroxyl group at C_9. PGE has four sub-groups while PGF has three subgroups, thus forming in all 14 prostaglandin groups.

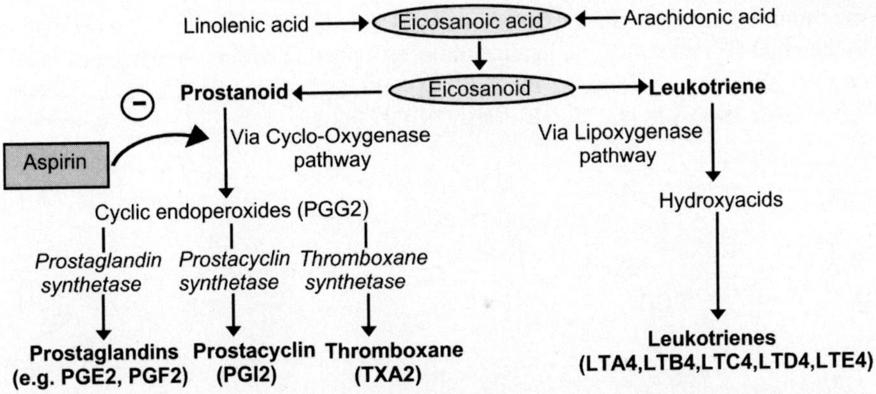

Figure 6.2: Synthesis of prostanoids and leukotriene.

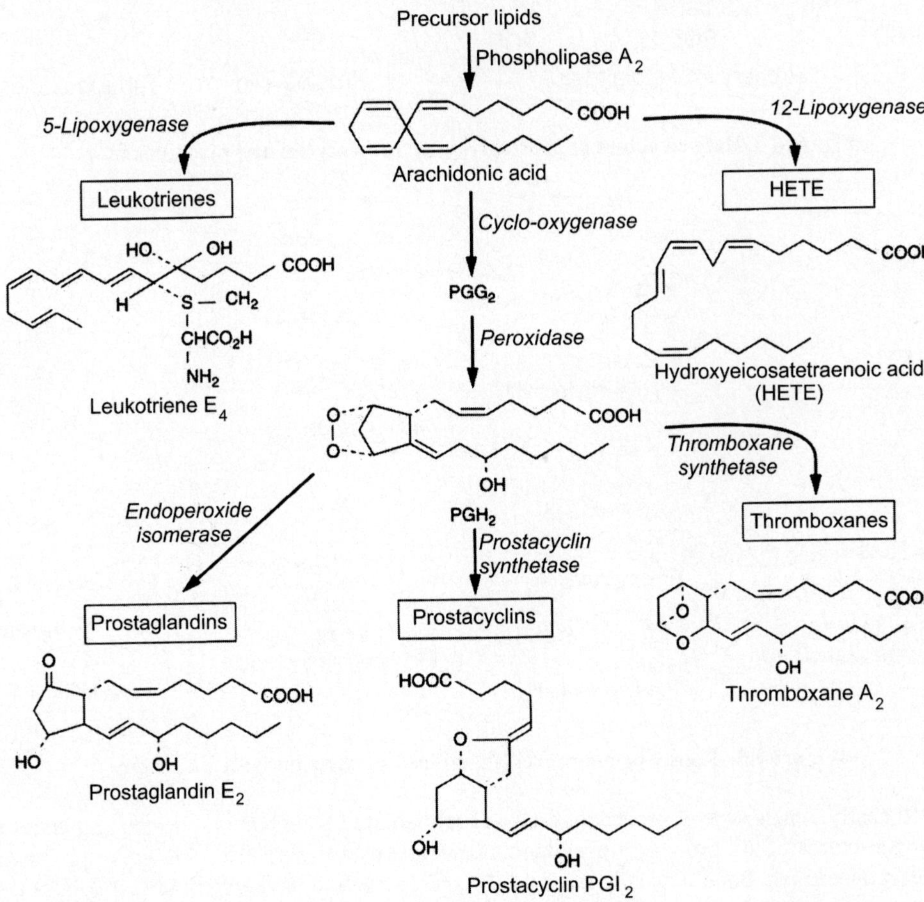

Figure 6.3: Formation of prostaglandins, prostacyclin, thromboxanes and leukotrienes.

The six prostaglandins PGE_1, PGE_2, PGE_3, $PGF_1\alpha$, $PGF_2\alpha$, and $PGF_3\alpha$ are called **primary prostaglandins** (Figure 6.5) as these can be converted into other types of prostaglandins, which in turn are called **secondary prostaglandins**. The six primary prostaglandins occur in most cells and can be converted to the eight secondary prostaglandins. Fourteen prostaglandins have been isolated from male reproductive tract and these are PGA_1, PGA_2, PGB_1, PGB_2, $PGEA_1$, $PGEA_2$, PGE_3, $PGF_1\alpha$, $PGF_2\alpha$, $PGF_3\alpha$, 19-OH PGA_1, 19-OH PGA_2, 19-OH PGB_1, 19-OH PGB_2.

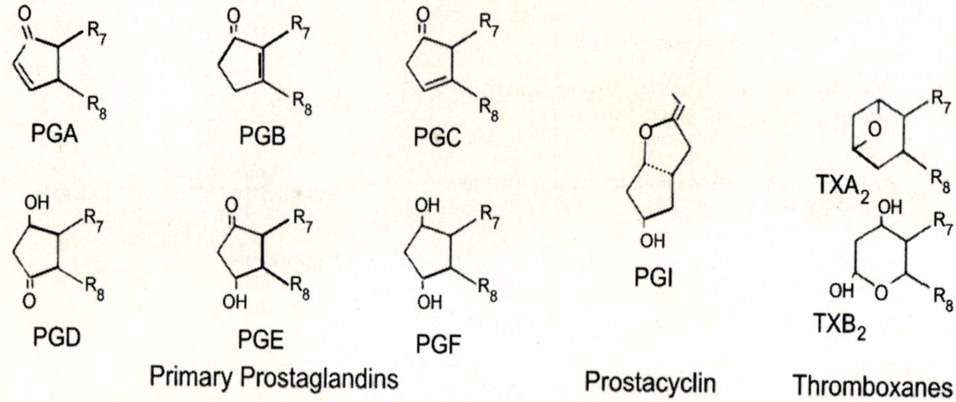

Figure 6.4: Ring structure of prostaglandins, prostacyclin and thromboxanes.

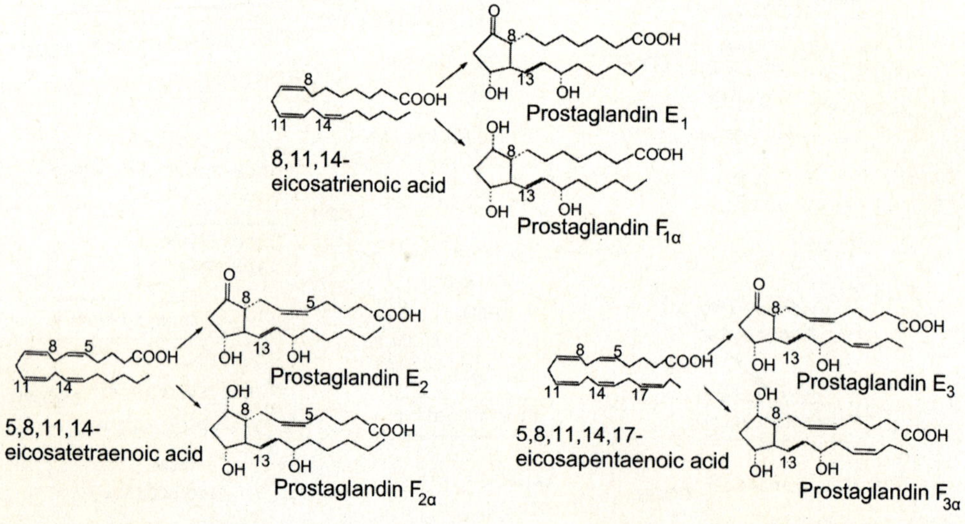

Figure 6.5: The six primary prostaglandins and their biosynthetic origin.

Recently, a new type of prostaglandin has been isolated from human plasma, and is designated as $\mathbf{PGX_1}$. Structures of six primary prostaglandins are given in Figure 6.5. All active prostaglandins have at least one double bond between positions 13 and 14. Some have two double bonds, the second being between positions 5 and 6, while some have three double bonds, the third one between positions 17 and 18. All prostaglandins have a hydroxyl group at position 15 and some have another hydroxyl group at position 19. When 5-carbon ring has two hydroxyl groups, their positions give rise to α or β isomers.

6.3 Prostacyclin and Thromboxanes

Prostacyclin (PGIs) and thromboxanes (TXAs) are structurally related compounds that arise from a nascent prostaglandin. Both are derived from a fatty acid, the arachidonic acid (Figures 6.2 and 6.3). However, in both of these, the cyclopentane ring is interrupted with an oxygen atom (oxane ring) to form the six-member ring, in contrast to prostaglandins, where a five-member ring is formed (Figure 6.4).

Prostacyclins are found in the walls of blood vessels. Endothelial cells and vascular smooth muscle produce them. They facilitate flow of blood in vessels by inducing vasodilation and prevent thrombosis by inhibiting aggregation of platelets. PGI_2 is known to be the most potent natural inhibitor of blood platelet aggregation. It binds to a specific platelet receptor and activates adenylate cyclase to result in an increase in the intracellular levels of cyclic AMP. These in turns are inhibitory to platelet aggregation and thus prevent blood clot formation. Prostacyclins have a short half-life (3 minutes).

Thromboxanes are secreted by blood platelets. They help in blood clotting by promoting aggregation of platelets at the place of injury. They also bring about vasoconstriction at places of injury to prevent excessive loss of blood. The effects of thromboxane are opposite to those of prostacyclin (Figure 6.6). Thus, prostacyclin and thromboxanes display a critical balance required for the normal functioning in the body in the regulation of vascular blood flow and blood clotting. Thromboxane A_2 is a specific product of the blood platelet while thromboxanes B_2 is a breakdown product of thromboxanes A_2. In response to stimuli which are known to induce clotting (collagen substrate, thrombin, epinephrine), platelet thromboxane levels are elevated to result in increased concentrations of cyclic AMP. This causes release of free cytosolic Ca^{2+}, which in turn is responsible for inducing the cellular shape changes associated with the platelet aggregation phenomenon.

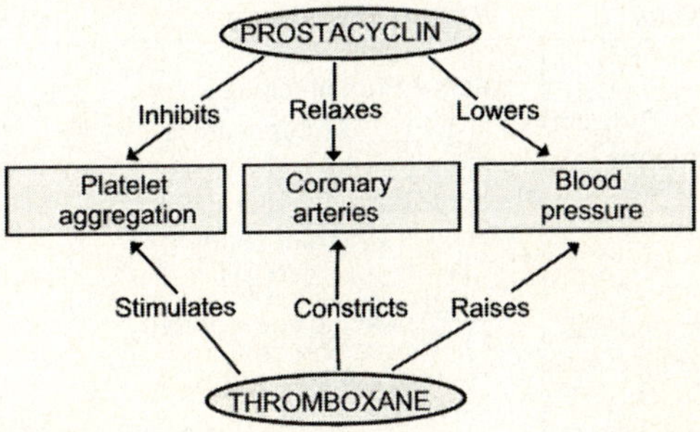

Figure 6.6: Effects of prostacyclin and thromboxane on cardiovascular system.

6.4 Leukotriene

Leukotrienes (LTs) are also derived from a fatty acid, the arachidonic acid but contain three conjugated double bonds (Figure 6.7). These eicosanoid derivatives are formed via the lipoxygenase pathway rather than cyclization of the fatty acid chain (Figure 6.2). Oxygen is inserted into 5,12 and 15 positions of arachidonic acid to give rise to hydroperoxycicosatetraenoicacid (HPETE) by three different **lipoxygenases (dioxygenases)**. Only 5-lipoxygenase forms leukotrienes. A_4 leukotriene is formed first and this in turn is metabolized to either leukotriene B_4 or leukotriene C_4. Subsequent removal of glutamic acid and glycine generates leukotriene D_4 and leukotriene E_4 (Figure 6.7).

Leukotrienes are so named because they are made by leukocytes. Thus, most cells of connective tissues (leukocytes, mastocytoma cells, platelets and macrophages), and eosinophils of blood secrete leukotriene. They are released in response to allergens acting on most cells and therefore, their effects are those observed in allergic reactions. Leukotrienes induce bronchoconstriction,

constriction of arterioles and also induce migration of neutrophils and eosinophils towards the place of inflammation. Their over-production serves as mediators in inflammatory and allergic reactions. They can cause asthma, arthritis, colitis etc.

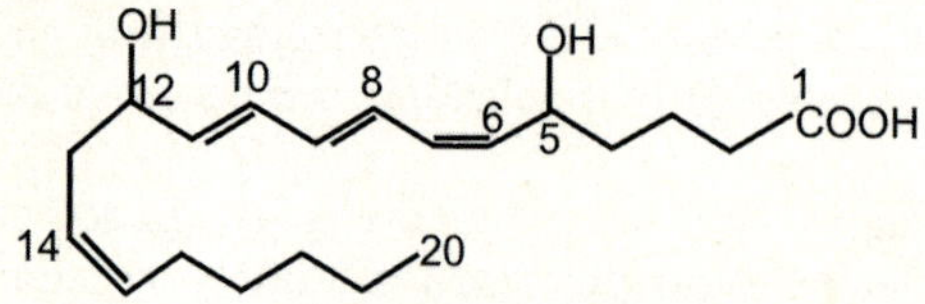

Figure 6.7: Structure of a common leukotriene.

6.5 Mechanism of Action of Prostaglandins and other Eicosanoids

Extrinsic stimuli such as hormones, pH, hypoxia etc. stimulates the formation of active phospholipase enzyme from its inactive form, which in turn results in the synthesis of arachidonic acid and eicosanoid hormones from phospholipids (Figure 6.8). These eicosanoids exert their effects by binding to receptors on the target-cell plasma membranes and inhibit or stimulate the synthesis of second messengers such as cyclic AMP. PGE_2 and PGI_2 invariably stimulate adenylate cyclase, while some PGF_2 receptors may be associated with a specific guanine nucleotide regulatory protein (GTP regulatory protein) linked to activation of phospholipase C. Leukotrienes and PGI_2, and thromboxane A_2 are released from their cells of origin to act as humoral messengers.

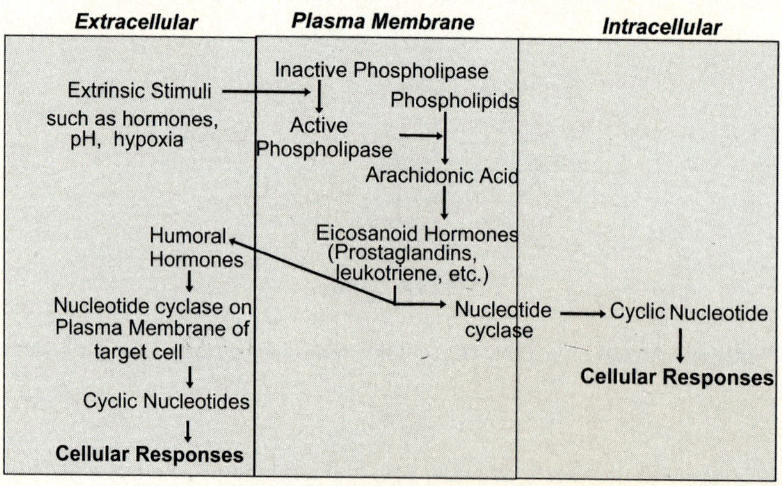

Figure 6.8: Mechanism of action of eicosanoid hormones.

6.6 Functions of Prostaglandins

Prostaglandins exhibit hormone-like activity and have multiple targets and effects. Some prostaglandins regulate cellular responses to hormones, while others can modulate the action of hormones. They can also act as secondary messenger. Biological effects of prostaglandins are as follows:

1. Prostaglandins in most of the tissues stimulate adenyl cyclase activity, thereby controlling production of cAMP and altering the cell's response to a hormone. By increasing the level of cyclic AMP, prostaglandins stimulate the formation of steroid hormones and the secretions of catecholamine. In the pancreas, it stimulates the release of insulin, and in the thyroid, synthesis of iodothyronine.
2. Prostaglandins stimulate secretion of hormones from adrenal cortex.
3. Prostaglandins are involved in the regulation of hypothalamic releasing factor release.
4. Prostaglandins lower cAMP in adipose tissue.
5. Prostaglandins inhibit secretion of hydrochloric acid from the wall of stomach thereby controlling the formation of acid-induced gastric ulcers.
6. Some prostaglandins help regulate blood pressure. They relax smooth muscle in the airways of the lungs and in the blood vessels, dilate these passageways, and thus lower down the blood pressure.
7. Prostaglandins also influence movements of sodium ions and water in the kidneys.
8. Prostaglandin inhibits the aggregation of blood platelets and the clot reaction.
9. Prostaglandins in low doses have been reported to elevate plasma free fatty acids (FFA) concentration whereas its high doses decrease FFA concentrations.
10. Prostaglandins have a sedative and tranquilizing effect on the nervous system.
11. Recently, it has been shown that prostaglandins are involved in the inflammatory reaction and pain. When tissues are injured, prostaglandins promote inflammation. Anti-inflammatory drugs such as aspirin in part act by inhibiting the synthesis of prostaglandins (Figure 6.2).
12. Prostaglandins have powerful effect on both male and female reproductive physiology. Prostaglandins can contract smooth muscle in the walls of the uterus, causing menstrual cramps and labor contractions. At the time of birth, certain cells of the fetus begin to produce oxytocin, which in turn acts on the placenta, causing it to release prostaglandins. This is evident from high concentration of prostaglandin $F_{2\alpha}$ in amniotic fluid during labor. Both oxytocin and prostaglandins are essential for initiating labor in humans. As umbilical cord contain high concentration of prostaglandins, they may have some role in regulation of placental blood flow. Prostaglandins are also involved in spermatogenesis, sperm maturation and their transport in female genital tract. Human semen is rich in prostaglandins, which when deposited in vagina during coitus, facilitates conception as a result of retention of the ovum within the tube and also may act locally on the cervix and body of the uterus to help in transport of sperm to the egg. Low levels of prostaglandins in seminal fluid may produce infertility in male.

6.7 Clinical Applications of Prostaglandins and other Eicosanoids

Prostaglandins have also proved their value in clinical practice. The following are some of the clinical applications based on the knowledge of the biosynthesis and the biological effects of prostaglandins and other eicosanoids.

Prostaglandins exert stimulatory effect on contractions of the human uterus. Therefore, it is given intravenously (PGE_1, PGE_2, and $PGE_2\alpha$) or orally (PGE_2 and $PGF_2\alpha$) to induce abortions so as to terminate pregnancy. Inhibitors of prostaglandin synthesis are used in treatment of dysmenorrhea (painful menstrual period). Prostaglandins are also used as contraceptives to prevent conception. Prostaglandins are of help in treating peptic ulcer patients as they increase gastric mucosal resistance to acid. They are used as vasodilator to lower blood pressure. PGE_1 by inhalation produces improvement in asthmatic patients. Prostacyclin is used as an inhibitor of platelet aggregation in cases of renal dialysis and cardio-pulmonary bypass. Steroidal anti-inflammatory agents, such as cortisone inhibit the release of arachidonic acid from cell membrane phospholipids and thus formation of all eicosanoids (prostaglandins, thromboxane, prostacyclin and leucotrienes).

Anti-inflammatory drug such as aspirin, act by inhibiting the synthesis of prostaglandins. **Aspirin** (acetylsalicylate) is a nonsteroidal anti-inflammatory drug (NSAID). It inhibits the cyclooxygenase activity of the enzyme prostaglandin synthetase by acetylating the terminal amino group of one of its subunits (Figure 6.9). Most other NSAIDs, such as indomethacin and ibuprofen, inhibit cyclooxygenase by competing with arachidonate. Aspirin in small doses, nearly 300 mg/day, inhibits thromboxane synthesis but not of prostacyclin. It blocks cyclo-oxygenase in platelets but not in the walls of blood vessel resulting in a decrease in platelet aggregation and a decrease in the risk of intravascular clotting and hence may be used in patients with coronary heart disease. Therefore, it spares the leukotriene synthesis pathway. Indomethacin is a more selective, non-steroidal anti-inflammatory drug, and it inhibits cyclo-oxygenase but not lipoxygenase. Thus, these drugs may be used selectively to inhibit prostaglandins, prostacyclin and thromboxane formation without a concomitant effect on leukotriene formation.

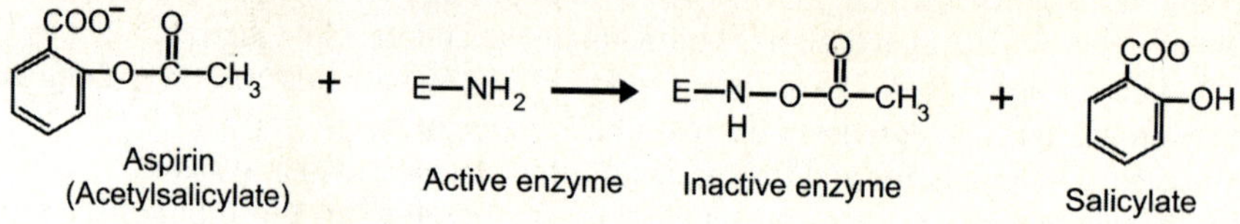

Figure 6.9: Inhibition of prostaglandin biosynthesis by aspirin.

It is also possible to affect the eicosanoid production by some food constituents such as garlic, onion, ginger, vitamin C, vitamin E, alcohol etc. These food constituents modulate the precursor fatty acid component in cell membrane phospholipids, and in turn alter the types of eicosanoids formed endogenously.

Summary

Prostaglandins are eicosanoids belonging to a category of local hormones (tissue hormones) and are paracrine. Three classes of eicosanoids are prostaglandins, prostacyclin & thromboxanes and leukotriene.

Prostaglandins are group of molecules derived from fatty acids found in all cell membranes. They have diverse effects, including stimulation of uterine contractions, regulation of blood pressure, control of gastrointestinal motility, and secretory activity. They are also involved in inflammation.

Prostacyclins (PGIs) and thromboxanes (TXAs) are structurally related compounds that arise from a nascent prostaglandin. Prostacyclins are found in the walls of blood vessels. They facilitate flow of blood and prevent thrombosis. Thromboxanes are secreted by blood platelets. They help in blood clotting and also bring about vasoconstriction at places of injury.

Leukotrienes are also derived from fatty acid. These are secreted by most of the cells of connective tissues, and eosinophils of blood. They induce bronchoconstriction, constrict arterioles and induce migration of neutrophils and eosinophils towards the place of inflammation.

Questions

1. What are eicosanoids? Give various classes of eicosanoids along with their functions.
2. What are the functions of prostaglandins and leukotrienes?
3. What are prostaglandins? Give their chemical structure.
4. What kind of effects do prostaglandins produce?

Chapter 7

Hormone Action

The endocrines form a vital coordinating system within the body of the vertebrates including humans. They secrete hormones that exert their effects by altering metabolic processes in the body. For example, a hormone might alter activity of an enzyme necessary for synthesizing a particular substance, or alter the rate at which particular chemicals are transported through cell membranes. The function of different hormones ultimately is to control the activity levels of target tissues. After exerting its action, hormone is degraded by the liver or kidneys.

In late fifties, analysis of effects of hormones showed some general features. These were: i) compared to the amounts injected, the hormonal effects were highly amplified; ii) some hormonal effects were metabolic while others were related to growth and development; and iii) given hormone showed a certain degree of specificity by affecting only its target tissue. Based on these observations, hormones were classified arbitrarily into two classes depending on the effects they produced. These were metabolic hormones and growth and developmental hormones. Recently much attention has been focused on to explain the ways by which the hormones mediate their action at the cellular level. To understand the mechanisms involved in exerting action by a hormone, it is essential to know first some of the characteristics of the hormones and the specific combinations they make at the cellular level.

7.1 Characteristics of Hormones

Hormones are present at very low concentrations in the extra cellular fluid (10^{-15} – 10^{-9} mol/L). Therefore, the organs or tissues on which a hormone will exert its action must be able to recognize and distinguish between different hormones. Cell-associated recognition molecules provide this high degree of discrimination. These molecules are called **receptors**. Such_cell or tissue, which is able to recognize the hormone, is called a_**target cell**. A target cell is thus defined by its ability to bind selectively with a given hormone via such a receptor. Use of radiolabelled hormones led to the discovery of receptors.

7.2 Receptors and Target Cell

Hormones initiate their biological action by binding to specific receptors present in the target cell. For example, hormones such as neurotransmitters, influence their target cells by binding chemically to specific protein or glycoprotein, which act as receptors. Only the target cells for a given hormone have receptors that bind and recognize that hormone. All receptors whether for polypeptide hormones or steroid hormones have at least two functional domains. A **recognition domain** binds the hormone and a second region generates a signal that couples (**coupling domain**) hormone recognition to some intracellular function. Coupling or signal transduction occurs in two general ways. Polypeptides and protein hormones and the catecholamines bind to receptors located in the plasma membrane, thus generating a signal that regulates various intracellular functions, often by changing the activity of an enzyme. On the other hand, thyroid and steroid hormones interact with intracellular receptors forming a complex, which provides the signal for exerting an action. Thus, receptors may be **membrane bound**, e.g. peptide hormone receptors or **cytosol receptors**, e.g. thyroid and steroid hormone receptors, as these occur either in cytosol or on the nucleus. The membrane bound receptors partly protrude in the extra-cellular fluid and partly remain within the cell membrane. The dual functions of binding and coupling ultimately define a receptor. The coupling of hormone binding to signal transduction is called **receptor-effector coupling** and it provides the first step in the amplification of the hormone response. This binding and coupling also distinguishes the target cell receptor from the plasma carrier proteins that bind hormone but do not generate a signal. The concept of receptors in hormone action also solved the mystery of why hormone action could not be demonstrated in cell free preparations.

Generally, a target cell has 2000-100,000 receptors for a particular hormone and receptors, like other cellular proteins, are synthesized and broken down constantly. When a hormone is present in excess, the number of target –cell receptors may decrease. This is called **down- regulation**. In contrast, when a hormone or neurotransmitter is deficient, the number of receptors may increase and this is called **up-regulation.** This makes a target tissue more sensitive to hormone. An effective control system in the target cell provide a means of stopping hormone-induced actions, called **responses** by dissociating effector from the receptor. Thus, hormones themselves regulate their own receptors.

7.3 Hormonel Action at Cellular Level

Considerable progress has been made in the last 4-5 decades to understand the hormone action at the cellular level and the research work in this direction has led to many Nobel Prizes. E.W. Southerland, an American pharmacologist and physiologist and his colleagues have made important contribution in the field of hormone action. He was awarded Nobel Prize in 1971 for his discoveries in cellular signal transduction. By now it is well established that the hormones act at the cellular level only after forming specific combination with receptors. Since any effective control system also must provide a means of stopping a response, hormone-induced actions generally terminate when the effector dissociates from the receptor. Change in the concentration of hormone in circulation or bound to receptors constitutes the hormonal signal. Recent evidences suggest that there are possibly three modes by which a hormone exerts its action on the target cell or organ. These are I) action at gene level, 2) alteration in permeability of cell membrane, and 3) action as co-enzymes.

Action at gene level: Hormones influence the genes of the cells of the target organs and exert their action, example steroid hormones.

Alteration in permeability of cell membrane: Hormones alter the permeability of the cell membranes, thereby, altering the metabolism of the cell by blocking or accelerating the entrance of certain substrates into the cell. For example, ADH increases the permeability of the cells of the distal renal tubules to water, or aldosterone promotes Na+ influx in them.

Action as co-enzymes: Certain hormones work by functioning as co-enzymes.

7.4 Classification of Hormones on the Basis of Location of Receptors

Hormones may be classified in several ways such as according to chemical composition, solubility properties (Chapter 3), location of receptors and the nature of signal used to mediate their action within the cell. Table 7.1 illustrates the classification of hormones based on these properties. Chemically hormones are either lipid-soluble or water-soluble. On the basis of location of receptors, hormones are categorized into two groups. These are:

- Hormones that bind to intracellular receptors, and
- Hormones that bind to cell surface receptors.

However, the coincidental sub cellular location of receptors on plasma membrane in the case of metabolic hormones and intracellular receptors in case of growth and developmental hormones validates the arbitrary classification.

Table 7.1: Classification of hormones on the basis of solubility and type of receptors

Chemical Class of Hormone	Binding With Receptor (Second Messenger)	Hormone	Where Produced
A. Lipid Soluble 1. Steroids	**Intracellular Receptors**	Androgens	Testes
		Estrogens	Ovary
		Progestins	Ovary
		Glucocorticoids	Adrenal Cortex
		Mineralocorticoid	Adrenal Cortex
2. Thyroid Hormone		Triiodothyronine (T_3) and Thyroxin (T_4)	Thyroid Gland
3.Gas (NO)	**Cell Surface Receptors** or **Membrane Bound Receptors** (cGMP)	Nitric Oxide(NO) Atrial Natriuretic Factor (ANF)	Endothelial Cells lining the blood vessel
B. Water Soluble 1. Amines	**Cell Surface Receptors** or **Membrane Bound Receptors** (cAMP)	Epinephrine, Nor-epinephrine (Catecholamines) α_2 and β-adrenergic	Adrenal Medulla
2. Peptides and Proteins	**Cell Surface Receptors** or **Membrane Bound Receptors** (cAMP)	TSH, ACTH, FSH, LH, MSH Parathyroid Hormone ADH HCG Glucagon	Anterior Pituitary Parathyroid Hypothalamus Placenta Pancreas
	Cell Surface Receptors or **Membrane Bound Receptors** (Calcium or Phosphatidylinositol or both)	Gonadotropin-releasing hormone Thyrotropin-releasing hormone Acetyl Choline ADH/Vasopressin Oxytocin	Hypothalamus
	Cell Surface Receptors or **Membrane Bound Receptors** (Kinase or Phosphatase Cascade)	Erythropoietin (EPO) Epidermal Growth Factor (EGF) Growth Hormone Insulin Prolactin (PRL) ? Prostaglandins and Leukotriene	Kidney Skin epidermis Ant. Pituitary Pancreas Ant. Pituitary All cells except RBC

7.5 Mechanism of Action of Hormones

Hormones have to bind to their specific receptors to exert their action and the series of these events will depend on the location of two types of receptors in the cell.

Hormones that bind to intracellular receptors: The hormones that **bind to intracellular receptors** are lipophilic (Table 7.1) in nature and have receptors inside the cell either in the cytosol or on the nucleus. Hormones belonging to this category are steroid-thyroid-retinoid family. With the exception of thyroid hormones, all steroid hormones such as androgens, estrogens, progestins, glucocorticoids and mineralocorticoids are derived from cholesterol. Once secreted, these hormones diffuse through the plasma membrane of all target cells but only encounter their specific, high affinity receptors. The receptor of these hormones is specific soluble, oligomeric transport protein present either in cytosol or in the nucleus (usually in the nucleus) of target cells and therefore, is called as **mobile receptor**. The hormones associate themselves with the receptor and form **hormone-receptor complex** (Figure 7.1). This is to prolong their plasma half-life and also to increase their solubility. The hormone-receptor complex undergoes a temperature and salt-dependent "activation" reaction, which causes changes in size, conformation, and surface charge, to render it to bind to specific region of DNA (called the **acceptor site** on chromatin). A spectrum of proteins with variation in affinity for a particular hormone is involved in the binding, transport and response to any given steroid hormone. These are the serum binding and transport proteins, the cytoplasmic binding proteins in the target cell, the membrane binding protein in certain cases, and the nuclear binding and responsive receptor proteins of the target tissue. The specificity involved in the control of transcription requires that regulatory protein bind with high affinity to the correct region of DNA, called **promotors**. These are generally located 5′ from-and adjacent to- the coding segment of a gene. Much has been learned by now about how protein contact DNA and a number of classes of such interaction have been described that account for many of these specific protein-DNA interactions. Structural analysis of these proteins show that they have three unique supra secondary structural motifs that appear to be characteristic of DNA binding proteins. These are 1) helix-turn-helix (helix-loop-helix), 2) zinc (Zn) finger and 3) the leucine zipper. Comparisons of the binding activities of the proteins that contain these motifs show following characteristics. 1) Binding must be of high affinity to the specific site and of low affinity to other DNA. 2) Small regions of proteins make direct contact with DNA. Rest of the protein provide the trans-activation domains and may be involved in the dimerization of monomers of binding protein, may provide a contact surface for the formation of heterodimers, or may provide a ligand-binding site. 3) Hydrogen bonds and Van der Waals forces maintain the protein-DNA interactions.

Interaction of the receptor with the hormone on one hand and DNA on the other at the molecular level has been studied in detail in many cases. Rates of synthesis of target tissue macromolecules including that of protein, RNA and sometimes of DNA are found to increase following hormone administration. For example, estrogen action on hen oviduct leading to egg formation, androgen action on accessory gland of reproduction of male such as seminal vesicle, or action of glucocorticoid on thymus leading to its involution. Although, the final picture is not very clear, yet a conceptual account of action of steroid hormone is possible. Thus, steroid on entering the cell, combines with and activates its specific receptor and this complex translocates to the nucleus, binds to the acceptor site on chromatin and results in RNA synthesis to produce hormone effects. After dissociating from the acceptor site, both, the steroid and receptor are degraded. Analogues of steroid hormones (artificial steroids) that function as **anti-steroids**, for example **anti-androgens** (cyproterone) and **anti-estrogens** (clomiphene, tamoxifen and nafoxidene) prevent natural steroids from binding to receptors and thus block their action. However, these anti-steroids bind to the receptor but fail to activate its translocation to the nucleus. Further, in testicular feminization condition in which patient is phenotypically female but genetically have XY-chromosome and abdominal testes secreting almost normal levels of androgens in blood with no masculine effects, there is deficiency or no androgen receptors on the target tissues and thus, they appear normal female in behavior, external genitalia and well-developed breasts. In case of some steroids, only transitory binding to acceptor site is permitted as seen with steroid hormone estriol for estrogen receptors. These steroids produce no or low estrogenic activity themselves but act as anti-estrogenic by competing with 17β estradiol.

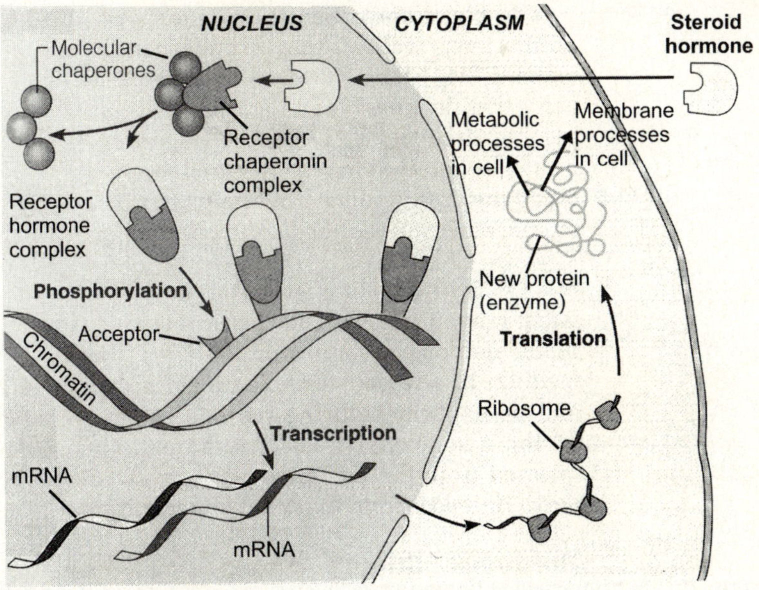

Figure 7.1: Hormone action through mobile receptor (e.g. steroid hormones).

Once the steroid hormone enters the cytoplasm of the target cell, it encounters specific receptors with high-affinity. It binds with the receptor protein and a hormone-receptor complex is formed (Figure 7.1). This complex then diffuses into or is transported into the nucleus where it reacts with the nuclear chromatin. Somewhere along this route, hormone-receptor complex undergoes a temperature, and salt-dependent "**activation reaction**" to enable it to bind to nuclear chromatin. The hormone-receptor complex binds to a specific region of DNA, known as "**hormone response element**". This activates or inactivates specific genes to affect selective gene transcription, to form messanger RNA (mRNA). The mRNA diffuses into the cytoplasm where it accelerates the translation process at the ribosome to synthesize new proteins, thus influencing the metabolic processes (Figure 7.2).

The effect of each of these hormones is quite specific and evidence suggests that steroid hormones exert their effect on gene transcription by interacting with specific cis-acting elements called **enhancers** or **silencers**. This influences the basic transcriptional machinery of the target cell and results in **up regulation** (enhanced) or **down regulation** (silenced) of specific gene transcription. However, these genes must be in region of "open" or transcriptionally active chromatin as defined by their susceptibility to digestion by the enzyme DNase 1. The genes show the presence of two separate **control sites** or **regulatory elements** in the DNA sequence immediately 5′ of transcription initiation site. The first of these is **the promotor element** (PE), and the second is the **hormone response element (HRE)** (Figure 7.3).

The promotor element is generic, as it is present in all genes in some form or the other. It specifies the site of RNA polymerase II attachment to DNA. This results in accurate initiation of transcription. The hormone response element is located slightly farther 5′ than the promotor element. It may consist of several discrete elements. It modulates the frequency of transcript initiation and is less dependent on position and orientation, thus resembling the transcription enhancer elements found in other genes. HRE has been identified in many genes regulated by steroid hormones. Its precise location varies from gene to gene and genes controlled by several hormones have a corresponding number of HREs. Although initial reactions of peptide hormones are different, yet they exert their effects on transcription through HREs. For example, hormones that use cAMP as a second messenger affect transcription.

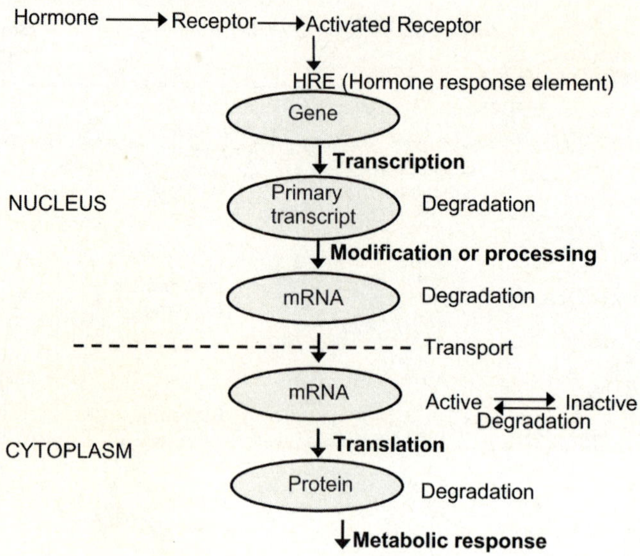

Figure 7.2: The "Information Pathway"- hormones can affect any of these steps.

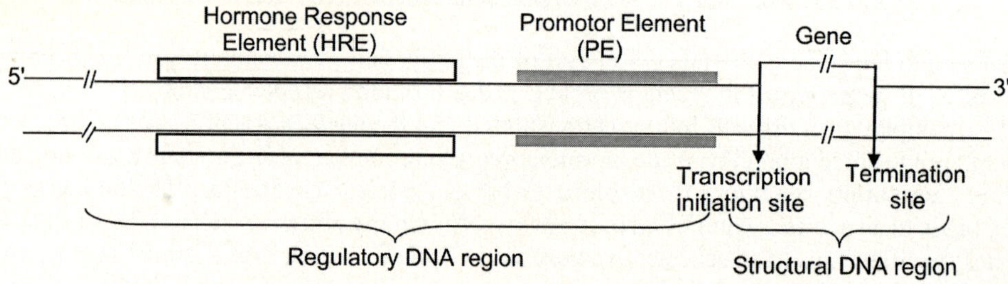

Figure 7.3: Promotor element (PE) and hormone response element (HRE) on gene.

The identification of HRE requires that a) it binds the hormone-receptor complex more avidly than does surrounding DNA, and b) it must confer hormone responsiveness. Recent evidence suggests that although simple HREs do transmit a hormone response yet in many genes, HRE must associate with other elements or binding proteins to function optimally. Such assemblies of *cis*- acting DNA elements and *trans* –acting factors are called hormone-response units (HRUs). The hormone response unit is an assembly of DNA elements and bound proteins. An essential component is the hormone response element with ligand-bound receptor and the important accessory factor elements with bound transcription factors. More than two dozens of the accessory factors have been linked to hormone effects on transcription. These factors can interact with each other or with the nuclear receptors. Thus, an HRU consists of one or more HREs and one or more DNA elements with associated accessory factors. The components of the HRU communicate with the basal transcription machinery through a co-activator complex and one or more of a class of co-regulator molecules accomplishes this. Several hormone response elements (HREs) of various hormones or effectors are known as: Glucocorticoids-GRE, Progestins-PRE, Androgens-ARE, Estrogens-ERE, Retinoic acid-RARE, cAMP-CRE etc. The first of these described was the CREB-binding protein, known as CBP (calcium binding protein). Through an amino terminal domain, CBP binds to phosphorylated serine 137 of CREB and mediates transactivation in response to cyclic AMP. It is therefore described as a co-activator. Co-activator interact with a number of signaling molecules such as activator protein I (AP-I), signal transducers and activators of transcription (STATS), nuclear receptors etc. Role of many co-activators is still evolving and it appears that certain combinations are responsible for specific ligand-induced actions through various receptors. Recent view holds that the **histone acetyltransferase** (HAT) activities, which also show assembly specificity, acetylate histones and result in the remodeling of chromatin into a transcription-efficient environment. Histone de-acetylation has been found to be associated with the inactivation of transcription. In certain instances, removal of a co-repressor complex through a ligand-receptor interaction results in the activation of transcription. For example, in the absence of hormone, the thyroid or retinoic acid receptors (TRE/RARE) are bound to a co-repressor complex containing nuclear receptor co-repressor (NCoR) or silencing mediator for RXR and TR (SMRT) and associated proteins, some of which have histone de-acetylase activity. The target gene is repressed until binding of hormone to the thyroid receptor results in the dissociation of this complex, and gene activation then ensues. Table 7. 2 list some mammalian co-regulator proteins. In addition to CBP and p300, three other families of co-activator molecules with about 160 KDa molecular mass have been described.

Table 7.2: Mammalian co-regulator proteins

300-kDa family of Co-activators		**CBP**	**CREB-binding proteins**
		P300	**Protein of 300 kDa**
160-kDa family of Co-activators	A	SRC-1	Steroid receptor co-activator 1
		NcoA-1	Nuclear receptor co-activator 1
	B	TIF2	Transcriptional intermediary factor 2
		GRIP1	Glucocorticoid receptor-interacting protein
		NcoA-2	Nuclear receptor co-activator 2
	C	p/CIP	p300/CBP co-integrator-associated protein 1
		ACTR	Thyroid activator & retinoic acid receptors
		AIB	Amplified in breast cancer
		RAC3	Receptor-associated co-activator 3
		TRAM-1	TR activator molecule 1
Co-repressors	NCoR		Nuclear receptor co-repressor
	SMRT		Silencing mediator for RXR and TR

Two complications have been met in the understanding of steroid hormone action. These are i) activation of a receptor without the ligand (**agonist**), and ii) presence of **orphan receptors** (receptors that have no known ligand). Orphan receptors have been discovered by reverse endocrinology approach. In addition, a number of diet derived small molecular weight organic compounds such as simple fatty acid derivatives when administered into recipient animals, could produce developmental effects probably through activation of such orphan receptors. Therefore, at present, a third group of hormones/factors, called, '**permissive**' hormones may be required in the body to permit other hormones to act. In their absence, when experimentally induced, other hormonal effects are attenuated. What exactly is the molecular basis of permissiveness is not clear at the moment.

Hormones that bind to cell surface receptors: The hormones that **bind to cell surface receptors** have receptors on the outer surface of the plasma membrane or cell membrane, and are water-soluble and not lipid-soluble. Examples of such hormones are peptide and protein hormones such as Gonadotropin releasing hormone (GnRH), Follicle stimulating hormone (FSH), luteinizing hormone (LH), thyroid stimulating hormone (TSH), adrenocorticotropic hormone (ACTH), vasopressin, oxytocin, prolactin, insulin, atrial natriuretic factor etc. These hormones cannot diffuse through the lipid bilayer of the plasma membrane to attach to receptors inside target cells. They have no transport proteins and therefore, are also categorized as having **fixed receptor**. Because of this, these hormones have a short plasma half-life. But they can induce their effects at very low concentrations as the cascade of chain reactions, which they initiate, amplifies the initial effect at each step. Discovery of adenosine-3', 5' cyclic monophosphate (cAMP) has been a major step in understanding the exciting details of action of these hormones. This also led to the concept of primary and secondary messengers in hormone action. Subsequently involvement of other second messenger systems like Calcium (Ca++), Phosphatidyl inositols (IP_3) or both, and adenosine and guanosine were also discovered. It was realized that the response of the hormone of this category is initiated by its binding to a receptor located in the plasma membrane and protruding into the interstitial fluid. Because water-soluble hormone binds to a receptor at the extra-cellular surface of the plasma membrane, it acts as the **first messenger**. First messenger then induces the release of **second messenger** inside the cell, where hormone-stimulated responses can take place. **Cyclic AMP** (e.g. FSH, LH, TSH, ACTH, TRH, hCG, CRH, LPH, MSH, glucagon, somatostatin and vasopressin); **cyclic GMP** (e.g. atrial natriuretic factor and nitric oxide); **calcium** or **phosphatidyl inositols** or **both** (e.g. oxytocin, vasopressin, acetylcholine, GnRH, TRH) or **a kinase** or **phosphatase cascade** (e.g. prolactin, insulin, growth hormone) may act as **intracellular second messengers** to exert hormone action. Cyclic AMP and other second messengers alter cell's function in specific ways to produce hormone action. A given hormone may use different second messengers in different target cells to induce its action

a) cAMP as second messenger

Cyclic AMP (cyclic adenosine 3′,5′ monophosphate) is the common second messenger seen in the action of many peptide hormones. It is synthesized from ATP (Figure 7.4). This reaction is catalyzed by enzyme adenyl cyclase, which is attached to the inner surface of the plasma membrane. Cyclic AMP plays an important role in the action of number of hormones especially peptide hormones. These receptors regulate the activity of an adenyl cyclase molecule. The series of actions are as follows.

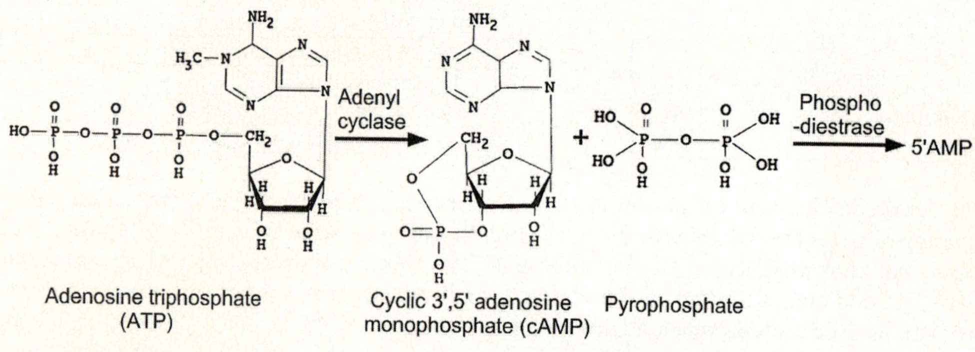

Figure 7.4: Conversion of ATP into cyclic AMP by adenyl cyclase and to 5′-AMP by phosphodiesterase.

A water-soluble hormone (First messenger) diffuses from the blood and binds to its receptor in a target cell's plasma membrane (Figure 7.5). The hormone receptor complex formed in this category of hormones combines with GTP-dependent trimeric nucleotide regulatory complex of the cell membrane. This binding activates or inactivates adenyl cyclase mediated by at least two GTP-dependent regulatory proteins, designated as Gs (stimulatory) and Gi (inhibitory). Each of these G proteins is composed of three subunits: α, β, and γ. Gs contain α_s β γ, while Gi contains α_i β γ. The α subunit is bound to GDP. Binding of hormone to receptor results in a receptor-mediated activation of G and GDP is exchanged for GTP (Figure 7.6). The α subunit separates from the combined β and γ subunits. The resultant GTP- α_s activates effectors, such as adenyl cyclase. The intrinsic GTPase activity of the α subunits then converts GTP and GDP leading to the reassociation of α with β γ subunits. In contrast, α_I -GTP inhibits adenyl cyclase by binding with it, thus lowering the intracellular concentration of cAMP. Adenyl cyclase converts ATP into cAMP in the cytosol of cell. In prokaryotic cells, cAMP binds to a specific protein, called "**catabolic regulator protein (CRP)**", which binds directly to DNA and influences gene expression. In eukaryotic cells, cyclic AMP activates one or several protein kinases by combining with a regulatory subunit of the kinase and promotes dissociation of the catalytic subunit. A protein kinase is an enzyme that phosphorylate i.e. adds a phosphate group to cellular proteins and the donor for this is ATP, which in turn is converted to ADP. A protein kinase is a heterotetrameric molecule consisting of 2 regulatory subunits (R) and 2 catalytic subunits (C). Cyclic AMP binding results in this reaction.

$$4\ cAMP + R_2C_2 \leftrightarrow R_2 + (4\ cAMP) + 2C$$

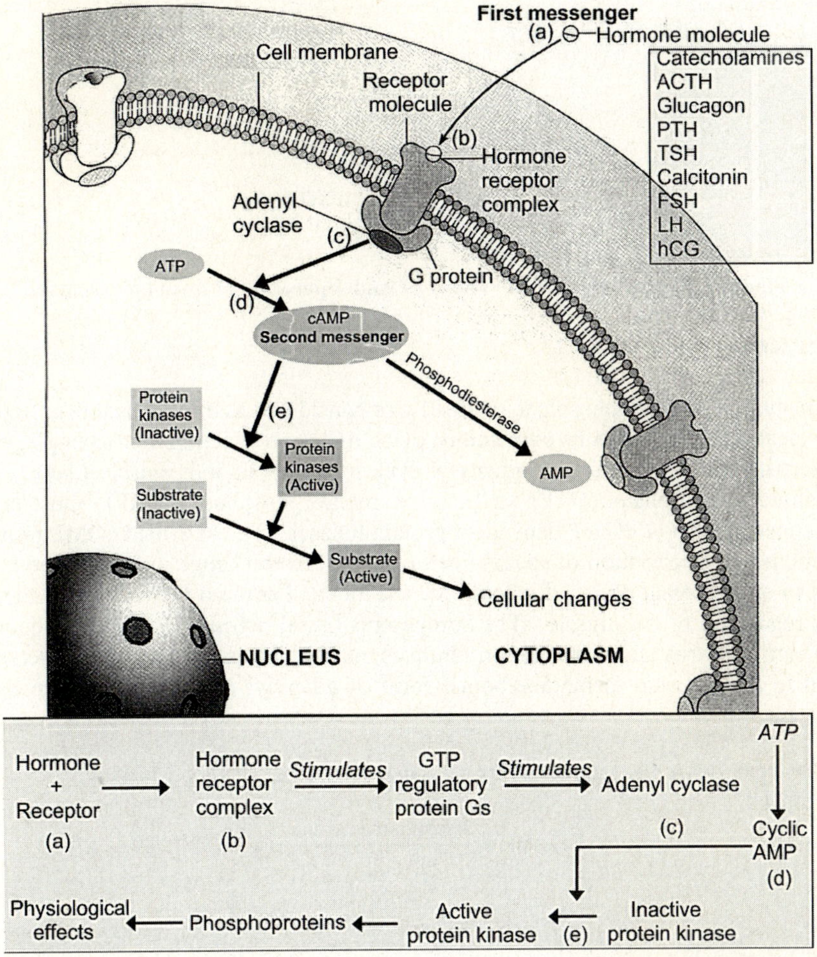

Figure 7.5: Action of hormones that bind to cell membrane receptor, mediated through second messenger.

The R_2C_2 complex has no enzymatic activity, but the binding of cAMP by R dissociates R from C and in turn activates the latter (Figure 7.7). Activated protein kinase catalyzes the transfer of γ phosphate of ATP (Mg^{++}) to a serine or threonine residue in a variety of proteins. This phosphorylates one or several other enzyme, which catalyze a cascade of reactions that result in secretion, protein synthesis, or a change in plasma permeability etc. to produce physiological responses. Different protein kinases exist within different target cells and within different organelles of the same target cell. Thus, one protein kinase may trigger triglyceride breakdown, a second glycogen synthesis, a third protein synthesis, and so on and so forth. After a brief period of time, **phosphodiesterase** enzyme inactivates cAMP converting it to physiologically inactivated 5′-AMP and cell's response is turned off. Many hormones such as TSH, ADH, ACTH, FSH, LH, hCG, PTH, MSH, ADH, epinephrine, glucagon, and hypothalamic releasing hormones exert their physiological effect through increased synthesis of cAMP (Figure 7.4). The level of cAMP decreases in response to the binding of hormone to its receptors in certain cases such as, growth hormone inhibiting hormone (GHIH), acetylcholine etc.

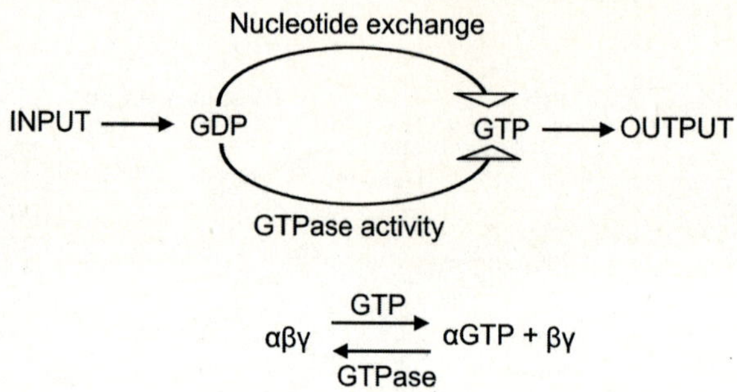

Figure 7.6: Exchange of GDP and GTP and separation of α subunit from βγ.

b) cGMP as second messenger

Initially cyclic guanosine monophosphate (cGMP) was considered as a functional counterpart of cAMP but now it is clear that cGMP has its own unique place in hormone action. For example, nitric oxide is known to exert its effect by activating guanylyl cyclase inside smooth muscle fibers. This enzyme converts guanine triphosphate (GTP) to guanine mono phosphate (GMP), thus increasing the intracellular concentration of cGMP dependent protein kinases. The activated cGMP protein kinase in turn brings about phosphorylation of specific cellular proteins to change their activation. This causes calcium ions to enter storage areas of smooth muscle fiber. Lowered Ca++ level in the cytosol as a result causes relaxation of the muscle. The atriopeptins (atrial natriuretic factor) produced in cardiac atrial tissues causes natriuresis, vasodilation, diuresis, and inhibition of aldosterone secretion. These peptides bind to and activate membrane-bound form of guanylyl cyclase resulting in an increase of cGMP.

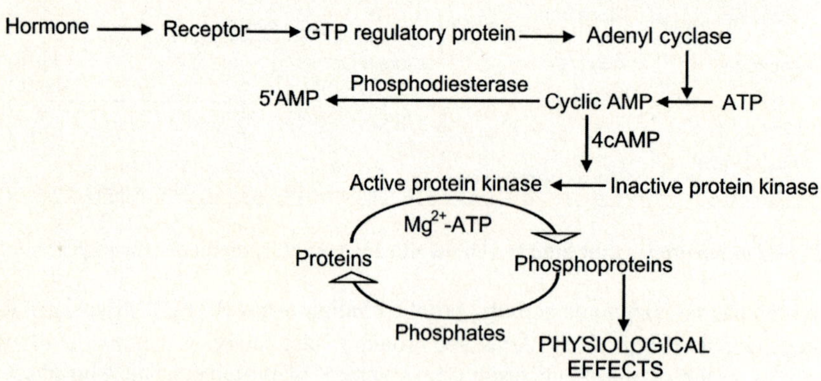

Figure 7.7: Hormone action through cAMP dependent protein kinase.

c) Calcium or posphatidylinositols or both as second messengers

Ionized calcium is also considered as an important intracellular messenger in hormone action (Figure 7.8). It regulates many cellular processes such as muscle contraction, stimulus-secretion coupling enzyme activity, membrane excitability and blood clotting cascade. A role for ionized calcium in hormone action has been suggested by the studies on pituitary, salivary glands, blood platelets and smooth muscle. It appears that Ca2+ free media blunts the effect of many hormones i) or when intracellular calcium is depleted, ii) or can be mimicked by agents that increase cytosolic Ca^{2+}, and iii) or influences cellular calcium flux.

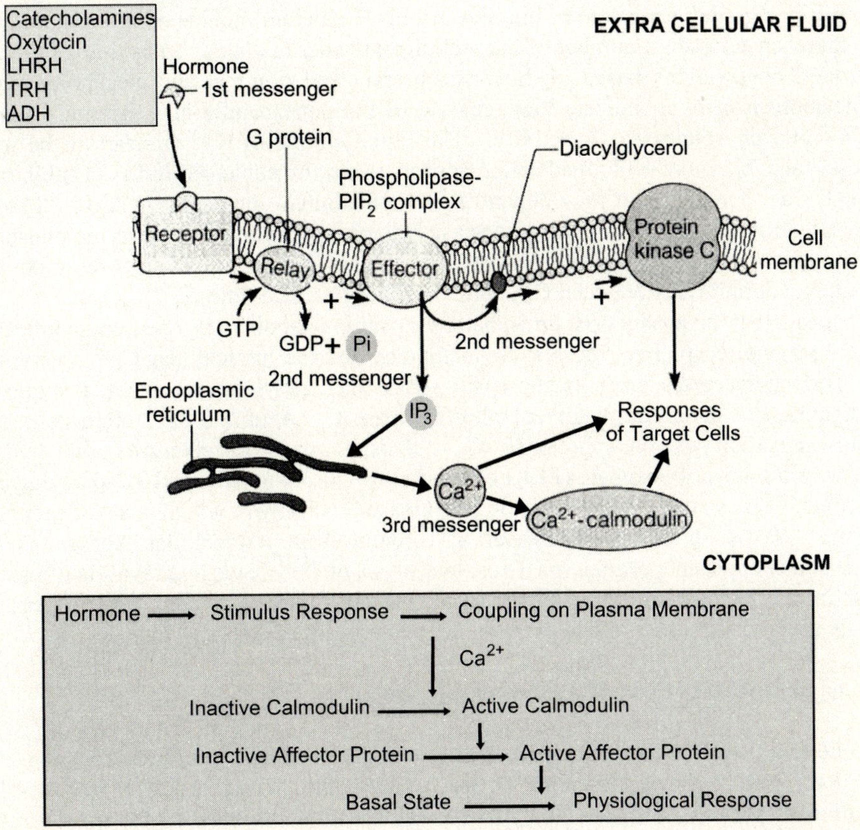

Figure 7.8: Action of hormones mediated through mechanisms that utilize Ca^{2+} , PIP_2- phosphatidylinositol 4,5-biphosphate, IP3-inositol triphosphate.

The extra cellular calcium concentration is about 5mmol/L and intracellular concentration is only 0.1-10 μmol/L. In spite of the many fold concentration gradients, Ca^{2+} is restrained from entering the cell and its levels are very rigidly controlled. The hormones that bind cell membrane receptor enhance membrane permeability to Ca^{2+} influx. This is accomplished by Na^{+} – Ca^{2+} exchange mechanism that has a high capacity but a low affinity for Ca^{2+}. Also, there is a Ca^{2+} – 2H+ ATPase-dependent pump that extrudes Ca^{2+} in exchange for H+. This has a high affinity for Ca++ but a low capacity and may be responsible for fine-tuning cytosolic Ca^{2+}. Finally, Ca^{2+} can be mobilized or deposited from/into the mitochondria and endoplasmic reticulum pool.

Calcium (Ca^{2+}), serving as second messenger in hormone action is better understood now. This is due to availability of variety of techniques that can quantitate the rapid changes of intracellular Ca^{2+} concentrations, and also due to the discovery of a Ca^{2+} dependent regulator of phosphodiesterase activity in the interaction of Ca^{2+} and cAMP within cells. The calcium-dependent regulatory protein is now referred to as **calmodulin**, a 17-kDa protein, homologous in structure and function to muscle protein troponin C. It has 4 Ca^{2+} binding sites. The interaction of Ca^{2+} with calmodulin is conceptually similar to the binding of cAMP to protein kinase and subsequent activation of this molecule. A number of enzymes are known that are, regulated directly or indirectly by Ca^{2+} through calmodulin (Figure 7.8). In addition to its effects on enzymes and ion transport, Ca^{2+} -calmodulin regulates the activity of many structural elements in cells such as actin-myosin complex of smooth muscle. Though calmodulin contains four binding sites for calcium, binding of only 3 calcium molecules are required to activate calmodulin that then activates a number of intracellular enzymes to alter cell physiological responses.

Further, observations based on how vasopressin and α-adrenergic catecholamines regulate glycogen metabolism in liver indicate that removal of hormone results in a prompt decline of both cytosolic Ca^{2+} and phosphorylase A activity. The initial source of Ca^{2+} appears to be intracellular organelle reservoirs, but more prolonged action appears to require enhanced influx or inhibition of Ca^{2+} efflux through Ca^{2+} pump, which may depend upon concomitant increase of cAMP. Phosphorylase activation results from conversion of phosphorylase B to phosphorylase A by enzyme phosphorylase B kinase. This enzyme contains calmodulin as its δ subunit and its activity increases with increase of Ca^{2+}, suggesting a definite link between Ca^{2+} and phosphorylase activation.

It appears that the products of Phosphatidylinositol metabolism provide communication signal between the hormone receptor on the plasma membrane and the intracellular Ca^{2+} reservoirs (Figure 7.8). Cell surface receptors such as those for ADH and acetylcholine, when occupied by their respective ligands, are potent activators of phospholipase C. A unique G protein couples receptor binding and activation of phospholipase C. Phospholipase C catalyzes the hydrolysis of phosphatidylinositol 4,5-bisphosphate (PIP_2) to inositol triphosphate (IP_3) and 1,2-diacylglycerol. The diacylglycerol is itself capable of activating protein kinase C activity of which is also dependent on free ionic calcium. IP_3 is an effective releaser of calcium from intracellular storage sites such as mitochondria and endoplasmic reticulum. Thus, hydrolysis of PIP_2 leads to activation of protein kinase C resulting in an increase in cytoplasmic calcium ion. The activated protein kinase C can phosphorylate specific substrates and alter physiological processes.

d) Kinase or phosphatase cascade as second messenger

Some hormone receptors like those for epidermal growth factor (EGF), insulin and insulin-like growth factor-1 (IGF-1) have intrinsic tyrosine kinase activity and activation of which results in the phosphorylation of protein substrates on tyrosine residues to show insulin action. Tyrosine kinase activation can also initiate a phosphorylation and dephosphorylation cascade that involves the action of several other protein kinases to counter balance actions of phosphatase. To initiate this cascade, two mechanisms are employed: i) growth hormone, prolactin, cytokines and erythropoietin activate tyrosine kinase to initiate their action, but this activity is not an integral part of the hormone receptor. The hormone-receptor interaction activates cytoplasmic protein tyrosine kinases. These kinases phosphorylate one or more cytoplasmic proteins, which then associate with other docking proteins through binding to Src homology 2 domains. These peptide segments are referred to as SH2 domains. One such interaction results in the activation of a family of cytosolic proteins called **signal transduction and activators of transcription** (STATs). The phosphorylated STAT protein dimerizes and translocates into the nucleus, binds to a specific DNA element like interferon response element or serum response element, and activates transcription. ii) Other SH2 docking events may result in the activation of PI 3-kinase, the MAP kinase pathway or G protein-mediated activation of phospholipase

C (PLCγ) with the attendant production of diacylglycerol and activation of protein kinase C. There is a potential for crossover when different hormones activate these various signal transduction pathways.

7.6 Termination of Hormone Action

Hormones that act at the plasma membrane are degraded within the blood by serum enzymes and their declined circulating level result in a decrease in further stimulation of membrane adenylate or guanylate cyclase activities. In the absence of cyclic nucleotide production, the residual intracellular cyclic nucleotides are destroyed rapidly by cytosolic phosphodiesterase action, and the cellular activity returns to basal levels. On the other hand, effects of hormones that act through intracellular receptors, such as steroid and thyroid hormones are of longer duration, involving DNA, RNA, and protein synthesis. In the case of these hormones, absence of further hormone stimulation results in degradation of newly synthesized RNA species and proteins by cytoplasmic enzyme actions. Evidences suggest that receptor modulation (down and up regulation) by circulating hormone concentrations is an important physiological adaptation in hormone action.

Summary

Endocrine glands secrete hormones that affect target cells possessing specific receptors. The concentration of each hormone in the body fluids is precisely regulated.

The number of hormone receptors may decrease (down-regulation) or increase (up-regulation) to maintain homeostasis in the body. Hormones only regulate their own receptors.

Chemically hormones are lipid-soluble, such as steroids, thyroid hormones and nitric oxide, or water-soluble, such as amines, peptides, proteins, glycoprotein and eicosanoids.

Water-soluble hormones circulate in free form in the blood, while lipid-soluble steroids and thyroid hormones attach to specific transport proteins synthesized by the liver.

Actions of hormones at the cellular and sub-cellular level require its binding to a receptor. Receptors have a high affinity for the hormone and their binding is highly specific and readily reversible. Receptors can be a component of plasma membrane, e.g. peptide hormones or may be located within the cell, i.e. intracellular as for steroid and thyroid hormones.

Sequence of steroid hormone action involves diffusion of hormone through target cell membrane to enter the nucleus. It combines with a receptor molecule to form steroid hormone-receptor complex. This binds to DNA and promotes synthesis of messenger RNA; mRNA enters the cytoplasm and directs protein synthesis, and newly synthesized proteins produce hormone's specific effects.

Hormone-receptor complex bind to specific regions of DNA, called hormone response elements (HRE). Several DNA elements in addition to receptor-binding element are necessary in many cases for a hormone response and this assembly is called a hormone-response unit (HRU)

The interaction of peptide hormones with receptors located on cell membrane results in the expression of specific genes, secretion of various molecules, activity of intracellular proteins, and regulation of ion and channel activity. Second messengers such as cAMP, cGMP, Ca++, phosphatidylinositides, and protein kinase cascades mediate these effects. The hormone itself is the first messenger. Thus, sequence of nonsteroid hormone action is as follows: endocrine gland secretes nonsteroid hormone; body fluid carries hormone to its target cell; hormone combines with receptor site on membrane of its target cells, activating G protein; adenylate cyclase molecules are activated within target cell's membrane; adenylate cyclase converts ATP into cyclic AMP; cAMP activates protein kinases; these enzymes activate protein substrates in the cell that change metabolic processes; cellular changes produce the hormone's effects.

There are two types of G proteins. The first turns off adenylate cyclase and is called an inhibitory G protein while the other turns on adenylate cyclase and is called a stimulatory G protein.

Calcium receptor is called calmodulin. It contains four binding sites for calcium. However, binding of only 3 calcium molecules are required to activate calmodulin. Calmodulin then activates a number of intracellular enzymes to alter cell physiology.

The cellular response to a non-steroid hormone is amplified because the enzymes induced by a small number of hormone-receptor complexes can catalyze formation of a large number of second messenger molecules.

Different hormones can cause production of the same second messenger when their receptors activate the same membrane protein (e.g. adenylate cyclase). There is a potential for crossover when different hormones activate various signal transduction pathways.

Questions

1. Describe the two major mechanisms by which hormones bring about their effects on target tissues.
2. How does a steroid hormone act on its target cells?
3. How does a nonsteroidal hormone act on its target cells?
4. What is a second messenger?
5. Explain how the cellular response to a hormone operating through a second messenger is amplified.

Part II

Biology of Reproduction

- Development of Genital System
- Biology of Sex
- Germ Cells and Gamete Formation
- Puberty, Adolescence and Menopause
- Male Reproductive System
- Physiology of Male Reproduction
- Female Reproductive System
- Reproductive Cycles
- Ovulation and Fertilization
- Implantation and Pregnancy
- Parturition and Lactation

Chapter 8

Development of Genital System

Genital system includes:

i) Gonads, the testes and ovaries,

ii) Genital ducts, efferent ductules, duct of epididymis and ducts of vas deferens in males, and oviducts or fallopian tubes and uterine tubes in females,

iii) The structures associated with the transmission of sperm from the male (penis) to their reception in the female (vulva and vagina), and

iv) That part of female duct system, (the uterus) which is highly modified for the reception and nourishment of conceptus.

Developmental history of the genital system is particularly complex owing to i) the origin of its different components from diverse and disparate primordia, ii) variation in the contributions from the primordia in two sexes, and iii) contribution by all the three germ layers in its formation. In the 'pregonadal stage', the embryo lacks any specific gonadal structures but the ultimate development of a male or female gonad is predetermined by its chromosomal sex.

8.1 Development of gonads

The development of the genital system proceeds with the development of gonads from an indifferent stage in which the sex of the gonad is not yet determined and in which both, mesonephric and paramesonephric duct systems are present. Genetically however, the sex of the normal embryo is determined at the time of fertilization depending on whether or not the Y- chromosome is present in the fertilizing sperm.

The indifferent stage: Genital system makes its appearance during the 5th - 6th weeks (5-12 mm embryo) of intrauterine life. This is the **'indifferent period'** because sex cannot be determined either by gross inspection or by study of sections of gonads. It is only at 8 weeks that sex can be determined by inspection of gonad or external genitalia.

The male and female gonads are derived embryologically from the same site, an area called **the urogenital ridge**. Until 6th week of uterine life, there is no differentiation in this site in male or female fetuses. In the genetic male, the testes begin to develop during 7th week. A single gene on the Y chromosome (the SRY gene, the sex determining region of the Y chromosome) is expressed at this time in the urogenital ridge cells and triggers this development. In the absence of a Y chromosome, and hence, the SRY gene, testes do not develop and instead ovaries begin to develop in the same area at about 11 weeks.

The early development of the gonad proceeds in the same manner in both males and females. In both sexes the gonads are derived from two distinct tissues: **somatic mesenchymal tissues** which form the matrix of the gonad, and the **primordial germ cells** (derived from the yolk sac endoderm) which migrate into and colonize this matrix to form the gametes (Figures 8.1 and 8.2). Two important events occur simultaneously and form the specific feature of the initial gonadal development. These are:

i) Migration of the primordial germ cells into the coelomic epithelium and underlying mesenchymal tissue covering the mesonephros, and

ii) Release and migration of mesonephric cells into the same zone.

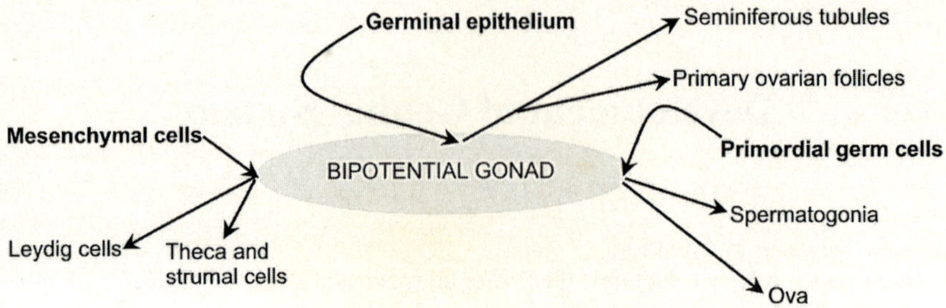

Figure 8.1: Origin of bipotential gonad and structures derived from it.

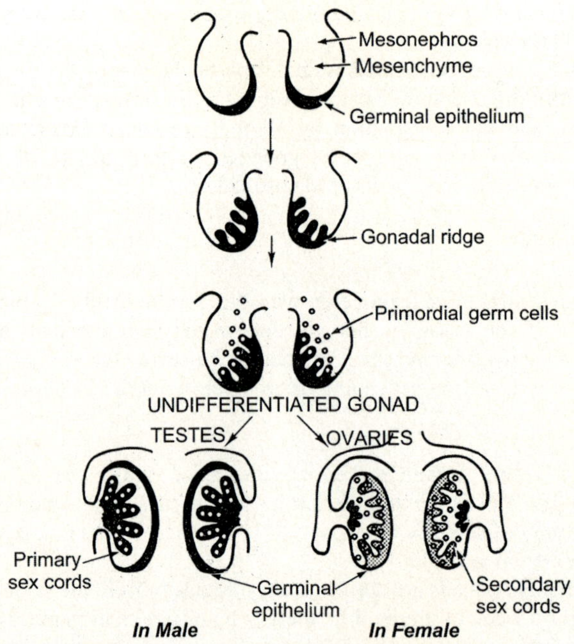

Figure 8.2: Relationship of mesonephros, mesenchyme and germinal epithelium in gonadal development.

The primordia of primitive gonad (term used as long as it is structurally indistinguishable into male or female) makes its appearance in embryos of 4-5mm as thickenings within a localized region of the mesodermal mesenchyme, called the **urogenital ridge** (Figure 8.3). It is located on the posterior wall of the embryo, on either side of the central dorsal aorta in the lower thoracic and upper lumbar region. This ridge contains the primordia of both, the genital and the nephric systems. It is superficial and medial to the developing **mesonephric tissue**. On the ventro-median surface of the urogenital ridge, the peritoneal epithelium begins to thicken in 6mm embryo and rapidly becomes several layers thick. Proliferation causes this region to bulge into the coelom. This is called the **genital ridge** (Figure 8.4). This gonadal primordium originate as paired mesenchymal structures, projecting on each side of the dorsal mesentery from the medial aspect of the mesonephros and consists essentially of mesodermal cells of coelomic epithelium origin. The mesonephros is the second of the three (pronephros, mesonephros and metanephros) consecutive primordial kidneys that form during fetal life. Each genital ridge shows a mesenchymal core composed of simple stellate or spindle-shaped cells that are covered by rapidly multiplying coelomic epithelium and surface epithelium. Genital ridges are first seen in dog embryos at 24 days, pig embryos at 26 days and bovine embryos at 28 days. Soon however, cells of a special type become apparent interspersed in the substance of the gonadal primordium. These are spherical and are distinctly larger than the surrounding mesenchymal cells. They possess large vesicular nucleus and their abundant cytoplasm is less eosinophilic than that of mesenchymal cells and it is difficult to fix them properly. These special cells are called **primordial germ cells or gonocytes**. They originate extragonadally from yolk sac endoderm near the developing allantois and are first identifiable in the human embryo at about three weeks (Figure 8.4 A). The "germ layer hypothesis" is put forth to suggest that primordial cells make their first appearance in and may arise from the extra embryonic endoderm. As early as 4mm embryonic stage, these cells are seen to proliferate by rapidly multiplying coelomic epithelium and migrate by way of the endodermal gut and dorsal mesentery into the region of the future genital ridge (Figure 8.4 B and C). Alkaline phosphatase activity is used to study the migration of germ cells. It indicates that by 13-20 somite stage of human fetus, the primordial germ cell population, expanded by mitosis, can be observed migrating to the connective tissue of the hind gut and from there into the gut mesentery.

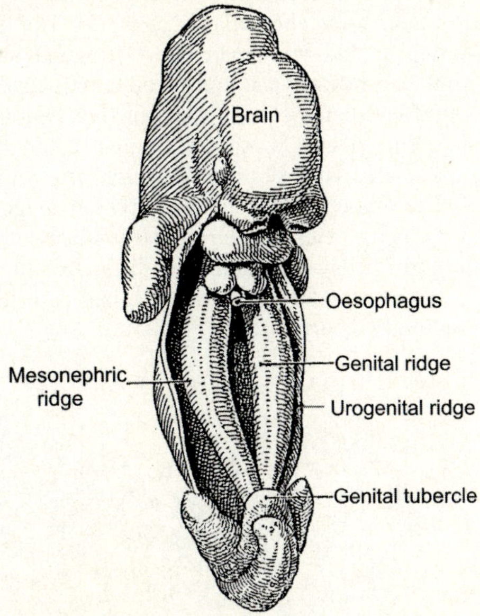

Figure 8.3: Human embryo (9 mm) dissected to show urogenital ridge.

From about the 25-somite stage onwards (30 days or so after fertilization) the majority of cells have passed into the region of developing kidneys and hence into the adjacent gonadal primordia where they come to lie between and within the developing sex cords. Migration of primordial germ cells occurs by their own amoeboid movement known as **diapedesis**. It is believed that the genital ridges may produce a chemotactic substance that attracts the primordial germ cells, and so gives direction to their movement. In reptiles and birds, primordial germ cells pass into the genital ridge by circulation. When the primordial germ cells arrive at the coelomic epithelium covering gonadal ridges, they appear to be "trapped" by processes from the epithelial cells. The motile properties of primordial germ cells are switched off when they colonize the genital ridges and this property of germ cells cannot be reawakened.

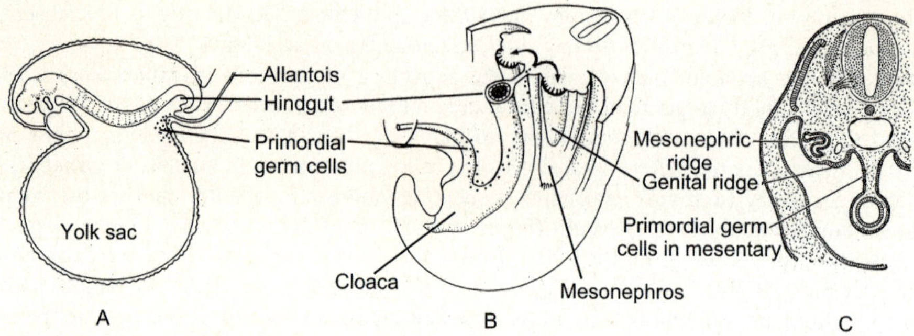

Figure 8.4: Three-week Human embryo showing, A-origin of primordial germ cells, B- route of their migration and C- embryo in transverse section at 7mm stage to show primordial germ cells in mesentery.

Structure of primordial germ cells: Primordial germ cells of rat are large, round and have a darkly stained cytoplasm than the surrounding somatic cells (Figure 8.5). The morphological features of the migrating germ cells in mammals including human show irregular shape of the cytoplasm with pseudopodia-like extensions, spherical nucleus and conspicuous reticulated nucleoli. The cytoplasmic organelles are specific to an undifferentiated cell. **Nuage** (active regions) appears to form a unique feature in both male and female germ cells. It consists of regular or spherical electron dense masses of fibrous to granular substance associated with ribosomes, which often forms a close association with mitochondria of the nucleus. The amount of nuage is increased in germ cells (may be related to increased mitotic activity of germ cells) with age during early stages of gonadal development and is greater in female than in male germ cells, suggesting the difference in RNA transcripts, because of differences in sex chromosomes. Presence of nuage in germ cells is considered to be a structural marker that supports the germ plasm continuity theory.

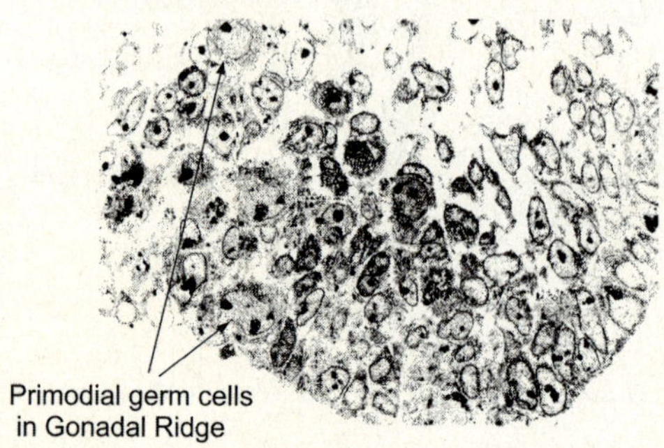

Figure 8.5: Light micrograph showing appearance of gonadal ridge on day 13 of development in Rat, with migrated primordial germ cells.

During settlement phase, germ cells become spherical and develop cytological features that are indicative of their increased differentiation. The primordial germ cells continue to divide mitotically during their migration and settlement in the gonad, thus increasing their number rapidly. Some growth factors may be involved in their proliferation. Once the primordial germ cells are settled in the gonad, they get enclosed in specific germ cell compartments where their further multiplication and differentiation are controlled by the surrounding somatic cells depending upon the composition of sex chromosomes of such cells. The patterns by which the germ cells form association with somatic cells in the gonadal folds differ greatly from those specific of the migratory phase as they get completely surrounded by the somatic cells rather than only locally as during migration. Further, fetal germ cells appear to retain a pattern of gene expression resembling that in early pluripotent embryonic cells and this may be important for the maintenance of genetic totipotency. The intercellular bridges connecting developing germ cells in both male and female gonads appear to regulate the developmental synchrony seen between germ cells within a single cluster.

It is generally believed that germ cells are unable to differentiate into somatic elements and those that fail to reach the gonadal primordia degenerate and disappear. Embryonic studies clearly indicate that the primitive genital ridges are unable to differentiate into anything resembling gonads unless adequate numbers of germ cells are incorporated into them. With the arrival of primordial germ cells, the genital ridges are transformed into indifferent or undifferentiated gonads in both the sexes. The arrival of primordial germ cells to the genital ridges coincides with the intense proliferation of the somatic cells and profound tissue organizational alterations.

In addition to the germ cells, indifferent gonads are composed of three different types of somatic cells. These are the proliferating coelomic epithelium, mesenchyme and mesonephric tissue. The genital ridge is covered with surface or coelomic epithelium, called the germinal epithelium, which is continuous with the mesothelium of the coelomic cavity forming the peripheral cord-like structures and the central mesenchymal tissue that vascularizes and develops as **stromal tissue** with in which specific endocrine cells condense in clusters later known as interstitial cells of Leydig. At the end of the 6th week, the sexless gonad, therefore, consists of a superficial **germinal epithelium** and somewhat loosely arranged stromal tissue or the **blastema** (Figure 8.6). As the genital ridge thickens and moves away from the mesonephros, it develops its own mesentery, known as **mesorchium** in the male and **mesovarium** in the female. This mesentery attaches the gonad to the body wall.

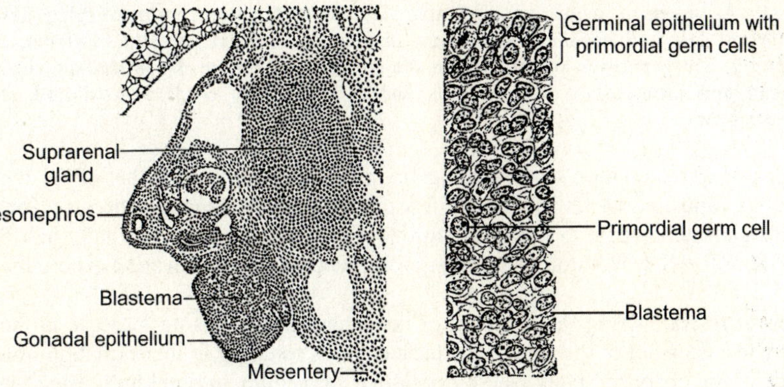

Figure 8.6: Transverse section of Human embryo at 12-mm stage to show primordial germ cells and blastema in indifferent gonad.

The coelomic epithelium initially becomes cuboidal, and later when the testis shows a rapid increase in volume it becomes flattened. The thickened coelomic epithelium that covers the genital ridge is separated from underlying mesenchyme by a basement membrane which soon disappears and cells are actively proliferated from the epithelial surface into the underlying mesenchyme (Figure 8.7 A and B). This finally results in the formation of a gonadal blastema containing gonocytes. It is constructed from mesenchyme and proliferation from the coelomic epithelium. The basement membrane reappears around 6th week and germ cells are incorporated into the epithelial layer. This structure, which has bisexual potential, is termed as **gonad** (Figure 8.7 C). It can potentially differentiate into a male or female system, thus having **embryonic bisexuality**.

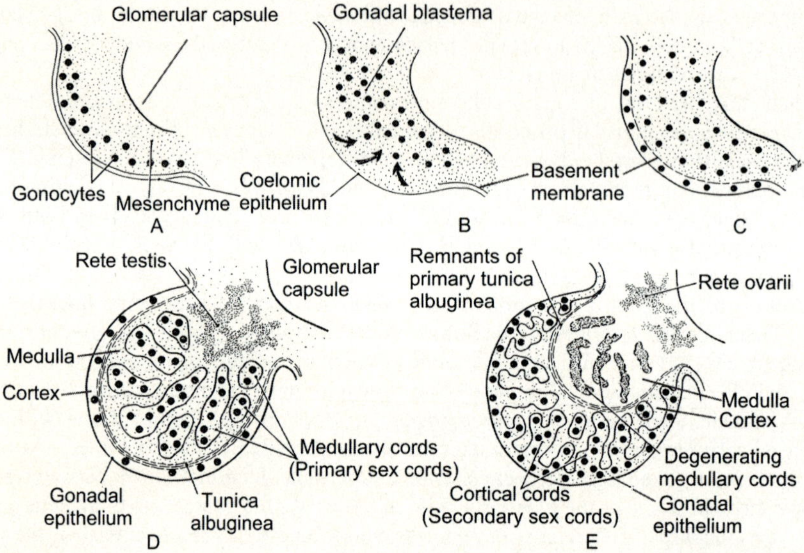

Figure 8.7: Embryogenesis of Mammalian gonad from indifferent stage (A, B, C) to the development of testis (D) and ovary (E), A- basement membrane separates coelomic epithelium from underlying mesenchyme, B- basement membrane lost and coelomic epithelium proliferate to form gonadal blastema, C- basement membrane restored, and gonocytes are present in the gonadal epithelium, D- medullary cords arise from gonadal blastema and differentiate into a testis and E- medullary cords regress and cortical cords proliferate to form ovary.

The sexual differentiation of the male gonad in mammals precedes that of the female and the time taken for this varies from a few hours to a few days depending upon the species. Throughout this time, the female gonads continue to show the structural organization of the sexually indifferent period and the lack of Sertoli cell differentiation of testis is regarded as a sign of ovarian differentiation.

Differentiation of testes:.During the 6th week of development, there is an increase in the size of the gonadal tissue and a decrease in the size of the mesonephros resulting in the formation of an elongated gonad suspended from the dorsal body wall by coelomic epithelium, mesorchium. By 7th week, certain histological changes occurs which result in the features characteristic of testis but distinctive ovarian features resembling the adult organ do not appear until 4th month.

The gonad at 6-7 weeks has bisexual potencies and consists of outer **cortex** of mesenchyme and a **medulla** of sex cords, rete cords and mesenchyme. In embryos 15mm long destined to be males, gonads begin to show two characteristics that mark them as testes. i) The appearance of prominent, branched and anastomosing strands of cells known as the **sex cords** or **testis cords**, and ii) the occurrence of a layer of connective tissue sheath known as the **tunica albuginea** or **fibrous capsule** between germinal epithelium and centrally located testis cords that is in the cortex region (Figure 8.7 D). The source of formation of testicular cords is the common blastema or central gonadal blastema. It functions as a source for all sorts of testicular cells and is similar to the primary gonadal blastema. The size and distribution of gonadal blastema differ among species. Various studies indicate that the mammalian gonad remains morphologically at a sexually indifferent stage until the testicular cords and tunica albuginea differentiate in the male gonad, and the first sign of primary sex differentiation is the appearance of Sertoli cells in the fetal gonad. These cells aggregate to form testicular cords, which later on enclose the germ cells.

Germinal epithelium, including primordial germ cells invaginates deep into the medullary or center region of the genital ridge and forms **primary (medullary) sex cords**. These become continuous with **rete cords** that arise from the blastema at a deeper level (Figures 8.7 D and 8.8 A and B). In the cortex of the gonad, the cords lose contact with the coelomic epithelium. The mesenchyme in that area forms a fibrous layer, known as the **tunica albuginea**. The cells of the sex cords first incorporate primordial germ cells within their columns, which cease mitotic division, and secrete an outer basement membrane. They are then known as the **seminiferous cords,** the forerunners of the seminiferous tubules of the adult. Their peripheral ends join in looping arches. The main portion of the seminiferous cords near the tunica elongate into highly twisted tubules known as **tubuli contorti.** However, nearer the mediastinum or rete testis, they remain straight and are known as **tubuli recti** (Figure 8.8 C). The cords of cells which constitute the testis cords are originally continuous with the germinal epithelium but by the end of the 7th week, a dense layer of fibrous tissue separates the cords from the germinal epithelium. The germinal epithelium loses the primordial cells, which apparently pass into the testis cords and regresses, becoming identical to other coelomic epithelium, and with its associated mesenchyme become distinct tunica albuginea. Cortical or secondary cords may begin to form in the human testes and in certain other species but such proliferation are normally abortive. The disappearance of the surface epithelium with its primordial germ cells removes all potentiality for cortical development. During maturation of testis, the cords of differentiating testis are changed into seminiferous tubule consisting of germ cells and Sertoli cells.

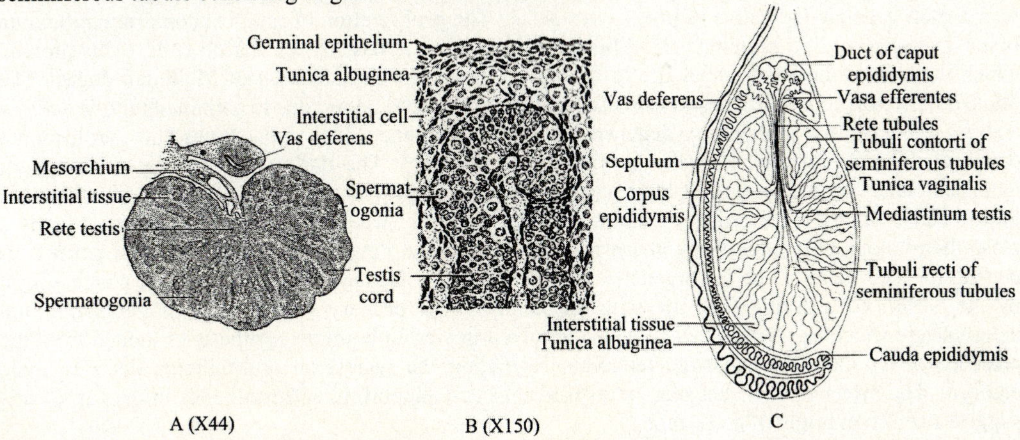

Figure 8.8: Advancing differentiation of Human testis, A and B are transverse sections at fourteen weeks, and C is schematic representation of adult testis.

The mesenchymal cells originate into the connective tissue fragments of testis and form testis lobules. The 200 lobules of the testis, each containing 3-4 seminiferous tubules derived from a primitive testis cords become isolated by partitions called **septula**. The septula form the framework of mesenchymal connective tissue. They extend to the tunica albuginea at the periphery and to the mediastinum testis in the interior (where the rete tubules lie). The septula divide the testis into **lobules**. Certain inter-tubular mesenchymal cells specialize into large pale elements lying between the seminiferous tubules and are designated as the **interstitial cells** (Figure 8.8). It is now well established that the interstitial cells differentiate from the fibroblast-like stromal cells. They are the precursors for **Leydig cells** and various **other interstitial cells**. The **Myoid** cells containing the microfilament typical of smooth muscle cells originate from mesenchymal precursor cells, which contain desmin and vimentin and then develop actin in increasing amounts. These cells organize into a continuous sheet in which adherent junctions connect the cells. In their distribution and organization, the myoid cells show variations in different regions of the testis. The myoid cells responding to androgens are believed to participate interactively in the histological and biochemical differentiation of Sertoli cells.

By the 5th month, the interstitial cells form a large portion of the gonad i.e. a greater proportion than that exists at any subsequent time in an individual's life. Various changes in the structural organization of interstitial Leydig cells during differentiation and maturation of mammalian testis are closely indicative of some changes in their function involving steroid hormone synthesis. The morphological and ultra structural differentiation of the fetal Leydig cells as well as their gonadotropin responsiveness is closely related with steroidogenic activity. Various enzyme systems related to steroid hormone synthesis are closely demonstrated histochemically in the Leydig cells of fetal and postnatal testes. However, at birth, interstitial cells are reduced to small clusters of cells due to atrophy that occurs during the later part of fetal life. In the pubertal years they again increase in number.

The steroidogenic activity appears earlier in the testis than in the ovary during embryogenesis of the reproductive organs.

Of the two populations of cells within the early testis cords, the primordial germ cells give rise to **spermatozoa,** while the mesodermal cord cells or somatic elements now known as the **sustentacular cells**, give rise to **Sertoli cells**. After the Sertoli cells are formed from the somatic cells of the developing gonad, they undergo morphological, chemical and metabolic changes during the fetal and postnatal development of mammalian testis. These changes are related to the establishment and support of specific compartment in which spermatogenesis can occur. All the developing cytological features of fetal Sertoli cells are indicative of protein synthesis. The proliferation of rough endoplasmic reticulum is for the secretion of a protein, **anti –Mullerian hormone (AMH)** by the Sertoli cells. This protein, which is secreted during the fetal life of the male, causes the degeneration of Mullerian ducts. The number of Sertoli cells continues to increase throughout the fetal period due to continual mitotic activity and are generally not affected by degeneration. But the human fetal testis during the fourth month develops dark staining Sertoli cells besides the light ones. The dark cells showing shrinkage of cytoplasm and unequal folding of their nuclear envelope appear to present the degenerative forms of Sertoli cells. Such Sertoli cells are present until the end of 27 weeks. These cells develop gradually a close morphological relationship with germ cells during fetal development indicating that germ cells depend for their nutrients on the organelles rich Sertoli cells. Degenerated germ cells are phagocytized by the Sertoli cells during fetal life with the help of their primary lysosomes, and autophagic and heterophagic vacuoles. Sertoli cells are also involved in steroid hormone synthesis as judged from the presence of agranular endoplasmic reticulum regulating the regression of Mullerian ducts in male embryo. The direct contacts between interstitial cells and supporting or Sertoli cells in the early testis suggest a common origin of these cells.

Gonadotropins (FSH and LH) and steroid hormones (especially androgens) play a key role in Sertoli cell development and function. Insulin, insulin-like growth factor, glucagon, and calcitonin are also known to play some important roles in the regulation of Sertoli cell structure and function. FSH binds specifically to Sertoli cells rather than to Leydig cells and also increases cAMP formation in Sertoli cell and not in Leydig cell preparations. LH however does not show this effect. Besides FSH, androgens also affect the metabolism of Sertoli cells.

Primordial germ cells or gonocytes remain small in number until the onset of puberty after which they begin to proliferate and produce spermatogonia in large numbers. The primary sex cords also get canalized at the time of puberty when their central cavities unite with the rete cord cavities.

When the testicular cords differentiate, the developing testis gets well vascularized with capillaries of variable diameter, confined to the mesenchyme and interstitium. Capillaries grow between the arches of the testicular cords. The blood vessel in the developing tunica albuginea show conspicuous development soon after the sex of the gonad is differentiated. Most peripheral capillaries lie below the gonadal surface. The coelomic epithelium, primitive cords, and the testicular cords themselves are not vascularized, but the blood capillaries characterize the blastema proper that has differentiated into testicular cord like structures and interstitium. The overlapping of vascular area and the area of its testicular cord like structures and interstitium in the embryonic testis is indicative of some regulatory relationship between its vascular pattern and differentiation of gonadal blastema in the Pig. An extra cellular space of varying width generally separates interstitial cells from the capillaries. However, the vascular wall in most blood vessels of the fetal testicular interstitium consist of one layer of endothelial cells which are connected to each other by adherent junctions. The permeability of the blood vessel wall as well as of their basement membrane permits transport of hormones and nutrients between the blood and testicular tissues. Some mesenchymal cells in the vicinity of blood vessels elongate and develop smooth muscle myosin. The testicular cords seem to differentiate first in the periphery where the vascularization develops first. The precise role of vascularization in differentiation of testicular components remains to be determined, but the blood vessels remain in the interstitium and do not invade the cords at any phase.

Soon after gonadal sex differentiation, the testis starts producing two types of hormones, steroid hormone and anti-Mullerian hormone (AMH). By producing androgens, fetal testis regulates the growth and differentiation of the internal and external genital organs, whereas regression of Mullerian ducts is regulated by AMH (Figure 8.9). Also, androgens play an important role in priming the brain tissue in the male direction. Any defect in genes involved in the expression of enzymes related to production of androgens can lead to abnormalities in the development of male reproductive system and brain. Testosterone is the main steroid hormone produced by the fetal testis. Its synthesis starts shortly after testicular differentiation or at about the time of Leydig cell differentiation. Steroidogenic capacity of fetal Leydig cells is higher than that of the adult cells and this can be attributed to the absence of many of the negative influences. The development and differentiation and maintenance of fetal Leydig cells in the testis of different mammalian species depend upon LH or chorionic gonadotropin. LH acts on the Leydig cell, which is the only testicular cell that binds labeled LH specifically, and causes a rapid increase in cAMP production in Leydig cells, resulting in an increase in androgen production.

Differentiation of the ovary: Whilst the male gonad shows these marked changes in organization, the female gonad continues to appear indifferent. This gland does not exhibit any distinctive ovarian features until several weeks after the gonad of the male has differentiated as a testis. The indifferent gonad can only be recognized as a potential ovary by the absence of development of the seminiferous cords and the lack of Sertoli cell differentiation.

In the 8th week, the gonadal blastema begins to show clusters of small indifferent cells and one or more primordial germ cells. Soon, a denser **primary cortex** beneath the germinal epithelium may be distinguished from the internal, looser **primary medulla** (Figures 8.7 E and 8.10). In addition, a compact cellular mass bulges from the medulla into the mesovarium to form the **rete ovarii**, a homologue of the rete testis. At this stage, neither epithelial cords nor tunica albuginea are developed as in the testis. In the 3rd month, like the testis the ovary gains a mesentery, called the **mesovarium** and settles to a more caudal position. At about 4 months, two important changes take place. 1) The ovary enlarges rapidly, due to deposition of a definitive cortex upon the original blastemal mass. This is the **secondary cortex**. It arises by the division of primordial germ cells and other cells of the superficial blastema already present, and also through the renewal of proliferation by the germinal epithelium. 2)

Ingrowth of connective tissue accompanied by blood vessels from the region of the rete ovarii. This produces supporting structures similar to the septula and mediastinum of the testis. The septula isolate the cortical substance into cord like masses (sometimes referred as **Pfluger's tubules**) (Figure 8.10). During the seventh month, septula spread out at the periphery of the ovary, forming a connective tissue layer called **tunica albuginea.** The primordial germ cells continue to proliferate mitotically, and the primitive sex cords of the developing ovary get replaced by a vascular fibrous stroma. This gives rise to a permanent **medulla**. Thus, the first generation of cords, called medullary or primary cords developed from a cellular blastema of mesonephric origin, degenerate and disappear shortly after their formation, instead, a second generation of cords, derived from the coelomic epithelium and giving rise to follicles then arises in the more cortical regions of the gonad, called the **cortical cords** or **secondary sex cords**. This is possible since there is no development of a dense fibrous connective tissue capsule isolating the germinal epithelium of the ovary. Thus, an ovarian cortex richly populated with germ cells and a medulla consisting mainly of mesonephric cells are thereby formed. The cord cells are somatic elements which give rise to granulosa or follicular cells of the follicle, while the germ cells which by now ceases their mitotic proliferation, give rise to **oogonia**.

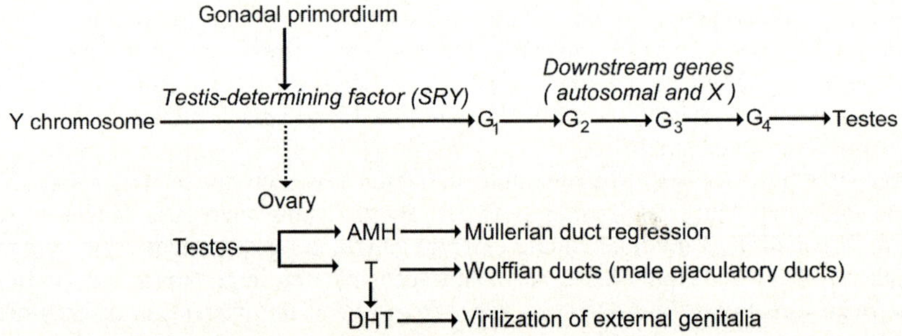

Figure 8.9: Diagrammatic representation of the cascade of genes involved in determination of testes and hormones involved in male sex differentiation.

The embryonic ovary after its sexual differentiation does not appear to receive more primordial germ cells. Those placed in the sexually differentiated ovary divide mitotically to form numerous germ cells, now called oogonia. The rate of mitosis during the time preceding meiosis shows species variation. Meiosis generally begins shortly after sex differentiation. The cells, which immediately surround the germ cells or oogonia in the ovarian cords, are called **pregranulosa cells**. After the formation of follicles, these are called **granulosa cells**. Pregranulosa cells form a close association with the germ cells. Stromal cells extending from ovarian medulla separate the germ cells and pregranulosa cells grouped in cords earlier, into individual primordial follicles. The formation of primordial follicles first starts in the ovarian cords of deeper cortical regions where oocyte first reach diplonema. During ovarian maturation, **folliculogenesis** (process of formation of follicles) spreads towards the surface. Species differences are seen in the initiation of folliculogenesis and this may be due to the time difference in the production of hormones by the pituitary and ovary.

The neighboring cells of germinal epithelium origin surround the primordial germ cells (young cortical oogonia) entrapped in the cortical cords. This initiates the formation of **primordial follicles**, a characteristic of the ovary in the later fetal months and even after birth. In these follicles, the cord cells secrete an outer basement membrane called the **membrana propria**. Follicular cells and Sertoli cells are homologous to each other since they originate from the somatic elements within the cortical and medullary cords respectively. The interstitial cells of the ovary and thecal layer of follicles arise from inter-tubular components. The earlier germ cells present in the primary medulla regress and are replaced by a **vascular fibrous stroma** to form the permanent **medulla** of the ovary (Figure 8.10).

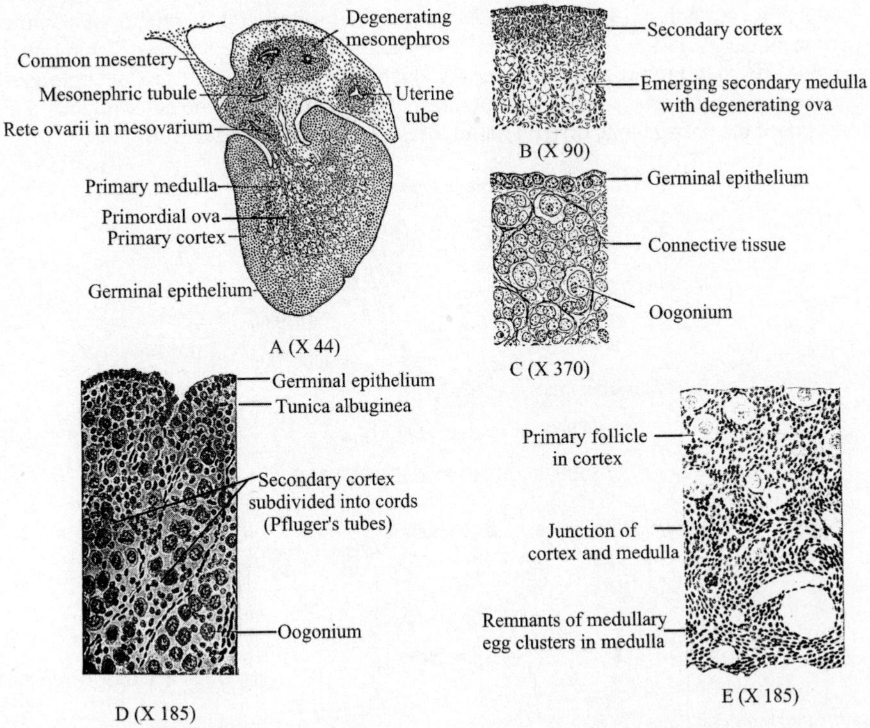

Figure 8.10: Transverse sections of Human embryo showing differentiation of ovary, A-general organization of structures at 3 months, structural details of cortex- B at 14 weeks, C at 4 months, D at 6 months and E-junction of cortex and medulla at 8 months.

8.2 Development of genital ducts and accessory glands of reproduction

Like the gonads, the duct system also passes through an undifferentiated stage. However, unlike gonad the fetus possesses the basic duct system for both sexes (Figure 8.11) and it is only with continued development that one system gains ascendancy and become definitive while the other regresses and can be demonstrated only as vestigial remnants.

During undifferentiated stages (15mm), two ducts appear on either side of mid ventral line. These run backwards and are known as **pronephric duct**, which drain the pronephros. This pronephros disappears in higher vertebrates and instead **mesonephric duct** draining the **mesonephros** is present. This is functional only in the embryonic stage and afterwards it disappears leaving the mesonephric ducts. Therefore, of the potential genital ducts, the first to be observed is the **mesonephric duct** also called **Wolffian duct** and associated **mesonephric tubules**. The mesonephros begins its degeneration as the gonad starts developing and the degeneration is almost complete shortly after the gonad begins to differentiate sexually. As the mesonephros degenerates, its tubules are liberated for possible use by the developing gonad. The testis is the only organ that forms a functional connection with the mesonephric tubules and the duct. Details of this development are given in Figure 8.12

The **paramesonephric duct or Mullerian duct** is observed at 37 days lateral to the cranial end of the mesonephric duct. At the caudal end, the two ducts fuse and in later stages they form a swelling at the point where they touch the urogenital sinus. This swelling is the **Mullerian tubercle**. At the caudal end of the fused mullerian ducts, the lamina of the ducts is separated by a septum that breaks down at 8th week to establish a common cavity. The cranial end of the mullerian duct retains its communication with the peritoneal cavity and forms the ostium of the uterine tube in the female. Commonly only one type of the duct persists giving rise to accessory ducts and glands while the heterologous system disappears except for unimportant vestigial structures. This regression of the heterologous duct system does not occur until the post-genetic differentiation of the gonad is well advanced.

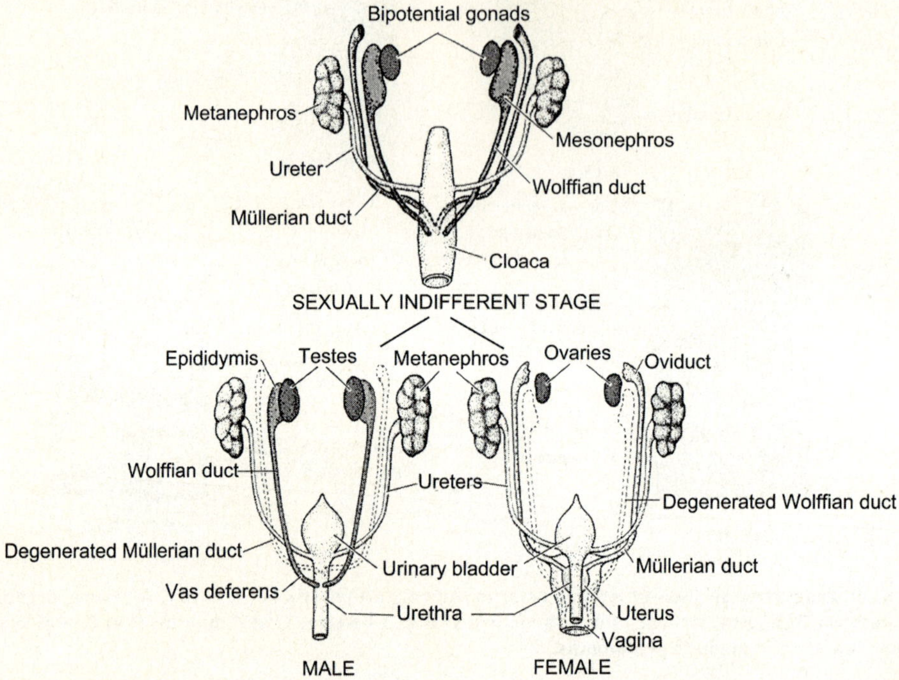

Figure 8.11: Bisexual potential of genital ducts at undifferentiated stage developing later into a male/female.

Development of the Male genital ducts and accessory glands:

As the metanephros develops and mesonephros degenerates (Figure 8.12), certain tubules of the mesonephros undergo reduction since the testis is not as large as the mesonephros. It is overlapped at the cranial and caudal ends by mesonephros and mesonephric tubules. Those tubules located opposite the rete testis unite with the rete tubules and establish a link between the seminiferous tubules and the mesonephric duct (6 months). These tubules are known as **efferent ductules of the epididymis or vasa efferentia**. The mesonephric tubules retained at the cranial end are called **ductuli aberrentes superiors** or **cranial aberrant ductules** and the ones at the caudal end are called **ductuli aberrentes inferiors** or **caudal aberrant ductules**. Some of the ductuli aberrentes inferiors are retained as **paradidymis**. These structures are vestigial and have no functional importance. The cephalic end of the mesonephric duct, which is joined by efferent ductules, undergoes extreme convolutions and becomes **ductus epididymis**. And the caudal portion extending from the epididymis to urogenital sinus remains relatively straight and becomes the **vas deferens** or **ductus deferens** and eventually gets surrounded by a muscular wall developed from the surrounding mesenchyme. The terminal end of the mesonephric duct, which joins the urogenital sinus becomes the **ejaculatory duct**. As the mesonephric duct undergoes specialization, the mullerian duct degenerates leaving two remnants. The cranial most portion is retained as **the appendix of the testis** and is located at the upper most (cephalic) tip of the testis. The terminal portion is probably represented in the adult male by a portion of **prostatic utricle** (Table 8.1).

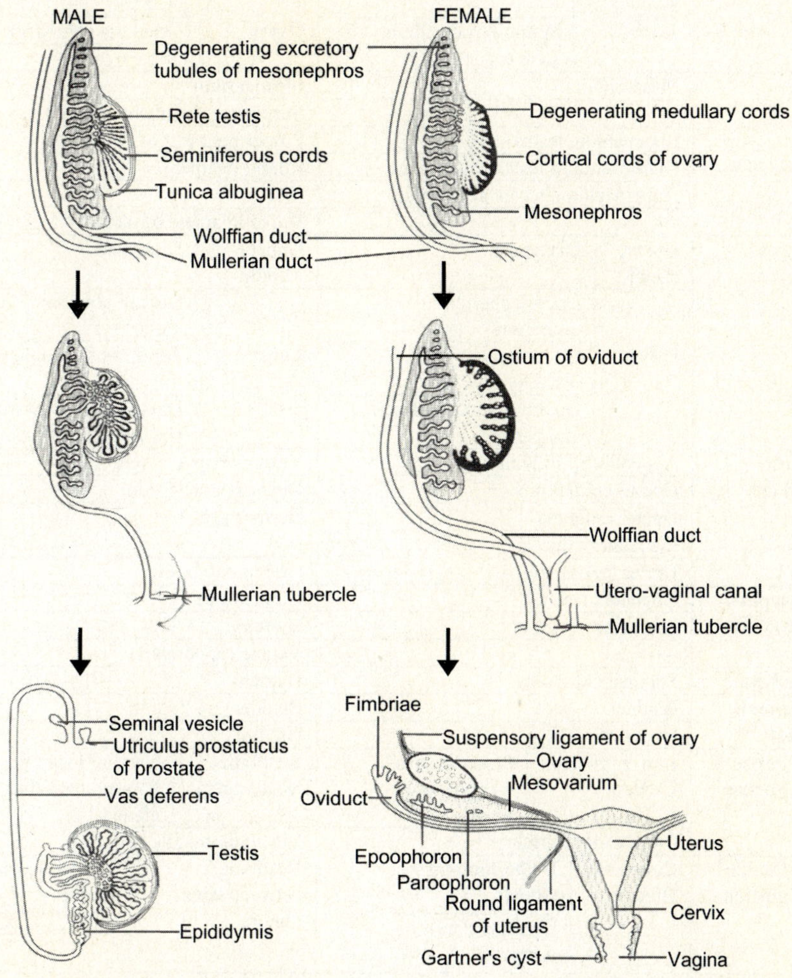

Figure 8.12: Differentiation of the genital ducts in Human male and female.

The accessory organs of the reproductive system are derived from evagination of certain segments of the urogenital tracts. These are homologous organs in both sexes although those in the male are more developed than those in the female (Figure 8.13). These glands are derived from each of the germ layers and may be classified on the basis of their origin. The glands derived from lower ductus deferens (and therefore are of mesodermal origin) are **ampullary glands** and **vesicular glands**. Those derived from the lower endodermal part of urogenital sinus are **prostate, membranous** and **penile urethra**. Those derived from proximal ends of mullerian ducts are **prostatic utricle**. And those derived from the ectoderm of prepubertal or inguinal region are **preputial** and **inguinal glands**.

Table 8.1: Developmental homologues of male and female genital systems

Indifferent stage		Male		Female	
Pronephros		Disappears		Disappears	
Gonad		Testes	----	Ovary	Cortex
			Seminiferous tubule		Medulla (primary)
			Rete testes		Rete ovarii
Genital ligaments		Mesorchium		Mesovarium	
		---		Suspensary ligament of ovary	
		Ligamentum testes		Proper ligament of ovary	
		Gubernaculum testes-caudal part		Round ligament of uterus	
		Gubernaculum testes-as a whole		---	
		---		Broad ligament of uterus	
Mesonephros Collecting Tubule		Upper, middle	Disappear	Upper, Middle	Disappear
		Lower	Ductuli aberrant Superiors	Lower	Ductuli aberrant Superiors
			Efferent ducts of Epididymis		Tubules of epoophoron
			Ductus aberrant inferior and paradidymis		Ductulus aberrant inferior and ductules of paroophoron
Mesonephric (Wolffian) duct		Appendix epididymis		Vesicular appendage	
		Ductus epididymis		Duct of epoophoron	
		Ductus deferens		Gartner's duct	
		Ejaculatory duct			
		Ureter, pelvis, etc.		Ureter, pelvis, etc.	
Paramesonephric (Mullerian) duct		Appendix testes		Uterine tube	
		Uterus musculinus		Uterus	
		---		Vagina (upper part)	
Muller's tubercle		Seminal colliculus		Hymen	
Vesico urethral primordium		Bladder		Bladder	
		Upper prostatic urethra		Urethra	
Uro-genital Sinus	Pelvic Portion	Lower prostatic Urethra	Prostatic utricle and prostate gland	Vestibule-Near vagina	Vagina (lower part), Para-urethral ducts and Urethral glands
		Membranous urethra		Vestibule-middle part	
	Phallic portion	Cavernous Urethra	Bulbo-urethral Glands	Vestibule-between labia minora	Vestibular glands of Bartholin
			Urethral glands of Littre		Lesser vestibular glands
Phallus	Glans	Penis	Glans penis	Clitoris	Glans clitoris
	Lips of urogen		Urethral surface of penis		Labia minora
	Shaft		Corpora cavernosa penis Corpus cavernosum urethra		Corpora cavernosa clitoridis and vestibular bulbs
Genital swellings		Scrotum and scrotal raphe		Labia majora, posterior commissure	

Ductus deferens may expand into **ampullary glands** before its junction with urethra. It develops an evagination caudal to the ampullary glands around 13 weeks of intrauterine life known as **seminal vesicles** (Figure 8.13). The portion of the ductus deferens lying between the diverticulum and the union of the ductus deferens and urogenital sinus becomes the **ejaculatory duct**. The **prostate** arises from the endodermal part of male urethra. These outgrowths, which arise from the urethra near the opening of the prostatic utricle, form five lobes, which are named according to their relation to the urethra. These are **dorsal prostate**, **ventral prostate**, and **ventro-lateral prostates** (or **coagulating gland**). The **bulbourethral or Cowper's glands** arise as evagination of the proximal end of the penile urethra. These are endodermal in origin. The **urethral glands of Littre** arise as multiple and simple outgrowths from the epithelial lining throughout the length of the urethra.

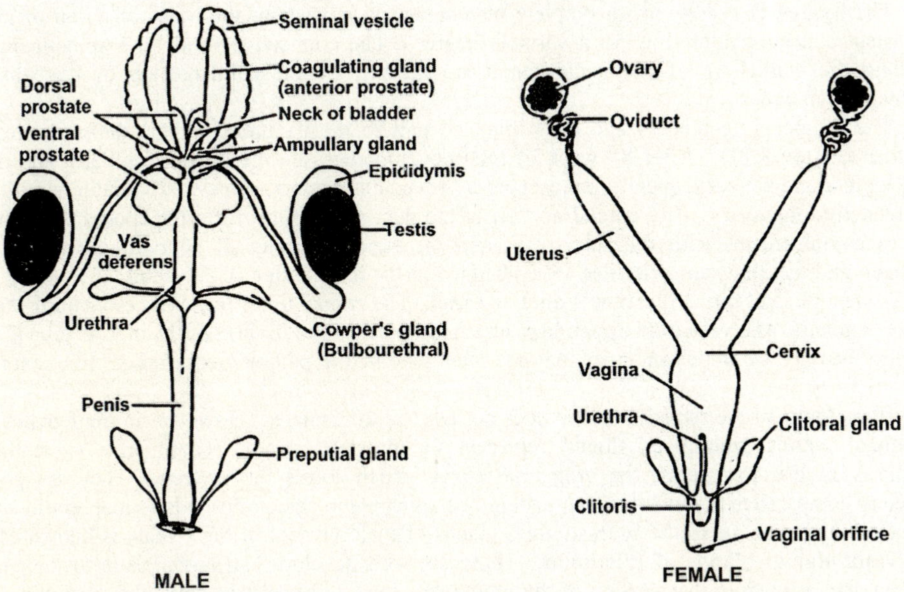

Figure 8.13: Reproductive systems of adult male and female Rat.

Development of female genital ducts and accessory glands: As indicated above, the mullerian or paramesonephric duct appears in embryo of approximately 37 days. This duct is destined to form virtually the entire reproductive tract of the female whereas the mesonephros or Wolffian duct and associated mesonephric tubules remain only as scattered vestiges. The paramesonephric duct lies lateral and parallel to mesonephric duct throughout most of its course (Figures 8.11 and 12). At its caudal extremity it crosses the mesonephric duct ventrally and fuses with the duct of the opposite side in the mid-line (undifferentiated stage) (Figure 8.12). As the mesonephros completes its degeneration leaving only the ducts and tubules as indication of its former position, the fold of peritoneum, which suspended it from the dorsal body, becomes the **mesosalpinx**. This contains the enlarging **paramesonephric duct** or **uterine tube** and degenerated mesonephric duct or tubules. The communication of the cranial end of the mullerian duct with the coelom is retained as the ostium of the uterine tube. The caudal ends of the paramesonephric ducts get fused and form a single cavity, the **utero-vaginal canal** (10th week), the blind end of which projects on the posterior wall of the **urogenital sinus** where it forms a swelling, the **mullerian tubercle** (Figure 8.12).

Mass of the cells laid down between urogenital sinus and utero-vaginal canal occurs in a cranio-caudal direction and is completed by 5th month. The unfused portions of the paramesonephric ducts form the uterine tubes, known as **oviducts** or **fallopian tubes**, whereas the fused portions of the ducts give rise to the **uterus** and four-fifths of the **vagina**. Separation of uterus and vagina is not well marked until 5th month, though uterus is marked little earlier due to its slightly thicker wall. The uterus is divided into a larger caudal portion, the **cervix** and a **smaller fundic** portion at the junction of the **uterine horns** (Figure 8.13). The fundus remains relatively small until puberty. During the last trimester, when it gains the adult condition, the epithelium of the uterine lumen and adjacent mesenchyme become the endometrium. By birth, it develops characteristic yet small uterine glands.

The uterine tube or oviducts become coiled and acquire differentiated epithelia and fimbriae. Just before birth, signs of epithelium differentiation include increased mucosal height, pseudostratification, and presence of peg cells and evidence of secretory activity.

The **hymen** is usually an incomplete membrane. It persists at the point of union of utero-vaginal canal and urogenital sinus to a variable degree. The connective tissue and smooth muscle surrounding the epithelium of the genital tract are derived by the condensation of the adjacent mesenchyme (6 months).

The mesonephric tubules and ducts play no part in the formation of the definitive female genital tract (Figure 8.12). After 8th week of fetal development, the mesonephric tubules and ducts begin to regress and are subsequently represented by several structures, somewhat variable in size and closely related to the ovary. The cranial portion of the duct and tubules form the epoophoron, which sometimes communicates with the rete ovarii and the superior group of aberrant ductules. The **epoophoron** and the **aberrant ductules** are embedded in the mesovarion of the adult. The lower part of the mesonephric duct forms **Gartner's duct or canal**. The cranial tip of the paramesonephric duct is present occasionally as a **vesicular appendage** attached to one of the fimbria of the uterine tube (Table 8.1). These vestiges are important since they are often involved in pathological changes like **cysts** and **tumors.**

Homologue of the seminal vesicle does not exist in the female. However, in the females, the **paraurethral glands (glands of skene**) represent the prostate gland. These arise as epithelial diverticula from that portion of the urogenital sinus, which forms the urethra. They are poorly developed as compared to the prostates but undergo enlargement in cases of pseudohermaphroditism. A pair of glands homologous to the bulbourethral glands of male present in the female is known as the **greater vestibular** or **glands of Bartholin**. These are well developed in comparison to their male homologue, and arise from that portion of the urogenital sinus destined to become the vestibule. The lesser vestibular glands are diverticula's from the anterior portion of the vestibule hence considered to be homologous to the glands of Littre of the male.

8.3 Development of External genitalia

The primordia of the external genitalia, unlike those of the internal genitalia are bipotential (Figure 8.14). In the female, the urinary and the genital openings remain separate while in the male, there is only one opening for both and is called the urogenital opening.

At the end of the 5th week (8mm in size) a conical **genital tubercle** is present in midline on ventral side between umbilical cord and tail. It bears a shallow **urogenital groove** whose sidewalls are slightly elevated and known as **urogenital folds**. During 7th week, genital tubercle elongates into a somewhat cylindrical phallus. Lateral to the base of the phallus a rounded ridge makes its appearance on each side known as the genital swellings (to be later designated as labial or scrotal swellings). From this indifferent stage, the external organs of male and female are formed in later weeks.

During 8th week, the sex of an embryo begins to be grossly indicated by certain characters chief among which are erectness of phallus, length of urethral groove and relation of urogenital folds to genital swellings. At three months, the external genitalia show changes recognizable as distinctively male or female (Figure 8.14).

External Genitalia in Male: At 10 weeks, genital swellings become the **scrotum**. The two-scrotal sacs are separated by a **scrotal septum** marked superficially by **scrotal raphe**. Phallus and urethral folds becomes **penis** enclosing the urethra (Figure 8.14). The genital tubercle forms the tip of the penis or **glans penis** and the two urethral folds fuse giving rise to the **shaft** or **body** of the penis.

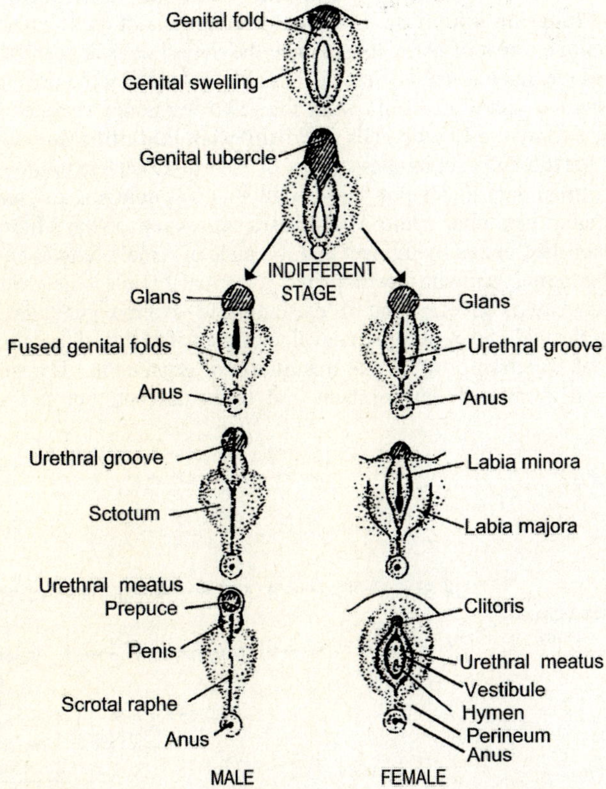

Figure 8.14: Development of external genitalia in Human male and female from an indifferent stage.

External Genitalia in Female: Changes to form the external genitalia are slower in females in comparison to male. The phallus lags in development and becomes the **clitoris**. The urogenital groove is shorter than that in the male, never invading the clitoris. It opens permanently to the exterior, since the floor of the groove (the urogenital membrane) ruptures and fails to reclose. After this, the combined shallow cavity is called the **vestibule** into which open both the urethra and the vagina. The urogenital folds which lie on either side of the urogenital groove becomes plate-like but do not fuse and are retained as **labia minora**. The genital swellings grow caudally and enlarge into the **labia majora** (Figure 8.14).

Thus, embryogenesis of gonad show that the testis develops predominantly from the medulla of the sexually undifferentiated gland while the ovary arises primarily from its cortex. It starts with the formation of indifferent genital ridge. The primordial germ cells arise extra-gonadally, migrate into the genital ridge and get enclosed in the sex or gonadal cords. Then under the influence of Y-chromosomal or SRY antigen, an indifferent gonad is converted into a testis, whereas its absence results in an ovary. **Genetic maleness** leads to **gonadal maleness** and the main role of the sex chromosomes in sexual determination is completed with the establishment of the fetal gonad. Male development pathway leads to the invasion of the genital ridge by mesenchymal endothelial cells from part of the degenerating mesonephros. This is the first event that begins to distinguish a testis from an 'indifferent gonad'. Then the genital ridge enlarges and gonadal cords become more pronounced first in the medullary region, may be as a result of some epithelial-stromal interaction. Some time later, identifiable Sertoli cells appear, and they secrete **Mullerian inhibiting hormone (MIH)**. In addition to its named function, it is also said to induce the mitotic arrest of germ cells. Once the Sertoli cells appear, differentiation of the Leydig cells occur around the gonadal cords. This is possibly induced by the presence of Sertoli cells. Leydig cells start testosterone secretion. Following this, two hormones secreted by the developing testis, the **androgens** secreted by the **Leydig cells**, and **Mullerian inhibiting hormone (MIH)** secreted by the **sustentacular** or **Sertoli cells** act as messengers of masculine differentiation of the ducts. The androgens induce the Wolffian duct to develop into epididymis, vas deferens and seminal vesicles, and also development of external genitalia, while MIH causes regression of the Mullerian ducts (Figure 8.15). This has been established in rats by the fact that if a male or female fetus is castrated (removal of gonad), its internal and external genitalia develop into a normal female type. Further, exposure of female fetuses to androgens causes development of 'masculinized' external genitalia, and suppression of endogenous androgens in the male fetus results in development of 'feminized' external genitalia. There is a link between postnatal secretion of MIH and maturation of germ cells. It appears that MIH may have additional effects on germ cell development and testis descent, but not on primary gonad differentiation.

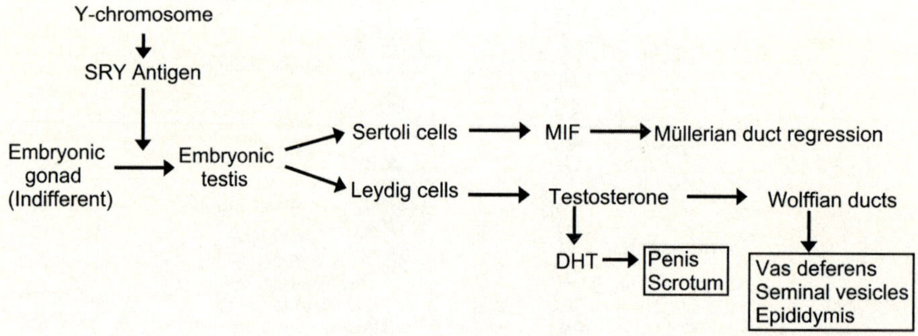

Figure 8.15: Role of Y chromosome or SRY antigen in the development and differentiation of males.

In the female 'default' pathway, there is no mesenchymal or endothelial invasion of the genital ridge. It remains small. The germ cells enter mitosis, then meiosis, and then they are arrested in prophase. The oocyte then induces development of follicular cells and split up the gonadal cords. Stromal invasion of the gonad and differentiation of granulosa and theca interna cells of the primordial follicle follow this.

Figure 8.16 represents a schematic sequence of sexual differentiation, indicating that testicular differentiation precedes all other forms of differentiation. Thus, the sex of an animal depends on three distinct but related phenomenon: i) inherited genes, ii) gonadogenesis, and iii) formation and maturation of accessory reproductive organs. Genes basically determine the sex of an embryo but an expression of the gametic sex is a developmental process depending upon the function of the fetal gonad and occasionally the adrenal cortex. Estrogen and androgen can cause sex reversal in male and female embryos respectively, only during a brief period early in fetal life. In contrast, the accessory reproductive organs remain sexually labile for a much longer time and hormone treatment late in development can induce considerable reversal in these structures. However, the age at which this bisexual potential is completely lost varies with the species.

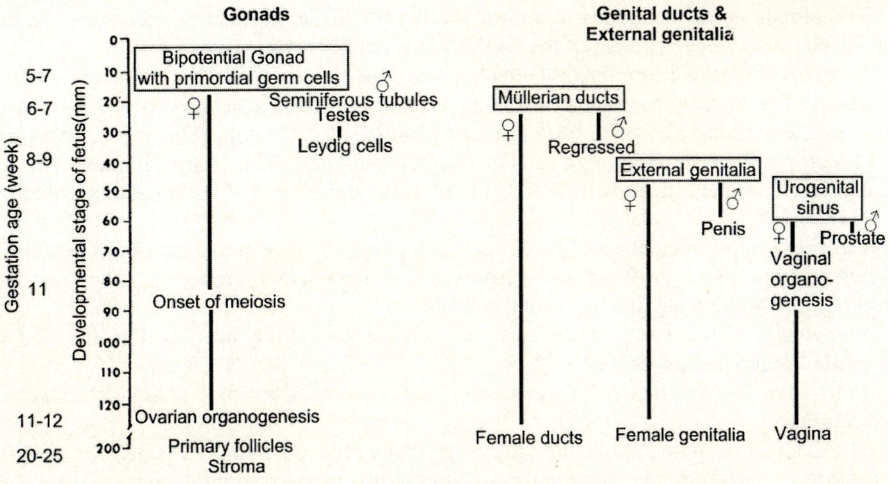

Figure 8.16: Schematic sequence of sexual differentiation in Human fetus.

Summary

Genital system consists of gonads (testes in male and ovaries in female), associated ducts and glands, and the external genitalia.

The early development of the gonad proceeds identically in both males and females and in both sexes, the gonads are derived from two distinct tissues: somatic mesenchymal, forming the matrix of the gonad and the primordial germ cells which form the gametes.

The first indication of gonadal development is the appearance of a protuberance called gonadal ridge, located medially to each mesonephros at about 3-4 weeks of intra-uterine life in human.

The gonadal ridge enlarges from the periphery to the center of the mesenchyme, forming primary sex cords upon which primordial germ cells that migrate along the dorsal mesentery are deposited. This is the indifferent stage of the bipotential gonad.

The development of the undifferentiated gonad is completed by the sixth week.

Testicular development from the indifferent gonad occurs during the seventh week, while development of ovaries starts during the sixteenth week

Testis develops from the medullary region of the indifferent gonad, and the ovary from the cortex.

Columns of coelomic epithelium penetrate into the underlying mesenchymal tissue to form the primitive sex cords. Primordial germ cells migrate and colonize these cords.

The Y-chromosomal determination of gonadal sex manifests itself only when colonization is completed during the sixth week in human embryo.

In male embryo, at this time, the primitive sex cords proliferates and organize in the medullary center of the mesenchymal mass, and establish contact with rete blastema. The cords in the cortex of gonad lose contact with the coelomic epithelium, and the mesenchyme there forms a fibrous tunica albuginea. The cells of the sex cords incorporate primordial germ cells in their columns and constitute the seminiferous cords and later seminiferous tubules of the adult testes. The enclosed primordial germ cells give rise to spermatogonia while the mesodermal cord cells, now called as sustentacular cells, give rise to Sertoli cells. The loose mesenchyme vascularizes to form stromal tissue, and the specific endocrine cells-the interstitial cells of Leydig.

The female gonad continues to appear indifferent so far and can be recognized as potential ovary by the absence of development of the seminiferous cords.

In the ovaries, the seminiferous cords become less prominent and are replaced by a vascular, fibrous stroma, thus forming permanent medulla. Instead, a second generation of cords arise in more cortical region. The primordial germ cells released from the degenerating primary sex cords, move to the cortical cords and start forming egg cells or oogonia and later, the primary follicles. The cord cell secretes an outer basement membrane, membrana propria, and gives rise to the granulosa cells of the follicle.

Development of internal genitalia of ducts and glands in male and female shows that instead of one indifferent primordium, there are two separate sets of unipotential primordia. These are Wolffian (mesonephric) and Mullerian (paramesonephric) ducts.

In males, Wolffian duct persists and gives rise to the epididymis, vas deferens, and seminal vesicles, while Mullerian ducts regress.

In females, the Wolffian ducts regress and Mullerian ducts give rise to oviducts, uterus, cervix and upper vagina.

The external genitalia, unlike the internal genitalia are bipotential. In males, the urethral folds fuse to enclose the urethral tube, the genital swellings fuse in the midline to form scrotum, and the genital tubercle expand to form the penis. In females, the urethral folds and genital swellings remain separate and form labia minora and majora, while genital tubercle diminishes to form the clitoris.

The development of fetal gonad into testis or ovary is dependent on chromosomal sex, but after that, hormones of the fetal testis, androgens and MIH directs the development of internal and external genitalia.

Questions

1. Describe the development of testis from indifferent stage.
2. Describe the development of ovary from indifferent stage.
3. Describe the development of genital ducts and accessory sex glands in male and female.
4. Describe the development of external genitalia in male and female.
5. Describe the role of hormones in differentiation of the gonads, the mesonephric ducts, the paramesonephric ducts and the external genitalia.
6. The male homologue of the female clitoris is **a) the penis**, b) the scrotum, c) the penile urethra, d) the testis.
7. The sex of a child is determined by a) the sex chromosome contained in the oocyte, **b) the sex chromosome contained in the sperm**, c) the number of sperm fertilizing the oocyte, d) position of fetus in the uterus.

Chapter 9

Biology of Sex

This chapter deals with a variety of topics that have to do, in one way or another, with sequential changes in reproductive development or function.

Modern genetics and experimental embryology made it clear that, in most species of mammals, the multiple differences between the male and the female depend primarily on a single chromosome (the Y chromosome), and a pair of endocrine structures, the testes in the male and the ovaries in the female (Table 9.1). Genetic inheritance sets the sex of the individual, known as **sex determination** and is established at the time of fertilization. This is followed by **sex differentiation**, which involves the multiple processes resulting in the development of reproductive system in the fetus. The developing and differentiating mammalian testis and ovary undergo a long series of successive morphological, histochemical, biochemical and physiological changes during the embryonic, prenatal, postnatal and prepubertal periods to become structurally and functionally mature for the cyclic production of gametes and steroidal and non-steroidal substances. However, in mammals, sex is not influenced by environmental factors.

Table 9.1: Major differences between a male and a female

Character	Male	Female
Sex Chromatin	XY	XX
Gonad	Testis	Ovary
Hormones	Testosterone	Estrogen and Progesterone
Puberty	Spermatogenesis cannot be induced	Ovulation can be induced
Gametes number and formation during reproductive phase in life	Number of sperms not fixed. Therefore, spermatogenesis continues throughout life	Number of oocyte fixed. Therefore, menopause occurs
Pattern of hormone secretion	Acyclic	Cyclic

9.1 Sex Determination

Sex is determined genetically by inheritance of two chromosomes called the **sex chromosomes**. Besides this one pair of chromosomes, the remaining pairs are called **somatic chromosomes** or **autosomes**. In humans and many other mammals, the sex chromosomes are the X and the Y-chromosomes. The larger is the X chromosome and the smaller is the Y chromosome. **Males** possess one X and one Y (**XY pattern**) whereas **females** have two X- chromosomes (**XX pattern**). Thus, the genetic difference between male and female is simply the difference in one chromosome. This results in the development of various distinguishing characters between males and females, such as gonads, external genitalia, body size, behavior etc., since the chromosomal and gonadal sex is mirrored by the phenotypic sex. The sex determining genes located on the sex chromosomes of the embryo play an important role in the differentiation and transformation of the embryonic gonad into a testis or ovary, depending upon the genetic sex of the individual. Thus, during the process of formation of gametes (**gametogenesis**) as a consequence of meiosis, each normal ovum contains a single X chromosome, but half the normal sperms contain an X chromosome and half Y chromosome. When a sperm containing a Y chromosome fertilizes an ovum, a XY pattern results and the zygote develops into a **genetic male**. When fertilization occurs with an X containing sperm, a XX pattern and a **genetic female** result. Interestingly, however, the sex ratios at birth are not exactly 1:1 but, for unclear reasons, there tends to be a slight preponderance of male births.

9.2 Human Chromosomes

Human chromosomes can be studied by the following technique: Human cells are grown in tissue culture and are treated with drug colchicines (which arrests mitosis at the metaphase). They are exposed to a hypotonic solution that makes the chromosomes swell and disperse. Then the chromosomes are "squashed" on to the slide. With the help of fluorescent and other staining techniques, individual chromosomes can be identified and studied in detail.

There are 46 chromosomes in humans-22 pairs of autosomes and one pair of sex chromosomes, which may be an X, and Y chromosome in case of males or two X-chromosomes in females. Autosomes provide the genetic information for the development and differentiation of most of the cells in the body. And the sex chromosomes provide the genetic information that directs the differentiation of gonadal cells into ovaries or testes. The individual chromosomes are usually arranged in an arbitrary pattern called **karyotype**. Figure 9.1 gives the karyotype of human female (homogametic) and male (heterogametic). On the basis of their morphological characteristics, the numbers 1-22 identifies individual autosome pairs. In the sex chromosome pair, human Y chromosome is smaller than the X chromosome and the sperms containing the Y chromosome are lighter and able to "swim" faster up the female genital tract, thus reaching the ovum more rapidly. This may account for the fact that the number of males born is slightly greater than the number of females. Visualization of all the chromosomes in a karyotype technique is also important in revealing a group of genetic sex abnormalities characterized by unusual chromosomal combinations such as 45-XO (**Turner's syndrome**), 47-XXY (**Klinefelter's syndrome**), 48-XXXY and 49-XXXXY. The end result of such combinations is usually the failure of normal anatomical and functional sexual development.

9.3 Sex Chromatin

An easy method, known as the **Barr** or **sex chromatin** test exists for determining whether a person's cells contain two X-chromosomes, i.e. the normal female pattern or not. When two X-chromosomes are present, only one function, and the non-functional X chromosome condenses to form a nuclear mass called **sex chromatin**. In normal cells, the inactive X chromosome condensation can be seen in various types of cells, usually on the inner surface of nuclear membrane (also called Barr body). Thus, there is a **Barr body** for each X chromosome in excess of one in the cell (Figure 9.2). The single X chromosome in male cells rarely condenses to form sex chromatin or Barr body. The Barr test is now widely used in analyzing sex abnormalities in man. This is readily observable with a light microscope. Leukocytes, skin biopsies, exfoliate cells from the vagina, or scrapings from oral or nasal epithelia, all provide readily available material for execution of the test. The genetic sex of very young embryos can be determined long before this would be possible by studying histology of the gonad. The sex chromatin is even present in the gonocytes, or primordial germ cells even before they reach the gonadal primordia. The choice of which X chromosome remains active is random, so normally one X chromosome remains active in approximately half of the cells and the other X chromosome is active in the other half. The selection persists through subsequent divisions of these cells, and consequently some of the somatic cells in adult female contain an active X chromosome of maternal origin and some contain an active X chromosome of paternal origin.

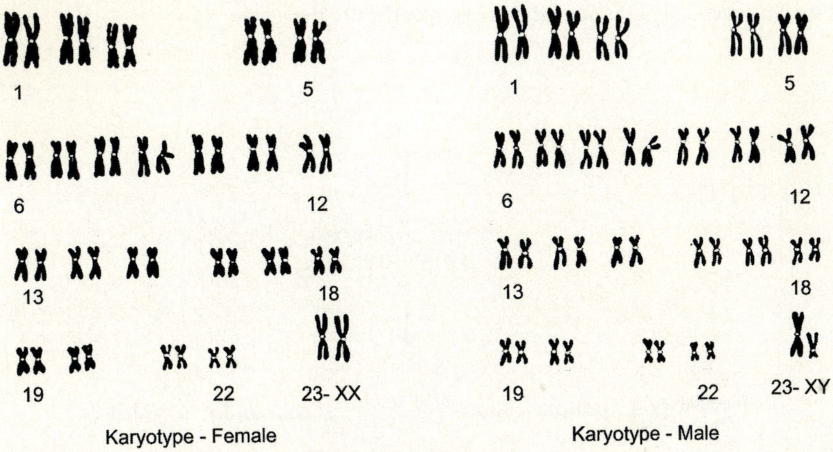

Figure 9.1: Karyotype of Human female (homogametic) and male (heterogametic).

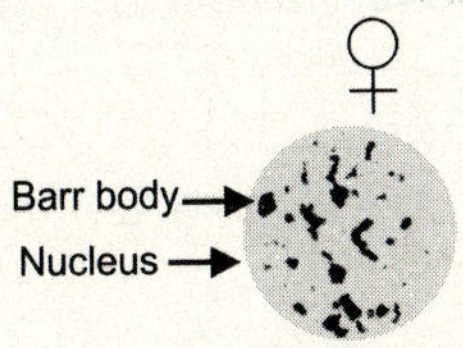

Figure 9.2: X Chromatin (Barr body) in the nucleus of buccal mucosal cell of a normal Human female.

9.4 Sex Differentiation

It is surprising to note that embryos of both sexes, male and female are identical during the first six weeks of life inspite of the fact that the genetic sex is fixed at the time of fertilization. This is because the sex determining mechanism established at fertilization directs and controls all the later ontogenic processes involved in male and female differentiation. Both male and female potentialities exist in every embryo. Most individuals differentiate in accordance with their chromosomal sex, but all degrees of expression of the genetic sex occur. Furthermore, individuals may differentiate toward the sex contrary to chromosomal sex, resulting in intersexuality if a genetic male have testes and female internal genitalia (vagina and uterus). Such people are termed male pseudohermaphrodites. Genetic sex is unalterably fixed at fertilization but factors such as evacuators, hormones, temperature extremes, and probably other agents influence phenotypic sex differentiation.

Sexual differentiation, like the differentiation of the systems, proceeds in steps: **Chromosomal** or **genetic** or **genotypic sex** is determined at fertilization. The genetic information contributed to the zygote determines whether the primitive/indifferent gonad will differentiate into testes or ovaries. This constitutes the **gonadal sex** of the individual. The establishment of gonadal sex is followed by differentiation of the Mullerian or Wolffian duct system into female or male accessory genitalia respectively. Secondary sex characteristics, and endocrine profiles constitute the **phenotypic**

sex of the individual. The final step is the establishment of the **somatic** and **psychic sex** with the characteristics of male/female sex characteristics and behavior (Figure 9.3). It is important to remember here one essential generalization that the genes directly determine only whether the individual will have testes or ovaries. All the rest of sex differentiation depends upon the presence or absence of substances produced by the genetically determined gonads, specifically the testes.

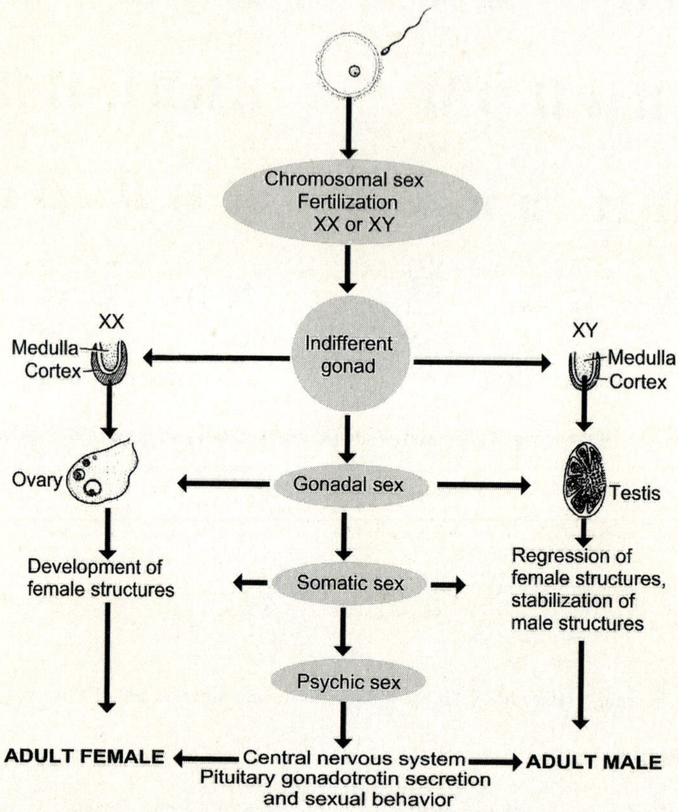

Figure 9.3: Four consecutive steps of sexual differentiation.

The primitive gonad has all the cellular elements to give origin to a testicle or ovary. The differentiation of sexual characteristics depends upon the relationship between male and female determining genes and their interaction with the internal environment. Genes associated with female characteristics are located on the X chromosomes. Homologous (XX) chromosomes appear to be necessary for differentiation of the normal ovary. In Turner's syndrome, XO, the adult gonad is an elongated mass of connective tissue. Genes for male development are located on autosomes and on the Y chromosome. The Y chromosome or some X-Y interaction is responsible for the differentiation of the testes. In man, individuals with 45, XO syndrome is a female, whereas those with 46,XY; 47,XXY; 48,XXXY and 49, XXXXY are all males. Normally, the female being homozygous for X has an abundance of female determining genes and develops as a female. Conversely, in the male, genes for masculinity on the autosomes and Y-chromosomes predominate over the female determining genes in the single X chromosome, and thus male characters differentiate. The Y chromosome bears factors, which determine the morphological differentiation of the testes, but its presence does not guarantee normal testicular development and its functioning either in the fetus or in the adult. Despite the male determining side of the Y chromosome in mammals, a gene in the X chromosome appears to be necessary for testosterone secretion. The genes directly determine only whether the individual will have testes or ovaries; virtually all the rest of sexual differentiation depends upon this genetically determined gonad.

9.5 Theories of sexual differentiation

Various theories have been proposed by many scientists to explain sex differentiation. These are given one by one.

Hormone theory: Lillie has proposed Hormone theory in 1957. Based on **freemartin** studies, Lillie proposed that certain aspects of development of the genital system are actually brought about by sex hormones. Freemartin is a genetic female, which is associated, *in utero* with a male co-twin and has been modified, in the male direction to varying degrees (Figure 9.4). Lillie proposed that partial masculinization of external and internal sex organs of the female partner (freemartin) are the result of the effect of humoral factors transmitted by blood exchange with the male twin. The condition results only in those cases where there is an early fusion of the two placentae and a consequent intermingling of blood between the two fetuses. The external genitalia of the freemartin are generally female in type but the clitoris is often enlarged. The accessory sex organs usually consist of both Wolffian and Mullerian duct derivatives. The gonads are **hypoplastic** (defective development) and may contain sterile seminal tubules with practically no cortical development; in other instances both cortical and medullary components may be present to form the equivalent of an ovotestis.

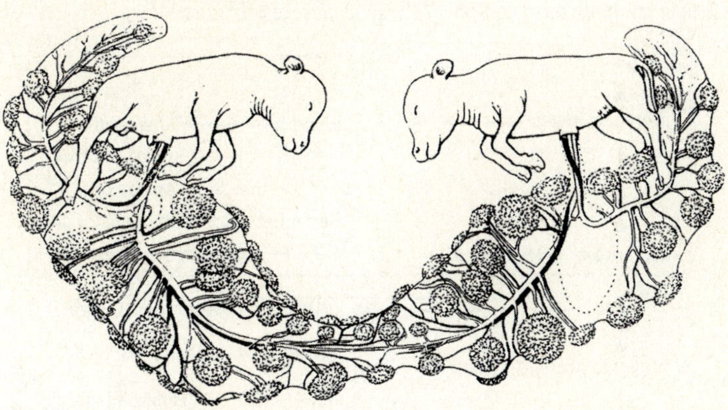

Figure 9.4: Twin Calves removed from the uterus to show chorionic fusion and anastomosis between major blood vessels, left-male twin and right-freemartin.

Masculinizing factors from the male twin enter the blood vascular system of the female co-twin and exert their influence before the development of ovary and Mullerian system have occurred in the female. Hence the sexual apparatus of the freemartin is stimulated to develop male structures. All degrees of masculinization are observed presumably due to variable amounts of male morphogenic substance reaching the reproductive system of the female co-twin. Similar anomalies have been reported in sheep, goats and pigs. Dominguez *et al* (1990) have investigated the steroid hormone correlates of ovarian alteration in bovine freemartin fetuses. The discovery of anastomosis between the twins placentas supports the production of some substances by the male twin, which are transported to the female twin via the blood circulation (Short 1970). This suggestion is further supported by the fact that the masculinization of the female co-twin is prevented after ligation of the common blood vessels.

Placental fusion may also occur in cats, rabbits, marmosets and human beings, but without resulting in any sexual anomaly. These negative findings do not necessarily invalidate the hormone theory. They do suggest that vascular anastomosis must occur at a very early age in order to modify the sexual development of the female fetus.

In many species, it is possible to remove or damage the area from which the gonads derive without interrupting the pregnancy. When this is done, regardless of the genetic sex, the gonad less embryo develops the female duct system, i.e. Mullerian ducts persist and form oviducts and uterus, whereas Wolffian ducts degenerate. This signifies that normally the presence of functioning testes represses the development of the female duct system and induces development of the male organs; in contrast, a female gonad need not be present for the female organs to develop. The primitive testes exert their effect by secreting two substances, both of which act locally. Mullerian regression factor (MRF) or Mullerian inhibiting substance (MIS) or anti-Mullerian hormone (AMH) is a protein made by Sertoli cells and causes regression of Mullerian duct; and testosterone is secreted by Leydig cells and induces differentiation of Wolffian duct into epididymis, vas deferens, seminal vesicles. It was found that bovine AMH can induce a secretion of testosterone instead of estradiol in fetal ovine ovaries. Various observations suggested the possibility that MRF or AMH may function as an autocrine factor to influence gonadal differentiation towards a testicular pathway. As Mullerian ducts and ovaries lose their responsiveness to AMH early in development, exposure to AMH is deleterious to female differentiation only in the young fetus and not later. A similar analysis holds for the later development of external genitalia, vagina, and prostate etc. In other words, absence of functioning testes, results in female development, whereas presence of testes through the inducing effects of testosterone, results in male differentiation of these structures (Figure 9.5).

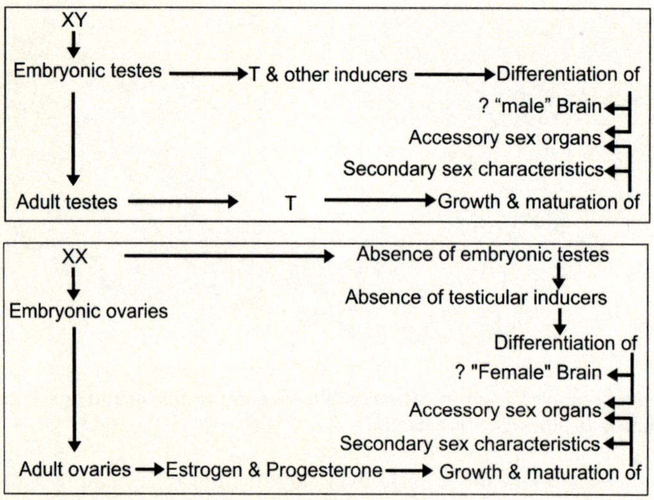

Figure 9.5: Sex organ differentiation in male and female as proposed by Lillie, T- testosterone.

Theory of Cellular Chimarism: It is the most recent theory proposed by Ohno in 1969, advanced as an explanation of freemartin in cattle. Ohno and collaborators reported presence of XX cells, possibly primordial germ cells from the freemartin lodged in the testes of male co-twin. XY cells could be transmitted by the blood in a reverse direction thus suggesting that freemartin are **chimerie** (XX/XY). They proposed the cellular theory of free martinism stating that XY cells carry the 'H-Y antigen', which may play an important role in male development. Some years ago, a testis-determining substance was proposed to be identical to the male-specific H-Y antigen (Wachtel *et al* 1975, 1991), also called as the classical histocompatible Y antigen. This hypothesis is attractive as until recently, it was observed that almost all mammals having a testis were H-Y positive independent of their karyotype. Based on their concept, it is suggested that H-Y antigen produced by the XY cells of fetal testis of male co-twin would act directly to masculinize the freemartin ovary and genital ducts. A relatively small number of XY cell may exert a disproportionate effect. Fewer than 10 % male cells are found in extensively **virilized (masculinized)** ovaries. It has been proposed that **H-Y** antigen is released from the surface of XY cells, coats the surface of majority of genetically XX cells of the medulla and by doing so, induces them to form a testis. In the presence of H-Y antigen, XX cortical cells degenerate. This proposal for action of H-Y antigen is speculative and evidence is largely circumstantial. Other substances may be implicated in sexual development but may not determine it. It seems however, that some gene product of a Y-linked gene must participate and must have many of the properties possessed by H-Y antigen.

Cortico-medullary Induction theory: E. Witschi proposed this theory in 1957. It is based on the fact that the early gonads of vertebrates are composed of discrete primordia, medulla and cortex, which are determined genetically to form testes or ovaries respectively. There is no transformation of one primordium into the other, but rather a development of one is accompanied by the recession of the other (Figure 9.6). Witschi theorized largely on the basis of his amphibian studies, that the medulla and cortex might be the source of special substances called **medullarian** and **corticin/cortixin** respectively, which act as embryonic inductors. These postulated diffusable substances are believed to be mutually antagonistic although it may not be necessary to involve the secretion of cortixin in the absence of medullarian. The medullarian is not present to cause the medulla to develop. Several facts should be kept in mind with respect to the hypothetical gonadal inductors.

- There is necessarily much vagueness in the use of the term "**inductors**".
- Such materials have never been isolated and chemically identified.
- There is no information on the biochemical mechanisms, which intervene between sex genes and characters, they determine.

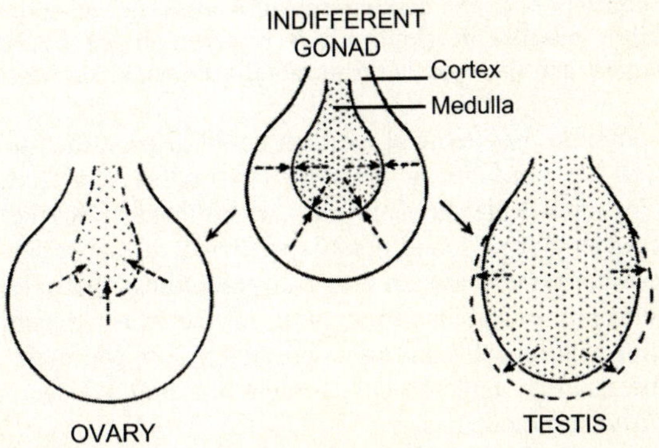

Figure 9.6: Diagrammatic representation of medulla and cortex in indifferent gonad, broken arrows indicate mutually antagonistic actions of these two components in course of sexual differentiation as proposed by Witschi.

Further, there is no doubt that steroid hormones and gonadal grafts can modify or completely reverse gonadal differentiation in certain vertebrates. It is not known whether steroid hormones act directly in these cases as "inductors" or produce their effects secondarily by modifying some kind of an inductor system.

In the male toad, at the cranial end of each testis is present a cortical deposit or rudimentary ovary. This is called **Bidder's organ**. When the testes are removed, this organ enlarges and slowly develops into a functional ovary capable of producing fertile eggs.

Among amphibians it is relatively easy to graft gonad primordia and also animals can be united parabiotically (Figure 9.7). **Parabiosis** is joining together side by side or laterally of two individuals. The two animals are sutured together so that their vascular systems join and these parabionts then share a common circulation. When heterosexual combinations are made, one sex is suppressed and partial/complete reversal of this suppressed sex results. Typically the male gonad is dominant. Removal of the dominant gonad graft or separation of the parabionts may permit the transformed individual to return to the type of sexual development typical for its genetic constitution. Parabiosis is also accompanied by compensatory organ hypertrophy following removal of the same organ from one of the parabiont animals as shown in rat in Figure 9.7.

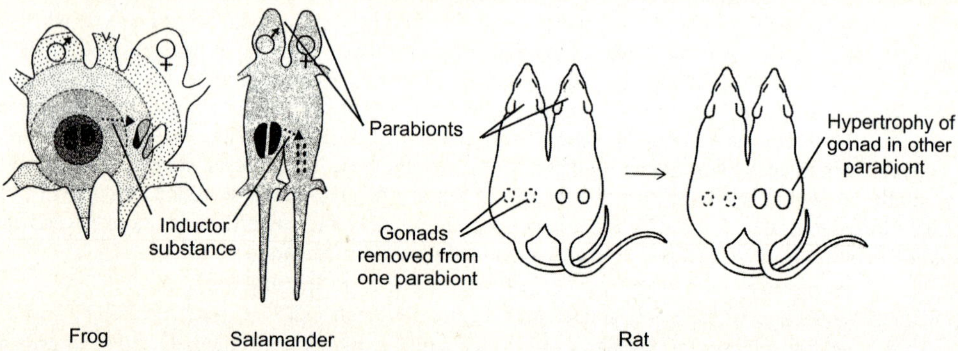

Figure 9.7: Parabiosis-in Frog some inductor substance manufactured by the testes passes across into female and partially interfere with the development of ovaries, in Salamander male gonadal inductor substance completely inhibits ovarian development; it is accompanied by compensatory hypertrophy following removal of the same organ from one of the parabiotic animal as shown in adult rat.

In humans it is possible that hermaphroditism could also be due to hormonal imbalance. In these cases, the source of the hormone is probably the mother, e.g. there may be an excessive production of androgens by adrenal glands of the mother and these affect the male fetus. The estrogen produced by the mother under normal conditions is sufficient to cause any profound effect on the testes. Nevertheless, these hormones have an effect on the uterus- that is enlargement of cervix; on vagina- resulting in hypertrophy of vaginal epithelium; on the ovary- resulting in stimulation of the follicles; on breast- causing enlargement and pseudosecretion. In the male fetus during intrauterine life, it is noted that the breasts may undergo enlargement and produce secretion. These changes are probably due to estrogen from the mother.

These theories clearly indicate that presence of Y chromosome and androgens result in the development of male fetus while their absence causes development of female fetus. However, once sexual differentiation of any particular structure has taken place, its development cannot be reversed. Hormonal aberration present at a critical stage of development could result in differentiation in an abnormal direction. For example, a temporary excess of estrogens in a genetic male could cause a modification or reversal of the portion of the system undergoing differentiation at that time.

9.6 Chromosomal Sex Determination in Mammals

Chromosomal sex determination can be **primary** and **secondary**: **Primary sex determination** involves the formation of either an ovary or a testis from the bipotential gonad, and it is strictly the function of sex chromosomes. On the other hand, **secondary sex determination** affects the bodily phenotype outside the gonads. For example, a male mammal has seminal vesicle, prostates, penis etc, while a female mammal has uterus, cervix, vagina, and mammary glands. Hormones secreted by the gonads usually determine these secondary sex characteristics.

Recent views on the mechanisms of mammalian sex determination suggest the involvement of several genes whose function is necessary for normal sexual differentiation (Figure 9.8).

In humans, the major gene in primary sex determination for the testis-determining factor resides on **the short arm of Y chromosome**. It is necessary and sufficient for the production of testes and is called the **SRY** gene (sex-determining region of the Y chromosome). It is expressed at the time of differentiation of the gonad in the urogenital ridge cells and triggers the development of testes in the seventh week of uterine life. SRY contains a DNA-binding domain and probably acts as a cascade of genes necessary for testicular differentiation. In the absence of a Y chromosome, and hence, the SRY gene, testes do not develop. Instead, ovaries begin to develop in the same area at about 11 weeks. Recent studies (Capel *et al* 1999) suggest that SRY work via an indirect mechanism. SRY in the genital ridge cells induces the cells to secrete a chemotactic factor that permits the migration of mesonephric cells into the XY gonad. These mesonephric cells induce the gonadal epithelium to become Sertoli cells with male-specific gene expression patterns. Another protein that may be directly or indirectly activated by SRY is the transcription factor **Sf1** or **SF1 (Steroidogenic factor 1)**. SF1 is necessary to make the bipotential gonad, and it appears to be active in masculinizing both the Leydig and the Sertoli cells. In the Sertoli cells, SF1, working in collaboration with SOX9 (one of the autosomal genes involved in sex determination), is needed to elevate the levels of AMH transcription. In the Leydig cells, SF1 activates the genes encoding the enzymes that make testosterone. It is believed that SRY directly or indirectly activates the SF1 gene, and the SF1 protein then activates both components of the male sexual differentiation pathway, Sertoli AMH and Leydig testosterone (Figure 9.8 A and B). Secondary sex determination (hormonal regulation of the sexual phenotype) involves the development of the female and male phenotype in response to hormone secreted by the ovaries and testes. Formation of the male phenotype involves the secretion of two testicular hormones. The first of these is **AMH (Anti-Mullerian duct hormone, also referred to as Mullerian regression factor, MRF or Mullerian-inhibiting-substance, MIS)**. The Sertoli cells make this hormone, and it causes the degeneration of the Mullerian duct. The second is the **steroid testosterone**, which is secreted from the fetal Leydig cells. This hormone causes the Wolffian duct to differentiate into the epididymis, vas deferens, and seminal vesicles, and it also causes the urogenital swellings to develop into the scrotum and penis. If the bipotential gonads are removed from the embryo, the female phenotype is realized, thus, the Mullerian ducts develop and the Wolffian ducts regress.

Figure 9.9 summarizes the major events occurring in determination of sexual differentiation towards a male and a female. The findings indicate that development of a male reproductive pattern is determined by the presence or otherwise of a testis during a critical period. In its absence, a cyclic female pattern results. The presence or absence of an ovary is immaterial for this differentiation and also later removal of testes does not permit a male to revert to a female reproductive pattern.

9.7 Aberrant Sexual Differentiation

Abnormalities of sexual development could be caused by genetic (chromosomal) defects, enzyme defects or hormonal defects or due to some other nonspecific teratogenic influences. These can be dealt separately in females and males. The major classes of abnormalities are listed in Table 9.2.

(i) Chromosomal Abnormalities

Chromosomal Abnormalities in the Females: As discussed earlier, the normal female embryo has 23 pairs of chromosomes (22 autosomal pairs and one pair of sex chromosomes, XX). Both of the X-chromosomes are essential for normal differentiation of the ovaries, but only one X is necessary for the differentiation of the Mullerian ducts and the female external genitalia. One chromosomal abnormality that has been identified in the female is the presence of only one X sex chromosome, designated as XO, which is termed **gonadal dysgenesis** or alternatively **ovarian agenesis** or **Turner's syndrome** (Table 9.2). This chromosomal deficiency is characterized by impaired development of the female gonads, which results in the appearance of an incompletely formed gonad, termed a **vestigial gonadal streak**. The uterus, fallopian tubes, and female external genitalia develop normally. The XXX ("**super female**") pattern does not seem to be associated with any characteristic abnormalities (Figure 9.10).

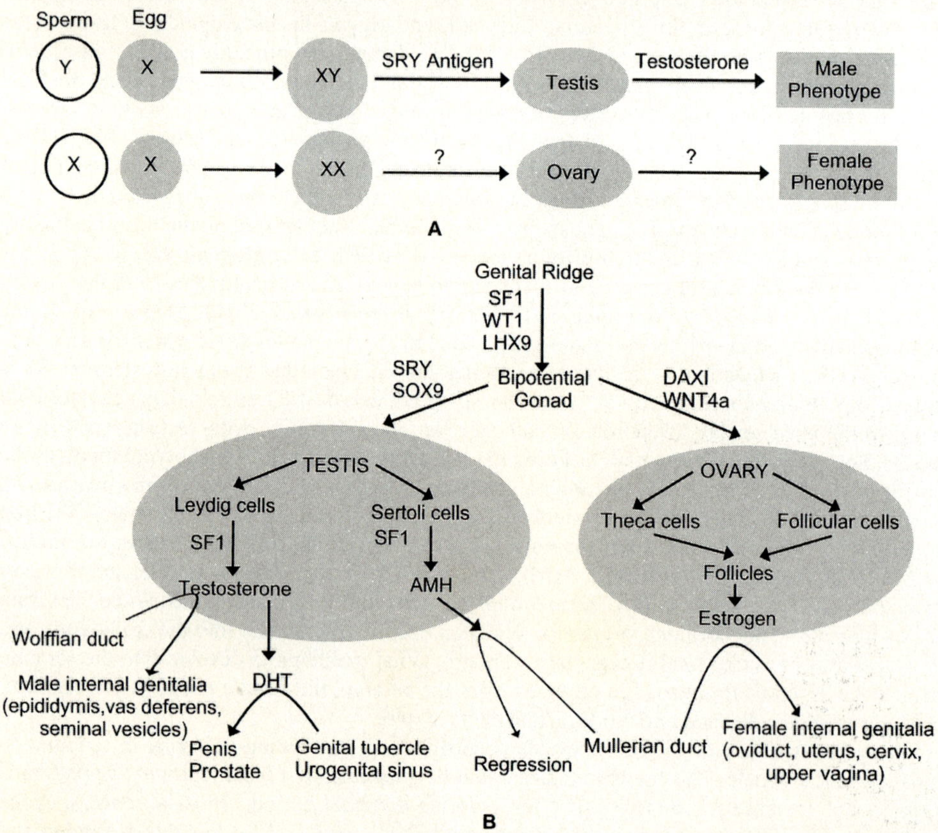

Figure 9.8: Mechanism of sex determination in Mammals, A-role of SRY antigen in primary sex determination and B-formation of sexual phenotype.

Chromosomal Abnormalities in the Males: The normal male embryo has 23 pairs of chromosomes (22 autosomal pairs and one pair of sex chromosomes, XY). Some genetically male individuals receive an extra X chromosome (XXY), which results in **Klinefelter's syndrome** (Table 9.2). In these cases the presence of the Y chromosome directs differentiation of the testes, but they are reduced in size. As in normal males, testosterone secretion from the testes in XXY males stimulates development of the Wolffian duct system and development of the male external genitalia, while MIS secretion from the testes induces Mullerian regression. However, the presence of the extra X chromosome leads to testicular dysfunction owing to impaired development of the seminiferous tubules and a deficiency in spermatogenesis **(seminiferous tubule dysgenesis)**. YO combination is probably lethal (Figure 9.10).

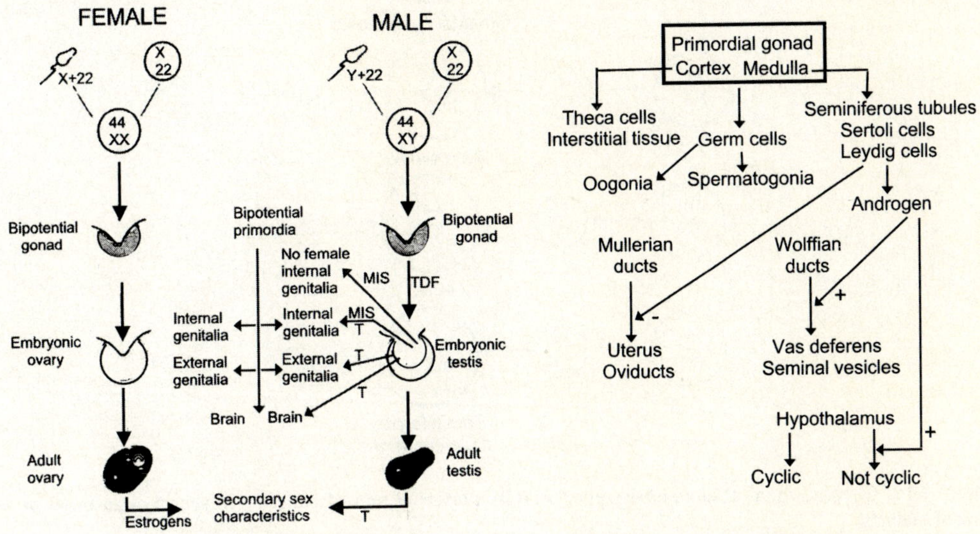

Figure 9.9: Summary of major events in determination of sexual differentiation.

Table 9.2: Abnormalities of sexual differentiation

Chromosomal complement	Abnormality	Enzyme or receptor defect	Gonads	Internal genitalia	External genitalia
XO	Turner's syndrome	-	Ovaries with impaired development (streak gonads)	Female	Female
XXY	Klinefelter's syndrome	-	Testes with impaired development of seminiferous tubules and deficient spermatogenesis	Male	Male
XX	Adrenogenita l syndrome	Adrenal 11- or 21-hydroxylase deficiency	Ovaries	Female	Male/ Female
XY	Testicular feminization	Lacks androgen receptors	Testes	None	Female
XY	-	Lacks ability to synthesize testosterone	Testes	Male with impaired development	Female/ Male
XY	-	5-α reductase deficiency	Testes	Male	Female/ Male

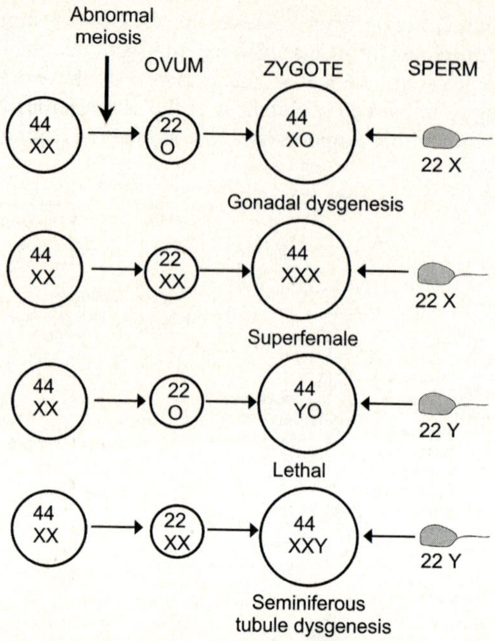

Figure 9.10: Chromosomal abnormalities produced by maternal non-disjunction of sex chromosomes at the time of meiosis.

ii) Abnormal sex differentiation due to defects in Enzyme

Enzyme deficiencies in the female: Some genetic females' (XX) lack the enzymes 11-hydroxylase or 21-hydroxylase in their adrenal glands. These enzymes are necessary for the synthesis of gluco- and mineralo- corticoids. In the absence of these enzymes, the adrenal glands use the steroid precursor cholesterol to synthesize androgens. Hypersecretion of adrenal androgen results in the development of the adrenogenital syndrome also called congenital adrenal hyperplasia (Table 9.2). These individuals have normal ovaries, owing to a full chromosomal XX compliment. The absence of a Y chromosome in these individuals precludes the development of the Mullerian duct system (including the uterus and fallopian tubes). However, hypersecretion of adrenal androgens can result in masculinization of the external genitalia. The degree of masculinization depends on the severity of adrenal enzymatic deficiency; it can range from mild hypertrophy of the clitoris to fusion of the urethral folds and labio-scrotal swellings, which then resemble a penis and scrotum. Severe masculinization of the female external genitalia, a condition termed " **female pseudohermaphroditism**" can lead to mistakes in identifying the gender of the infant.

Enzymes deficiencies in male: Genetic males (XY) who lack androgen receptors cannot respond to testosterone or dihydrotestosterone, which results in a condition known as **testicular feminization syndrome** (Table 9.2). In these individuals, the presence of the Y chromosome results in the development of the testes, and testicular secretion of MIS induces regression of the Mullerian ducts. However, androgen insensitivity results in a lack of development of the Wolffian duct system and the absence of masculinization of the external genitalia. Therefore, these individuals have no internal genitalia at all, because MIS induces regression of the Mullerian ducts while the lack of androgen receptors precludes development of the Wolffian ducts.

iii) Abnormal differentiation due to Hormones

It is known that androgen receptor concentrations are about three times higher in genital tissues than in for example forearm skin. How is this "geographical" distribution of receptors regulated during fetal development remains to be elucidated? The development of the male external genitalia occurs normally in genetic males in response to androgens secreted by the embryonic testes, but male genital development may also occur in genetic females exposed to androgens from some other sources during the eighth to the thirteenth weeks of gestation. The syndrome that results is called **female pseudohermaphroditism**. A pseudohermaphrodite is an individual with the genetic constitution and gonads of one sex and the genitalia of the other. After the thirteenth week, the genitalia are fully formed, but exposure to androgens can cause hypertrophy of the clitoris. Female pseudohermaphroditism may be due to congenital virilizing adrenal hyperplasia, or it may be caused by androgens administered to the mother. Conversely, development of female external genitalia in genetic males (**male pseudohermaphroditism**) occurs when the embryonic testes are defective. Because the testes also secrete MIS, genetic males with defective testes have female internal genitalia.

Another cause of male pseudohermaphroditism is **androgen resistance** in which, as a result of various congenital abnormalities, male hormones cannot exert their full effects on the tissues. One form of androgen resistance is a 5α-reductase deficiency in which the enzyme responsible for the formation of dihydrotestosterone, the active form of testosterone, is decreased. Other forms of androgen resistance are due to various mutations in the androgen receptor gene, and the resulting defects in receptor function range from minor to severe. Mild defects cause infertility with or without gynecomastia. When the loss of receptor function is essentially complete, the testicular feminizing syndrome results. In this condition, MIS is present and testosterone is secreted at normal or even elevated rates. The external genitalia are female, but the vagina ends blindly because there are no female internal genitalia. Individuals with this syndrome develop enlarged breasts at puberty and usually are considered to be normal women until they are diagnosed when they seek medical advice because of lack of menstruation.

It is worth noting that genetic males with congenital blockade of the formation of pregnenolone are pseudohermaphrodites because testicular as well as adrenal androgens are normally formed from pregnenolone. Male pseudohermaphroditism also occurs when there is a congenital deficiency of 17α-hydroxylase.

Summary

There are 46 chromosomes in humans-22 pairs of autosomes and one pair of sex chromosomes. Primary sex determination (the determination of gonadal sex) is the function of the sex chromosomes.

Sex is determined by two sex chromosomes: XY for males and XX for females. XX and XY mammals both have a bipotential gonad. The Y chromosome plays a key role in male sex determination. In humans, the SRY gene is the testis-determining factor on the Y chromosome.

Secondary sex determination involves the hormones produced by the developing gonads.

SRY activates directly or indirectly the SF1 gene, which is believed to activate the SOX9 gene, as well as several other genes, involved in synthesizing steroid hormones and anti-Mullerian duct hormone (AMH or Mullerian inhibiting substance, MIS or Mullerian regression factor, MRF).

AMH produced by the Sertoli cells causes degeneration of Mullerian duct, while the testosterone produced by the Leydig cells enables the Wolffian duct to differentiate into the vas deferens and seminal vesicles etc.

Lack of testosterone in females causes degeneration of Wolffian duct.

Only one X chromosome is required for differentiation of Mullerian ducts and female genitalia. Testosterone, secreted by Leydig cells of the testes, has no effect on Mullerian ducts.

The absence of ovaries will not preclude development of the Mullerian ducts or the female external genitalia.

Exposure of the genetically female embryo to androgens during early development results in variable degree of masculinization of the external genitalia depending on when during development the exposure occurs. Exposure to androgens does not alter development of the ovaries or the Mullerian ducts.

Testosterone is converted to Dihydrotestosterone (DHT) in tissues of the external genitalia where it stimulates its differentiation. An absence of DHT formation results in reduced masculinization of the external genitalia but does not affect normal development of Wolffian ducts, which respond directly to testosterone.

Sexual differentiation takes place in a series of stages. First the sex of gonad is determined, then that of the genital tract, and finally the pattern of gonadotropin release and sexual behavior. Initially, the presence or absence of a Y chromosome is decisive but later, the presence or absence of a male gonad. X chromosome, and ovaries, is not relevant.

Abnormalities of sexual development could be caused by genetic or hormonal or developmental defects.

Questions

1. Discuss various theories of sex differentiation.
2. What are the mechanisms of mammalian sex determination?
3. Discuss aberrant sexual differentiation in male and female.
4. The normal diploid number of human chromosomes is a) 48, b) 47, **c) 46**, d) 23.

Chapter 10

Germ Cells and Gamete Formation

Eggs and sperms are very special cells formed to perform a very specific purpose of forming a new individual of the next generation. The developmental history of these reproductive cells (gametes) is a complex period of preparation for this special function. Discussion on the formation of gametes is an appropriate way to begin a study on physiology of reproduction.

The definitive germ cells, the egg and spermatozoa, are derived solely from the primitive sex cells found early in embryonic development. Male germ cells (spermatogonia) are produced in the testis and female germ cells (oogonia) in the ovary. The position of the germ cells within the gonad affects their development and thus, the female germ cells that enter the medulla usually degenerate or remain dormant as ovary is derived from the cortical portion of the gonad primordium. There is no evidence that they ever become male gamete cells in mammals. Similarly, the male germ cells that persist in cortex never become oogonia.

Towards the end of sex differentiation, the number of primordial germ cells increases sharply by mitosis. The first spermatogonia appear in the human testis during the 5th month of the intrauterine life and in other species sometimes after birth. The testes of rats have been shown to contain more sex cells at this early stage than do the ovaries. However, the situation rapidly reverses since the male germ cells become relatively undifferentiated gonocytes, which rarely undergo division.

The ovarian germ cells also rapidly become transformed into oogonia. The population of oogonia increases greatly in a relatively short period of time. For example in rat, the number of germ cells increases from 11,500 to 75,500 during the period of oogonial division. In man, there are about 1700 germ cells during migration into gonad, 600,000 during the 2nd month of pregnancy, 7 million at the 5th month, and this number drops to 2 million at birth and 100,000 at age 20. Figure 10.1 shows fluctuations in number of germ cells in the ovaries of fetus and infant of human, monkey, rat and guinea pig. All the oocytes from about 5th month of intrauterine time onwards, are incapable of increasing their numbers, and the population of germ cells reduces with increasing age due to the processes of atresia and ovulation. Thus, stem cells of the ovary proliferate very rapidly for several months and then stop dividing prior to birth, and the maximum number of egg cells or ova that a woman will ever have are present three or four months before she is born. In contrast, stem cells in the testes continue to divide throughout life of an individual and thus in the testis, mitotically active spermatogonia persist throughout adult life. The germ cells get transformed into gametes for the first time at puberty, through the process that represents the culmination of events that begins early in embryonic life.

10.1 Gametogenesis

The production of **reproductive cells** or **gametes** from germ cells is called **gametogenesis**. Two types of gametes produced during gametogenesis are **spermatozoa** (*singular*: **spermatozoon**, usually shortened to **sperm**) in males and **ova** (*singular*: **ovum**) in females. The process by which male gametes are formed is termed as **spermatogenesis**, and the other resulting in the formation of female gametes is called **oogenesis**.

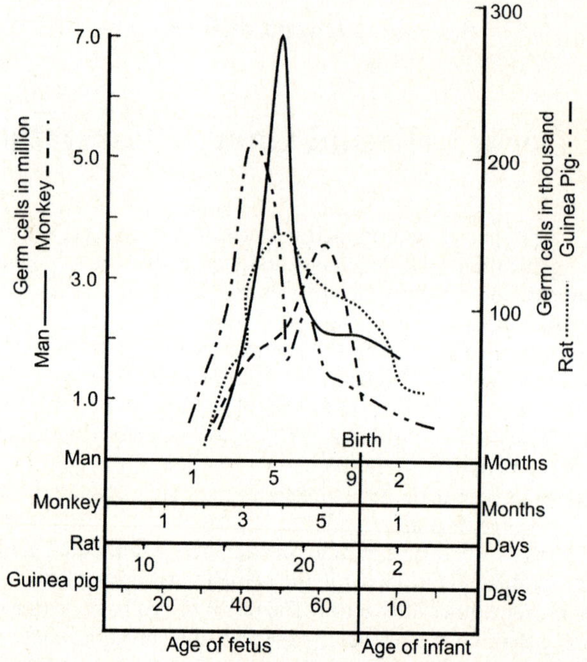

Figure 10.1: Number of germ cells in ovaries of fetus and infant of Human, Monkey, Rat, and Guinea pig.

General principles of gametogenesis are essentially the same in males and females. Broadly speaking, gametogenesis consists of **three phases** or **stages**. The **first stage** is the **proliferation of the primordial germ cells** by mitosis to produce **gametogonia**. In mitosis, all the dividing cells having 46 chromosomes are replicated, and each of the two daughter cells resulting from the division receives a full set of 46 chromosomes identical to those of the original cell. Thus, each daughter cell receives identical genetic information. In this manner, mitosis of primordial germ cell provides a supply of identical germ cells for the next stage. The timing of mitotic activity in germ cells differs greatly in females and males. In the female, mitosis of germ cells occurs exclusively during the individual's embryonic development. In the male, some mitosis occurs in the embryo to generate the population of germ cells present at birth, but mitosis really begins in earnest at puberty and usually continues throughout life.

The **second stage** of gametogenesis is the **growth phase**, during which the **gametogonium** formed after mitotic divisions of germ cells, increases markedly in size, and become **gametocytes**. The growth phase is more important and marked in females than in males, resulting in many fold increases in the size of gametogonium in females.

The **third phase** of gametogenesis is the **reduction phase**. This involves **meiosis**, in which each resulting gamete receives only 23 chromosomes from a 46-chromosome germ cell, one chromosome from each homologous pair. Because a sperm and an about-to-be fertilized egg, each has only 23 chromosomes, their union result once again in a cell with a full compliment of 46 chromosomes.

The **final phase** of gametogenesis is the **maturation phase** in which the resultant haploid cells mature to form a functional gamete ready for fusion in fertilization to produce a zygote.

10.2 Meiotic Division during Gametogenesis

Meiosis is a type of nuclear division restricted to gametes, i.e. spermatocytes and oocytes, wherein the number of chromosomes characteristic of somatic cells, the diploid number (2n), is halved to the haploid number (1n). For this reason, meiosis is termed as reduction division (Figure 10.2). The gametes with haploid number of chromosomes unite during fertilization and the diploid number of chromosomes is restored. The fertilized ovum and all its descendents except the gametes divide by mitotic division, and the diploid number is therefore, maintained in somatic cells. Meiosis has the second major function of providing genetic variation by the exchange of segments of homologous chromosomes and random selection of one of the two homologues during the reduction division.

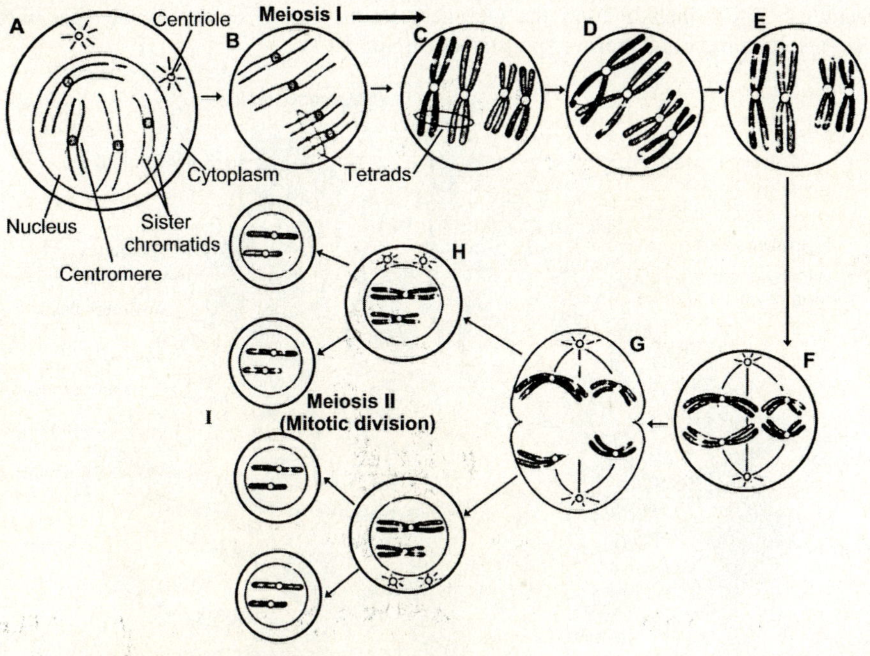

Figure 10.2: Stages of meiosis in a generalized germ cell, A-Interphase, B to H-First meiotic division and H to I-Second meiotic division (mitotic).

Initiation of meiosis is controlled by meiosis inducing substance (MIS) and meiosis preventing substance (MPS) that is present in reproductive organs of both sexes of mammals. The MIS: MPS ratio may influence the continued spermatogenesis. It was observed that around the time when the gonads are being morphologically sex differentiated, the rete system of both sexes secretes MIS, which triggers the germ cells to enter preleptotene chromosome condensation. It was found that only those gonocytes of developing testis, which are not enclosed in testicular cords, and lie close to or within the rete system, enter the leptotene and zygotene stages, while gonocytes placed within the testicular cords are prevented from entering meiosis by MPS. The enclosure of gonocytes within the cords together with MPS prevents action of MIS. MPS is believed to be the product of Sertoli cells. Recently, the meiosis inducing substance is termed as MAS (meiosis activating sterol) to avoid confusion with Mullerian inhibiting substance (anti-Mullerian hormone). MIS shows steroid-like properties and may regulate meiosis by the plasma membrane associated inositol-secondary messenger pathway. Both male and female germ cells can enter meiosis under the influence of the rete system.

10.3 Spermatogenesis

The process of formation of sperm is called spermatogenesis. It takes place within the coiled seminiferous tubules of the testis with the transformation of gonocytes into spermatids and thus results in the production of haploid male gametes. This transformation proceeds in a very progressive way, apparently occurring at random throughout the testis.

The seminiferous epithelium is composed of two population of cells: i) **nonproliferating population of supporting cells**, known as the **Sertoli cells**, and ii) a **proliferating population of germ cells** that migrate continuously from the periphery of the tubules to luminal free surface. The germinal elements consist of successive generations of cells arranged in well-defined concentric layers within the epithelium. These include from the periphery to the lumen of the tubule **spermatogonia**, **spermatocytes**, **immature** and **mature spermatids** (Figure 10.3).

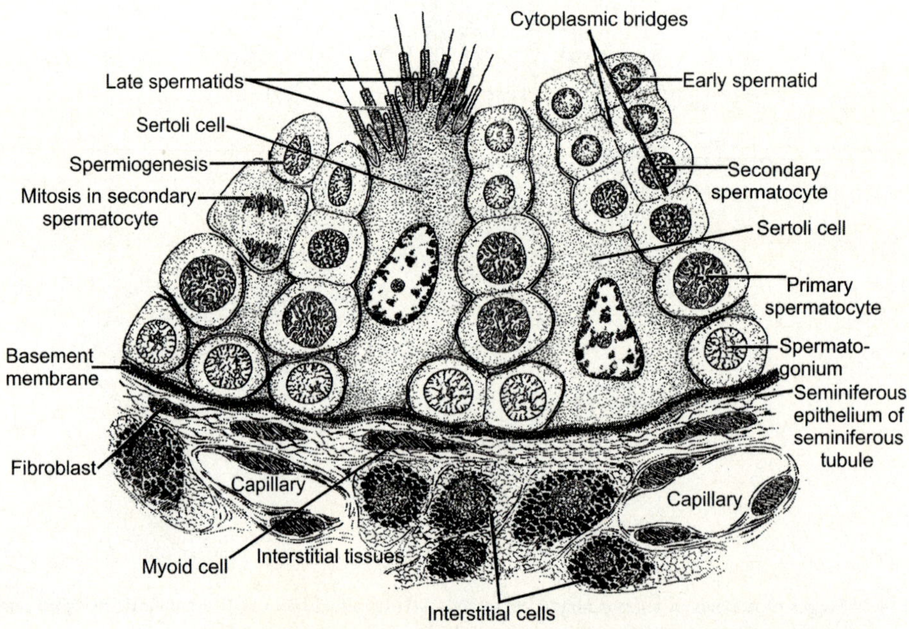

Figure 10.3: Structural organization of the Human seminiferous tubule and interstitial tissue.

Spermatogenesis lasts several weeks in all mammals. It may be subdivided into three phases: the **first phase** is the **mitotic multiplication** and growth of spermatogonia, and the **second** is the **reduction phase** involving **meiosis**. The third and the final phase is the **spermiogenesis** or **spermateleosis** that involves the **transformation of spermatids** into **spermatozoa**. Spermatogenesis process begins at puberty. Figure 10.4 illustrates various steps in spermatogenesis.

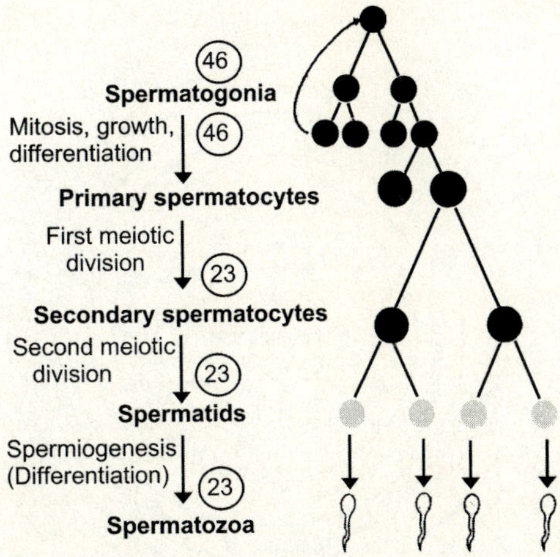

Figure 10.4: Events in the process of spermatogenesis.

In rat, spermatogenesis begins on the 4th day after birth and by 45-50 days the first set of spermatozoa are produced. The duration of the cycle of the seminiferous epithelium is about 12 days in adult rat, and spermatogonia divide to initiate spermatogenesis at fixed intervals of 12 days in rat. It is of 16 days in man. Spermatogenesis takes 5-8 weeks to get completed depending on the species. However, its duration is fixed and is constant for a given animal species (Table 10.1, and Figure 10.5). The duration of spermatogenesis starting from the division of stem cell spermatogonium is about 49 (45-50) days in rat and 74 (65-75) days in man.

Table 10.1: Duration of spermatogenesis and seminiferous epithelium cycle

Mammalian Species	Time for completion of Spermatogenesis (days)	Duration (in days) of the Cycle of Seminiferous Epithelium
Cow	56	14
Man	64	16
Monkey	70	10.5
Mouse	34	8.6
Pig	32	8
Ram	49	10.4
Rat	48	12
Sheep	40	10

Differentiation of Germ Cells: Although primordial germ cells are present in the testes from an early age, active spermatogenesis does not begin until puberty. Once begun, the process of sperm production continues into old age. Spermatogenesis is constantly being repeated and all stages of sperm cell development are present in the seminiferous tubules at the same time.

The early development and differentiation of germ cells before the initiation of spermatogenesis is described as prespermatogenesis. This includes: a) initial fetal stages of multiplication, b) a quiescent period during which germ cell mitosis possibly stops, and c) a second mitotic stage (postnatal) just before the start of spermatogenesis with the more marked alterations appearing at the time of initiation of spermatogenesis.

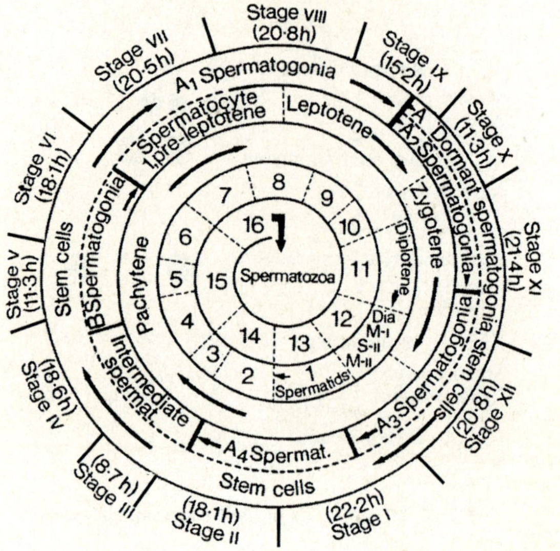

Figure 10.5: Dynamics of spermatogenesis (Mouse), Dia-Diakinesis, M-I and M-II First and Second Meiotic Division, S-II Secondary spermatocyte, and 1-16 Spermiogenesis Stage.

Prespermatogonia can be distinguished from spermatogonia by their large size, more uniform spherical shape, and looser distribution of chromatin (Figure 10.6). Narrow strips of intervening Sertoli cell cytoplasm separate the prespermatogonia from the tubular periphery and thus they are not directly placed against the basal lamina. The spermatogonia, in contrast, lie very close to the basal lamina (Figure 10.6).

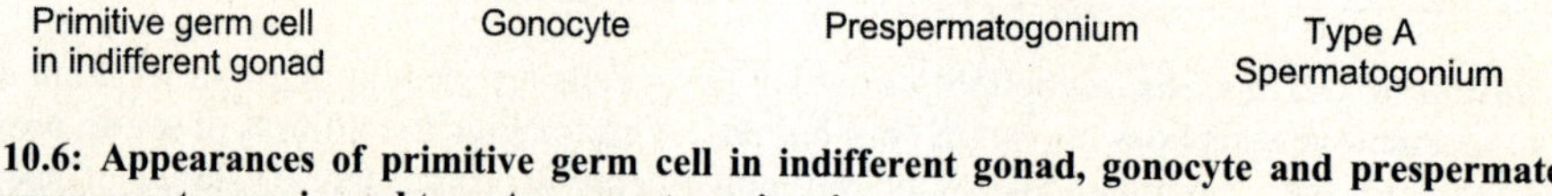

Figure 10.6: Appearances of primitive germ cell in indifferent gonad, gonocyte and prespermatogonium during prespermatogenesis, and type A spermatogonium in spermatogenesis.

Mitotic Divisions during Spermatogenesis: Spermatogenesis begins at puberty with the transformation of prespermatogonia into **spermatogonia** (*singular*: **Spermatogonium**), which contain the diploid (2n) number of chromosomes. The development of type A spermatogonia is related to the resumption of mitosis and onset of spermatogenesis.

Spermatogonia are **stem cells** because when they undergo mitosis, some of the daughter cells remain near the basement membrane of the seminiferous tubule in an undifferentiated state to serve as reservoir of cells for future mitosis and subsequent sperm production. The rest of the daughter cells lose contact with the basement membrane and divide mitotically for a specified number of division cycles so that clones of spermatogonia are produced for each original spermatogonium. Some growth and differentiation occurs in addition to cell division. The cells that result from the final mitotic division and differentiation in the series are called **primary spermatocytes**. The primary spermatocytes, like spermatogonia, are diploid (2n), i.e., they have 46 chromosomes and these are the cells that will undergo the next phase of spermatogenesis, called **reduction phase**, which involves reduction division.

Several types of spermatogonia can be identified in testicular sections on the basis of nuclear staining techniques (Figure 10.7). Three classes of spermatogonia have been described in man: i) **dark type A (Ad)**, ii) **pale type A (Ap)**, and iii) **type B spermatogonia**. In rodents, four successive generations of type A spermatogonia have been described-A_1, A_2, A_3, A_4. The type A_1 cells divide by mitosis to give rise to type A_2; the type A_2 in turn yields type A_3, which finally produce type A_4 spermatogonia. Type A_4 spermatogonia divide and give rise to intermediate (In) spermatogonia, which in turn yield type B cells. The later spermatogonia (B) are the differentiated elements, committed to the production of spermatocytes. Clermont and co-workers in 1968 proposed the sequence of these divisions for rat and man (Figure 10.8). In addition, a group of spermatogonia is present in the seminiferous epithelium, which rarely divide or have a long cell-cycle time. These have been referred to as "**reserve stem cells** (A_0).

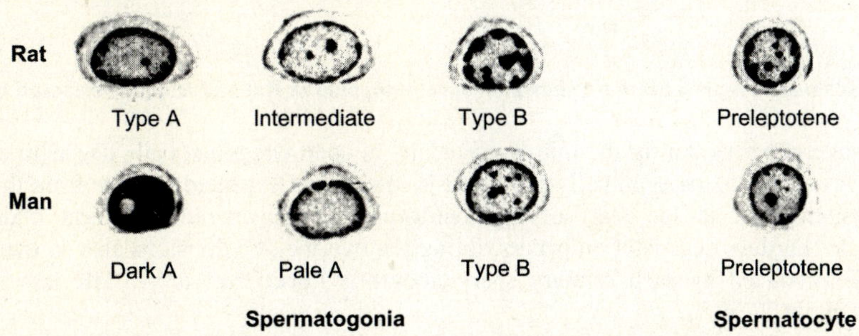

Figure 10.7: Types of spermatogonia and preleptotene spermatocyte in Rat and Man.

It must be emphasized here that if all the cells in the clone produced by each original spermatogonium followed the pathway of division together, the spermatogonia would get exhausted and disappear-that is, all spermatogonia would be converted into primary spermatocytes. Therefore, for spermatogenesis to continue indefinitely, without exhausting the supply of spermatogonia, at an early point, one of the cells of each clone "drops out" of the mitosis-differentiation cycles and reverts to being a primitive spermatogonium that, at a later time, will enter into its own full sequence of divisions. Again, one cell of the clone it produces will do likewise so that the supply of undifferentiated spermatogonia does not decrease. Thus, some type A spermatogonia serve as "stem cells". Some investigators believe that the undifferentiated type A_4 spermatogonia serve as stem cells while others believe that the long cycling population of cells, known as the type A_0, act as the stem cell spermatogonia (A_s). In primates, A_d spermatogonia may act as the reserve stem cells.

The process whereby during each cycle of spermatogonial multiplication, new stem cells arise to replace those that differentiate into spermatocytes is called "**renewal of stem cells**". The time during the multiplication cycle of type A spermatogonia, when these renewing stem cells arises, varies in different species.

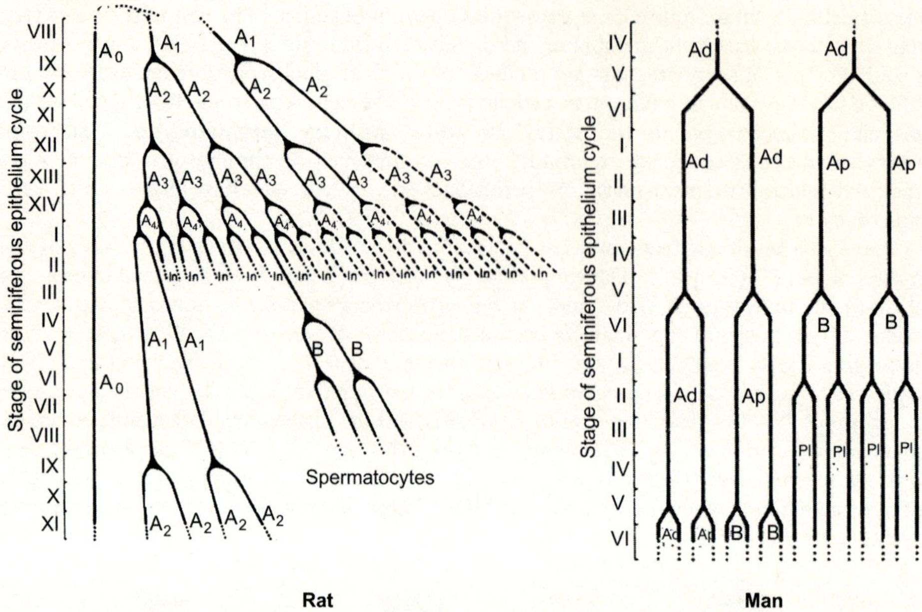

Figure 10.8: Schematic representation-renewal of spermatogonia in Rat and Man as proposed by Clermont.

At several points during the mitotic divisions of spermatogonia, cells degenerate, so that the total number of spermatozoa eventually produced is lower than expected to arise from the number of type A spermatogonia at the start of spermatogenesis. Degeneration affects mainly type A spermatogonia. Further, degeneration occurs during the two meiotic divisions also so that the number of spermatids produced by each primary spermatocyte is lower than four. The loss in spermatid production is about 27-30 %.

The spermatogonia are approximately 12 μm in diameter and border the limiting membrane of seminiferous tubules. Their nuclei are round or slightly ovoid and 6-7 μm in diameter with nucleoli usually attached to the nuclear envelope. The A_d spermatogonium has deeply stained dust-like chromatin while A_p spermatogonium possesses a nucleus showing a finely granulated and lightly stained chromatin in humans. Type A spermatogonium, e.g. rodents, bull, ram and boar has an ovoid nucleus containing very fine chromatin granules distributed along the nuclear envelope and a centrally located nucleolus. Type B spermatogonia are characterized by spherical nuclei containing large clumps of chromatin adjacent to nuclear envelope and a centrally located nucleolus. Some spermatogonia exhibit morphological features that are intermediate between those of type A and B cells. Fine chromatin granules attached to nuclear envelope characterize these intermediate type spermatogonia (In).

Reduction Phase of Spermatogenesis: Each **spermatogonium** increases in size during the growth phase of spermatogenesis, and differentiates to become **primary spermatocyte**. The primary spermatocyte enters the next phase of spermatogenesis called the reduction phase, involving meiosis. During meiotic division, there is a random assortment and recombination of maternal and paternal chromosomes. In addition, homologous chromosomes (similar chromosomes, one of maternal origin and other of paternal origin) exchange chromosomal segments in a process known as "crossing over". This process ensures that genetic material is recombined in an infinite number of ways. DNA synthesis increases within the primary spermatocyte, and each of the 23 maternal and 23 paternal chromosomes in the cell are duplicated. The homologous maternal and paternal chromosomes pair with each other to form 23 four-stranded (tetrad) chromosomes. The primary spermatocyte undergoes two very rapid divisions, the **first meiotic division** results in the formation of two **secondary spermatocytes**, each of which contains 23 two-chromatid chromosomes. Each secondary spermatocyte then **undergoes the second meiotic division**, which is **mitotic**, resulting in the formation of two **spermatids**. Thus, each primary spermatocyte, containing 46 chromosomes, gives rise to four spermatids, each containing 23 chromosomes.

The **final phase** of spermatogenesis is the **differentiation of the spermatids** into spermatozoa. This process involves extensive cell remodeling, including elongation, but no further cell division. The total number of stages during the entire development of spermatids varies in different species. These are 19 in rat, 16 in mouse, and 14 in monkeys.

10.4 Spermiogenesis

As primary spermatocytes differentiate into spermatids, they migrate away from the basement membrane of the seminiferous tubule towards the fluid-filled lumen of the tubule. Near the lumen, the spermatids undergo the final phase of spermatogenesis called the **spermiogenesis** or **spermateleosis** during which spermatids undergo many changes that lead to the formation of spermatozoa or sperm. The sperms are then released into the lumen of the testis by a process called **spermiation**. From the lumen, the sperm leave the seminiferous tubule and enter the epididymis.

During spermiogenesis, the spermatids do not undergo cell division but rather go through a complex series of cytological changes, which are divisible into a number of **steps** on the basis of morphological differences and are numbered by Arabic numerals. These steps can be grouped in **four-phases**: **Golgi phase, cap phase, acrosome phase,** and **maturation phase** (Figure 10.9). The number of steps varies in different species. They are characteristically associated with different stages of the cycle as seen in Figure 10.10. Morphology of spermatid development can be studied using the periodic acid-Schiff (PAS) reaction, which stains deeply red, the glycoprotein material in the acrosomal structures (Figure 10.11).

Golgi Phase: The early spermatid has a small spherical nucleus 5-6 μm in diameter with a finely dispersed chromatin and several darker chromatin masses. The cytoplasm contains a Golgi apparatus near the nucleus and two centrioles at its periphery, as well as other organelles. During **Golgi phase**, small granules known as **proacrososmal granules**, which are stained intensely by PAS, appear in Golgi apparatus. Each granule is enclosed within a membrane-limited vesicle of the Golgi complex. As development progresses, the proacrosomal granules unite to form a single **acrosomal granule**, with its **acrosomal vesicle**. Later other vesicles from the Golgi apparatus contribute to the growth of the structure. The enlarged acrosomal vesicle becomes adherent to the nuclear envelope at the future anterior pole of the sperm nucleus. In the mean time, one of the two centrioles, located at the opposite pole of the cell, gives rise to the flagellum, which grows out of the cell though still enclosed within the plasma membrane. Golgi phase includes steps 1-4 in rat and steps 1-3 in man (Figure 10.11).

Cap Phase: The acrosomal vesicle spreads over the surface of the nucleus, forming a **cap**, which covers the anterior half or two-thirds of the nucleus. The two centrioles migrate from the periphery of the cytoplasm inward toward the nucleus. One of them, the proximal centriole becomes localized at the posterior pole of the nucleus, opposite the acrosome. The other, the distal centriole acts as a basal corpuscle for the flagellum, which has in the meantime elongated. This phase includes steps 5-7 in rat and steps 4-7 in man (Figure 10.11).

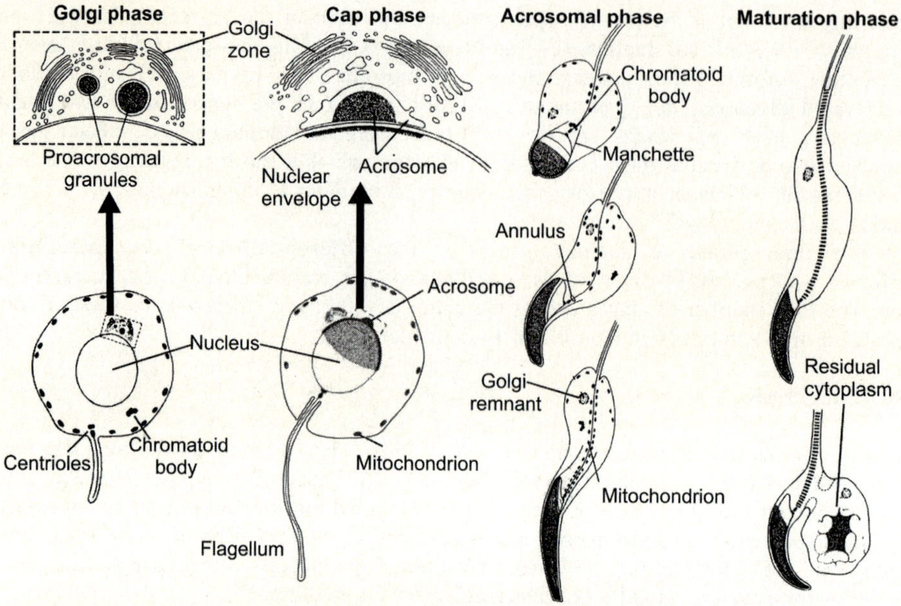

Figure 10.9: Phases of spermiogenesis in Rat.

Acrosomal Phase: This phase is characterized by profound modifications of the acrosome, the nucleus and the flagellum. It includes steps 8-14 in rat as seen in Figures 10.10 and 10.11. The nucleus moves from the canter to the periphery of the cell, becomes elongated and slightly flattened. Its chromatin condenses progressively into coarse dense granules. The spermatid now rotates so that the acrosome becomes directed toward the wall of the seminiferous tubule. The acrosomal apparatus adapts to the shape of the nucleus, and so varies in shape and size in different species according to the form taken by the elongating nucleus; it also becomes condensed in appearance. The mitochondria distributed at the periphery of the cytoplasm, migrate toward the portion of the flagellum inside the cytoplasm and surround it. These will develop later into the mitochondrial sheath of the sperm middle piece.

Maturation Phase: During this, the spermatid completes its transformation into a spermatozoon. The main features of this phase are the pinching off and phagocytosis of the residual spermatid cytoplasm by the Sertoli cells. A small portion of the cytoplasm, called the **cytoplasmic droplet**, remains attached to the mature spermatid around the initial part of the flagellum. The nucleus and acrosome take on the shape characteristic of the species. For example, in rat and mouse, nucleus is sickle shaped while in man, nucleus takes a flattened pyriform shape and acrosome surrounds $2/3^{rd}$ of its anterior portion. The annulus, which surrounds the flagellum a certain distance from the distal centriole, marks the limit between the middle piece and the principal piece of the flagellum. At the proximal part of the flagellum, the mitochondria arrange themselves helically forming the mitochondrial sheath of the middle piece. This phase includes steps 15-19 in rat (Figure 10.10). However, in man no clear-cut separation can be made between acrosome and maturation phases (Figure 10.11).

With the completion of the spermiogenesis, most of the excess cytoplasm is cast off in the form of a **residual body of Regaud**. Soon after the shedding of the residual bodies, the sperm heads are released from the Sertoli cytoplasm, which has so far tightly embraced the developing spermatids, and the spermatozoa are set free in the lumen of the seminiferous tubule. This process is called **spermiation**.

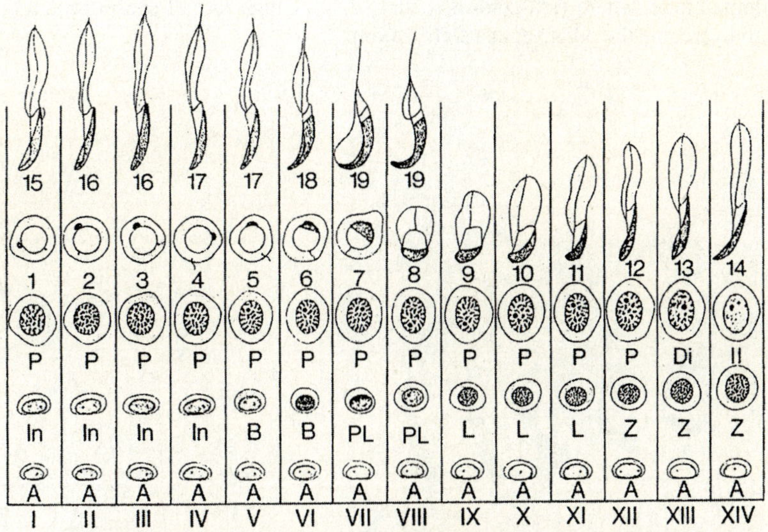

Stage (I-XIV) of the cycle in Rat (Numbers represent steps of the cycle)

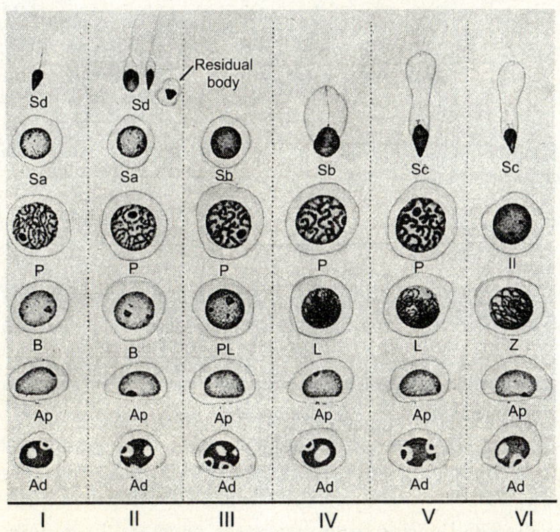

Stage (I-VI) of the cycle in Man

Figure 10.10: Cellular associations of the 14 stages in Rat and 6 stages in Man of the cycle in the seminiferous epithelium, A, In, B. Ad, Ap, B-Type A, Intermediate, Type B, Dark Type, Pale Type and B Spermatogonia, PL, L, Z, P and II-Preleptotene, Leptotene, Zygotene, Pachytene and Secondary Spermatocyte, 1-19 and Sa-Sd represent successive stages of Spermiogenesis in Rat and Man respectively.

The entire process of spermatogenesis, from primary spermatocyte to sperm formation, takes approximately 64 days in man. The normal human male manufactures approximately 30 million sperm per day. However, of this enormous number, only a few hundred may reach the distal portion of the female fallopian tube, where fertilization occurs. A very high rate of sperm production appears to be necessary to overcome the odds against fertilization.

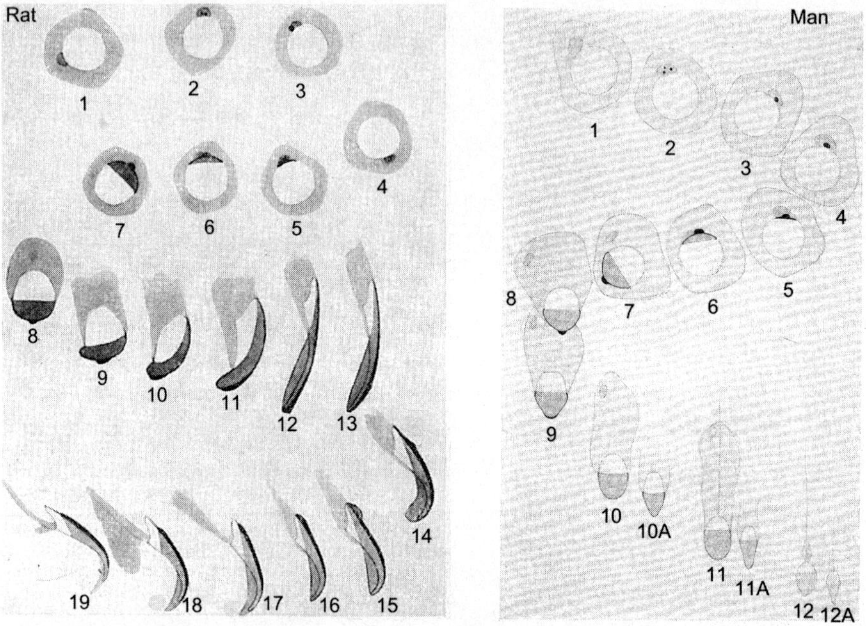

Figure 10.11: Spermiogenesis in Rat and Man as seen with Periodic-Acid-Schiff staining, drawings labeled A in Man show the spermatid in lateral view.

10.5 Spermatozoa

After leaving the seminiferous epithelium, the spermatozoa move slowly forward into the tubuli recti and the rete testis, and then through the efferent ducts to reach the epididymis.

Morphology of Spermatozoa: The mature human spermatozoa, is approximately 60 µm long and may be subdivided into two major parts, the **head** and the **tail** (Figures 10.12 and 10.13). The principal components of the head are the **acrosome**, and the **nucleus**. Segments of the tail, in order of their proximity to the head are designated as the **neck**, the **middle piece**, the **principal (main) piece** and the **end piece** (Figure 10.13).

The shape of the head varies from species to species. In human, it has a flattened pyriform shape and is 4.5 µm long, 3.0 µm wide and 1 µm deep. Head consists of two parts-nucleus and acrosome. The nuclear chromatin appears extremely condensed. The acrosome overlies the anterior 2/3rd of the nucleus like a cap and contains glycoprotein and numerous lysosomal enzymes that are probably important in fertilization.

The neck region consists of a pair of centrioles and nine segmented columns (connecting piece) that appear to merge with the nine outer dense fibers of the rest of the tail. The middle piece 5-7 µm long and nearly 1 µm thick extends from the neck to the annulus. It contains proximal portion of the characteristic 9+2 flagellum. The nine coarse fibers and the mitochondria adhering tightly to the coarse fibers are packed in a helical arrangement. The principal piece, extending from the annulus to the end of the tail forms main portion of the flagellum and is approximately 4.5 µm in length. The end piece is simply the terminal segment (5 µm) of the flagellum. It is composed of the axial filaments enclosed only within the plasma membrane.

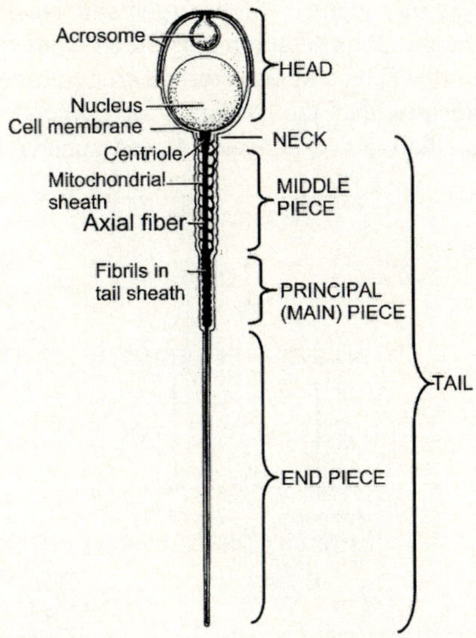

Figure 10.12: Structure of Human spermatozoon.

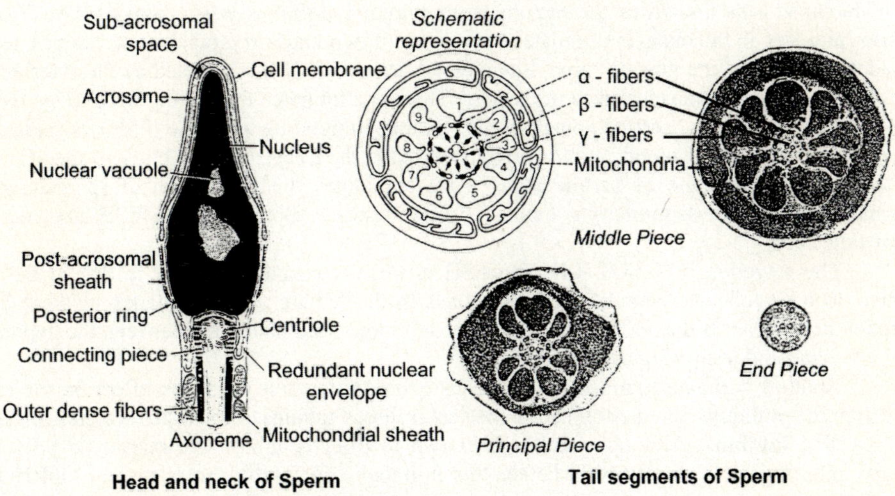

Figure 10.13: Sagittal section of head and neck region, and cross sections of the segments of tail of Human spermatozoa to show detailed structure.

10.6 Hormonal Control of Spermatogenesis

Very divergent views exist about the mechanism of action of gonadotropins and steroids in the onset of first spermatogenic cycle. The effect of gonadotropins on spermatogenesis is mediated by the Sertoli cells, which produce a variety of proteins important in spermatogenesis. Sertoli cells surround-developing spermatids with their cytoplasmic processes and nurture and coordinate the completion of sperm maturation in the seminiferous tubule. Steinberger and Ducket (1965) have suggested that hormones are not required for the initiation of spermatogenesis from early spermatogonial steps up to those of late pachytene stage and that FSH and testosterone are required only for the final stages of the spermatogenic cycle. This indicates that the initiation of spermatogenesis in the rat is possibly mediated by testosterone or other androgens and does not need gonadotropins.

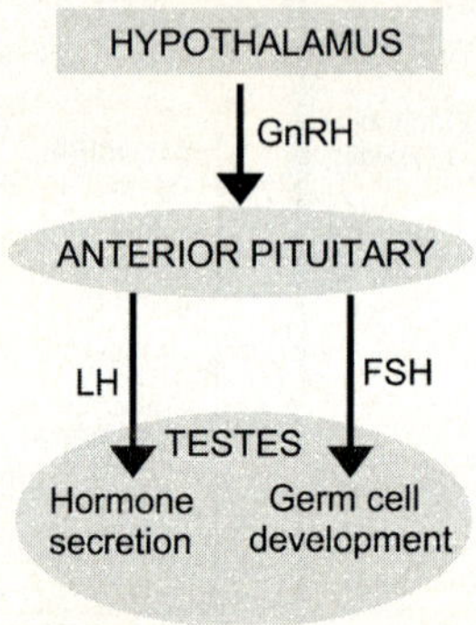

Figure 10.14: Relationship among the hypothalamus, pituitary and testes.

Neuroendocrine Control: The hypothalamus secretes a releasing factor called gonadotropin releasing hormone or GnRH (Figure 10.14). GnRH is transported to the anterior pituitary gland via a complex set of blood vessels known as the hypothalamic-pituitary portal vessels. When GnRH reaches the anterior pituitary in the male, it stimulates the release of two major reproductive hormones, termed the gonadotropins. The first gonadotropin, luteinizing hormone or LH, is secreted by the anterior pituitary into the blood, and is transported to the testes. There it stimulates the Leydig cells to synthesize and secrete testosterone. The second gonadotropin, follicle-stimulating hormone (FSH), is secreted by the anterior pituitary into the blood, and is also transported to the testes, where it binds to specific receptors on the plasma membrane of Sertoli cells. FSH stimulates the conversion of spermatogonia into spermatocytes in the seminiferous tubules of the testes. Both LH and FSH are required for spermatogenesis.

The secretion of GnRH, LH, and FSH is fairly constant from day to day in the male, in contrast to the cyclic secretion of these hormones in the female. The constancy of these hormones secretion in the male is due to the presence of a continuous feed back loop between the hypothalamus, pituitary gland and testes (Figure 10.15).

Another hormone secreted by the testes exerts a negative feedback effect on the release of FSH from the pituitary. The Sertoli cell in the seminiferous tubules of the testes secretes this hormone, and is called **inhibin**. Although inhibin is known to directly inhibit the release of FSH from the anterior pituitary, it is not known whether this hormone can inhibit the release of GnRH from the hypothalamus.

Sensory Stimuli: The hypothalamus receives neural inputs from a variety of brain areas involved in processing sensory stimuli. The amount of GnRH released by the hypothalamus is controlled by the excitatory and inhibitory neural signals that the hypothalamus receives. Visual, olfactory, or tactile stimuli are capable of altering GnRH release and hence the release of LH, FSH, and testosterone. In addition, thoughts, moods, and stress can also alter the secretion of these sex hormones. Figure 10.16 gives the concentrations of LH, FSH and testosterone during the seasonal sexual cycle of the ram, with different phases of testicular development. There is increase in frequency of the episodic peaks in LH during reactivation of the testes and vary marked increase in the concentrations of testosterone when the testes are fully developed.

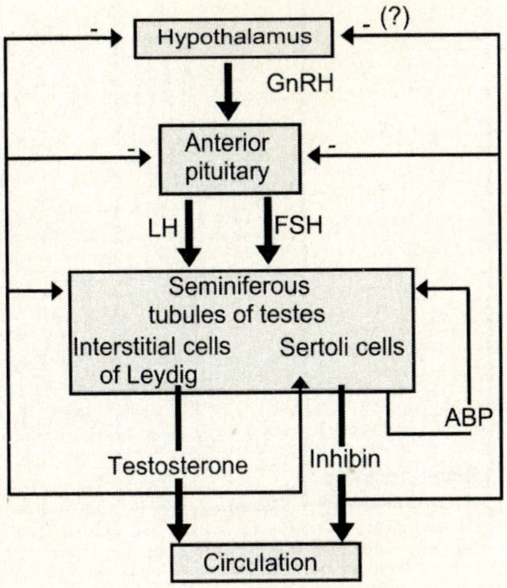

Figure 10.15: Hormonal feedback loops within the hypothalamus-pituitary-testes.

Effects of testosterone on spermatogenesis: Spermatogenesis requires the presence of high levels of testosterone in the seminiferous tubules. A decrease in testosterone production can result in sterility. Testosterone is thought to stimulate both the formation of spermatogonia and the second meiotic division that results in the formation of spermatids in the seminiferous tubules (Figure 10.17).

An interesting interdependence exists between testosterone and the Sertoli cells. Testosterone stimulates protein synthesis and fluid secretion from Sertoli cells, and the Sertoli cells in turn secrete androgen binding protein (ABP), which binds testosterone and keeps testosterone levels high in the seminiferous tubules.

10.7 Cycle and Wave of Seminiferous Epithelium

Investigations on the manner in which germ cells are associated in the seminiferous epithelium of mammals led Von Ebner (1871) and Regaud (1901) to define two important concepts, one dealing with the evolution of germ cells in time (called it **cycle**) and the other with their arrangement along the length of the seminiferous tubule (called it **wave**). Thus, examination of the seminiferous epithelium in all mammals, including human reveals that the germ cells are not arranged at random but are organized into well-defined cellular associations. For example, in a particular region of the seminiferous tubules, late spermatids at a given step in spermiogenesis occur only in specific combinations with early spermatids, spermatocytes and spermatogonia at respective steps of their development. These grouping of cells succeed one another in any given area of the seminiferous tubules and the sequence repeats itself indefinitely. Each recognized cell grouping represents a stage in the cyclic process and the series of successive stages occurring between two appearances of the same cellular association, in a given area of the seminiferous tubule represents the cycle of the seminiferous epithelium. Thus, the **cycle** of seminiferous epithelium is defined as the time interval between two successive appearances of the same cellular association in any given area of the seminiferous tubule.

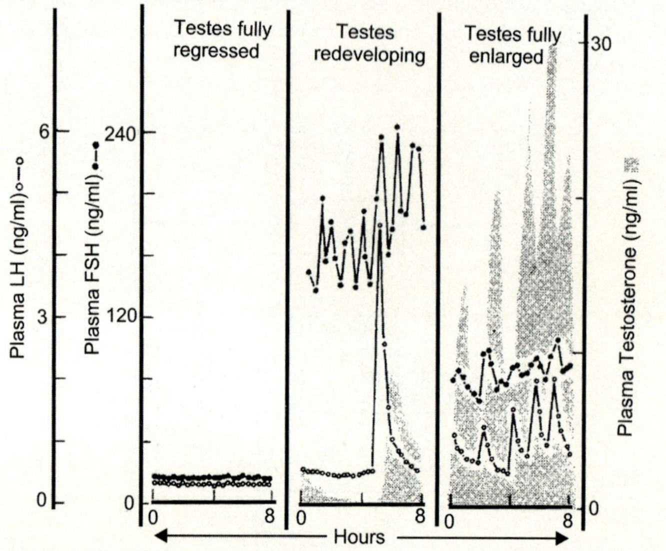

Figure 10.16: Concentrations of LH, FSH and Testosterone in plasma during the seasonal sexual cycle of Ram in different phases of testicular development.

The number of such stages in a cycle is constant for any given species. For example, rat has 14 stages in a cycle, the guinea pig and monkey has 12, and man has 6. The stages are designated by **Roman numbers** such as I, II III…XIV (Figure 10.10).

Whereas the cycle refers to changes occurring over a period of time in a given area of the seminiferous tubule, the concept of **wave** refers to the arrangement of the cellular associations in space at any given movement along the length of the seminiferous tubule (Figure10.18). Each complete series of adjacent segments containing the typical cellular associations of the cycle is defined as a wave of the seminiferous epithelium. In rat, each seminiferous tubule contains 12 waves measuring 2.6 cm on average (range is 0.7 to 6 cm). However, in man, comparable wave of seminiferous epithelium like that of rat etc. does not exist. Instead, different cell associations occupy different portions of the circumference in seminiferous tubule, forming a mosaic pattern in contrast to the linear pattern seen in subhuman primates and in lower species such as rodents (Figure 10.19). But the fundamental pattern of the cycle of the seminiferous epithelium is as characteristic of man as of other mammalian species.

In some places, the orderly sequence of the stages of the cycle along the tubule, called **'continuity of the segmental order'**, is disturbed by local reversal in the order of the consecutive stages.

The irregularities are termed "**modulations**" of the segmental order or simply a modulationTable 10.2 compares the characteristics of cycle and wave of seminiferous epithelium taking rat as an example.

10.8 Oogenesis

The whole process involved in the transformation of an oogonium into an oocyte and then into a haploid ovum is called **oogenesis** (Figure 10.20). It starts either during fetal development or shortly after birth.

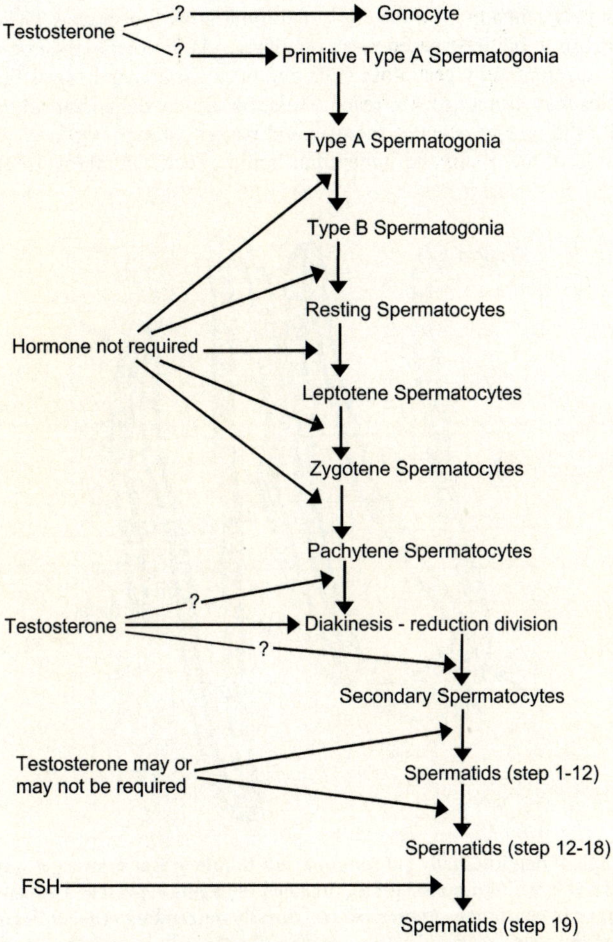

Figure 10.17: Schematic representation of hormonal control of spermatogenesis.

During early fetal development, primordial or primitive germ cells migrate from the endoderm of the yolk sac to the ovaries. These germ cells differentiate within the ovaries into **oogonia** (singular-**oogonium**). These are diploid cell (2n) and like spermatogenesis involve meiosis later in the process to form female gamete called **ova** (singular-**ovum**). These oogonia divide mitotically to produce millions of germ cells. Before birth, most of these germ cells degenerate through, a process known as **atresia**. A few, however, grow and develop into larger cells called primary oocytes. At birth, 200,000-2,000,000 oogonia and primary oocytes remain in each ovary. Of theses, about 40,000 remain at puberty, and only about 400 mature and ovulate during a woman's reproductive lifetime, while the remainder undergoes atresia.

The growth of oocyte is arrested during the last phase of meiotic prophase, i.e. the diplotene stage. The meiotic oocytes remain in this suspended state of meiotic arrest until meiosis is resumed shortly before either ovulation or atresia. The duration of meiotic arrest differs among species depending upon the length of the interval separating birth from start of reproductive life, as well as among individual oocytes depending on the start of follicle growth or atresia. The factors involved in meiotic arrest still remain to be determined more precisely. At diplotene, the oocyte nucleus shows 2n chromosomes. It is surrounded by granulosa cells and basal lamina and forms the primordial follicle. The primordial follicles may either grow to reach ovulation or may degenerate at various stages of their growth. At ovulation, the oocyte resumes meiosis and passes through two unequal meiotic divisions, leading to the formation of the ovum and three polar bodies, each containing 1n chromosomes (Figure 10.20).

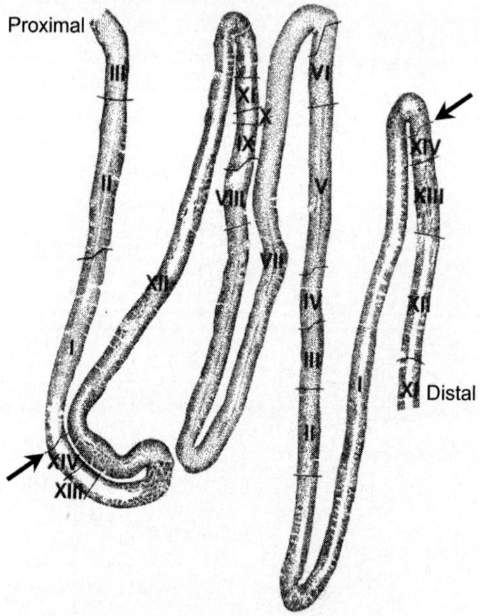

Figure 10.18: Photograph of longitudinally cut seminiferous tubule of Rat showing a wave (limits of the wave are indicated by arrows, it is without modulation), fourteen segments represent 14 stages of the seminiferous epithelium cycle arranged in continuous numerical and distally descending order to form a wave.

After the oogonia cease to divide, they enter reduction division phase and are called oocytes. The synthesis of DNA occurs during the last premeiotic interphase of the oogonium. The premeiotic DNA synthesis is an important event because this DNA persists throughout the lifetime of the oocyte, lasting until fertilization or atresia.

The germ cells, present in the central parts of the embryonic ovary close to the mesonephric connection, are the first ones to enter meiosis. Formation of follicles also starts in the same central part. Further formation of meiotic germ cells and follicles progressively extends towards the surface epithelium, as the outermost oogonia are the late ones to enter meiosis and form follicles. Estradiol is believed to interfere with the secretion of MIS (meiosis inducing substance) and MPS (meiosis preventing substance). Regulation of meiosis in fetal gonads is possibly dependent on enclosure of germ cells in compartments, on relative concentration of MIS and MPS within the germ cell compartment, and on the influence of steroid hormones. Two different cell types, namely the meiosis inducing (MI) cells and the meiosis preventing (MP) cells in fetal gonads of human and rabbit are believed to function antagonistically in regulating the gonadal sex differentiation and meiosis. Inversion of the MI cells is much more vigorous in developing ovary than that of MP cells and this leads to induction of meiosis.

Table 10.2: Comparison between cycle and wave of seminiferous tubule (example Rat)

Cycle	Wave
Similarities	
Cycle consists of 14 stages succeeding one another in time in any one area of the seminiferous tubule.	Wave consists of 14 segments following one another in space along the length of the seminiferous tubule.
Each stage is characterized by the presence of one of the 14 cellular associations.	Each segment is characterized by the presence of one of the 14 cellular associations.
Differences	
Duration of stage is constant, e.g. stage VIII lasts for 21 hours.	Length of segment is variable, e.g. segment VIII varies from 0.2 to 6.2 mm.
Transition between stages is gradual.	Boundaries of segments are sharp.
Sequence of stages is irreversible.	Series of segments may be altered by modulations.
Duration of cycle is constant, for example it is 12 ± 0.2 days in rat.	Length of wave is variable, the extremes being 0.7 and 6.0 cms.

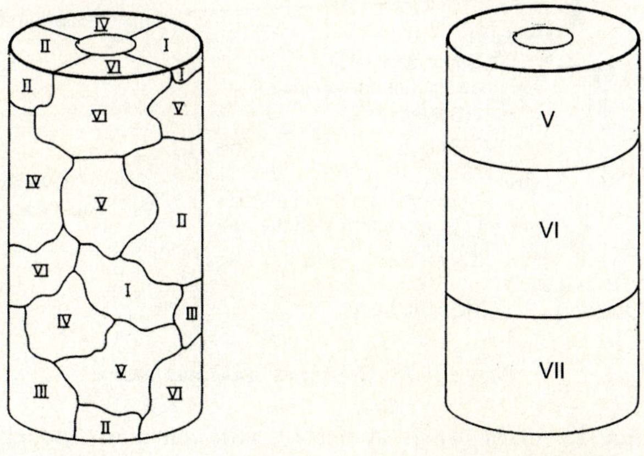

Man
Cell associations occupy small patch-like areas along the length of tubule

Subhuman species
Each cell association occupies a more extensive area along the length of tubule

Figure 10.19: Diagrammatic representation of distribution of stages of spermatogenic cycle in seminiferous tubule of Man and Sub-human species, Man-cell associations show mosaic pattern of distribution of stages.

Although meiosis shows similar events in male and female germ cells, the time schedule and the resulting number of haploid germ cells formed during spermatogenesis and oogenesis in testis and ovary respectively show great differences. The meiosis in the female germ cells initiates during early stages of ovarian development, often during fetal life. The first oogonia to start meiosis always occupy the inner parts of the ovarian cortex. But the meiosis is arrested in late prophase stage of the first meiotic division and further divisions are delayed until maturity (puberty time), and are completed around ovulation time. In contrast to female germ cells, the meiosis in the male germ cells starts at puberty and completes without delay. Also, the meiotic divisions are unequal in oocytes, thus leading to the formation of a single functional gamete (ovum/egg) and three abortive cells, known as the polar bodies. This is in contrast to the formation of four functional male gametes (sperms) from each spermatocyte.

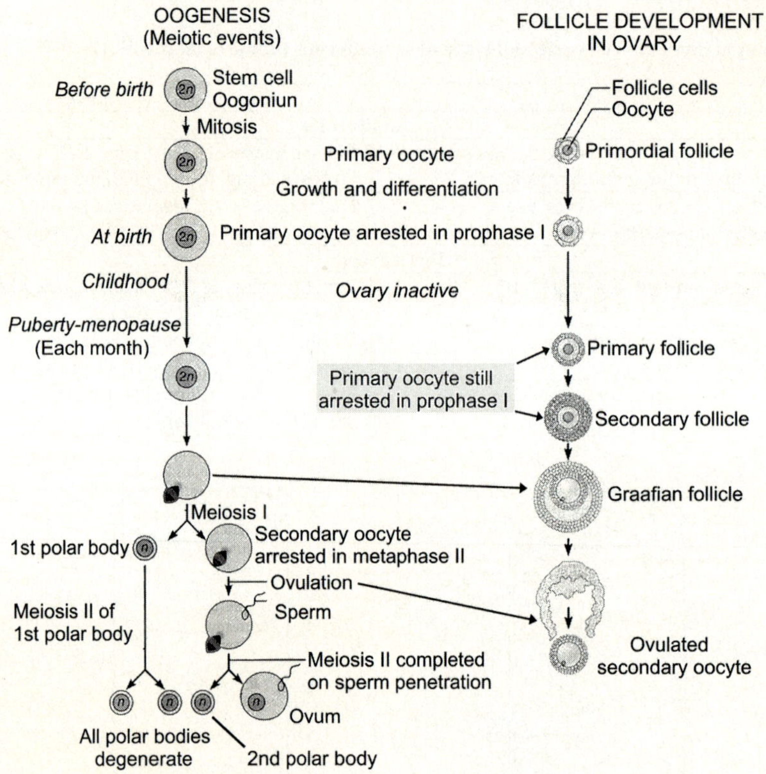

Figure 10.20: Oogenesis in Human ovary.

Gamete production in males begins at puberty and continues throughout life. However, situation is different in females. A female's total supply of eggs is determined at birth and the time span during which eggs are released at each cycle at ovulation extends only from puberty to menopause period in female life. Like spermatogenesis, oogenesis is divided into three phases: **the proliferation, growth** and **maturation.**

Proliferation Phase: The initial mitotic divisions resulting in the formation of large number of oogonia constitute the multiplication phase. This is followed by the growth phase in which the oogonium increases in size tremendously due to accumulation of lots of food material.

Growth Phase: At the start a human oogonium measures 0.02mm in diameter and its follicular covering consists of single layer of flattened epithelial cells. Through growth the oogonium increases in diameter seven-fold (0.14 mm) and is then called primary oocyte. In company with such enlargement on the part of the primary oocyte, the follicle cells become cuboidal, proliferate and form several cells thick encasement and form a cavity called the antrum. As the growth of the follicle continues to form mature or Graafian follicle, the oocyte becomes located more and more eccentrically. Growth of the follicle is slow at the start, but a rapid increase occurs in the last day or two before rupture (ovulation). The full-grown human follicle, that is, the primary oocyte is million time bulkier than the primary follicle, and its final diameter reaches to nearly 15 mm.

Maturation Phase: After a primary oocyte has finished its growth, the succeeding stages of oogenesis are devoted to the important process of maturation. The principal feature of maturation is two specialized nuclear divisions, the first one of which is the reduction division. Beginning at puberty, a small number of primary oocytes are activated each month. However, only one is "selected" to continue meiosis I, ultimately producing two haploid cell, each with 23 replicated chromosomes but of dissimilar size. The smaller cell is called the **first polar body** and the larger cell, which contains nearly all the cytoplasm of the primary oocyte, is the **secondary oocyte**. This is because, the spindle forms at the very edge of the oocyte (Figure 10.20). A little "nipple", into which the polar body chromosomes will be cast, appears at the edge to ensure that the polar body receives almost no cytoplasm or organelles.

The first polar body usually undergoes meiosis II producing two even smaller polar bodies. However, in humans, the secondary oocyte arrests in metaphase II and it is this cell (which is not a functional gamete yet) that is ovulated. If a sperm does not penetrate an ovulated secondary oocyte simply deteriorates, but if sperm penetration does occur, it quickly completes meiosis II, yielding one large **ovum** and a tiny **second polar body** (Figure 10.20). Therefore, at the end of oogenesis, **three tiny polar bodies**, nearly devoid of cytoplasm, and one **large ovum** are produced. All of these are haploid, but only the ovum is a **functional gamete.** This is quite different from spermatogenesis, where the product is four viable functional gametes-spermatozoa. Also, the unequal cytoplasmic divisions in oogenesis ensure that a fertilized egg has ample nutrient for its seven-day journey to the uterus. Without nutrient-containing cytoplasm, the polar bodies degenerate and die. The processes of male and female gamete formation are compared in Table 10.3 and Figure 10.21.

Table 10.3: Comparison between spermatogenesis and oogenesis in mammals

Spermatogenesis	Oogenesis
Spermatogenesis occurs in testes or male gonad.	Oogenesis occurs in ovaries or female gonad.
Four functional gametes are produced per meiosis called spermatozoa.	Only one functional gamete is produced per meiosis called ovum.
Growth phase is short, so increase in size of spermatogonium to form primary spermatocyte is little only.	Growth phase is prolonged with many fold increases in the size of oogonium to form primary oocyte.
Meiosis is initiated continuously in a mitotically dividing stem cell population.	Meiosis is initiated in a finite population of cells.
Meiosis is completed in days or weeks and there is no meiotic arrest.	Completion of meiosis is delayed for months or year and it is arrested at first meiotic prophase to allow the egg to grow.
Differentiation of gamete occurs while haploid, that is after meiosis ends.	Differentiation of gamete occurs while diploid, in first meiotic prophase.
Sex chromosomes are excluded from recombination and transcription during first meiotic prophase.	All chromosomes exhibit equivalent transcription and recombination during meiotic prophase.

Summary

The process of formation of gametes is termed as gametogenesis. In testis, it results in the formation of male gametes called spermatozoa by the process of spermatogenesis. In ovary, female gametes called ova are produced by oogenesis.

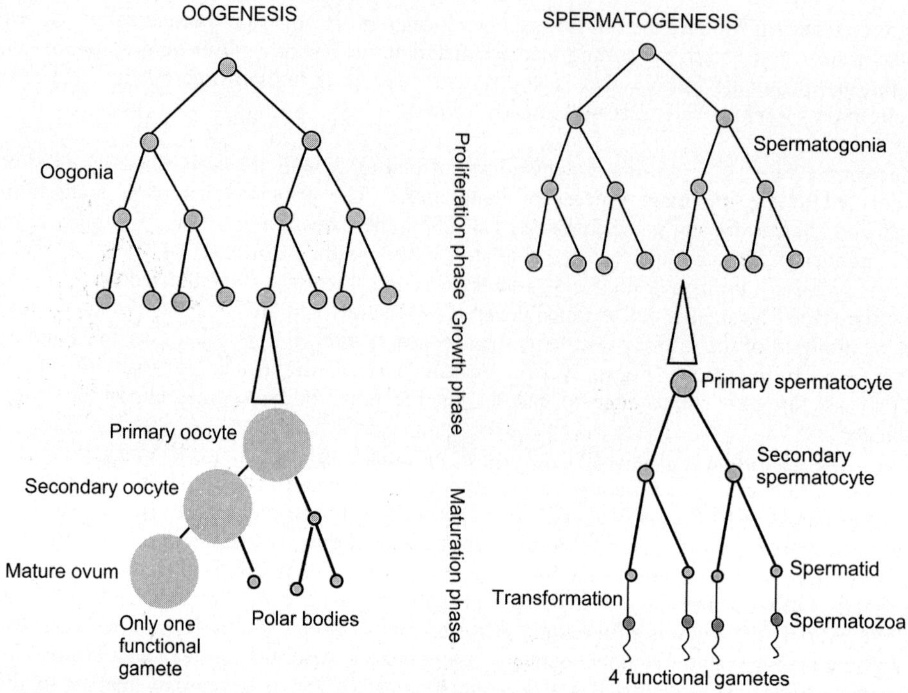

Figure 10.21: Comparison between spermatogenesis and oogenesis.

Meiosis is the basis of gamete production. It consists of two consecutive nuclear divisions without DNA replication in between. Meiosis reduces the chromosomal number by half and introduces genetic variability. Events unique to meiosis include synapses and crossover of homologous chromosomes. Meiosis inducing substances (MIS) and meiosis preventing substances (MPS) ratio regulates meiosis.

Spermatogonia divide by mitosis to maintain germ cell line and a few are kept as reserve while others enter the process of gamete formation. Spermatogenesis begins at puberty. It is divided into three phases, namely a) the division of spermatogonia leading to the formation of primary spermatocytes, b) the primary spermatocytes undergo meiosis I to produce secondary spermatocytes, which undergo meiosis II leading to the formation of four haploid (n) spermatids, and c) the differentiation of spermatids to form functional spermatozoa by spermiogenesis. During spermiogenesis, superfluous cytoplasm is stripped away and an acrosome and a flagellum or tail are produced. Sustentacular or Sertoli cells nourish spermatogenic cells and move them toward the lumen of the tubules. They secrete fluid for sperm transport and form the blood-testis barrier.

Gonadotropins, especially follicle stimulating hormone (FSH) regulates spermatogenesis and testosterone acts at the meiotic and post meiotic stages. The receptors for androgens occur in interstitial cells and Sertoli cells. The function of Sertoli cells is important for initiation and maintenance of spermatogenesis. The effect of FSH on androgen binding protein (ABP) synthesis by Sertoli cells resulting in local concentrations of androgen may be particularly related to the initiation of spermatogenesis. The transformation of testosterone into estrogen under the influence of FSH in Sertoli cells may also be important in the regulation of spermatogenesis.

Oogenesis begins in the fetus. Oogonia, the diploid stem cells of female gametes are converted to primary oocytes before birth. The female infant ovaries contain about 400,000 primordial follicles, each containing a primary oocyte arrested in prophase of meiosis I. At puberty, meiosis resumes, and each month, one primary oocyte completes meiosis I producing a large secondary oocyte and a tiny first polar body. Meiosis II of the secondary oocyte produces a functional ovum and a second polar body. However, it does not occur unless a sperm penetrates the secondary oocyte. The ovum contains most of the primary oocyte's cytoplasm. The polar bodies are nonfunctional and degenerate.

Questions

1. Describe spermatogenesis.
2. What is the importance of meiosis?
3. Describe the process of spermiogenesis.
4. Describe the structure of a spermatozoon.
5. Define cycle and wave of seminiferous epithelium. How do they differ from each other?
6. Give the hormonal control of spermatogenesis.
7. Describe the major events of oogenesis.
8. How is polar body formation beneficial to an egg?
9. How does oogenesis differ from spermatogenesis?

Chapter 11

Puberty, Adolescence and Menopause

The function of the reproductive system is to produce offspring. The gonads produce gametes (sperm and ova) and sex hormones, while all other reproductive organs are accessory structures assisting in reproduction. Most organ system of the body starts functioning from birth and function almost continuously throughout life to maintain the well being of an individual. The reproductive system, however, appears to "slumber" for initial few years after birth. It remains in a juvenile state during the first decade of life and at about ten years of age, hormone-directed changes start to occur in both sexes until puberty is reached.

11.1 Puberty and Adolescence

Puberty means a ripe age. In Latin, puberty is written as *pubescere* meaning to be covered with hair. It is the period of life, usually occurring sometimes between the ages of 10 and 15 years, when the reproductive organs grow to their adult size and become functional. It is the period when secondary sexual characteristics begin to develop and the potential for sexual reproduction is reached. The events of puberty occur in the same sequence in all individuals, but the ages at which these occur varies widely. During puberty, the reproductive organs, having differentiated many years earlier *in utero*, mature and start producing gametes. This period of final maturation is known as **adolescence** (Latin *adolescere* means to grow up). As such, adolescence is the period between childhood and adult life, but generally, it is considered to start with the development of secondary sex characteristics and to end when physical growth of the body stops. For example in humans, ages 11 to 20 for boys, and 10 to18 for girls is the adolescence period while puberty is the period in adolescence when sexual maturity is reached.

Thus, **puberty** is defined as the state at which the gonads come to maturity relative to their endocrine and gametogenic potential for reproductive function. These changes occur in response to rising levels of gonadal hormones, testosterone in males and estrogen in females. As such, the very first signs of puberty are due not to gonadal steroids but to increased secretion of adrenal androgens. The onset of this increase in steroids from adrenal is called **adrenarche**. The biological role and cause of adrenarche is unknown, and puberty can occur in the absence of adrenarche. Adrenarche occurs at the age of 8-10 years without any change in the secretion of cortisol or adrenocorticotropic hormone (ACTH). It may be due to a change in the enzyme systems in the adrenal so that more pregnenolone is diverted to the androgen pathway. In both sexes, these androgens cause the very early development of pubic and axillary (armpit) hair and also, the early stages of the total body growth spurt. All other puberal (pubertal) development however, reflects increased activity of the hypothalamic-anterior pituitary-gonadal system of hormones.

11.2 Onset of Puberty

The age at the time of onset of puberty is variable. It is generally attained any time between the ages of 8 to 15 years. In general, puberty starts one or two years earlier in girls than in boys (Figure 11.1). In Europe and USA, the age at the time puberty has been declining at the rate of approximately 1 to 3 months per decade in last 175 years. The statistic records show that in girls the age of puberty has decreased from about 16.5 years in 1850 to 13.5 years in 1970. In USA, it has been noticed that puberty occurs between the age of 8 and 13 in girls, and 9 and 14 years in boys. This is due to improvements in socioeconomic conditions, nutrition and general health amongst general public especially children. However, this trend has ceased during last few decades in the "developed world", suggesting the attainment of optimal conditions in terms of health to allow puberty to begin at a genetically determined age.

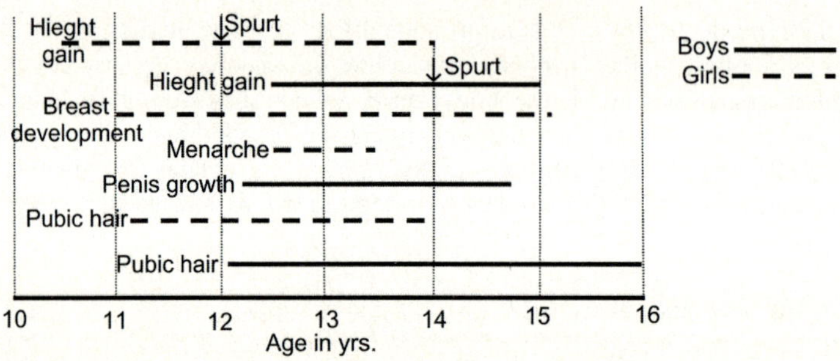

Figure 11.1: Comparison of the age between Boys and Girls at the onset of puberty.

Species-wise differences are noticed with regard to the age and body weight at puberty. It is believed that age of the animal is not the criterion in attaining the puberty but relative growth and body weight influence the onset of puberty. The period of puberty also varies in different breeds and is associated with nutritional status of the individual. The average age at puberty in exotic cows and in Indian cows of well-defined breeds ranges between 8-18 months and 24-50 months respectively. Buffaloes reach puberty between 24-48 months depending on the breed and environmental conditions. Mares reach puberty at about 18 to 25 months, while in ewes, puberty is reached by 8-12 months, and in goats at an average age of 6-18 months. Sows attain puberty between 6-12 months, cats between 6-15 months, bitches between 6-12 months and hens start laying eggs on an average at the age of 6 months.

In addition to the general state of nutrition and health of the individual, a number of other factors such as geography and genetics also influence both the onset and the course of puberty. Nutrition, specially increased protein intake, is the chief factor in attaining earlier sexual maturity. Malnutrition and chronic illness often delays puberty. Moderate obesity is associated with an earlier onset of puberty, while severe, morbid obesity delays onset of puberty. Genetic factor may also affect sexual development and attainment of puberty. There is a significant correlation of age at attainment of puberty between mother and daughter and also within ethnic populations, suggesting the influence of genetic factors. The effect of climate if any at all is slight on the onset of puberty, though higher altitude consistently seems to slow down sexual development.

11.3 Signs of Onset of Puberty in Female and Male

Onset of puberty is marked by the: i) structural and functional changes in the gonads, ii) onset of secretion of sex hormones, iii) development of functional interactions between hypothalamus, pituitary and gonads, iv) maturation of all reproductive organs, v) development of secondary sexual characteristics, and vi) a final spurt of growth in height (Figure 11.2).

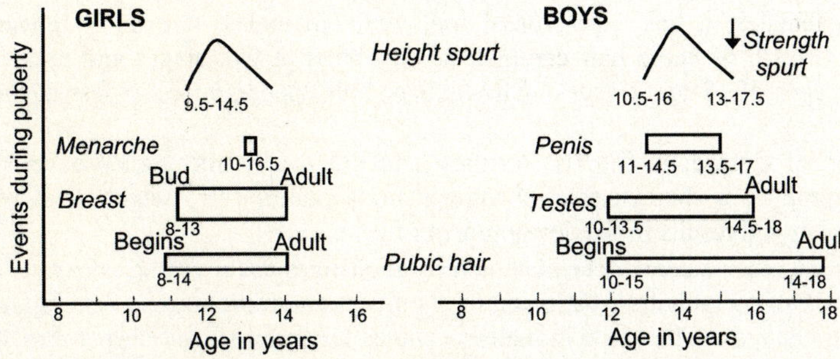

Figure 11.2: Changes associated with puberty in Girls and Boys, figures below each bar are the range of ages in years within which the event may begin and reach adult stage.

Changes occurring to attain puberty gradually take place over a period of 2-4 years. It begins in males with penile and scrotal growth and in females with breast development. Corresponding changes occur in different mammals, such as the development of mane in lions and antlers in deer. In small species such as rodents, which grow rapidly, puberty appears within a few weeks of birth, so that the young animals may be able to breed almost at once. But in large seasonal breeders e.g. deer, puberty may not be reached before the onset of winter, so the animals mature in the following year. Even larger mammals require from 3-7 years to reach puberty. Various somatic and sexual changes which occur during puberty are:

Growth of Reproductive Organs: Growth of reproductive organs during puberty occurs in both sexes. They increase in size and show functional manifestations. In females, the vulva takes an adult appearance, with growth of both labia majora and labia minora. The vagina takes a mature histological appearance with an increase in the thickness of its epithelial lining. The vaginal discharge becomes acidic (pH 4.5) as it contains lactic acid. The acid comes from the breakdown of glycogen present in the vaginal epithelium by Doderlein's bacilli, which invade the vagina at puberty and become normal inhabitants there. The increased thickness of the vaginal epithelium and the low pH of the secretions are protective mechanisms against ascending infection. The uterine body also grows during puberty so that it increases to about twice the length of the cervix and its muscle fibers also increase in bulk. The cervical glands start secreting a mucoid secretion. The lining of the uterus, and the endometrium proliferates under the influence of estrogens and subsequently respond to progesterone. These changes are responsible for the onset of menstruation.

Changes in the gonads, ducts, and accessory reproductive organs result in the attainment of reproductive capacity, so that sperm formation starts in male and ovulation begins in female.

Development of Secondary Sex Characteristics: A number of secondary sex characters develop in both the sexes that phenotypically define a male and a female. These changes are

- Distribution of Fat: The body shape (body contour) changes due to deposition of subcutaneous fat around certain areas, such as beneath the breasts, around thighs and hips and in the gluteal region. This change mainly occurs in the females.
- The Breasts: Development of breasts occurs in females and this takes place in five stages. The first stage is the infantile stage that persists from infancy until puberty. Further development of

breast occurs during puberal years and continues for 2-5 years (average 4 yrs.). Attainment of adult breast marks the fifth stage.

- Distribution of Pubic Hair: Distribution of hair in the pubic region shows a very characteristic pattern. In females, it has a horizontal top, while in males, it extends upward towards the umbilicus. Growth of pubic hair can also be described in five stages and is usually completed between the ages of 12 to 17 years. The axillary hair appears more or less at the same time as pubic hair.
- Development of Cutaneous Glands: Axillary and pubic apocrine glands develop and begin to function to produce a characteristic change in body odour. The secretion of sebaceous gland becomes thicker and results in the development of acne.
- In males certain other secondary sex characteristic changes occur during puberty. These are voice change, growth of facial hair, broadening of shoulders and more muscle development, in addition to behavioral changes. The voice in males becomes low-pitched and deeper due to growth of the larynx and elongation of vocal cords. Facial hair appears in males and the hairline recedes at the anterolateral aspects of the forehead, with a general increase of body hair. There is also an increase in skeletal growth and more muscle development. In behavior, boys become more aggressive and develop an interest in the opposite sex.
- Changes in Body Composition: This also is a prominent change during puberty. Prepubertal boys and girls start with equal lean body mass, skeletal mass, and body fat. But after attainment of puberty, men have nearly 1 ½ times the lean body mass, skeletal mass, and muscle mass of women, while women have twice as much body fat as men. Bone density also increases during pubertal development.

The Adolescence Growth Spurt: Around the age of puberty, growth of the body accelerates and becomes steep. This acceleration of growth is termed the puberty or adolescent growth spurt. In girls, the peak is reached around 12 years of age, while in boys, it is reached about two years later. In girls, the pubertal growth spurt begins in early puberty and is mostly completed by menarche (first menstruation), while in boys, it occurs toward the end of puberty. Total height attained during the pubertal growth spurt in girls is about 25 cm and in boys, it is about 28 cm. Also, the growth does not begin at the same time in all parts of the body.

Puberty in Girls: The first event associated with the onset of puberty in girls is **thelarche**, the development of breasts, followed by **pubarche**, the development of axillary and pubic hair, and then by **menarche**, the first menstrual period. Critical body weight or a critical amount of body fat is required for first ovulation or menarche. The initial periods are generally anovulatory and regular ovulation appears about a year later. In the female, gonadotropin releasing hormone (GnRH), the pituitary gonadotropins and estrogen are all secreted at very low levels during childhood. Accordingly, there is no follicle maturation beyond the early antral stage, and so menstrual cycles do not occur before puberty. Also, the female accessory sex organs remain small and non-functional, and there are minimal secondary sex characteristics. But as the age advances towards puberty, all the changes in ovaries, genital tract and secondary sexual characters become very evident. The average age of menarche is 13 years with a range of 10 to 16 years. Menarche is preceded by changes that begin around age 9-10. The ovaries begin to enlarge, young follicles start secreting estrogen, breasts enlarge and fat begins to accumulate between the glandular epithelium, pubic hair start appearing, the adolescent height spurt begins, and skin pigmentation becomes more apparent in vulva and areolae of the breasts. Once menarche occurs, changes in pelvis, internal organs such as uterus and vagina start to occur, axillary hair appears and pubic hair becomes dense. The uterus increases nearly tenfold in size between 10-15 years of age.

Puberty in Boys: Attainment of reproductive maturity in boys is also a gradual process but there is no dramatic change such as menarche or menstruation in female and for this reason, puberty is somewhat more accurately studied in girls than in boys. The changes at puberty in boys include growth of testes and seminiferous tubules (which were solid and dormant before puberty, but at the onset of puberty, start to become hollow), and increase in number of interstitial cells. The interstitial cells start synthesizing and secreting significant amounts of testosterone. Some viable sperm are produced early, yet full function of spermatogenesis develops slowly. The pubic hair develops. Adolescence growth spurt and growth spurt of penis and external genitalia begins. The voice deepens as the larynx enlarges and vocal cords thicken. The prostates and seminal vesicles mature and start secreting their characteristic secretions. Ejaculation is now possible. The appearance of spermatozoa in early morning urinary specimens is known as **spermarche** and it occurs at a mean chronological age of 13.4 years. If puberty starts earlier or later, the age of spermarche also changes accordingly. Axillary hair appears, sweat and oil glands enlarge, body fat decreases, and development of muscle progresses rapidly at this time.

11.4 Hormonal Control of Puberty

The onset of puberty is caused in large part, by an alteration in brain function that raises secretion of GnRH from the hypothalamus. Changing levels of gonadotropins (follicle stimulating hormone-FSH and luteinizing hormone-LH), Prolactin and the steroid hormones during development and maturation of gonads in both male and female (Figure 11.3) suggest maturation of hypothalamic-pituitary-gonadal inter-relationship.

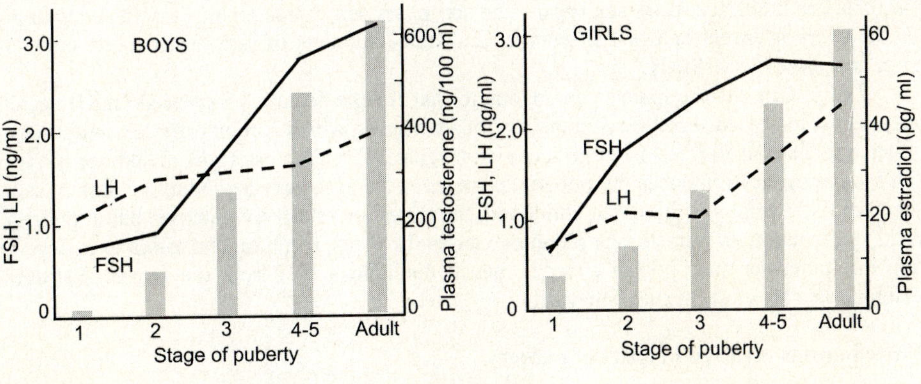

Figure 11.3: Changes in plasma hormone concentrations in Boys and Girls during puberty.

The male fetus shows lower gonadotropin levels than the female at mid gestation suggesting that the testis-pituitary axis starts functioning at this time in the male. Both morphological and biochemical initiation of germ cell division and Leydig cell differentiation at the time of sexual maturation in the male form the significant changes which are regulated by a variety of possible influences of intra-testicular and extra-testicular origin. For the onset of gonadotropic action on the testes, the pituitary initiates gonadotropin synthesis and secretion, testes develop functional gonadotropin receptors, and the hypothalamic regulation of gonadotropin secretion becomes functional. The initial source of gonadotropic stimulus in some species such as rat is the fetal pituitary whereas in others like human, it is the chorionic gonadotropin. The hypothalamic-hypophyesal testicular axis apparently becomes functional from birth onward and during pre-pubertal period. Testicular androgen production generally shows two active phases during development. The first occurs in the fetal-neonatal period, and the second in acquiring the adult condition. At least two factors including the plasma levels of pituitary gonadotropins and the testicular responsiveness to these hormones regulate the blood levels of the steroids during the fetal life of male. Depending on species, the mid- or late-gestational fetal testis produces large amounts of testosterone, which is known to induce masculinization of the male genitalia. The early pituitary-gonadal activity continues, or is reactivated during the first days or weeks of postpartum, but the physiologic role of this postnatal androgen production is not known. It may be involved in masculinization of certain region of the central nervous system, the testicular descent and priming of androgen dependent tissues for maturation in later life. The female differs in this regard from the male, as significant steroid production by the ovary does not begin until puberty. The postnatal activation of pituitary-gonadal function is due to the changed hormonal environment of the neonate and it eliminates the pituitary suppression by the high levels of placental steroid hormones at least in human. Besides the steroid hormone, the placental hCG (human chorionic gonadotropin) is also eliminated after birth. Many of the hormones produced by placenta are known to influence the development and function of the fetal-hypothalamic-pituitary gonadal axis in human. The serum levels of testosterone after showing a brief increase immediately after birth are decreased during the first week of life. This is due to the elimination of hCG, followed by a parallel increase in gonadotropin levels, which peak at 1-3 months of age to nearly adult male levels.

In the female rat and other mammals, a rise in estrogen concentration precedes the release of gonadotropins suggesting the requirement of this stimulating action of estrogen for normal release of gonadotropins. Effects of external and internal factors are transmitted to the hypothalamus, which in turn, regulate the release of gonadotropins during sexual maturation of the females. Thus, GnRH stimulates secretion of pituitary gonadotropins, which result in follicle development and estrogen secretion (Figure 11.3). Estrogen, in addition to its critical role in follicle development, induces the striking changes in the accessory sex organs and secondary sex characteristics associated with puberty. When the ovary is absent or when it secretes inadequate amounts of estrogen, puberty either fails to occur or progresses very slowly.

The picture for the male is analogous to that for the female. Increased GnRH secretion at puberty causes increased secretion of pituitary gonadotropins, which stimulate the seminiferous tubules and interstitial cells to start testosterone secretion (Figure 11.3). Testosterone, in addition to its critical role in spermatogenesis, induces the pubertal changes in the accessory reproductive organs, secondary sex characteristics, and sex drive. In childhood, the testes are relatively inactive, but at puberty (ages 11 to 13) until about 20, testosterone secretion causes the penis, scrotum, and testes to enlarge greatly. During this time, the male begins changes, which distinguish him from the female. Estrogens and testosterone also affect the sexual behavior.

11.5 Mechanisms involved in onset of puberty

A number of theories have been put forth to explain the mechanisms involved in the onset of puberty, but no single theory provides all necessary information. The **missing-link hypothesis** suggests that some component of brain-pituitary-gonadal axis is nonfunctional or missing before puberty. The **gonadostat hypothesis** suggests that there is a decrease in hypothalamic sensitivity to feedback inhibition by gonadal steroids before puberty. The **critical weight hypothesis** suggests that a young female cannot ovulate for the first time until she has accumulated a critical amount of fat relative to her lean body mass. However, there is no consensus of opinion as yet in either case. But, from all the available data, one thing seems clear that the central nervous system (CNS) is the structure, which receives the trigger to initiate and regulate the processes involved in attaining sexual maturity. It is assumed that areas of CNS concerned with onset of puberty, exerts their effects through the hypothalamic GnRH neurons. These neurons represent final common pathway of communication between the rest of the brain and the anterior pituitary gonadotropins (Figure 11.4).

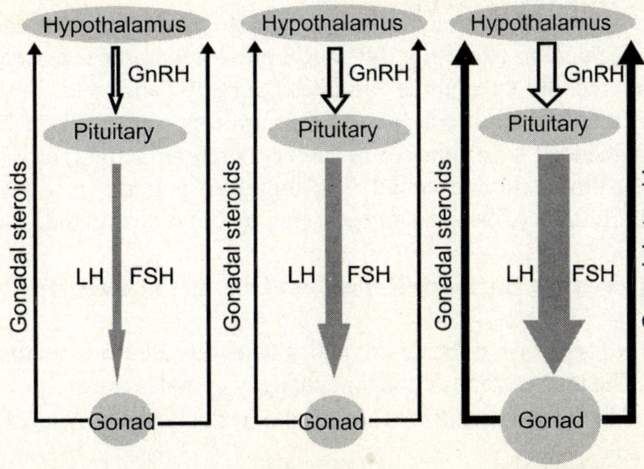

STAGE OF PUBERTY	Pre-pubertal stage	Onset of puberty	Adult stage
GONADOTROPHINS	Low	Increasing	Adult level
NEGATIVE FEEDBACK	Operative and sensitive	Decreasing in sensitivity	Operative at adult level
GONADAL STEROIDS	Low	Unchanged	Adult level

Figure 11.4: Gonadostat hypothesis of puberty illustrating the proposed decreasing sensitivity of the negative feedback mechanism to sex steroids during puberty which underlies increasing FSH and LH output, the latter then drives gonadal steroid production to reach adult level.

The mechanism of the brain change that results in increased GnRH secretion at puberty remains unknown. One important event is that, at the time of puberty, the brain becomes less sensitive to the negative-feedback effects of gonadal hormones. Also, the adipose-tissue hormone leptin is known to stimulate the secretion of GnRH and may play a role in the onset of puberty. This explains the accumulation of fat as energy stores in a girl's body during pubertal changes. The effect of leptin on GnRH could also explain why women who exercise extensively and become extremely thin lose their menstrual periods since such women would have low plasma concentrations of leptin. Whatever is the mechanism, the process is not abrupt but develops over several years, as evidenced by slowly rising plasma concentrations of the gonadotropins and testosterone or estrogen (Figure 11.3). In contrast to the situation in adulthood, removal of gonads during the period from soon after birth to puberty causes little or no increase in gonadotropin secretion, indicating that gonadotropin secretion is not being held in check by the gonadal hormones. In children between the ages of 7 and 10, a slow increase in estrogen and androgen secretion precedes the more rapid rise in the early teens.

Some children with brain tumors or other lesions of the hypothalamus may undergo precocious puberty, i.e. sexual maturation at an unusually early age. This is due to early secretion of increased amounts of GnRH. The youngest mother on records who gave birth to a full-term, healthy infant by Cesarean section (abdomen incision) has been 5 years, and 8 months.

11.6 Control of Onset of Puberty

Gonadotropins (FSH, LH or ICSH) are not secreted and are not found in the circulation in any significant amount prior to the beginning of puberty. However, the gonads of children can be stimulated by gonadotropins. In immature monkey, normal menstrual cycles can be brought on by pulsatile injection of GnRH, and these persist as long as the pulsatile injection is continued. In addition, GnRH is secreted in a pulsatile fashion in uteri. Thus, it seems that during the period from birth to puberty, a neural mechanism is operating to prevent the normal pulsatile release of GnRH. The nature of the mechanism inhibiting the GnRH pulse generator is unknown.

Since the hypothalamus initiates puberty and the brain controls the hypothalamus, environmental factors can affect puberty through this route. Thus, both, the onset and the course of puberty are influenced by a number of factors, such as geography, genetics, and the general state of nutrition and health of the individual. The timing of puberty in some mammals may be controlled by melatonin, a hormone synthesized and secreted by the pineal gland.

11.7 Male and Female Hormone Dependent Changes at Puberty

Changes at the onset of puberty in males and females are testosterone and estrogen dependent respectively. The testosterone dependent changes in males are:

- Growth of facial hair occurs. This results in the development of mustache and beard. The scalp line recedes.
- Hair appears on the chest, armpits, pubic region, and extremities.
- The testes, scrotum and penis begin to enlarge. The scrotum becomes pigmented with increased blood vessels and its skin becomes wrinkled. The penis enlarges in length and circumference. The prostate grows significantly at puberty.
- Vocal cords and larynx enlarge, thereby lowering the pitch of the voice. During pubertal changes, the voice is relatively hoarse and cracks, but gradually it changes into masculine bass voice.
- Skin thickness increases and deposition of melanin occurs thus making the skin take on a deeper color. The subcutaneous tissue becomes much stronger. Secretion from sebaceous glands on the face increase, and this result in the development of the acne. After a period of time, the skin adapts itself to testosterone's effect on the oil glands.
- Around age 13-14, a tender nodular plaque develops sometimes around the nipple on one or both breasts. This plaque disappears in 6-8 months, but sometime it may persist (a form of gynecomastia) and may cause a source of embarrassment to the boys.
- Muscle mass increases due to an increase of protein throughout the body.
- Growth of long bones increases to a rate of nearly 3 inches/year resulting in increase in size of bones. Strength of bone also increases due to increased calcium retention and quantity of bone matrix.
- Androgens produce a stimulatory effect on erythropoiesis (red blood cell production). Therefore, male has a higher red cell count and hemoglobin than female.
- Following puberty, aggressive behavior in males becomes pronounced.

The estrogen dependent changes in females are:

- It stimulates growth of internal reproductive organs, external genitalia, and breasts. Under the influence of female hormones, the vagina and the uterus increase their size and become thicker. Blood flow to the uterus increases, and muscle activity of the uterus becomes greater. The labia minora and majora enlarge and become pigmented. The breasts develop adult contours. Hips widen and pelvis takes on a contour more compatible with carrying a baby.
- It stimulates linear growth, and also accelerates early closure of the epiphyses of long bones. This results in a shorter height in women than in men.
- It stimulates the growth of body hair, but not to the extent it does in the male. Hair grows under the arms, and in the pubic area. Compared to male, more hair grows on the head.
- Skin changes are similar to male, with increased secretions of the sebaceous glands and a proneness to acne.
- It stimulates the "female pattern of fat distribution, that is, more fat in the hips, thighs, buttocks, and breasts.

11.8 Precocious and Delayed Puberty

Attainment of sexual maturity at an earlier than normal age is known as **true precocious puberty**. It may result from disorders of the hypothalamus (enhanced GnRH secretion) or may be of a constitutional or genetic nature. In addition, precocious gametogenesis and steroidogenesis can occur without the pubertal pattern of gonadotropin secretion. This represents the gonadotropin-independent precocity. It has been noticed in at least some such cases that the sensitivity of LH receptors to cells is increased because of an activating mutation in the G protein that couples it to adenyl cyclase. **Isosexual precocity** occurs in accordance with the phenotypic sex, and is due to estrogenic effects in a girl and androgenic effects in a boy. **Heterosexual precocity** is characterized by the development of sexual characteristics at variance with the phenotypic sex, and is due to androgenic effects in a girl and estrogenic effects in a boy.

Precocious pseudopuberty on the other hand is characterized by the development of secondary sex characters without the gametogenesis. This syndrome may arise due to abnormal exposure of immature males to androgen or females to estrogen, either of gonadal or of adrenal origin. High levels of circulating steroids exert a negative feedback inhibition of GnRH, resulting in a failure of gametogenesis, but secondary sex characters develop normally at puberty. In some girls breast development without other sexual characteristics can occur at an early age, and is called **premature thelarche**. Similarly, early appearance of axillary and pubic hair in association with increased androgen levels is called **premature adrenarche**. On the other hand, when appearance of hair is not associated with increased androgens, it is called **premature pubarche**. Girls with premature thelarche, adrenarche, or pubarche fall in the category of incomplete sexual precocity because menses, ovulation, and the ability to conceive do not exist.

Onset of puberty is considered delayed (**delayed** or **absent puberty**) if the menarche fails to occur by the age of 17 or testicular development by the age 20. It may arise due to panhypopituitarism, where all pituitary hormones including gonadotropins are absent, or due to defect at the level of hypothalamus, or an isolated deficiency in FSH or LH secretion. Delayed puberty due to deficiency in gonadotrpins as a result of GnRH deficiency is known as **Kallman's syndrome**. In some individuals, puberty is delayed even when the gonads are present and other endocrine functions are normal. This clinical picture is called **eunuchoidism in males**, and **primary amenorrhea in females**.

Causes of Precocious Puberty: In 85 % girls and 65 % boys, precocious puberty is **idiopathic** (when cause not found). Since premature activation of hypothalamic-pituitary axis is considered as the basic pathophysiologic mechanism in attaining precocious puberty, central nervous system (CNS) seems to be involved directly or indirectly in causing precocious puberty (Table 11.1). Although congenital anomalies, inflammatory processes, trauma, and tumors can lead to precocious puberty, no pathologic lesion is found in majority of cases. Pineal tumors rarely cause precocious puberty, however, lesions in the area of pineal gland may result in it. Primary hypothyroidism can cause precocious puberty in girls.

Table 11.1: Causes of precocious puberty

Involvement of Central Nervous System (CNS)		
Direct		**Indirect**
Congenital anomalies:	Hydrocephalus, Cysts	Hypothyroidism
Inflammatory processes:	Meningitis, Encephalitis, Brain abscess, Trauma	Neurofibromatosis (Von Recklinghausen's disease)
		Polyostotic fibrous dysplasia (Albright's syndrome)
Tumors:	Hypothalamic, Pineal	
Idiopathic		

Causes of precocious pseudopuberty are given in Table 11.2. Defects in the secretion of sex steroid is the main cause of precocious pseudopuberty in both males and females, and the sources of sex steroids are the testes, ovaries, adrenals, and non-endocrine organs such as liver or can be through exogenous administration. Testicular androgen production can be in Leydig cell tumors, or to a response to chorionic gonadotropin in choriocarcinoma, or in adrenal carcinomas/hyperplasia. Granulosa cell tumors of ovaries cause isosexual precocious pseudopuberty in nearly 60 % girls. Estrogen containing creams and vitamins, and ingestion of oral pills by a child may also lead to isosexual precocious pseudopuberty.

Table 11.2: Causes of precocious pseudopuberty

Isosexual		Heterosexual	
Males	**Females**	**Males**	**Females**
Testicular Tumors: Leydig cell Choriocarcinoma	Ovarian tumors: Granulosa cell Theca cell	Testicular tumors: Leydig cell Choriocarcinoma	Ovarian tumors: Arrhenoblastoma Hilar cell
Adrenal tumors: Arcinoma	Adrenal tumors: Carcinoma	Adrenal tumors: Carcinoma	Adrenal tumors: Carcinoma
Congenital adrenal Hyperplasia	Vaginal: Foreign bodies tumors, Trauma	Hepatocellular Carcinoma	Congenital adrenal Hyperplasia
Iatrogenic: Human chorionic gonadotropin Androgens	Latrogenic	Estrogen administration	Androgen administration

Clinical Manifestations, Diagnosis and Management: In girls, precocious puberty leads to development of breast and of pubic and axillary hair, and menstrual bleeding, and if androgens are involved, it will lead to voice changes, hirsutism, hypertrophy of clitoris, and short stature. In boys, it leads to early appearance of pubic and axillary hair, enlargement of phallus, voice changes, increased muscle mass, short stature, and also gynecomastia when chorionic gonadotropin or estrogen is involved.

Diagnosis and proper management of precocious puberty involves the correct identification of the cause with laboratory assistance and its elimination either surgically in case of tumors etc. or through administration of sex hormones.

11.9 Menopause and Climacteric

After puberty in females menstrual cycles continue at regular intervals into late forties or early fifties, when these usually become increasingly irregular. Then, in a few months or years, the cycles cease altogether. This period in life is called **menopause (female climacteric**). The phase of life beginning with menstrual irregularity and including the first year after cessation of menstrual flow is termed the **perimenopause,** the counterpart of puberty. Menstruation does not cease suddenly. A period or two may be missed from time to time over a year or more and finally, the actual menstrual flow becomes very scanty, occurs infrequently and ultimately ceases entirely. This is because ovaries become atrophied at this time and there are no mature follicles in them. The output of estrogen also becomes very low or absent altogether. In the absence of estrogen inhibition, follicle-stimulating hormone (FSH) is secreted in large quantities.

The term "climacteric" literally means running of a ladder". It is concerned with the stage of life when the gonads undergo degenerative or senescent changes. This applies to man and woman alike. If we view the ladder of life of the female, we learn that she matures sexually at about fourteen years of age when menstruation commences. Then at about the fiftieth year, another great change occurs called the climacteric. At this time menstruation ceases. This cessation is called the menopause. The two-term climacteric and menopause are not synonymous. The latter simply refers to the end of the monthly menstrual cycle while the climacteric embraces all the changes, which occur during this period. Psychologically, climacteric may be a very difficult period of life. Many women become highly irritable and emotional and start crying at the slightest provocation.

Menopause Age: Menopause begins before the age of 45 years in about 25 % of women, between ages 45 to 50 in 50 %, and after age 50 in 25 %. However, the general state of health and environmental factors may affect the time of onset of menopause.

Physiology of Menopause: The cause of menopause is aging of the ovaries. At birth, the ovary contains all the germ cells that have the potential to mature into ova during the reproductive life of a woman. From puberty, to about 35 years of cycling, few primary follicles remain to respond to pituitary gonadotropins. Consequently, the follicles no longer mature and ovulation does not occur. The hypothalamus and anterior pituitary function normally as evidenced by the fact that the gonadotropins are secreted in greater amounts (up to 10 times the levels in premenopausal women). This is due to diminished negative feedback effect of ovarian estrogens and progesterone on gonadotropin secretion. Thus, measurement of these gonadotropins from blood and urine can be used to confirm the onset of the menopause or climacteric (Figure 11.5A). A small amount of estrogen usually persists in plasma beyond the menopause, mainly from the peripheral conversion of adrenal androgens to estrogen, but the level is inadequate to maintain the estrogen-dependent tissues and therefore, cycle stops and menopause occurs.

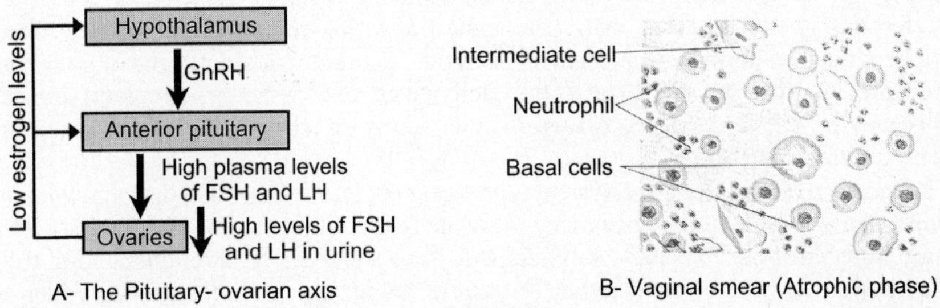

Figure 11.5: The Pituitary-ovarian axis (A) and Human exfoliated cells in vaginal smear (B) at menopause.

Symptoms and Signs of Climacteric/ Menopause: As a result of reduced estrogen concentration and lack of progesterone, the breast and genital organs such as vagina, uterus, and uterine tubes gradually atrophy to a large degree. The muscle of the uterus is gradually replaced by fibrous tissue. The vaginal smear during menopause is a typical "atrophic" smear. The dominant cells in this smear are rounded or oval basal cells of varied diameters, intermediate cells are scarce while neutrophils are abundant (Figure 11.5B). However, a vaginal smear from menopausal woman varies depending on the stage of menopause and levels of estrogen present in circulation. The vaginal epithelium may also disappear and the vaginal skin no longer contains glycogen. As a consequence of these changes, the bacteria (*Doderleins bacilli*), which are normally present in the vagina during reproductive span of a woman to act upon glycogen to produce lactic acid, also disappear. The vaginal pH thus rises from highly acidic to slightly alkaline (4.5 to 7.2) followed by a marked change in the vaginal flora and **vaginitis** becomes a frequent complaint of post-menopausal women. Thinning and dryness of the vaginal epithelium can also cause sexual intercourse discomfortable and painful (**dyspareunia**). Sex drive frequently stays the same and may even increase. This may be because the adrenal cortex continues to secrete small quantities of both male and female hormones, although it may also be influenced by the fact that a fear of pregnancy has been eliminated. The pubic and axillary hair becomes thin and the glandular tissue and ducts of the breast also atrophy as a result of estrogen withdrawal. Marked decrease in bone mass and strength, termed **osteoporosis** may also occur.

The hot flashes so typical of menopause are caused by periodic sudden increase in body temperature, which induces a feeling of warmth, dilation of the skin arterioles, and marked sweating. How estrogen deficiency causes this is unknown?

Another aspect of menopause is its relationship to cardiovascular diseases. Women have much less coronary artery disease than men until after menopause, when the incidence becomes similar in both sexes. This is due to the protective effects of estrogen, as it exerts beneficial actions on plasma cholesterol, and also exerts multiple direct protective actions on vessel walls. Atherosclerotic changes gradually occur due to a progressive increase in plasma concentration of cholesterol, triglycerides, and low and very low-density lipoproteins (LDL and VLDL). Some women also show emotional instability.

Most of the symptoms associated with menopause, as well as the increase in and death from coronary artery disease and osteoporosis can be reduced by administration of estrogen. This is called estrogen replacement therapy (ERT), which consists of estrogen delivered through a transdermal (skin) patch. The desirability of administering estrogen to post-menopausal women is controversial, because of the fact that long-term estrogen administration (more than 5 years) increases the risk of developing uterine endometrial cancer, and possible, breast cancer as well. The increased risk of endometrial cancer can be virtually eliminated by administration of a progestogen along with estrogen, but the progestogen does not influence the risk of breast cancer. However, numerous studies indicate that overall, hormone replacement therapy, definitely decreases mortality in post-menopausal women principally through estrogen's protective effects against heart disease. Recent development of certain substances, for example, **tamoxifen** that exert some pro-estrogenic and some anti-estrogenic effects seems to be beneficial in hormone replacement therapy. These drugs are collectively termed **selective estrogen receptor modulators (SERMs)** as they activate estrogen receptors in certain tissues but not in others. This may be due to existence of two distinct forms of estrogen receptors, which are affected differently by different SERMs.

Changes in male reproductive system with aging are less drastic than those in women. There is no "male menopause" similar to that occurring in women. Once testosterone and pituitary gonadotropin secretions are initiated at puberty, they continue, at least to some extent, throughout adult life. There is a steady decrease, however, in testosterone secretion, beginning at about age 40, which apparently reflects slow deterioration of testicular function. Along with the decreasing testosterone levels, both sex drive and capacity diminish and sperm become much less motile. Despite these events, many men continue to be fertile in their seventies and eighties. With aging, some men manifest increased emotional problems such as depression, and this is sometimes referred to as "**male menopause**" or **male climacteric**. However, what role hormone changes play in this phenomenon is not yet very clear.

Summary

Puberty is a stage in development characterized by sexual maturation, somatic growth, psychological changes and ability to reproduce. It is accompanied by physical and hormonal changes.

The age at the onset of puberty is variable. Puberty is generally attained any time between the age of 8 to 15 years.

Onset of puberty is marked by the: i) structural and functional changes in the gonads, ii) onset of secretion of sex hormones, iii) development of functional interactions between hypothalamus, pituitary and gonads, iv) maturation of all reproductive organs, v) development of secondary sexual characteristics, and vi) a final spurt of growth in height.

Puberty in males is marked by increase in testicular volume, increase in size of penis and external genitalia, appearance of facial, axillary, pubic, and body hair, growth spurt, and increased muscle mass.

In females, puberty is associated with breast budding followed by development of mature breasts, appearance of axillary and pubic hair, fat deposition, beginning of menses, growth spurt, and uterine, endometrial, and vaginal changes.

Puberty appears to develop as a result of a decrease in the sensitivity of the feedback mechanism controlling the secretion of the gonadotropin releasing hormone, thus, leading to an increase in plasma FSH, and LH concentrations, gonadal stimulation, and subsequent maturation.

Pubertal changes are dependent on testosterone in males and on estrogen in females.

Precocious puberty is the development of sexual characteristics with maturation of gonads and adult sexual function such as menses or spermatogenesis before the expected age of 8 years for girls and 10 years for boys respectively

In precocious pseudopuberty, sexual development occurs, steroid sex hormones are overproduced, but gonadal maturation does not occur. It is usually caused by adrenal or ovarian abnormalities. It is caused by regression of the ovaries. There is a progressive decrease in the number of follicles and therefore, progressively less estrogen.

Around the age of 50, a woman's menstrual periods become less regular and ultimately disappear. This is called menopause. It is the period of reproductive senescence in women. The cause of menopause is a decrease in number of follicles and their hypo responsiveness to gonadotropins. The physical symptoms of menopause are those produced by a lack of estrogen, and therefore, most of the effects of estrogens induced during attainment of puberty are slowly reversed during menopause.

Men show a steady decrease in testosterone secretion after nearly forty years of age but there is no complete cessation of reproductive functions as seen in females and they remain fertile. This is because changes in male reproductive system with aging are less drastic than those in women and thus there is no male menopause similar to that seen in women.

Questions

1. What is puberty? How does it differ from adolescence?
2. What are the factors and signs of onset of puberty in male and female?
3. Which hormone initiates the changes associated with male sexual maturity?
4. Describe the male secondary sex characteristics.
5. What are the estrogen-dependent changes in the females at the onset of puberty?
6. What are the causes of precocious and delayed puberty?
7. List three secondary sex characteristics of females.
8. Define menarche. What does it indicate?
9. What are the changes that may occur at menopause?

Chapter 12

Male Reproductive System

The organs of the male reproductive system are the **testes**, a **system of ducts**, **accessory sex glands** and the **several supporting structures** such as the scrotum and the penis.

Testes are the male gonads that produce sperm and secrete male hormones. These are located externally in the scrotum. The system of ducts of male reproductive system consists of in order from testis, the vasa efferentia (ductuli efferentes), the epididymis, the ductus deferens (vas deferens), and the urethra. The urethra opens to the outside at the tip of the penis. The duct system assists in the maturation and storage of spermatozoa in the epididymis and in transporting and conveying them to the exterior during ejaculation. The accessory sex glands in males are the seminal vesicles, prostate gland, the bulbourethral glands (Cowper's glands), the glands of Littre and the preputial glands. These glands secrete various secretions that contribute to the formation of seminal plasma of the semen. The accessory sex glands empty their secretions into the ducts and urethra during ejaculation. The male organ penis helps in depositing the semen through ejaculation during sexual intercourse into the female genital tract. Figure 12.1 presents a posterior view of reproductive system in man.

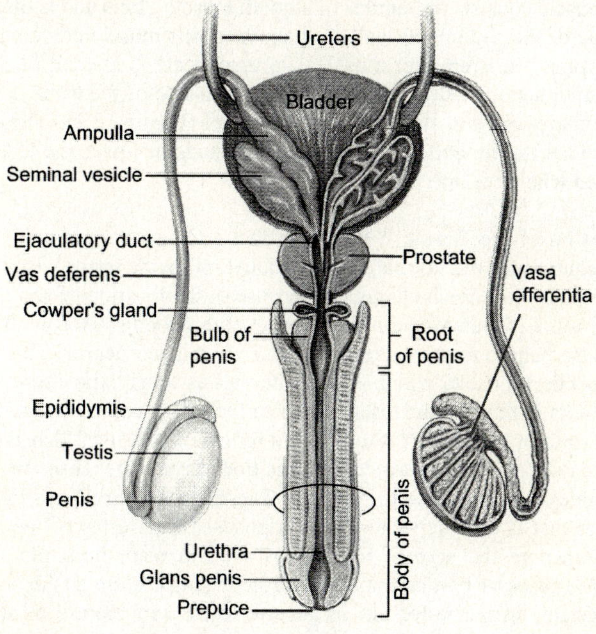

Figure 12.1: Reproductive system of Man in posterior view.

12.1 Scrotum

Scrotum literally means bag. It is a sac consisting of loose pouch of skin, muscle and superficial fascia (sheets of connective tissue) that hangs from the root or attached portion of the penis. The testes are located in the scrotum.

Scrotum is the supporting structure formed by an out pouching of the abdominal wall and therefore, lies externally below the abdomen. Externally, the scrotum looks like a single pouch of skin separated by a median ridge called the **raphe** into lateral portions, one for each testis. A **septum** divides the scrotum internally into two sacs. Each of these sacs contains one testis.

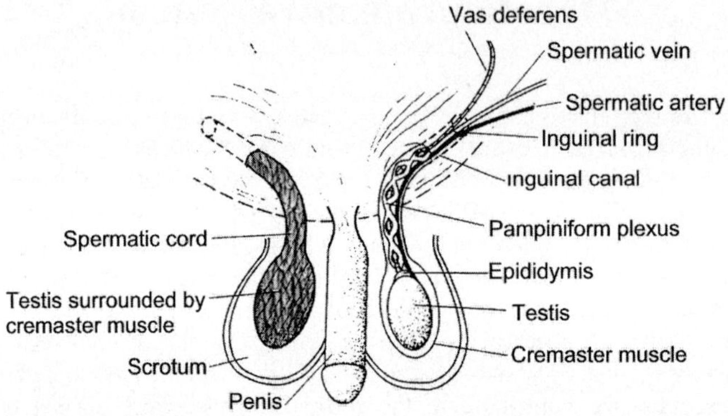

Figure 12.2: Scrotal structures, left side-superficial dissection and right side-internal details.

The scrotum consists of superficial fascia and muscle tissue called the dartos (skinned) muscle. The dartos muscle consists of bundles of smooth muscle fibers and is directly continuous with the subcutaneous tissue of the abdominal wall so that, when this muscle contracts, it causes wrinkling of the skin of the scrotum. The cremaster muscles, "a suspender" is a small band of skeletal muscles that arise and are in continuation with the internal oblique muscle of the trunk. The cremaster muscle extends down the spermatic cord and also surrounds the testes (Figure 12.2). These muscles elevate the testes bringing them closer to the abdomen in the cold periods or lower the testes by dropping them away from the abdomen when it is hot.

Temperature Regulation of the Testis: It is known that a temperature about 2-3 °C below the core body temperature is required for the normal sperm production by the testes. This lower temperature is maintained and regulated by two mechanisms. i) Because of the location of scrotum outside the pelvic body, the testis temperature is maintained at a lower level than body. And ii) the contractions of the scrotal muscle fibers also help to regulate the temperature to a lower degree. This is done with the help of the cremaster (suspender) muscle, which elevates the testes upon exposure to cold and also during sexual arousal, and results in moving the testes closer to the pelvic cavity, where they can absorb body heat. Exposure to warmth or during hot weather, the process is reversed that is the testes are moved away from the pelvic cavity and in turn away from the body heat. The dartos muscle also contracts in response to cold and relaxes in response to warmth. These muscular reflexes in the testes ensure and maintain a temperature that is conducive to spermatogenesis. The testes of mammals are not always held outside the abdomen in the scrotal pouches as seen in man, bull, ram, dog, rat etc. Also, abdominal testes are not necessarily maintained at the same temperature as the body owing to counter-current blood flow systems in the testes but in general lower temperature of scrotal testes does not appear to be the reason for their migration into scrotal sacs.

The blood supply of the scrotum is derived from the internal pudendal branch of the internal iliac artery, the cremasteric branch of the inferior epigastric artery, and the external pudendal artery from the femoral artery. The scrotal veins follow the arteries. The scrotal nerves are derived from the pudendal nerve, posterior cutaneous nerve of the thigh, and ilio-inguinal nerves.

12.2 Testes

The testis begins its appearance during the fifth-sixth week of fetal life from a primitive undifferentiated gonad (Chapter 8). It develops from three structures; **germinal or coelomic epithelium** (giving rise to the seminiferous epithelium), **mesenchymal cells** (giving rise to Leydig cells and the Sertoli cells), and **primordial germ cells** (giving rise to the spermatogonia).

Structure: The testes or testicles are paired oval glands located externally in the scrotal sacs (Figure 12.1). Each **testis (plural- testes)** in human measures about 4.5 cm in length, 2.5 cm in breadth, and 3 cm in the antero-posterior diameter and weighs 10-15 grams. The testes are surrounded anteriorly and laterally by a serous sac called the **tunica vaginalis** (*tunica* = sheath), derived from peritoneum (Figure 12.3). Posteriorly the serous sac is lacking and the testis lies behind and outside the tunica vaginalis. Immediately deep to the tunica vaginalis, the testis is covered with a thick white fibrous capsule called the **tunica albuginea** (*albu* = white). The inner aspect of tunica albuginea or underneath the tunica albuginea is the **tunica vasculosa**, which is a loose layer of connective tissue rich in blood vessels. The tunica vasculosa merges with the stroma of the testis known as the **intertubular** or **interstitial connective tissue**. At the posterior margin of the testis, the tunica albuginea thickens greatly and is projected into the interior of the testis as the **mediastinum testis** or **corpus Highmori**. Ducts, blood vessels, lymphatic, and nerves enter or leave the testis through the mediastinum and the interstitial connective tissue of testis becomes continuous with the connective tissue of the mediastinum. From the mediastinum, delicate connective tissue septa known as the **septula testis** (singular- septum of testis) radiate into the organ and blend with the tunica albuginea at various points (Figure 12.3). The septula subdivide the interior of the testis into a number of pyramidal lobules known as the **testicular lobules**, with bases directed toward the periphery and apices at the mediastinum. The septula do not form complete partitions, instead the tubules anastomose with each other in numerous places. There are about **250 testicular lobules**. Each testicular lobule contains several intricately sperm producing coiled tubules known as the convoluted **seminiferous tubules** (*semin* = seed; *fer* = to carry). These are surrounded and supported by intertubular connective tissue.

The seminiferous tubules are long, extremely convoluted and are seen therefore, sectioned in various planes (Figure 12.4). These are lined with several rows of highly specialized epithelium, which rests on a thin basement membrane. The seminiferous tubule epithelium contains inside the **spermatogenic cells** and the **supporting cells**, also known as the **Sertoli cells** (Figure 12.4). The spermatogenic cells are the elements of **spermatogenesis** at various stages of developent, and thus consist of **spermatogonia, spermatocytes, and spermatids** arranged in several concentric rows from periphery towards tubule lumen respectively. The intertubular or interstitial connective tissue is rich in blood vessels and fills the spaces occupying the intervals between the seminiferous tubules. It is filled with blood vessels, lymphatic, nerves, macrophages, fibrocytes, lymphocytes and groups of epithelioid cells known as the **Leydig cells** (the **interstitial cells** or **interstitial endocrinocytes**). The interstitial cells of Leydig are the endocrine cells and are responsible for the production of **male sex hormone** called **testosterone**.

The seminiferous tubule form coiled loops having single, double, or even triple arches. Both limbs of an arch are not always in the same lobule and lateral branches that pass through the incomplete interlobular septa establish communication between the tubules of adjacent lobules. Toward the apex of a lobule or at the junction of the testis and mediastinum, the **convoluted tubule** of each lobule converges to form a narrow **straight tubule**. The straight tubule has a short duct lined with cuboidal or low columnar epithelium. These tubules pass into a series of **rete testis tubules** that lie in the connective tissue of the mediastinum and empty their contents at both ends into the rete testis. Rete testis is a series of irregular anastomosing epithelial lined channels with broad lumens and thin walls of cuboidal or low columnar epithelium. The straight tubules and rete testis form the beginning of the male genital duct system.

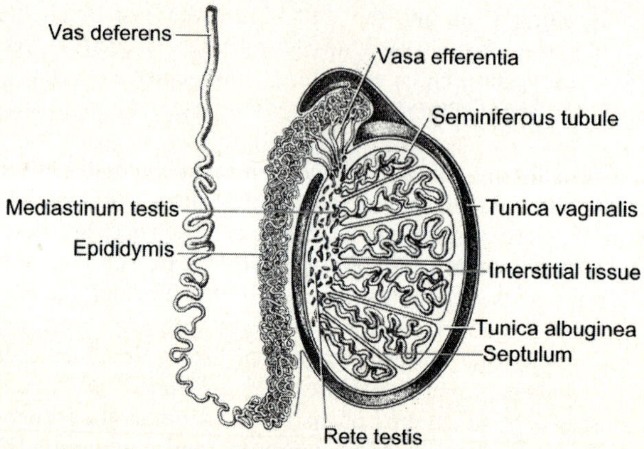

Figure 12.3: Diagrammatic section of Human testis.

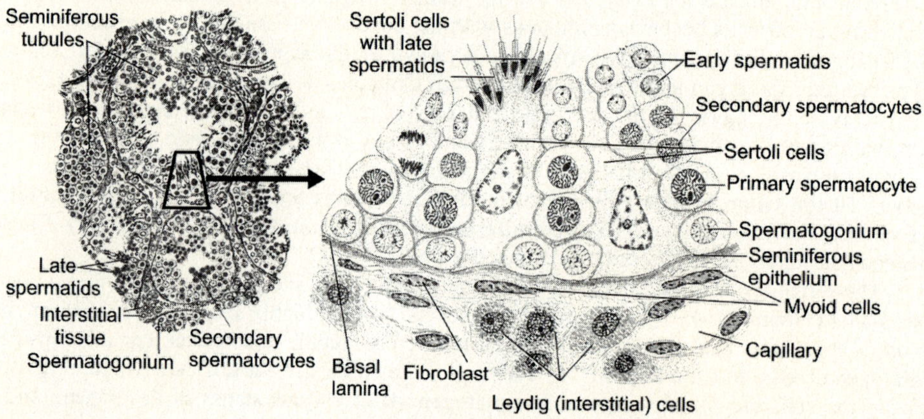

Figure 12.4: Transverse section of Human testis and enlarged view of a part of it.

From the rete testis arise eight to fifteen tubules known as the **ductuli efferentes (efferent ductules** or **vasa efferentia**). The rete testis tubules become wider as these approach the efferent ductules. The efferent ductules are straight tubules at their origin, but become highly convoluted as these pass into the **head of the epididymis**. **Spermatozoa** and **testicular fluid** produced within the testicular tubule pass into the **ductuli efferentes** and **epididymis** via the **rete testis** (Figure 12.3). Anastomosis and branching of the seminiferous tubules are common in man. When uncoiled, each seminiferous tubule can measure up to 80 cm in length and 150-250 μm in width.

Blood Supply to Testis: A distinctive feature of mammalian testis is the **testicular artery**, which becomes highly convoluted as it approaches the testis (Figure 12.5). A venous pampiniform plexus surrounds the testicular artery. It is a **thermo-regulatory device** for pre-cooling arterial blood. Therefore, in addition to the scrotal location and its cremaster muscles, pampiniform plexus also helps to maintain and regulate the testicular temperature to somewhat lower degree than the rest of the body, which is required for normal sperm production. Some branches of testicular artery enter the testis through the mediastinum while others pass over the periphery of the testis in the tunica vasculosa. Lymphatic vessels are numerous in the tunica albuginea and extend along the tubules. The testes have both a vasomotor and a sensory innervation. The blood vessels and nerves do not penetrate into the seminiferous epithelium.

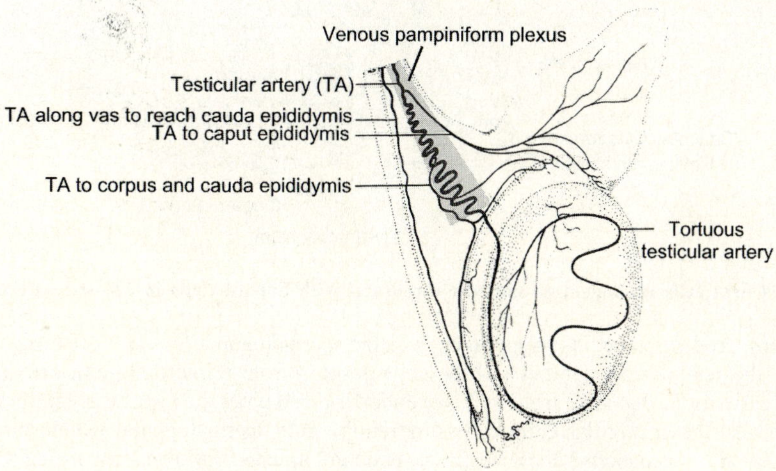

Figure 12.5: Blood supply to testis and epididymis.

The Seminiferous Tubule: The seminiferous tubules are bounded by a constant number of clearly defined acellular and cellular layers. The wall of the convoluted seminiferous tubule consists of an outer capsular layer called **tunica propria**. It is a fibro elastic connective tissue layer with flattened fibroblasts that closely invests the tubule (Figure 12.4). A thin homogeneous **basement membrane** and a lining of a **complex stratified epithelium** follow tunica propria. The tunica propria (the fibro-elastic layer) is the acellular layer forming a clear zone containing fibrils of varying orientation. On its periphery, a thin collagenous reticulum, which is a layer of flattened cells called the **myoid cells** is followed by lymphatic endothelial cells. The myoid cells constitute an important part of the boundary tissue or wall of the seminiferous tubules along with non-cellular material. Collectively, the structures surrounding the epithelium, mainly the myoid cells are responsible for the rhythmic movements of seminiferous tubules and may assist in the propulsive movements of sperm and testicular fluid from the seminiferous tubules to the rete testis. In many instances of male infertility, the boundary layers of the tubules become greatly thickened.

The seminiferous tubules are lined by a highly complex and specialized stratified epithelium forming the cellular layer. In adult, this epithelium is composed of two populations of cells: i) **nonproliferating** population of **supporting cells** known as the **Sertoli cells** and ii) a **proliferating** population of **germ cells** (**spermatogenic cells**) that migrates continuously from the periphery to the tubule lumen. The germinal element consists of successive generations of cells arranged in well-defined four to eight concentric layers occupying the space between the basement membrane and the lumen. These cells include from the periphery to the lumen of the tubules, spermatogonia, spermatocytes and immature and mature spermatids (Figure 12.6).

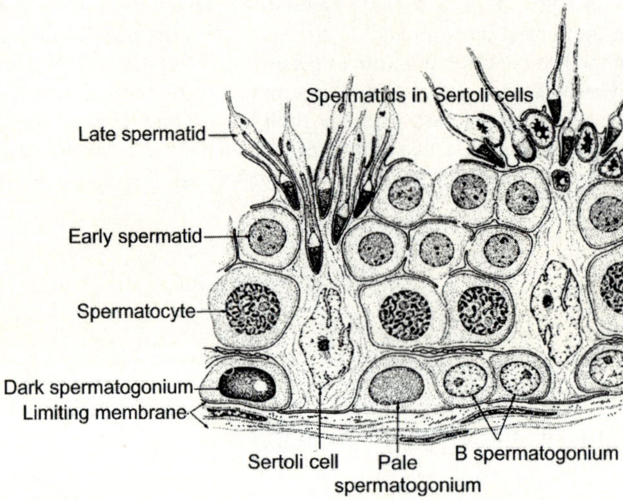

Figure 12.6: Germ cells arrangement and their relation with Sertoli Cells in the seminiferous tubule of Human testis.

Sperm production begins in sperm cells called spermatogonia (*gonia* = offspring) that line the periphery of the seminiferous tubules. These cells develop from primordial germ cells (*primordia* = primitive or early form) that arise from yolk sac endoderm and enter the testes early in fetal life. In the embryonic testes, the primordial germ cells differentiate into spermatogonia, which remain dormant during childhood. At puberty, they begin to undergo mitosis, followed by meiosis, and finally differentiate to produce sperm (Chapters 10 and 11). Once a sperm cell or spermatozoan (*zun* = life, sperm and spermatozoa are plural terms) is formed, it is retained in the lumen of the seminiferous tubule for a short time and is then released into the rete testis to reach the epididymis via vasa efferentia (ductuli efferentes) for its maturation and storage. The process of release of spermatozoa into the rete testis is known as **spermiation**.

Sertoli cells: The **Sertoli** or **sustentacular cells** are nondividing slender, tall irregular columnar elements, embedded among the spermatogenic cells inside the seminiferous tubules (Figure 12.6). The Sertoli cells occupy a pivotal position in the seminiferous epithelium as they extend from the basement membrane to the tubule lumen. The sides of Sertoli cells are markedly uneven, showing pits and depressions into which fit the adjoining germ cells. Each Sertoli cell consists of a basal portion, an intermediate portion and an apical portion. Basal portion of the cell is voluminous and contains an irregularly shaped nucleus. The nucleus is ovoid, pale staining, with finely dispersed chromatin. It usually contains one or more prominent nucleoli. The position of the nucleus varies in different Sertoli cells from the basal position to a considerable distance from the basement membrane. The intermediate portion of Sertoli cell provides lateral processes around which the spermatocytes and spermatids are arranged while the apical projection of Sertoli cells encloses the late spermatids just prior to their release into the tubule lumen. Thus, mature or nearly mature spermatozoa are frequently observed in the active tubule, with their heads in close attachment with the cytoplasmic processes of the Sertoli cells, and their tails extending out into the lumen. Free spermatozoa in the lumen of the tubules are relatively rare, because as soon as they are detached from the Sertoli cells, they pass into the epididymal tubules and are stored there.

The Sertoli cells are the only cells that extend from the basement membrane to the tubule lumen, thus giving a structural organization to the seminiferous tubule and also have contacts with all the other cell types in the epithelium. The Sertoli cells are joined to one another by specialized attachments called **tight junctions** (Figure 12.7). As a result, the Sertoli cells form a ring around the inner diameter of the seminiferous tubul. Pairs of Sertoli cells are also joined to one another by junction complexes that have an extremely intricate morphology. These complexes prominently bring the two cell surfaces very close together. The intercellular spaces between pairs of Sertoli cells are thus divided into a **basal compartment** between the boundary tissue and the junctions and an **adluminal (central) comapartment** above the junctions. All stages beginning with any given spermatogonium are present between the same two Sertoli cells. Spermatogonium A and B are found only in the basal compartment between the tight junctions of Sertoli cells and the basement membrane of the tubule. After several mitotic cycles (A to B spermatogonia), type B spermatogonia give rise to primary spermatocytes, which cross a tight junction and come in the central compartment, enlarge, divide and complete further development there. Because of this arrangement, the processes at the apical end of each Sertoli cell support and nourish the developing spermatids. The Sertoli cells have cytoplasmic processes that increase in number and size at the time when the spermatids are maturing. Thus, the Sertoli cells exhibit a cyclic activity that is correlated with the stage of spermatogenesis in any given region of the seminiferous tubule.

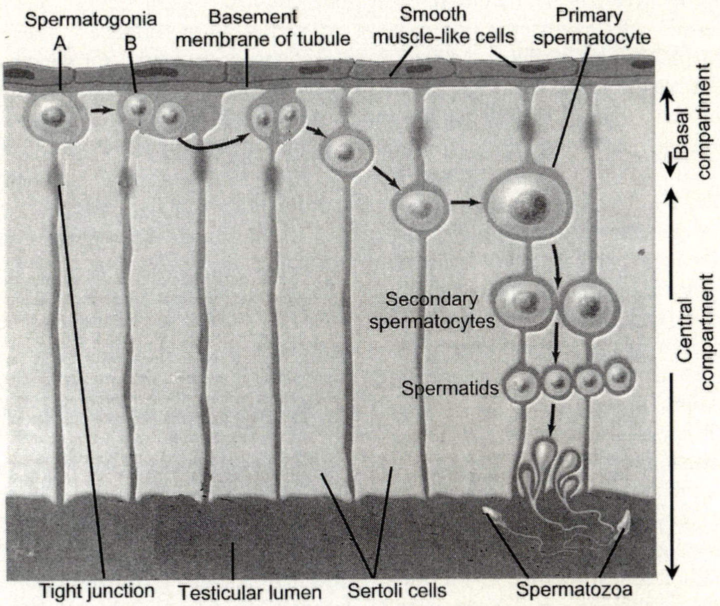

Figure 12.7: Tight junctions of Sertoli cells and their relation to germ cells, Sertoli cells form a ring as barrier around the entire tubule, all stages beginning with any given spermatogonium take place between the same two Sertoli cells.

Functions of Sertoli cells: Sertoli cells play many functions: I) They provide support and nutrition to the developing germ cells or sperm. 2) They release late spermatids into the tubule lumen. 3) Tight junctions join the neighboring Sertoli cells to one another and form the blood-testis barrier. The blood-testis barrier largely isolates developing germ cells metabolically and immunologically from the rest of the body. By isolating the spermatogenic cells from the blood, the barrier prevents an immune response against the spermatogenic cell surface antigens, which are recognized as foreign by body's immune system 4) Sertoli cells bring about cell-to-cell communication. 5) They secrete paracrine agents that influence the function of Leydig cells. 6) They synthesize and secrete luminal fluid, androgen binding protein (ABP) and a protein hormone called **inhibin**. 7) They phagocytize and remove damaged germ cells and defective sperms. 8) They secrete during embryonic life Mullerian inhibiting substance (MIS), which causes the primordial female duct system to regress.

One of the important functions of the Sertoli cells is to form a blood-testes barrier, which prevents many substances from entering or leaving the seminiferous tubule. For example, this barrier prevents a variety of hormones, proteins, ions, and drugs from entering the tubule, some of which could otherwise destroy the developing spermatogenic cells. Also, the barrier keeps the sperm in the tubules from diffusing into the blood. Mature sperms are very immunogenic, and if they enter the blood, they would be recognized as foreign proteins, and may result in the production of antibodies specific to them. The blood-testes barrier develops at the time of puberty, just before the beginning of spermatogenesis, and provides a protected environment in which sperm development and maturation can occur.

Further, the Sertoli cells secrete its fluid mainly in the lumen of the seminiferous tubules. This fluid is rich in enzymes, proteins, nutrients, androgens, and certain ions such as potassium and bicarbonates. These chemicals stimulate and nourish the developing sperm, and the fluid provides a drive for flushing sperm out of the tubules into the epididymis.

The Sertoli cells synthesize two proteins of particular importance. These are **androgen binding protein (ABP)** and inhibin. Both of these proteins are essential for spermatogenesis. The androgen binding protein is secreted into the seminiferous tubular fluid, where it binds to testosterone and increases the concentration of testosterone within the seminiferous tubules of the testes. Inhibin is secreted into the blood and transported to the pituitary gland, where it regulates the secretion of FSH.

Functions of the Testes: The testes contain two major components. These are the Leydig cells (interstitial cell) and the seminiferous tubules. The Leydig cells comprise the **major endocrine component** of the testes, and the primary secretory product of these cells is the male hormones mainly testosterone. Testosterone is responsible either directly or indirectly for embryonic differentiation of the internal and external genitalia along the male lines, secondary sexual developments of male at puberty, and maintenance of libido and potency in the adult male. On the other hand, the seminiferos tubules comprise the bulk of the testes and are responsible for the **production of male gametes**, spermatozoa. Approximately 30 million spermatozoa per day are produced during male reproductive life, i.e. from puberty to death.

Reproduction in males is achieved with the help of spermatozoa, which are produced within the seminiferous tubules. The steroids, which are of primary importance in male reproductive function, are testosterone, dihydrotestosterone, and estradiol, though testosterone is the most important androgen. The testicular Leydig cells secrete over 95 % of the testosterone and the remainder is derived from the adrenals. In addition to testosterone, the testes secrete small amounts of dihydrotestosterone (a potent androgen) and the weak androgen dehydroepiandrosterone (DHEA) and androstenedione. The Leydig cells also secrete small amounts of estradiol, estrone, and pregnenolone, and 17 α-hydroxypregnenolone and 17 α-hydroxyprogesterone. Details of steroid hormones and their functions are given in Chapter 5.

Control of Testicular Function: Hypothalamic-Pituitary-Testicular Axis: Both the above-mentioned components of the testes, the Leydig cells and the seminiferous tubules, are interrelated and also, both require the presence of an intact hypothalamic-pituitary axis for initiation and maintenance of their function.

Development and maintenance of genital ducts and glands, and the secondary sex characteristics in males is mediated by testosterone, which is a hormone secreted by the Leydig cells of the testis, under the influence of luteinizing hormone (LH) of the anterior pituitary. LH in males is also called as interstitial cell stimulating hormone (ICSH). Testosterone also plays an important role in the process of spermatogenesis. FSH is mainly responsible for the initiation of spermatogenesis, while full maturation of the spermatozoa appears to require both, FSH and testosterone.

The hypothalamus synthesizes a decapeptide, gonadotropin-releasing hormone (GnRH) and secretes it in pulses every 90 to 120 minutes into the hypothalamo-hypophyseal portal blood. After reaching the anterior pituitary, GnRH binds to the gonadotropes and stimulates the release of the gonadotropins, FSH and ICSH both into the general circulation (Figure 12.8). Secretions of these hormones are regulated by feedback mechanisms (Chapter 2). LH is taken up by the Leydig cells to result in the secretion of androgens. In turn, the elevation of androgens inhibits the secretion of LH from the anterior pituitary through a direct action on the pituitary and also exerts an inhibitory effect at the hypothalamic level. Both the hypothalamus and the pituitary have androgen and estrogen receptors. However, the major inhibitory effect of androgen on the hypothalamus appears to be mediated principally by estradiol that may be derived locally through the aromatization of testosterone.

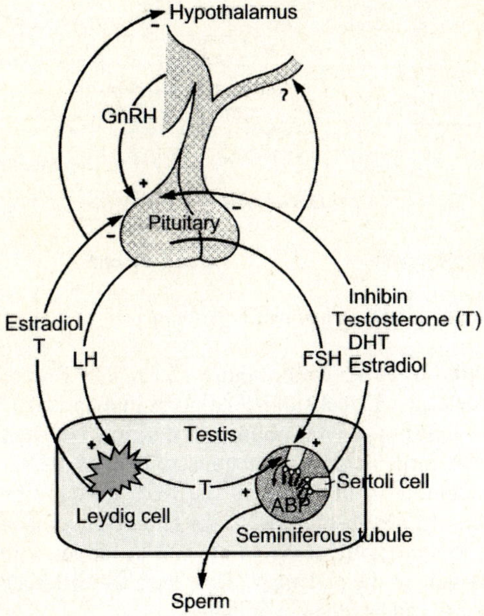

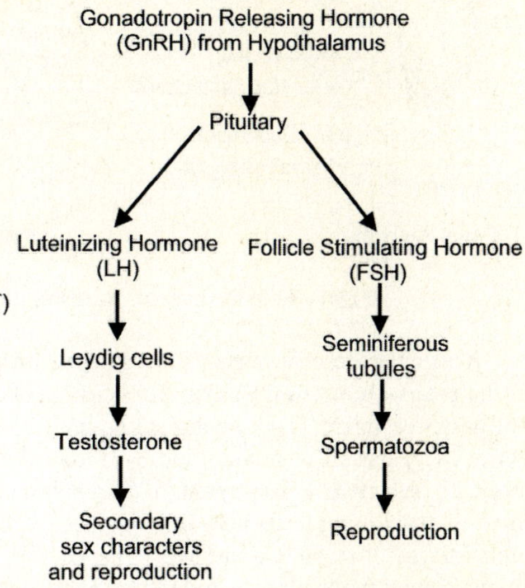

Figure 12.8: Regulation of testicular function by hypothalamus and pituitary, ABP-androgen binding protein, DHT-dihydrotestosterone.

After stimulation by GnRH, FSH is also secreted into the systemic circulation. This hormone binds to specific receptors in the Sertoli cells and stimulates the production of androgen binding protein (ABP). The major action of FSH on initiation of spermatogenesis is via this stimulation of ABP production. FSH secretion is inhibited by the hormone inhibin, which is also produced by the Sertoli cells of the seminiferous tubules. FSH directly stimulates the Sertoli cells to secrete inhibin, and therefore inhibin is probably a physiologic regulator of pituitary FSH secretion, possibly together with the gonadal steroids.

Descent of the Testes: Testis develops near the kidney, in the posterior portion of the abdomen. During fetal development, the testes are located in the abdomen, but in the adults, testes are located externally in the scrotum. Testes usually begin their descent into the scrotum during the later half of the seventh month of the fetal development. Thereafter, testes remain suspended in the scrotum. Descent of testes occurs through the inguinal canals, which are pathways in the anterior abdominal wall. During descent toward the scrotum, testes drag along their developing vas deferens, supplying blood vessels and nerves also behind them (Figure 12.9). These structures later take part in the formation of the **spermatic cord** by which the testis is suspended in the scrotum. The male sex hormone, testosterone, secreted by the developing testes stimulates the testes to descend into the scrotum. A fibro- muscular cord called the **gubernaculums** guides and aids the movement of the testes through the **inguinal canal**. This cord is attached to each developing testis and extends into the inguinal region of the abdominal cavity. It passes through the abdominal wall and is fastened to the skin on the outside of the scrotum. This descent is essential for the normal sperm production during adulthood, since sperm formation requires a temperature several degrees lower than the normal internal body temperature.

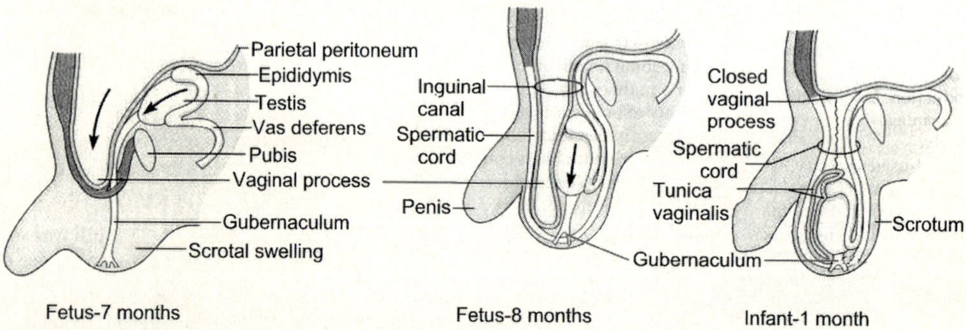

Figure 12.9: Descent of the testes during fetal development in Human.

Testicular descent occurs in **two separate phases** as shown in Figure 12.10. The first one is called the **trans-abdominal phase**. It occurs between 10-15 weeks of gestation in human and 15-19 days of gestation in rat. The second is known as the **inguino-scrotal phase** and it occurs between 26-35 weeks of gestation in human and 3-21 days after birth in rats. The trans-abdominal descent is produced by selective enlargement of the gubernaculums in the male as the fetus enlarges and it anchors the developing testis near the inguinal region. In contrast to this, in the female gubernaculum does not enlarge or swell and the ovary moves with the enlarging uterus in humans or moves with the ascending kidney in developing rodents and thus remains in the abdomen. However, the difference in gonadal position at the end of the first phase is greater in rodents than in humans.

12.3 Cryptorchidism

In most males the testes descend in the scrotum before birth. However, in a few males, testes fail to complete the descent into the scrotum. Such an abnormality is called **cryptorchidism**.

Cryptorchidism (*crypt* = hidden; *orchid* = testis) is the condition in which the testes (one or both) do not descend into the scrotum and remain in the abdominal cavity or remain lodged in the inguinal canal. It occurs in nearly 3 % of full-term infants and about 30 % of premature infants. The incidence of cryptorchidism decreases from 1 in 10 at birth to 1 in 50 by the first year of life and 1 in 250 at puberty time. **Unilateral Cryptorchidism** is the condition in which testis of one side only (a testicle) fails to descend into the scrotum. The term cryptorchidism is generally used for **bilateral cryptorchidism** (failure of testes descend of both sides). Unilateral Cryptorchidism is more common than bilateral type. Figure 12.11 illustrates the shrunken unilateral cryptorchid testis in comparison to the normal scrotal testis. Undescended testes may be located anywhere between the abdomen and the inguinal canal. The cryptorchid testes of nearly 80 % boys descend spontaneously during the first year of life.

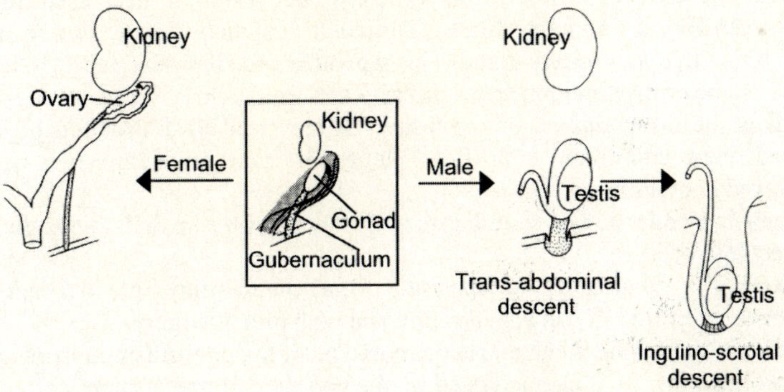

Figure 12.10: Testicular descent in Mouse showing two morphological phases.

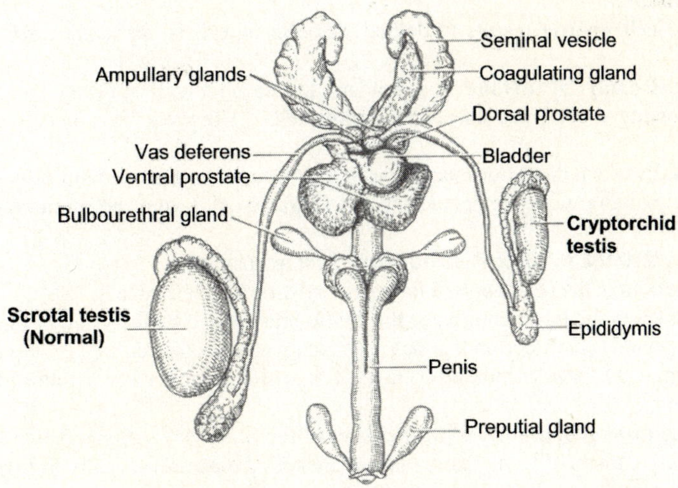

Figure 12.11: Unilateral cryptorchidism in adult Rat.

Untreated bilateral cryptorchidism results in sterility because the higher temperature of the pelvic cavity destroys the cells involved in the initial stage of spermatogenesis. It has been observed that the chance of testicular cancer increases 30-50 times more in cryptorchid testis in comparison to the normal scrotal testes. Surgical correction of cryptorchidism is known as **cryptorchidectomy**.

The reason for failure of testicular descent is either anatomical or mechanical. The former may be due to abnormal testicular development or due to short spermatic artery while the latter is generally due to the narrowing of inguinal rings and is called **hernia**. Cryptorchid condition can be corrected surgically which should be ideally done before 18 months of age to prevent permanent testicular damage. Since chances of testicular tumors are more in undescended testes, a testicular biopsy should be performed and repeated 2 years later following surgical descent.

12.4 Disorder of Testicular Functions

Testicular dysfunction may be mainly due to defects in the seminiferous tubules or in Leydig cell function. The former leads to infertility, while the later results in decreased libido, and lack of development of secondary sex characteristics. Testicular dysfunction may also be due to decreased gonadotropin secretion by the pituitary gland. This may affect the reproductive function, the hormonal function, or both. Some of the common testes diseases are listed below.

Orchitis is the inflammation of the testes. It may lead to destruction of the seminiferous tubules, decreased sperm count, and infertility. The testosterone production is normal since Leydig cells are not involved in orchitis.

Hydrocele is a collection of fluid between the layers of tissue that covers the testicles. Minor surgery can correct hydrocele.

Varicocele is a dilation of the spermatic vein (pampiniform plexus), and is sometimes associated with male infertility. It can also be corrected with minor surgery.

Klinefelter's syndrome is the most common type of hypogonadism in males and is caused by chromosomal abnormalities. It is characterized by the presence of one or more extra X-chromosomes (XXY or XXXY).

Testicular Agenesis is lack of testicular development in phenotypic males leading to sexual infantilism and infertility.

Germinal-cell aplasia results in defective spermatogenesis, testicular atrophy, and elevated serum FSH levels.

Sertoli Cell-Only Syndrome is secondary to Germinal-cell aplasia. It refers to severely affected testes showing a complete absence of germ cells. However, Sertoli cells morphologically appear normal.

Eunuchoidism is a condition occurring in males due to hypogonadism. Such individuals are sterile with small genitalia, no male secondary sex characteristics, and the pubic hair is of a female configuration.

Disorders Related to Male Reproductive System are:

Gynecomastia is the term applied to hypertrophy of the male breast.

Epididymitis is the inflammation of the epididymis caused by infection or physical trauma. It is often caused by gonorrheal infection that has ascended the vas deferens.

Prostatitis is the most common problem of the male organs, usually induced by an infection of the prostate gland.

The anatomy of the male genital tract and the nature of the accessory sex glands vary from species to species. Reproductive tracts of some mammals are illustrated diagrammatically in Figure 12.12.

12.5 Ducts of the Testis

The spermatozoa and fluid after their release into the lumen of convoluted seminiferous tubules are propelled toward the straight tubules due to the pressure generated by the continual release of sperm and fluid secreted by the Sertoli cells. The straight tubules lead to a network of ducts in the testis known as the **rete testis** (rete means network), from where the spermatozoa move through a series of coiled ducts called the **efferent ducts** (**vasa efferentia** or **ductuli efferentes**) and the **epididymis** (Figure 12.13). The epididymis empties its contents containing spermatozoa and secretions into a single tube known as the **vas deferens** (**ductus deferens** or **ductus epididymis**).

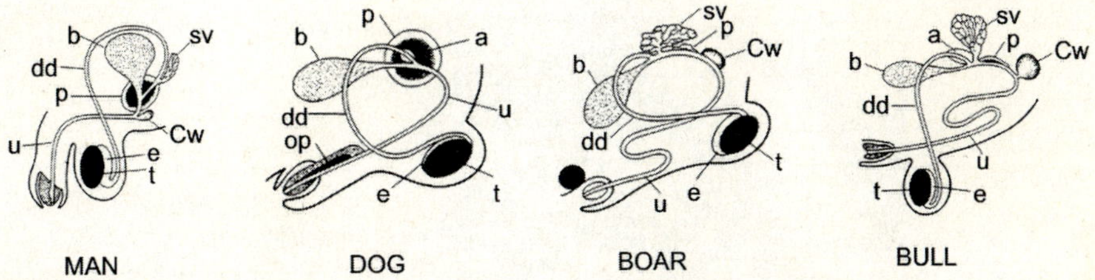

Figure 12.12: Diagrammatic representation of the male reproductive tracts of some Mammals: a-ampulla, b-bladder, Cw-Cowper's gland, dd-ductus deferens, e-epididymis, op-os penis, p-prostate gland, sv-seminal vesicle, t-testis, and u-urethra.

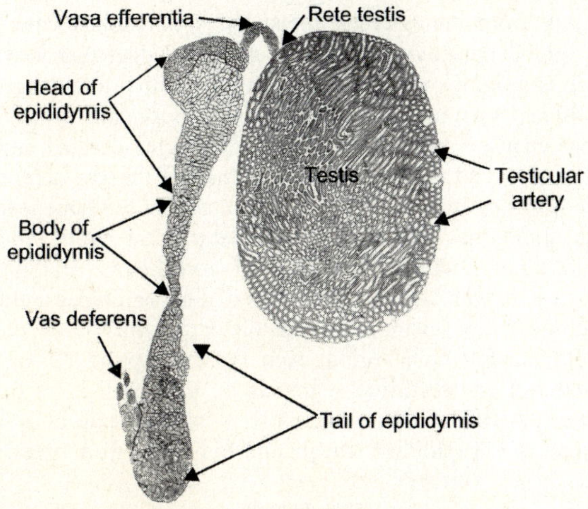

Figure 12.13: Ducts of testis- vasa efferentia, epididymis, and ductus deferens.

The **rete testis** is composed of wide anastomosing channels. These channels course upward toward the ductuli efferentes. The spaces of rete testis are lined by a simple epithelium, and some of these cells have a flagellum connected to the distal centriole. No secretion droplets are present here. There is no definite lamina propria on the tubules of rete and also there is no smooth muscle around the straight tubules or rete testis.

The epithelium of the **efferent ductules** (**ductuli efferentes** or **vasa efferentia**) is basically simple and consists of two types of cells. These are **tall columnar ciliated** cells and **non-ciliated cuboidal** cells, which are apparently absorptive. **Basal cells** may occasionally be present in the epithelium to give it a pseudostratified look in part. The lumen of the tubules thus appears folded or wavy due to varying heights of the cells (Figure 12.14). The epithelium rests on a **basement membrane**, which however, is not affected, and externally the tubules have a smooth contour. Beneath the basement membrane is a thin layer of dense connective tissue known as **lamina propria**. It contains many capillaries and smooth muscle fibers. Both types of cells, tall and low are secretory in function. Bleb-like secretion droplets can be seen adhering to the free surface of the non-ciliated cells. As the tubules approach the epididymis, the distal ends of the efferent ductules are lined with mainly tall (columnar) cells, so that the lumens have an even contour with very few pockets or folds.

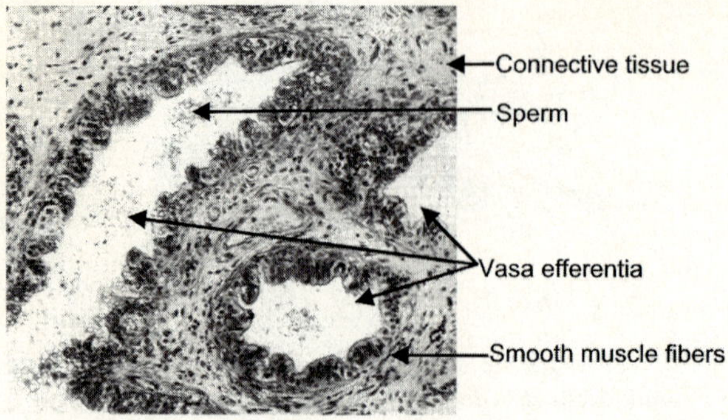

Figure 12.14: Transverse section of ductuli efferentes of adult Man.

Epididymis: On emerging from the efferent ducts, the spermatozoa enter the epididymis. The mammalian epididymis (plural **epididymides**) is an elongated duct that is derived embryologically from the Wolffian duct. It is a tightly coiled, thread like tube with a total length of about 20 meters in man, 60 meters in boar, 40 meters in bull and about 6 meters in rodents. Its lumen opens cranially into the testis via the efferent ducts, a group of six or more tubules derived embryologically from the persisting mesonephric tubules, and caudally into the lumen of the vas deferens (Figure 12.13). The duct has an even contour, as the entire epithelial cells end nearly at the same level.

Customarily the epididymis is divided into the **head** or the **caput epididymides**, **body** or the **corpus epididymides** and **tail** or **cauda epididymides** (Figure 12.15). But in fact, each of these three regions possesses sub-segments, which exhibit their own distinct cell types and functional peculiarities. Based on the serial histology, many scientists divided the epididymis of rat into six zones while those of rabbit and human epididymis into eight regions each. Further, epididymis has also been divided into **initial**, **middle (intermediate)** and **terminal** segments on the basis of its functional characteristics (Figure 12.15). However, the size of these regions from where head, body or tail and also initial, middle or terminal segments of the epididymis begin and end varies from species to species.

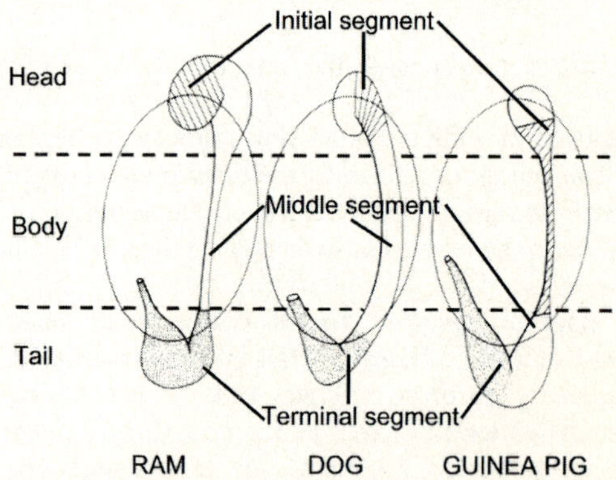

Figure 12.15: Anatomical divisions of the epididymis.

The transverse section of the rat epididymis is shown in Figures 12.16 and 12.17 for structural details. It shows convolutions of the epididymal tubule as varied size of individual sections surrounded by the connective tissue. The lining of the tubule consists of **pseudostatified columnar epithelial** cells with **nonmotile stereocilia** on their free surfaces. The stereocilia are supposed to assist in forming a pathway for the secretion of the epithelium into the lumen of the tubule. The height of the epithelial cells and the length of their stereocilia vary greatly in different regions of the epididymis. The initial segment (caput epididymis) of the mammalian epididymis is characterized by tall, columnar epithelium with long, straight stereocilia (Figure 12.16) while the middle segment shows the presence of supranuclear vacuoles in the epithelium and its stereocilia are usually bent. The epithelium of the tubules of terminal segments (cauda epididymis) varies from low columnar to cuboidal type with low stereocilia (Figure 12.17). The lumen of the tubule of initial segment is small and contains very few spermatozoa while that of the terminal segment is wide and is densely packed with spermatozoa. The epithelium rests on the basement membrane, which is distinct in each tubule. The lamina propria has circularly arranged smooth muscle fibers. It is thin but more pronounced than that of the ductuli efferentes.

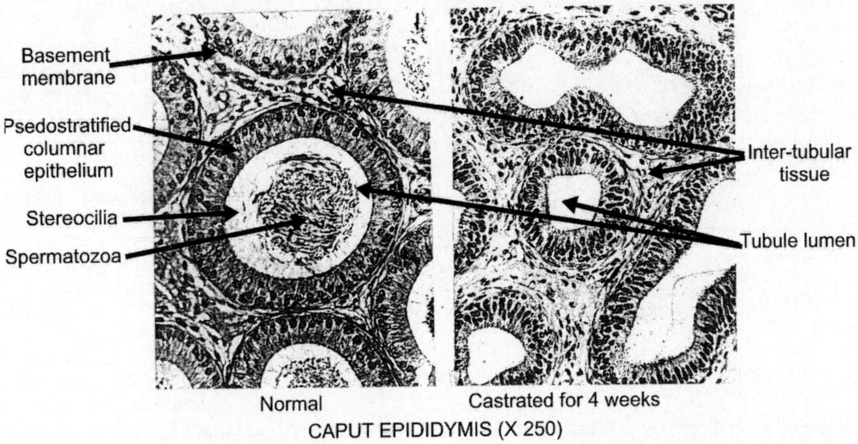

Figure 12.16: Transverse sections of the caput epididymidis of normal and castrated Rat.

The ultra structure of the epididymis shows various types of cells in its epithelium. These are **principal** and **basal** types in addition to **apical**, **halo** and **clear** cells. The principal cells are present along the entire length of the epididymal duct, extending from the basal lamina to the lumen of the epididymis and their free surfaces are provided with long stereocilia. Their nucleus is lobed and the cytoplasm contains lysosomes, multi-vesicular bodies and other cell inclusions. These cells are richly endowed with endoplasmic reticulum and Golgi complex and thus seem to be involved in synthetic activities. In addition, these cells have extensive pinocytotic vesicles, which may be involved in the reabsorption of fluid from epididymal lumen. The basal cells are also found throughout the length of the epididymis at the basal region of the principal cells and are variable in shape. Their cytoplasm contains few organelles and inclusions. The halo cells lie between the principal cells and are found more towards the apical region. These are amoeboid in appearance. The nucleus is small and stains more densely than that of the principal cells. The clear cells are vacuolated and columnar extending from the based lamina to the luminal surface of the epididymis. Their cytoplasm is filled with dense osmiophilic lipid droplets, mitochondria, free ribosome and short segments of endoplasmic reticulum.

Serial histology and ultra structure of the epididymis indicates regional differentiation in the pattern of innervation and distribution of morphologically distinguished types of smooth muscle cells in the human epididymis and vas deferens. There is a gradual proximal – distal increase in the thickness of the muscle coat of human epididymis. There are two sets of morphologically distinct smooth muscle cells. These cells receive different type of adrenergic inervation in the different parts of the epididymis.

This results in different motility behavior of its upper and lower parts. The proximal epididymis exhibits spontaneous local, slow, rhythmic, migratory contractions while the distal portion remains quiescent. Also there is a characteristic distribution of capillaries in the different parts of the epididymis. The cells lining the higher regions of the epididymis appear to be metabolically more active and have a higher blood flow per unit weight than those in the lower regions.

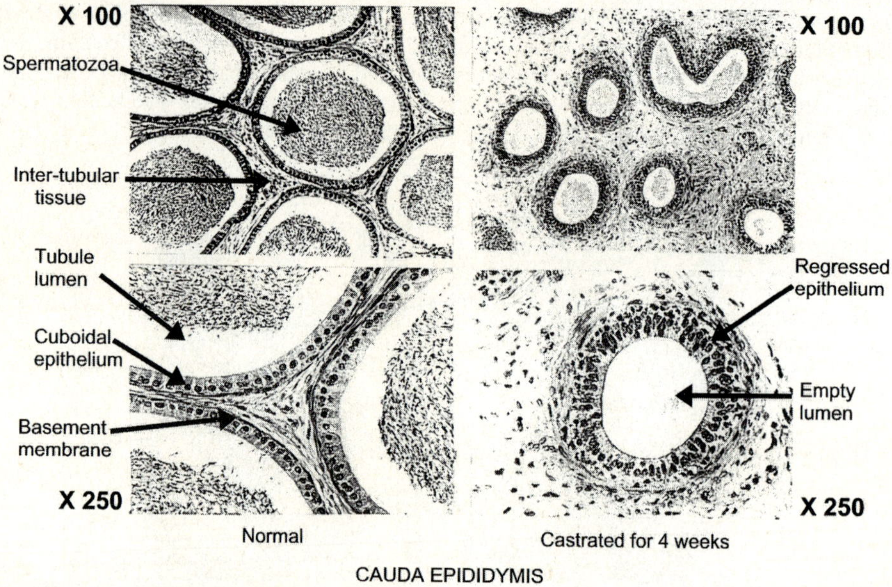

Figure 12.17: Transverse sections of the cauda epididymidis of normal and castrated Rat.

The time interval, which the spermatozoa require to pass along the entire length of the epididymal duct, varies from species to species, frequency of ejaculation and certain other conditions. Thus the journey of spermatozoa in the epididymis may take from a few days to several weeks. This is probably because of their dormant state to some extent in the epididymis. The spermatozoa are generally capable of surviving longer in the epididymis than in any other part of either male or female reproductive tract. In rabbit for instance, they retain their fertilizing ability for at least a month.

The major force that propels the spermatozoa along the epididymal duct is of neuromuscular origin and depends on spontaneous rhythmic contractions of the duct, which in turn are dependent on the presence of androgen. Thus, the spontaneous contractility of the duct ceases on castration and is restored with testosterone treatment. The cauda epididymis is particularly well supplied with adrenergic nerves. On denervation, its spontaneous contractions are inhibited. Catecholamines and oxytocin exert a stimulatory effect on contractility of this organ. However, there is no clear-cut evidence as yet that the spermatozoa themselves contribute to their advance within the epididymis or the epididymal plasma assists in their progress.

The epididymis influences the environment of spermatozoa by synthesis and/ or secretions as well as by reabsorption of fluid and macromolecules from the lumen. It produces various secretions and by way of absorption and secretion participates together with the accessory sex glands in the formation of seminal plasma. However, unlike the prostate and seminal vesicle, chief role of epididymis is not so much in sperm activation as in ripening and life prolonging of spermatozoa. It provides them a favorable milieu for acquiring the capacity to fertilize mature ova. The changes, which result in the acquisition of fertilizing capacity by the spermatozoa during their sojourn in the epididymis, are referred to as **maturational changes**.

The epididymis acts as a highly efficient storage organ also, enabling the spermatozoa to preserve their motility and fertilizing potential. Another important function of the epididymis is the disposal and phagocytosis of aging and abnormal spermatozoa by its epithelium and spermiophages. The secretory fluid of the epididymis assists this function. The initial and middle segments of the epididymis show micropinocytosis, characterized by absorption and secretion of certain substances while the terminal segment mainly store spermatozoa in its lumen at a high density.

Apart from high K+/Na+ ratio of epididymal plasma, a wide range of organic constituents form a characteristic feature of this organ. The major biochemical constituents synthesized and secreted by the epididymis include Glyceryl Phosphoryl Choline (GPC), Carnitine, Sialic Acid, Lipids, a variety of active enzymes, various Steroids and Steroid Hormones. However, one of the chemical characteristics of epididymal secretion is its complete deficiency of fructose and any other reducing glycolyzable sugar. Not all the substances present in the epididymal plasma are products of biosynthetic activity of its epithelium some are produced by the epididymal spermatozoa. For example, a small portion of epididymal glycerylphosphorylcholine is derived from the metabolism of sperm phospholipids. Also, other substances reach the epididymis via blood, lymph or testicular semen, for example most of the glutamic acid in bull semen originates in the testis. Further, the ability of the epididymis to synthesize and secrete various organic constituents differs characteristically between different regions of the epididymal duct.

Large amounts of **Glyceryl Phosphoryl Choline (GPC)** are secreted by the epididymis of a number of mammals including man. The epididymis of rabbit synthesizes GPC *de novo*, from ^{32}P and ^{14}C - labeled Choline. There seems to be regional differences in the synthesis of GPC in the epididymis. It is synthesized more in the caput than in the cauda epididymides of rats and guinea pigs. However, its biosynthetic pathways have not been worked out completely as synthesis of GPC does not seem to be localized to any particular cell type in the epididymal epithelium. The physiological role of GPC remains to be unknown. It may be involved in maintaining the osmotic balance in the lumen of the epididymis.

Carnitine is a compound that in other tissues is involved in the transport of certain fatty acids into mitochondria. Carnitine (β-oxo-α-butyrobetaine) together with acetylcarnitine is a major constituent of the epididymis. Further, carnitine has been found in high concentrations in the epididymal secretion. From this one might think that this substance is either synthesized in the epididymis itself or enters this organ from the peripheral circulation. No evidence of its local synthesis has been found so far. So unlike GPC, carnitine is not synthesized in the epididymis but is transported there via the blood. Carnitine concentration is highest in cauda and corpus epididymides. Testicular spermatozoa contain very low amounts of carnitine but they accumulate it, which reaches a maximum when they are in the cauda epididymides. This may be related to the maturation and consequent development of fertilizing ability of the spermatozoa. Carnitine may also be involved in deriving energy in metabolism of spermatozoa during their storage in the epididymis by oxidizing long chain fatty acids.

Sialic acids have also been identified in the epididymis of a number of mammals in the free as well as bound form. Sialic acids are a group of amino sugars containing carbohydrates associated with glycoproteins and glycolipids. There appears to exist an inverse relationship between the levels of bound sialic acid in the epididymal luminal plasma and that bound to spermatozoa in the epididymis. There have been a number of speculations but no satisfactory explanation of the significance of sialoprotein in epididymis is found so far. Optimum levels of sialic acid are regarded as essential for sperm maturation and survival in rat epididymis. Sialic acid may be involved in the:

- maintenance of ionic balance in the epididymis,
- antigenic interaction between the epididymis and spermatozoa, and

- maturation of spermatozoa and maintenance of structural integrity of the membranes of spermatozoa.

he concentration of sialic acid in the epididymis falls following castration while its secretion is stimulated by administration of androgen. In addition, evidences indicate that the level of bound sialic acid in the epididymal secretion is also controlled by androgens.

Lipids form another important constituent of the epididymal secretion and are thought to be the source of energy for spermatozoa. Lipids also form an important component of membranes of the spermatozoa as seen in a number of mammals such as boar, ram, bull and monkey. The concentration of total lipids and phospholipids is higher in caput than in cauda epididymides. The contents of these constituents in spermatozoa are also high in caput but these decreases as spermatozoa move to the cauda epididymidis. The phospholipids may serve as a substrate for spermatozoa during their epididymal maturation or may act as a source of epididymal GPC.

The **steroids**, testosterone and dehydroepiandrosterone are present in the epididymis. These steroids are transported to the epididymis in the fluid from the rete testis, but there is suggestive evidence that the epididymis itself may also have some capacity for the synthesis of these steroids. Various enzymes (hydroxy steroid dehydrogenase) that are essential for the synthesis of androgenic steroids have been demonstrated both histochemically and biochemically in the epididymis. It has been shown that mouse epididymis *in vitro* can synthesize cholesterol from acetate. *In vitro* synthesis of dehydroepiandrosterone from pregnenolone has also been demonstrated from rabbit epididymis. Synthesis of small quantities of testosterone, by cell free homogenates of rat epididymis from various substrates has been reported. To what extent epididymal steroid synthesis occurs *in vivo* and what is its physiological significance are the questions still unanswered?

Enzymes of various kinds are also found in the epididymal plasma. The enzymes that are wholly or partly produced and secreted by the epididymis itself include some of the **lysosomal enzymes** encountered in both the epididymal epithelium and the plasma. The formation and secretion of most of the enzymes of epididymis are androgen dependent. **Glycosidases** are more highly concentrated in epididymal plasma than in spermatozoa and their secretion is androgen dependent. The physiological role of glycosidases in the epididymis is somewhat uncertain; they may be involved in the degradation properties of the epididymis and also in the synthesis of mucoproteins in the epididymal semen. The other important lysosomal enzymes of the epididymis are **acid phosphatase**, **protease** and **deoxyribonuclease**. The action of the proteolytic and nucleolytic enzymes may be related to digestive processes leading to the disposal of the aging spermatozoa. Normal spermatozoa are protected from enzymatic attack by their own mucoprotein coating and also because some of these enzymes occur either as zymogens or are bound to inhibitors. Once the degrading enzymes remove the protective coating, the denuded sperm nucleus itself may become accessible to nucleolytic enzymes. In addition to acid phosphatase, epididymal plasma also contains **alkaline phosphatase** and is contributed by secretion of the cauda epididymidis.

In addition to secretion, the epididymis also shows **absorptive function**. It is capable of absorbing selectively fluid and particulate materials from its lumen. The epididymal epithelium exhibits an exceptionally high resorptive power so that much of the water comprising the testicular plasma is moved from the lumen of the epididymal duct to the interstitium of the epididymis, thus changing the dilute testicular semen to highly concentrated epididymal semen. It has been found that in a sexually active ram, approximately 40 ml testicular semen containing nearly 10^8 spermatozoa/ml enters each epididymis daily and only 0.4 ml epididymal semen with nearly 10^{10} spermatozoa/ml leaves the epididymis daily to enter the vas deferens. This means that the volume of fluid, which leaves the epididymis of ram each day, is only 1% of the total fluid produced daily by the testis. Use of a variety of experimental techniques, such as ligation of vasa efferentia, use of dye and spermatocrit and electrolyte measurement along the epididymal duct shows that most of the testicular fluid is absorbed in the caput epididymides. Other findings that epithelial cells took up injected dyes and carbon particles from the duct lumen placed more emphasis upon a possible absorptive function of epididymal epithelium. The relative importance of absorption and secretion in the epididymis remains unsolved.

Factors Regulating the Structural and Functional Integrity of the Epididymis

Both hormonal and non-hormonal factors regulate the structural and functional integrity of the epididymis.

Hormonal factors: The functional integrity of the epididymis, like the accessory glands of reproduction, is dependent on the levels of circulating androgens and is thus greatly affected by castration, hypophysectomy and exogenous administration of androgens.

Castration results in a marked reduction in the epididymal tubular diameter, epithelial height, length of stereocilia (Figures 12.16 and 12.17) and specific cellular components like smooth endoplasmic reticulum, Golgi bodies and mitochondria of the epididymis in comparison to the normal epididymis of rats and mice. Replacement of androgens by testosterone or dihydrotestosterone injections in castrated animals restores the histo-architecture of the epididymis to near normalcy. The secretory activity of the epididymis is also adversely affected by castration. Various enzymes like acid and alkaline phosphatases, glucose –6-phosphate, esterase, diphospho pyridine nucleotide diaphorase in the epididymis respond to changing levels of androgens. The regressive changes following castration can be prevented by administration of androgens. The content of sialic acid in caput and cauda epididymides of rat, hamster and monkey decreases markedly following castration. Further, low doses of anti-androgen, cyproterone acetate released from subcutaneous implanted capsule is found to result in marked reduction in the content of sialic acid of caput and cauda epididymides. This also results in loss of motility, viability and fertilizing ability of spermatozoa in rats. Androgen deprivation also results in a decrease in the contents of total phospholipid in caput and cauda epididymides of rats, hamsters and monkey. The incorporation of ^{14}C – acetate into cholesterol and the synthesis of steroids in the epididymis is also affected by castration. This suggests that the synthesis of steroids by the epididymis is dependent on androgenic hormones from the testis.

Non-hormonal factors: The physiological integrity of the epididymis not only depends on androgen levels in the peripheral blood but also on the normal flow of testicular fluid and/or spermatozoa. The testicular fluid entering the epididymis contains besides spermatozoa, various other substances like androgens, amino acids and electrolytes, which may influence the normal physiology of the different regions of the epididymal canal. Prevention from entering of testicular fluid and spermatozoa into the epididymis by efferent duct ligation results in cytological and biochemical changes such as reduction in content of sialic acid and phospholipids in the caput and cauda epididymides. These changes are more marked in the caput than in the cauda epididymides. Treatment with an androgen antagonist like cyproterone acetate affects both the caput and cauda epididymides of rat and the levels of sialic acid and phospholipids decrease in both the regions.

Thus it is clear that the functional integrity of the epididymis like all other accessory glands of reproduction is largely dependent on androgens. However, the threshold of androgens required for the maintenance of the functional integrity of the epididymis is much higher than that required for the maintenance of the accessory sex glands as reported in the rat, hamster, and monkey. In addition, the epididymis also exhibits regional differences in its responses to androgens. The cauda epididymides require a higher threshold of androgens than caput epididymides for maintenance of its functions. The differential sensitivity of the caput and cauda epididymides and of accessory sex glands to androgens may be due to differences in the availability of androgens to these organs. The epididymis receives androgens both from the peripheral circulation and also directly from the testicular fluid entering the epididymis through the efferent ducts. Testicular androgens may be transported into the epididymis either as free testosterone or bound to androgen binding protein (ABP). In contrast, the accessory sex glands get their supply of androgens only from the peripheral circulation. Testosterone is metabolized to 5 α dihydrotestosterone or 5 α–androstanediol in exerting its action in the epididymis. In addition, epididymis is also capable of synthesizing androgens from suitable precursors as seen in rat, mouse, ram and rabbit. However, the relative importance of these sources of androgens and differential sensitivity of the caput and cauda epididymides remains to be clarified.

Vas Deferens or Ductus Deferens: Each vas deferens (pl., *vas deferentia*), also called ductus deferens, is a muscular tube of about 45 cms in length and o.5 mm wide in internal diameter in human. It begins at the lower end of the epididymis and passes upward along the medial side of a testis to become a part of the spermatic cord. Each vas deferens enters the abdominal cavity through the inguinal canal, courses over the pelvic brim and extends backward and medially into the pelvic cavity to end behind the urinary bladder in the prostatic portion of the urethra. Vas deferens dilates at this point into an **ampulla** (Figure 12.18), then slender again and unites with the duct of a seminal vesicle to form **ejaculatory duct**. The two ejaculatory ducts penetrate the prostate gland and empty into the urethra on either side of the prostatic utricle.

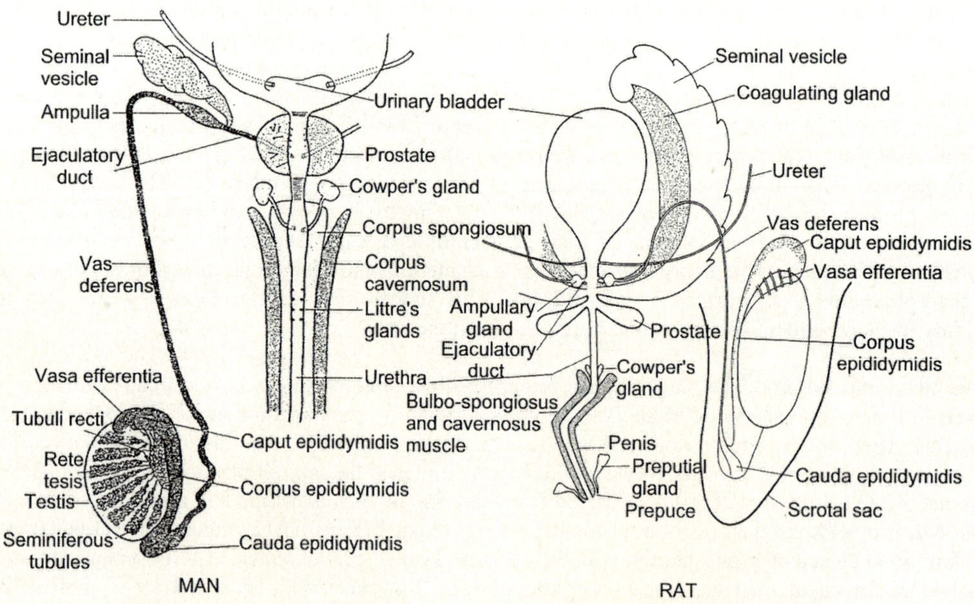

Figure 12.18: Diagrammatic outline of male reproductive tract in Human and Rat to show ducts and accessory glands of reproduction.

Histologically, the wall of the vas deferens consists of three coats-**mucosa**, **muscularis**, and **fibrosa** (adventitia). It has a narrow, irregular lumen, a thin mucosa, and a thick muscularis surrounded by adventitia. The adventitia contains abundant blood vessels and nerves. It merges with the surrounding connective tissue of the spermatic cord. The heavy coat of muscularis consists of three layers of smooth muscle, the inner (relatively thin) and outer layers are longitudinal while the middle layer is thick, and is made of circular muscles. The thin lamina propria is made of compact collagenous fibers with fine elastic networks. In transverse section, it has the appearance of papillae or crests.

Longitudinal folds of the lamina propria cause the irregularity of the lumen. The mucosa is lined by a pseudostratified columnar epithelium (Figure 12.19). The stereocilia are usually present, but their distribution varies, being absent on some cells and present on others. The secretory granules are not as numerous as found in the epithelial cells of the epididymis. The epithelium is surrounded by a stroma exceedingly rich in elastic fibers that form a compact lamina propria around the delicate basement membrane. In the deeper portion of the stroma are present numerous blood vessels. Owing to the abundant elastic tissue and strong muscularis the mucosa is thrown into four or five longitudinal folds, so that in transverse section, the lumen of the vas deferens appears star shaped. Castration affects the structure of the vas deferens.

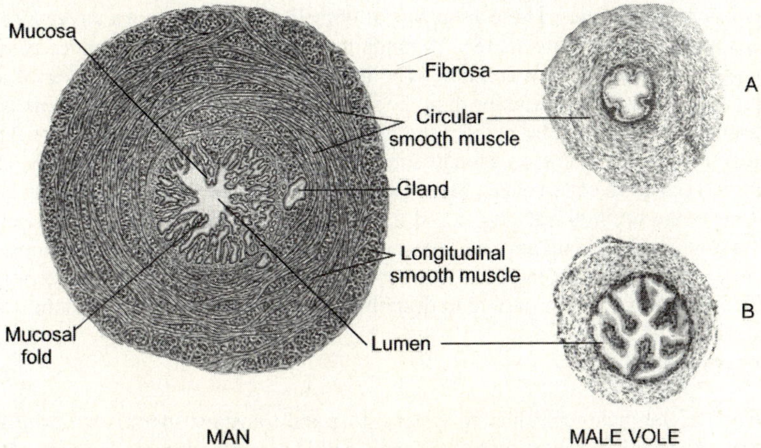

Figure 12.19:Transverse sections through the ampulla of vas deferens in Man and male Vole (A-sexually active normal adult and B-one month after castration).

The **ampullary glands (ampullae)** are glandular enlargements of the terminal portions of the vas deferentia. In some mammals, they are either small, or are not present as in the boar and pig. In other animals, e.g. stallion, their size can far exceed other accessory organs.

In the ampulla, the mucosa shows numerous folds forming crypts (recesses), many of which extend as tubular structures into the stroma (Figure 12.18). These are glandular structures lined by a cuboidal or columnar epithelium of a secretory nature. The epithelial cells frequently contain yellow pigment granules in yellowish-colored fluid having a high content of ergothioneine and phosphorus. The high phosphorus level of ampullae comes from glycerylphosphorylcholine, which is derived from the epididymides. Also, it contains ethanol-soluble materials, which are presumed to be free fructose and sialic acid. Fructose has been detected in the ampullary glands of rat, man, and bull but not in those of stallion.

Functionally, the vas deferens stores spermatozoa. These can remain viable in this duct for up to several months. Vas deferens conveys sperm from the epididymis toward the urethra by peristaltic contractions of the thick muscular coat. The spermatozoa that are not ejaculated ultimately are reabsorbed by phagocytosis.

The union of the duct from the seminal vesicle and the ampulla of the vas deferens form the **ejaculatory duct** (Figure 12.18). It is about 2 cm long and has a thin mucous membrane thrown into numerous fine folds, with glandular crypts like those of ampulla. The epithelium is simple, columnar or pseudostatified and becomes transitional near the urethral opening. Beneath the epithelium, there is a rich network of elastic fibers. A distinct muscularis is present only at the beginning of the ejaculatory duct. In the prostatic portion it disappears and the fibro-muscular tissue of the prostate gland takes its place. The ejaculatory duct terminates in the prostatic urethra, where it ejects sperm and seminal vesicle secretions just prior to ejaculation.

In males, the **urethra** is the shared terminal duct of the reproductive and urinary systems, and serves as a passageway for both semen and urine (Figure 12.18). It consists of **prostatic urethra** where prostate gland open, **membranous urethra** at the urogenital diaphragm, and the **spongy** or **penile urethra** at the corpus spongiosum of the penis. The spongy urethra ends at the external urethral orifice.

The **penis** is a cylindrical organ that conveys the urine as well as semen through the urethra to the outside. Penis consists of a **body**, **root** and **glans** penis. The **body** or **shaft** of the penis is made of **three columns** of **erectile tissue**. These are a pair of dorsally located **corpora cavernosa** and a single ventral **corpus spongiosum** (Figure 12.18). A tough capsule of white dense connective tissue known as **tunica albuginea** surrounds each column. The penis is enclosed in a thin layer of subcutaneous tissue, and a layer of connective tissue forming the **skin** of penis. The **root** of the penis is the attached proximal portion and consists of the bulb of the penis. It is the expanded portion of the base of the corpus spongiosum penis. The corpus spongiosum, through which the urethra extends, enlarges at its distal end to form a sensitive cone-shaped **glans penis**. The glans penis covers the ends of the corpora cavernosa and bears the urethral opening called the **external urethral orifice**. The skin of the glans penis is very thin, hairless and contains sensory receptors for sexual stimulation. A loose fold of skin known as the **prepuce** or **foreskin** is present just posterior to the glans extending anteriorly to cover it as a sheath. **Circumcision** is the term used to describe surgical removal of the foreskin.

12.6 Accessory Sex Glands

Whereas the ducts of the male reproductive system store and transport spermatozoa, the accessory sex glands secrete most of the liquid portion of the semen called seminal plasma. In man and several other mammals, various accessory sex glands are **seminal vesicles**, **prostate gland**, **urethral (Littre's) glands**, **bulbourethral** (**Cowper's**) **glands**, and the **preputial glands** (Figure 12.18). In some species additional organs exist, such as the **coagulating gland**. However, not every accessory sex gland is found in all mammals. For example, the cat and dog has no seminal vesicles, while the bull has large seminal vesicles but small prostate (Figure 12.12), and the rodents have coagulating glands (Figure 12.18) that can be considered as anterior developments of the prostate gland. Table 12.1 gives the comparative account of the principal accessory sex glands. Deprivation of testosterone has profound and rapid effects on the accessory sex glands. After castration, all the accessory sex glands such as seminal vesicles, prostate and others in various species involutes, their epithelia shrink and the secretory activity ceases. If the castrated animal is provided with exogenous testosterone, the involuted sex organs are fully restored, both in size as well as in secretory activity. These target organs (accessory sex glands) are found to possess cytoplasmic androgen receptors.

Table 12.1: Relative size of the male accessory sex glands in some Mammals

Species	Seminal Vesicle	Prostate	Coagulating Gland	Cowper's Gland
Cow	+++	+	—	±
Dog	—	+++	—	—
Horse	+	+++	—	±
Man	++	+++	—	±
Pig	+++	++	—	++
Rat	+++	++	++	++
Sheep	+	++	—	++

Seminal Vesicles: The seminal vesicles are paired, elongated (5 to 10 cm long) convoluted sacs, which lie closely, opposite to the ampullae. Each seminal vesicle is attached to the vas deferens near the base of urinary bladder. In man, boar, guinea pig, rat, and stallion, the seminal vesicles conform in shape to bags (Figure 12.18). However, in other mammals such as bull, they are more fittingly described as seminal or vesicular glands, since they consist of compact glandular tissue arranged in the form of multiple lobes, which surround tightly a system of ramified secretory ducts. In rat, seminal vesicles are large bag-like, flat with serrated edges (Figure 12.20) and lie somewhat in abdomen while in the guinea pig, they are long cylindrical tubes and lie in the cavity of the belly.

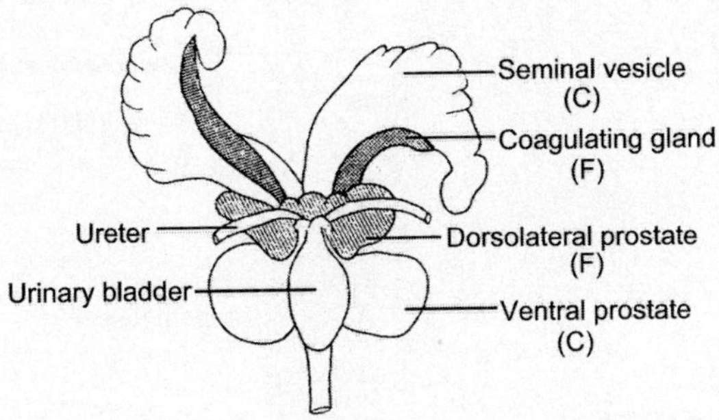

Figure 12.20: Arrangement of seminal vesicle, prostate and coagulating gland in male Rat along with the nature of their secretion, fructose (F) and citric acid (C).

Each seminal vesicle is provided with a highly convoluted, irregular lumen. Figure 12.21 depicts a section through the wall of seminal vesicle showing complex primary folds and innumerable thinner secondary folds frequently joined by anastomosis, forming many crypts and cavities. This arrangement increases the surface area of the secretory epithelium. The epithelium of the seminal vesicles appears simple. It is usually a low pseudostratified layer with basal cells and short columnar or cuboidal cells, which are secretory and not ciliated. The lamina propria is thin, rich in elastic fibers and forms a continuous layer around the vesicle. It extends around the bases of the folds and sends projections into them. Extensions of lamina propria form the core of the larger folds and the thin stroma of the smaller ones. The stroma of the folds is also rich in elastic fibers and contains some smooth muscle cells. Outside the lamina propria is the muscularis layer of smooth muscles. The muscularis is more or less in the form of an inner circular and an outer longitudinal layer. It is difficult to differentiate these layers in sections because of the convolutions of the vesicles. An adventitia in the form of an external sheet of loose connective tissue surrounds the muscularis layer.

Seminal vesicle is a highly glandular structure. Fluid secreted by the seminal vesicles normally constitutes approximately 60 % of the volume of semen. The abundant secretion formed in the seminal vesicle is a viscid material. It is a slightly alkaline fluid, which helps to regulate the pH of the tubular contents as sperm travel to the outside. The secretion of the seminal vesicle also contains fructose (Table 12.2), a monosaccharide that provides energy to the sperm, and prostaglandins, which stimulate muscular contractions within the female reproductive organs, aiding the movement of sperm toward the egg. Analysis of fructose in semen is used to evaluate the secretory activity of the gland. Prostaglandins were first discovered in sheep seminal vesicles and these glands are frequently used to study the mechanism of prostaglandin secretion. In addition to these constituents, secretion of seminal vesicles contains potassium, bicarbonate, acid-soluble phosphate and proteins. However, in rat, the seminal vesicle secretes citric acid and not fructose, while coagulating glands secrete fructose and not citric acid. Unlike in rat, the seminal vesicle of mouse shares the ability to secrete fructose with the coagulating gland. On the other hand, in the guinea pig, the seminal vesicles secrete both citric acid and fructose whereas the coagulating glands secrete only citric acid.

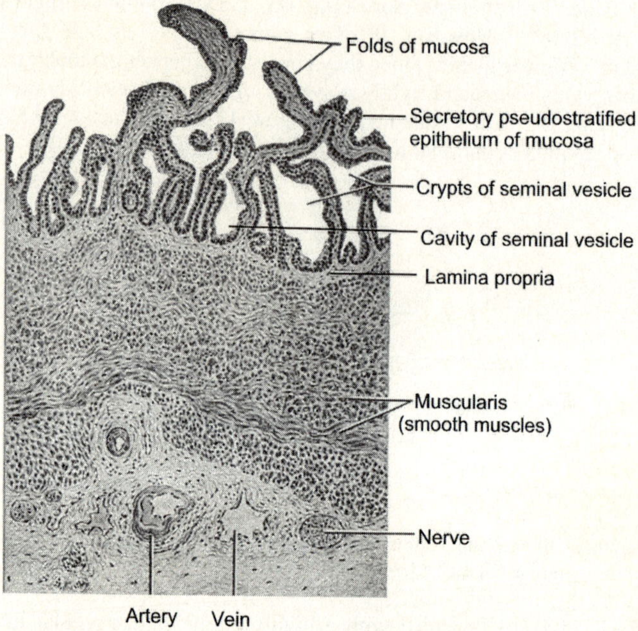

Figure 12.21: Transverse section through the wall of the seminal vesicle of Man.

The height of the epithelial cells and their functional activity are dependent upon the action of testosterone. Following castration, the seminal vesicles shrink, the epithelium is reduced to low cuboidal and cease forming fluid.

The normal vesicular secretion is yellowish but occasionally (in man and bull), it can be deeply pigmented, due to the presence of flavins that cause it to fluoresce strongly in ultraviolet light.

Table 12.2: Characteristic constituents of seminal vesicle secretion (mg/ml)

↓Constituents Species →	Man	Bull	Boar	Rat	Guinea Pig
Dry weight	1,200	1,370	15,670	975	965
Ascorbic acid	5	14	4	4	9
Citric acid	12.5	670	560	115	193
Fructose	315	970	52	0*	57
Inorganic Phosphorus	10	17	3	15	5
Acid-soluble Phosphorus	57	23	32	168	67
Ergothioneine	<1	<1	79	Trace	Trace

* In rat, the Coagulating Gland secretes fructose.

Prostate Gland: The prostate gland derives its name due to its anatomic location as the word prostate refers to "standing before or anterior to the bladder and vesiculae seminales in the supine position of the subject". It contains glandular structures, which form a considerable part of its tissues. The prostate gland has always been in the limelight because of its frequent pathology or hypertrophy in aging men.

A prostate gland or its equivalent is present in nearly all mammals with the exception of the monotremes. It is a chestnut shaped structure, nearly 4 cm across and 3-cm thick and surrounds the beginning of the urethra just inferior to the urinary bladder. It may consist of many lobes and rat prostate gland is notable for its complex structure. Rat prostate consists of ventral, dorsal and lateral lobes (Figure 12.20). The **'ventral prostate'** lies ventrally to the urethra and consists of two pear-shaped structures, whereas a **'dorso-lateral prostate'** encircles the urethra dorsolaterally and is made up of one clearly demarcated median portion and two lateral lobes, and a pair of lateral prostates known as **'coagulating glands'** previously called the anterior prostate. Ventral and dorso-lateral prostates and a pair of coagulating glands are also present in mouse, guinea pig and hamster and a lobed prostate is characteristic of the rabbit, mole and hedgehog.

Prostate gland is composed of many branched tubular glands enclosed in connective tissue (Figure 12.22). Septa of the connective tissue and smooth muscle extend inward from the capsule, thus separating the tubular glands. The gland is embedded in a distinctive fibromuscular stroma. Strands of smooth muscle course in various directions together with collagenous fibers and fine elastic networks. The prostate consists of many glandular alveoli (alveolus is singular) that vary in size. Their lumen is wide and frequently uneven in contour. The glandular epithelium in the prostate is usually simple columnar or pseudostratified (Figure 12.22), and the cells stain lightly in their superficial portions. Basal cells resting on the basal lamina are insinuated among the columnar cells. The alveoli may contain prostatic concretions, formed by concentric layers of coagulated secretions, which may become calcified. The ducts of prostate glands open into the urethra. The prostate releases its secretions into the urethra as a result of contraction of smooth muscles present in its capsular wall.

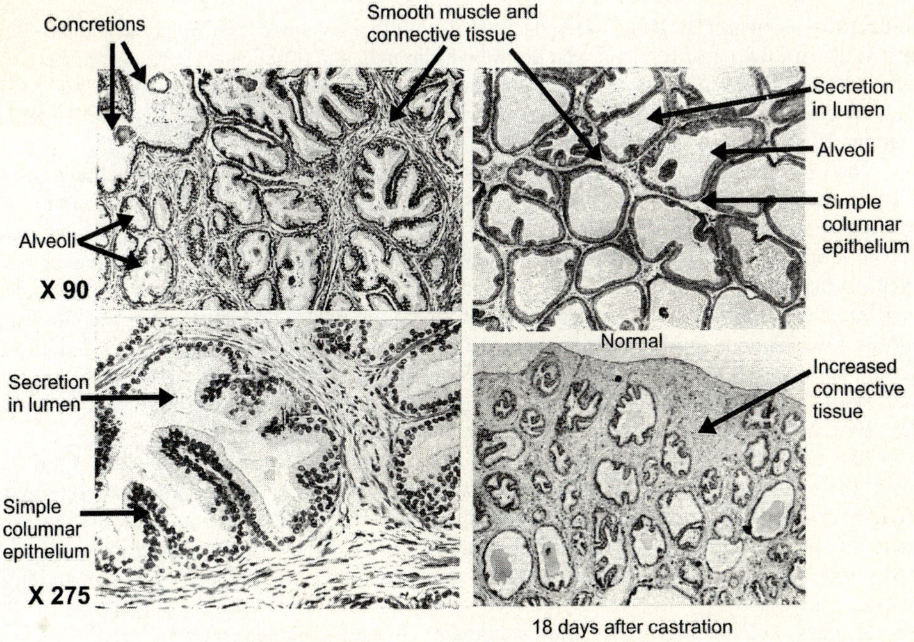

Figure 12.22: Sections through prostate.

Secretion from prostate gland is thin, milky or colorless and slightly acidic (pH about 6.5). Prostatic secretions make up approximately 25 % of the volume of the semen. The reducing sugars are almost completely absent in it. Prostatic secretion is the main source of citric acid and acid phosphatase of human semen; and the analysis of these two constituents provides a most convenient 'chemical indicator test' for the assessment of the functional state of human prostate. Spermatozoa use citric acid for the production of ATP via the Krebs's cycle. The prostatic secretion also contains phosphatase, zinc, several proteolytic enzymes, such as, prostate-specific antigen (PSA), pepsinogen, fibrinolysin, lysozyme, amylase, and hyaluronidase. The most potent proteolytic enzyme is fibrinolysin, which plays a role in the liquefaction of semen.

In the rat, ventral prostate has high concentrations of citric acid but completely lacks fructose whereas the dorso-lateral prostate and the lateral prostates (coagulating glands) produces fructose.

Coagulating Glands: The word-coagulating gland applies to all those organs, which produce the enzyme responsible for the phenomenon of coagulation of semen and formation of the 'vaginal plug'.

The coagulating glands lie immediately adjacent to the seminal vesicles and share a common peritoneal sheath between them. Walker first used the name-coagulating gland in 1910 in designating those accessory organs in small rodents, which occupy a position closely adjacent to the seminal vesicles (Figure 12.19). The position of coagulating glands is similar in rat, guinea pig and mouse. The coagulating glands are responsible for the secretion of the semen-coagulating agent, named 'vesiculase'. Apart from vesiculase, the coagulating gland secretes certain other highly potent proteolytic enzymes. In rat, coagulating gland along with the dorso-lateral prostate acts as a source of seminal fructose.

Bulbo-urethral (Cowper's) gland: Bulbo-urethral glands are named as Cowper's glands after the scientist William Cowper of England who described it in man and in the boar. These glands are placed on each side of the caudal portion of urethra a little above the bulbs of its cavernous body (Figure 12.18). They drain their secretion into the pelvic urethra in its bulbar region. Cowper's glands are enclosed by the fibers of the external urethral sphincter muscle.

The Cowper's glands are pea-sized compound tubulo alveolar glands whose tubules and ducts have a very irregular diameter. The end-pieces of these glands are rounded sacs or simple tubes. Cowper's glands are composed of closely adhering lobes called alveoli (Figure 12.23). The alveoli (lobule or tubules) are lined by a simple epithelium whose height varies from columnar to low cuboidal. In the resting state, the cells are columnar with granular cytoplasm and have a clear spherical nucleus, but at the peak of secretion, these cells get filled with mucus and their nuclei become flattened against the basal lamina. Basket cells may also be found. The Cowper's glands are divided into small lobules by septa. The stroma between the lobules consists of fibro-elastic tissue with few muscle fibers. Smooth and skeletal muscle fibers are however quite numerous in the septa between the lobules. Externally, a layer of skeletal muscle fibers encloses Cowper's glands.

The epithelial lining of Cowper's glands secretes milky white, mucus like fluid, which lubricates the end of the penis in response to sexual stimulation. This occurs in preparation for sexual intercourse or coitus as the secretion contains an alkaline substance that protects the passing spermatozoa by neutralizing acids from urine in the urethra. Also, the mucus that lubricates the end of the penis and the lining of the urethra helps in decreasing the number of sperm damaged during ejaculation.

In man, bull, stallion and other mammals, Cowper's glands are two small oval shaped structures nearly one cm in diameter, approximately the size of a pea. Boars have comparatively larger Cowper's glands that are cylindrical in shape and are filled with an extremely viscous, almost rubber-like white fluid, noticeable by a high content of sialoproteins. Cowper's glands of rat, hamster and monkey have also been shown to contain high amounts of sialic acid. The viscous secretion of Cowper's glands also contains besides sialic acid, galactose, galactosamine, galacturonic acid and a methyl pentose. It plays an important part in the process of 'gelation' which occurs in the boar seminal plasma at the time of ejaculation and immediately afterwards.

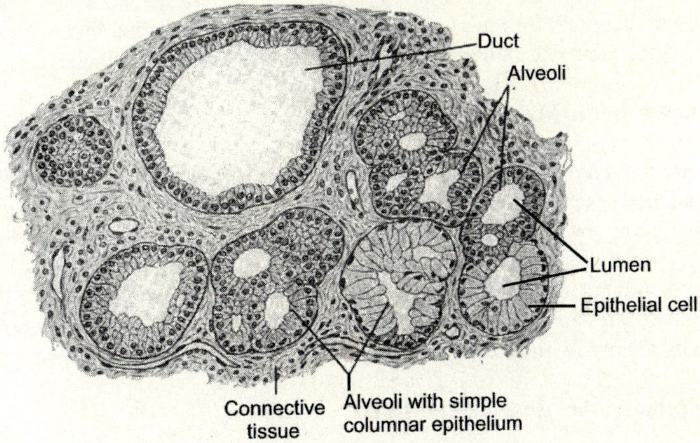

Figure 12.23: Section through Cowper's gland of Man

Urethral (Littre's) glands: There are numerous widely dispersed smaller glands in the urethral wall, which empty (void) their secretion into the urethra along its entire length (Figure 12.18). Alexis Littre of France called these as urethral glands. Urethral glands are also known as glands of Littre. These are found in man and other mammals. Their secretion is usually watery, clear and rich in mucoprotein. It constitutes the so-called pre-sperm fraction, which is emitted at the time of ejaculation prior to the spermatozoa.

Preputial Glands: Preputial glands are present at the tip of the penile urethra. These are paired, large modified sebaceous glands, which open to the surface on either side of the urethral meatus (Figure 12.18). These are analogous to the clitoral glands in the female. Their secretions seem to exert a great attraction in the opposite sex thus possessing pheromonal properties. These have been tentatively identified as C7 and C8 aliphatic alcohols. Preputial glands thus produce some specific substances and one of these is 7-dehydrocholesterol as it is found in the preputial glands and epididymis of male rats. Another is β-glucuronidase, which is found in unusually high concentration in the preputial gland of the female rat.

Inguinal glands: Inguinal glands are present in few mammals only such as rabbit. These are a pair of small compound tubulo-alveolar glands, which lie between the skin and abdominal wall on either side of the penis. Each gland opens by a single duct into skin folds near the end of the prepuce. Inguinal glands, however, does not contribute to the seminal plasma, but are sebaceous, odor-producing glands which are associated with sexual attraction.

12.7 Effects of Castration on Accessory Glands of Reproduction in Males

Surgical removal of testes is called castration. All the accessory glands of reproduction in males are maintained structurally as well as in their secretory activity by testosterone. Therefore, deprivation of testosterone either through **castration** or **hypophysectomy** or through treatment with **antiandrogens** such as cyproterone acetate has profound and rapid effects on all the accessory sex glands of the male genital tract. Following castration the seminal vesicles, prostate, Cowpers glands and epididymides or their equivalents in various species involutes, their epithelia shrink and their secretory activity ceases. If the castrated animal is provided with exogenous testosterone, the involuted organs are restored to near normalcy both in size and in secretory activity. All these accessory sex glands possess cytoplasmic androgen receptors for their androgenic activity. The seasonal breeders also depend on the actions of androgens for their seasonal appearance of secondary sexual characteristics.

12.8 Sperm Transport in the Male Genital Ducts

The spermatozoa are moved passively from the testis by the current of fluid secreted by the Sertoli cells and pass into a branched reservoir, the rete testis into which both ends of each testis tubule open. Vasa efferentia pass the sperm from rete testis to the epididymis and this is aided by the reabsorption of water in the ducts, which tends to pull spermatozoa in that direction. Sperm transport inside the epididymis is due to spontaneous, peristalsis-like contractions of the smooth muscle lining its wall and also due to hydrostatic pressure inside the tubule. Spermatozoa are transported from the epididymis into the vas deferens mainly by the steady flow of secretion through the epididymis.

12.9 Motility of Sperm in the Male Genital Ducts

Motility of sperm is very important and is correlated with its fertilizing ability. Spermatozoa acquire their full forward progressive motility as they travel down the length of the epididymis. A normal fertile male ejaculates 70 to 90 percent motile sperm and 5 to 25 percent abnormally formed sperm. The tail is the main propulsive unit of the sperm, pushing the head along by the propagation of waves. These waves pass distal along the length of spermatozoa and exert pressure on the surrounding medium. The contractile impulses arise from the inner fibers of the axial filaments at the level of the basal body of the neck and seem to coordinate the localized contractions in the outer fibers. Average frequency of the bending cycle in physiological solutions at 37 ^{0}C in case of bull sperm has been found as 9.1 per second and average forward movement with each contractile cycle has been measured as 8.3μ (Gray 1958). A complex series of biochemical events involving contractile protein elements and energy production and transfer are involved in the mechanisms responsible for sperm motility.

Spermatozoa recovered from the rete testis show only a weak vibrating movement of the tail. This is followed by slow circular swimming movements in the caput epididymis. These movements change to a vigorous unidirectional progression with longitudinal rotation of the head by the time spermatozoa reach to the cauda epididymis.

12.10 Erection, Orgasm and Ejaculation

Erection: During sexual stimulation, the parasympathetic nerve impulses from the sacral region of the spinal cord release the vasodilator nitric oxide. This results in the dilation of the arteries leading into the penis. At the same time, the increasing pressure of the blood entering the vascular spaces of the erectile tissue compresses the veins of the penis, thus reducing the flow of venous blood away from the penis. As a result blood accumulates in the erectile tissues, thus causing the penis to swell and elongate. This produces an **erection** of the penis.

Impotence: Impotence is the failure to achieve or to maintain an erection sufficient to accomplish intromission and coitus. If an erection is achieved, it usually subsides without ejaculation in impotence.

Emission: Emission is the movement of sperm cells from the testis and secretions from the various accessory glands of reproduction into the urethra, where they mix to form semen. Emission of semen occurs in response to sympathetic nerve impulses from the spinal cord, which stimulate peristaltic contractions in smooth muscles within the walls of the testicular ducts, epididymides, vas deferens, and ejaculatory ducts. Other sympathetic impulses stimulate rhythmic contractions of the accessory glands of reproduction. As the urethra fills with semen, sensory impulses are stimulated, pass into the sacral portion of the spinal cord and in response, motor impulses are transmitted from the cord to certain skeletal muscles at the base of the erectile columns of the penis. This causes them to contract rhythmically and increasing the pressure within the erectile tissues, thus aiding in forcing the semen through the urethra to the outside. This whole process is known as **ejaculation**.

Ejaculation: Ejaculation is the propulsion of semen out of the urethra at the time of orgasm.

The complete sequence of events during emission and ejaculation is coordinated in such a way that the secretion from the Cowper's glands is expelled at first, followed by the release of secretions from the prostate, the passage of spermatozoa and finally the ejection of secretion from the seminal vesicles. Immediately after ejaculation, sympathetic impulses constrict the arteries supplying the erectile tissue, thus reducing the inflow of blood. The veins of the penis also carry the excess blood out of its vascular spaces, and the penis gradually returns to its flaccid state. Usually, another erection and ejaculation cannot be triggered for nearly 10-30 minutes

Spontaneous emissions and ejaculations commonly occur in adolescent males during sleep. These are known as **nocturnal emissions**. Hormonal changes that accompany adolescent development and sexual maturation cause nocturnal emissions.

Coitus: Coitus is a sexual act by which the sperms are introduced into the vagina.

Orgasm: Orgasm is the culmination of sexual stimulation.. It is a pleasurable feeling of physiological and psychological release. In male, emission and ejaculation of semen accompany orgasm.

Circumcision: It literally means to cut around. Circumcision is a surgical procedure in which part or the entire prepuce is removed. It is usually performed just after delivery or 3-4 days after birth. As a part of a Jewish religious rite, circumcision is performed on the eighth day after birth. Some health-care professionals find no medical justification for circumcision, while others feel that it is beneficial in protecting from urinary tract infections and sexually transmitted diseases.

Summary

The male gonads or testes lie within the scrotum and produce sperm.

The testes are compound tubular glands. The bulk of the organ is composed of complex convolutions of seminiferous tubules.

The testis is covered externally by a tunica albuginea that extends internally to divide the testis into many lobules. Each lobule contains sperm-producing seminiferous tubules and interstitial cells that produce androgens.

During development, testes descend into the scrotum. The scrotum provides a temperature slightly lower than that of the body, as required for viable sperm production. Failure of descent of testes is known as cryptorchidism.

The male duct system from testis onwards consists of rete testis, vasa efferentia, epididymis, vas deferens, urethra and ejaculatory duct.

The epididymis is present close to the external surface of testis. It serves as a site for sperm maturation and storage. The vas deferens extends from the epididymis to the urethra and propels sperm into the urethra by peristalsis during ejaculation. The urethra extends from the urinary bladder to the tip of the penis and conducts semen and urine to the body exterior.

The accessory sex glands are seminal vesicles, prostates, coagulating glands, Cowper's glands, Littre's glands and preputial glands. Histologically, these glands have an outer adventitia followed by muscularis whose thickness varies with different glands, lamina propria and innermost layer of pseudostratified epithelium. The epithelium rests on basement membrane and is provided with stereocilia whose length varies in different regions. The epithelium is generally columnar, but may be low or cuboidal. The accessory sex glands secrete various secretions under the influence of male hormones and contribute in the formation of semen, for example, seminal vesicles secrete fructose, prostate secretes citric acid and phosphate and bulbourethral glands secrete mucus.

The penis is the male copulatory organ and is largely an erectile tissue.

Questions

1. What are the sex organs of the male reproductive system?
2. Describe the descent of the testes.
3. What happens if the testes fail to descend into the scrotum?
4. Explain the importance of testis location in scrotum.
5. Describe the structure of a testis. Which cells produce male sex hormones?
6. Explain the functions of the sustentacular cells.
7. Describe the structure and functions of the epididymis.
8. Where is the prostate gland located? Give its structure and functions.
9. Give the structure and functions of seminal vesicle.
10. What is circumcision?
11. Explain the regulation of secretion of male sex hormones.
12. Discuss the hormonal regulation of testicular function and the physiological effects of testosterone on male reproductive anatomy.

Chapter 13

Physiology of Male Reproduction

The transport of spermatozoa from the testis to the site of fertilization is indeed quite a journey. After leaving the testis spermatozoa pass into an exceedingly long tube that is twisted into a compact body called the epididymis and it lies next to the testis (Chapter 12). The contents of the epididymis consist of large numbers of spermatozoa suspended in the secretions of testis and of epididymis. This mixture moves slowly down the tube and takes many days to reach the vas deferens (Figure 13.1). Some of the suspending fluid is absorbed in the epididymis so that the mixture becomes somewhat concentrated by the time it reaches the end of the epididymis. Also the concentration of spermatozoa becomes remarkably dense in the vas deferens.

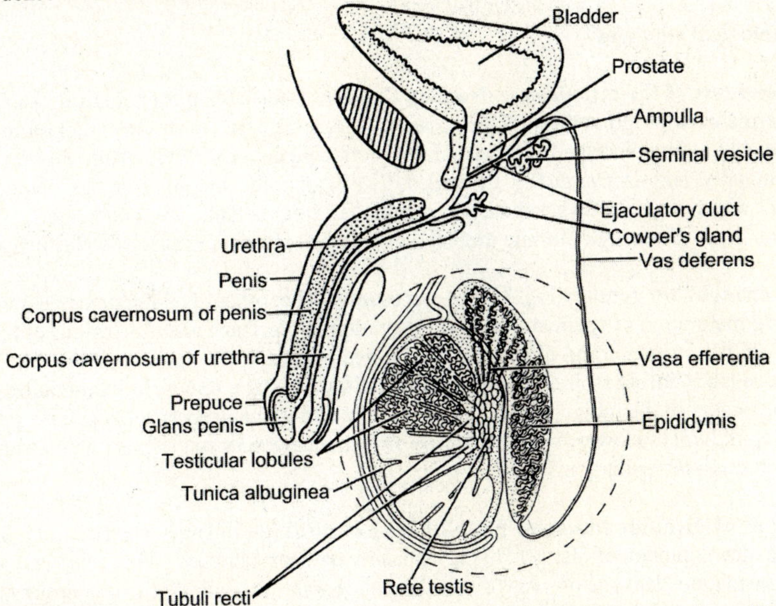

Figure 13.1: Reproductive system of Man in sagittal view, testis and epididymis, are enlarged in comparison to other parts to show structural details.

13.1 Maturation of Spermatozoa

When the spermatozoa leave the testis they are neither structurally nor functionally complete to perform their function. They do not show forward pattern of motility, which is a prerequisite in fertilization process and therefore, testicular spermatozoa are incapable of fertilizing an ovum.

Spermatozoa undergo several changes as they move through the epididymis. These changes render them to acquire characteristic pattern of forward motility and full fertilizing ability. This functional change in spermatozoa can be verified experimentally. The spermatozoa taken from the head of the epididymis show very little fertilizing ability, but on completing their journey through the epididymis, they show full fertilizing ability.

The epididymis provides a favorable internal milieu to spermatozoa in acquiring fertilizing ability and also for their storage until they are ejaculated or move down to the vas deferens. The duration for normal transport of spermatozoa through the epididymis is species dependent. It varies from 15 days in rat, 8 days in mouse, 14-18 days in guinea pig, 4-7 days in rabbit, 9-14 days in ram and 19-23 days in man (Bishop 1961). During their transit through the epididymis the spermatozoa undergo a series of changes that are collectively called as **maturational changes**. These changes result in the acquisition of characteristic patterns of motility and fertilizing ability in spermatozoa. Spermatozoa acquire their full fertilizing ability gradually as they are transported from the caput to the cauda epididymides. Orgebin and Crist have shown that in rat only 8 % of ova exposed to sperm suspensions from the caput epididymides were fertilized while spermatozoa from the cauda epididymides could fertilize 93 % of the ova. However, the exact region of the epididymis where maturation of spermatozoa occurs or is completed is variable in different species. In rat, majority of spermatozoa attains fertilizing ability on reaching the cauda epididymides while in rabbit and hamster maturation of spermatozoa occurs in the lower half of the corpus epididymides and the proximal segment of the cauda epididymides respectively. Changes in the spermatozoa during their maturation process can be broadly classified as morphological, physiological and biochemical.

A. Morphological Changes

Migration and loss of the cytoplasmic droplet: The most noticeable morphological change that takes place, as spermatozoa progress through the epididymis is the migration of the cytoplasmic droplet that surround the connecting piece and first part of the middle piece. The cytoplasmic droplet is gradually displaced caudally and is eventually discarded. Although the cytoplasmic droplet contains acid phosphatase, which may be lysosomal, its functional role is still not understood. However, a spermatozoon in which the cytoplasmic droplet was not shed shows no capacity to fertilize ova.

Structural changes or remodeling of the acrosome: The other well-documented morphological change during maturation of spermatozoa is the alteration in the shape and dimensions of the acrosome. Microscope studies in rabbit and ultrastructural studies in boar show that the size of the acrosome of spermatozoa reduces during their epididymal transit. Furthermore a remodeling (alteration of shape) of the acrosome occurs in the rabbit, guinea pig, chinchilla and monkey spermatozoa during their journey through the epididymis. However, the acrosome of human spermatozoa shows no modification during their transit through the epididymis.

Establishment of disulfide linkages: Establishment of disulfide linkages appears to be an important event in the development of the fertilizing capacity of spermatozoa. This was first revealed by reductive or oxidative cleavage of –s-s- (disulfide) linkages in the head of bovine spermatozoa and later by Feulgen staining technique. It has been shown that the molecular rearrangement of spermatozoa nuclear chromatin also occurs during the passage of spermatozoa through the epididymis. Calvin and Bedford (1971) found that major stabilization of the nuclear chromatin of mammalian spermatozoa occurs after spermiation by the formation of disulfide cross-links during the final stages of maturation of spermatozoa in the epididymis. It was noticed that spermatozoa of infertile animals stained either more or less intensely than normal spermatozoa. A correlation was found between abnormal nuclear morphology and infertility in human spermatozoa. Incomplete condensation of the nuclear chromatin in spermatozoa of certain infertile bulls was also detected under electron microscope.

B. Physiological and Biochemical Changes

Changes in the pattern of motility: The most striking physiological change during sperm maturation is the acquisition of characteristic pattern of progressive motility. Spermatozoa from the lower corpus epididymides of the rat exhibit a circular swimming movement while the development of complete forward movement by large numbers of spermatozoa occurs only as they enter the upper cauda epididymides. It was suggested that the non-progressive pattern of motility of spermatozoa from the caput epididymides inhibits them from going through the utereo-tubal junction and renders them infertile. Although the precise mechanism(s) that initiate (s) and regulate (s) this process is/are unknown but the observed shift in the ionic balance (K+ and Na+) in the epididymal secretion may be an important factor in the development of motility.

Increase in the net negative charge on the surface of the spermatozoa: The electrophoretic mobility and net negative charge on the surface of the spermatozoa increase as they move from the caput to the cauda epididymides. It was seen that the capacity to bind colloidal iron hydroxide (CIH) increases in the spermatozoa of rabbit, bull and hamster during their sojourn through the epididymis. Furthermore, human spermatozoa exhibited increasing affinity for the positively charged colloidal ferric oxide particles at pH 1.8 during their passage through the epididymis, thus indicating that the density of anionic groups present at the surface of sperm plasma membrane increases as sperm progress through the epididymis. However, the chemical identity of the residue (s), which are responsible for biding CIH, is not known but they appear to be neuraminidase resistant since digestion of rabbit and hamster spermatozoa with neuraminidase had no effect on CIH labeling.

Changes in sialic acid: The concentration of sialic acid in the spermatozoa of the rat, hamster and monkey is found to decrease during their transit from the caput to the cauda epididymis. These changes may be related to the maturation of spermatozoa.

The specific gravity and light reflection power: The specific gravity and light reflection power of spermatozoa increases during their migration through the epididymis. These changes have been attributed to progressive dehydration of spermatozoa and/or changes in the chemical composition of the cells.

Thermal and pH resistance: Resistance of spermatozoa to heat and cold and to variations in pH increases during their transit through the epididymis.

Changes in the permeability of membrane: Changes in the permeability of membrane are known to occur during maturation.

Changes in the metabolic pattern of spermatozoa: Various investigators have reported distinct metabolic differences between the epididymal and ejaculated spermatozoa. Factors like low partial pressure of oxygen, a high level of bicarbonates, metabolic overcrowding, a deficiency of glycolysable sugar, a high ratio of potassium to sodium and the presence of a metabolic inhibitor may contribute to the metabolic inactivity of epididymal spermatozoa. In addition, presence of steroids in the epididymal fluid has also been suggested to cause metabolic dormancy of epididymal spermatozoa. However, spermatozoa from the ampulla (the glandular enlargements of the terminal portion of the vas deferens) show an intermediate state of metabolism between the spermatozoa from the epididymis and that from the ejaculate, suggesting that the activation of spermatozoa take place in the vas deferens.

Earlier investigators believed that maturation of spermatozoa is primarily a temporal phenomenon. However, recent studies have established beyond doubt that a) intrinsic factors alone are not sufficient for sperm maturation to occur, and b) the epididymal environment plays a decisive role in this process. The development of motility and fertilizing ability are two independent phenomena. These conclusions were based on the fact that the rabbit spermatozoa when retained in the caput or corpus epididymides by ligature develop normal characteristic motility but do not acquire fertilizing ability. Hence a period of retention in the epididymal canal seems to be a pre-requisite for the culmination of maturational changes in the spermatozoa.

The epididymis may influence the spermatozoa by alterations of the tubular environment through secretion and reabsorption of various steroids and steroid hormones. The epididymis also has the capacity to metabolize androgens. 5 α-dihydrotestosterone and androstanediol appear to be in some way related to the metabolism and maturation of spermatozoa. The maturational changes in the spermatozoa are dependent on androgens and are affected by castration or hypophysectomy or by the administration of anti-androgens. Changes in the acrosome of guinea pig spermatozoa are inhibited during their transit through the epididymis by castration or administration of cyproterone acetate (an anti-androgen) and this inhibitory effect is prevented by treatment with testosterone. Further, Orgebin-Crist (1973) has shown that the spermatozoa from the distal cauda epididymides of rat lose their ability to fertilize ova within four days after castration and six days after hypophysectomy. It was found that loss in the fertilizing ability of spermatozoa precedes the loss in motility following castration or hypophysectomy. However, the motility and fertilizing ability of spermatozoa in castrated hamsters and rats can be maintained for a longer duration of time in the presence of testosterone or 5 α-dihydrotestosterone than in their absence. Androgens may influence sperm maturation through their effect on the epididymis since treatment of intact rats with cyproterone acetate result in a marked decrease in the content of sialic acid of the epididymis concurrent with the loss of integrity of the acrosome and motility, viability and fertilizing ability of spermatozoa.

13.2 Biochemistry of Semen

On emerging from the testis, the testicular contents containing secretions and yet immotile and infertile spermatozoa enter the epididymis. They complete their passage and maturation in the epididymal duct and pass into the vas deferens. In the course of the ejaculatory process, they encounter secretory fluids produced by several other accessory organs of reproduction located along the male tract. These secretions blend into seminal plasma at the time of semen emission.

Composition of semen: **Semen** is a milky white, somewhat sticky mixture, consisting of cellular component, the **spermatozoa** and the fluid component, the **seminal plasma**. Figure 13.2 gives the diagrammatic representation of the chemical composition of semen. The amount of semen propelled out of the male duct system during ejaculation is relatively small, only 2-5 ml but is very dense and contains between 50 and 130 million sperm per milliliter. Number of spermatozoa in one milliliter of semen represents the **density of spermatozoa**. Volume and sperm count in semen decreases with repeated ejaculation. In man, semen normally contains 20-40 million sperm per milliliter. Sperm count lower than 20 million per ml renders the semen sterile. The specific gravity of semen is 1.028 and its pH is 7.35-7.50. Seminal buffers such as phosphate and bicarbonate serve to protect the sperm against low pH of the vagina.

The accessory gland secretions exhibit marked species dependence and individual day-to-day variations in terms of both quantity and composition. There is also remarkable variation in the volume and composition of the individual gland secretions. In lower animals, bird and even among some of the mammals, seminal plasma may be so little that the emitted semen takes the form of a very thick lump of spermatozoa, closely packed together. But the higher animals, including man on the whole produce relatively dilute semen with seminal plasma representing a considerable proportion of the ejaculate. Also there is considerable variation in composition and volume of seminal plasma between species because the accessory glands, which vary from one species to another, contribute in its formation. The diversity in composition of semen is thus, one of the outstanding features of the ejaculate. Table 13.1 gives the sperm density and volume of ejaculated semen in different species.

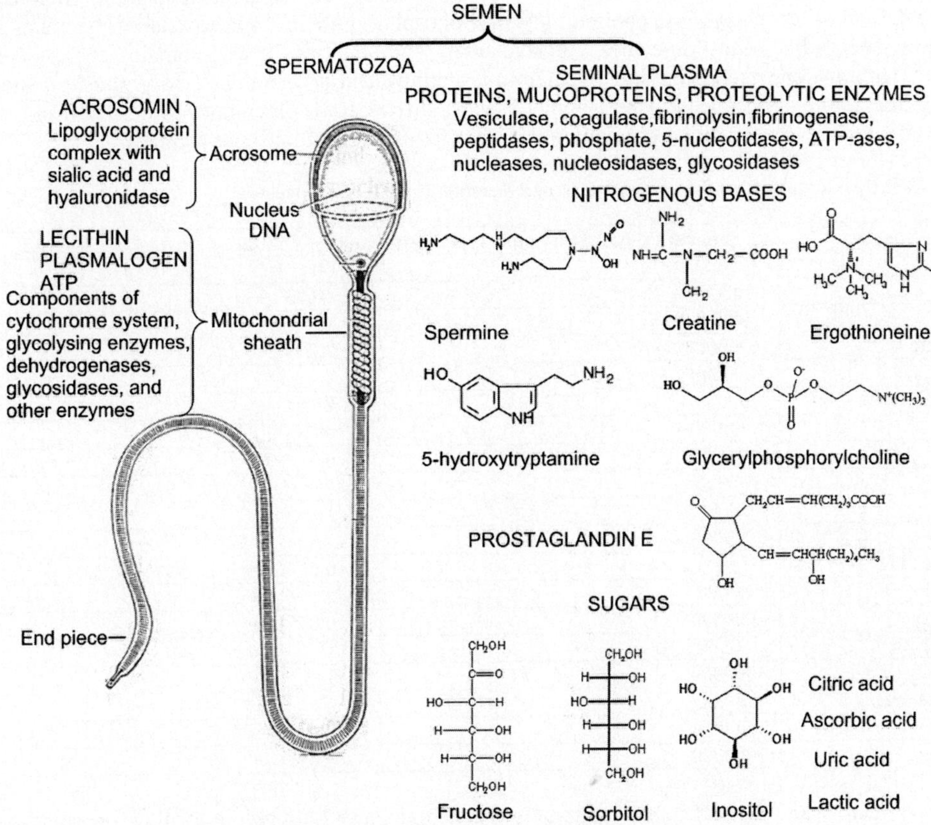

Figure 13.2: Diagrammatic representation of the biochemistry of semen.

Chemical Constituents: The seminal plasma is an extra-cellular fluid that provides the medium and vehicle for spermatozoa of the semen. It is a composite mixture of secretions coming from the male accessory glands of reproduction. The proportion of this fluid, which originates from various accessory secretory sex organs like epididymis, vasa deferentia, ampulla, seminal vesicles, ventral prostate, dorso-lateral prostate, coagulating glands, Cowper's glands and urethral (littoral) glands varies greatly from one species to another.

The chemical approach to the study of the accessory glands has received great importance from the pioneer studies of Thaddeus Mann. The secretion of the accessory glands of many species is a repository for huge quantities of substances, which are present only in trace amounts in other tissues and body fluids. It is obvious that the seminal plasma must provide a perfectly balanced and nutritive milieu suitable for the survival of sperm in the vagina and uterus. Therefore, two extraordinary features of male secretory glands are the following. i) The highly specialized chemical nature of the glandular secretion, and ii) close dependence of their development and secretory activity upon male hormones. Primarily hormones of testicular origin govern the functional activity of the accessory glands, and this in turn affects the composition of seminal plasma.

Since semen is a suspension of spermatozoa in the secretion of the epididymis, seminal vesicle, prostate, Cowper's glands etc, it contains various constituents contributed by each of these accessory glands. Thus, chemical analysis of seminal plasma of semen shows that it contains the following constituents- fructose, citric acid, ascorbic acid, uric acid, lactic acid, pyruvic acid, phosphates, inositol, phosphoryl choline, glyceryl phosphoryl choline, electrolytes, polyamines like spermine, spermidine, lipids, enzymes, prostaglandin, and inhibin. It also contains ergothioneine, sorbitol, carnitine and acetylcarnitine, hypotaurine, scyllitol, and glyceryl phosphoryl inositol, and N-acetylglucosamine. Chemically, the seminal plasma differs from other body fluids in being well endowed with free amino acids (especially glutamic acid) and small molecular peptides.

Table 13.1: Sperm density and volume of ejaculated semen in different Species

Species	Sperm Density in Semen (sperm/μl)	Volume of single ejaculate (ml)
Ass	300000	40
Bat	6000000	0.05
Boar	100000	25
Buffalo	600000	2.5
Bull	1000000	4
Camel	400000	8
Cat	1700000	0.03
Cock	3500000	0.8
Dog	300000	9
Fox	70000	1.5
Goat	3000000	1
Guinea Pig	10000	0.6
Man	80000	3
Pigeon	2000000	0.016
Rabbit	150000	1
Ram	3000000	1
Red Deer	200000	4
Stallion	120000	70
Turkey	7000000	0.3

Fructose and lactic acid are the principal metabolic substrates, while sorbitol, phospholipids, amino acids and fatty acids may be catabolized to a limited degree. The hydrogen ion concentration of seminal fluid is buffered at pH 7.0 by bicarbonate, citric acid, proteins and amino acids. The major electrolytes of seminal plasma are sodium, potassium, calcium, magnesium and chlorides. Various lipids, proteins and polypeptides present in seminal plasma may help to protect the spermatozoa membrane from the effect of dilution. An "antiagglutinin" is present and maintained in an active reduced state by ascorbic acid and ergothioneine in the seminal fluid to prevent agglutination of spermatozoa during dilution. A polysaccharide decapacitating factor (D.F.) coats the sperm and prevents them from penetrating the ovum until enzymes in the female genital tract remove it. Various enzymes of the seminal fluid are proteolytic enzymes, phosphatase, glycosidase, choline esterase, diamine oxidase and lactic dehydrogenase. Ascorbic acid, riboflavin and inositol are the vitamins, while epinephrine, norepinephrine, estrogens and androgens are the hormones of the seminal plasma.

Fructose: Fructose is present in semen of a large number of mammals like man, monkey, bull, boar, rat, guinea pig, dog etc. Seminal vesicles are the main source of fructose in higher mammals yet an additional small amount of sugar comes from the ampullary glands. In rat, the seminal vesicles are free from fructose. Instead, fructose is found in dorso-lateral prostate and coagulating glands. In mouse, fructose is present in both, coagulating glands and seminal vesicles.

Androgen and pituitary hormones regulate secretion of seminal fructose. Blood glucose levels also influence it since hyperglycemia results in an increase in the concentration of fructose in semen. The biosynthesis of seminal sugars involves a conversion of blood glucose into seminal fructose. In the extracts made from bull seminal vesicle tissue it was possible to demonstrate the synthesis of seminal sugars as per the reaction diagram shown in Figure 13.3.

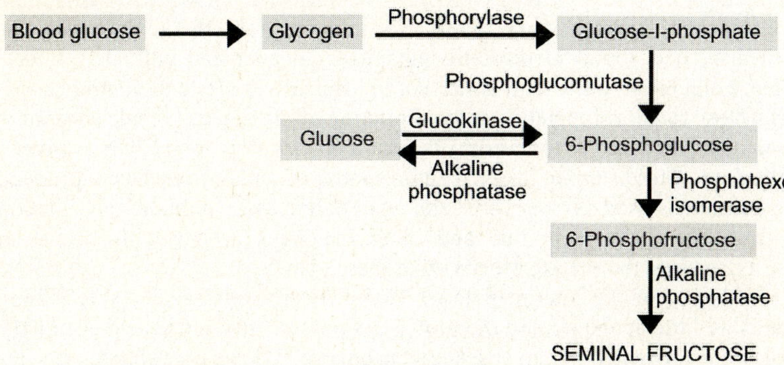

Figure 13.3: Biosynthesis of seminal sugars in Bull seminal vesicles.

The equilibrium mixture of 6-phosphohexoses acted upon by alkaline phosphatases yielded a mixture of free glucose and free fructose and these were present in the seminal plasma. Further studies in this field indicated that apart from the phosphorylative pathway of glucose metabolism, the accessory organs of ram and rat posses an alternative nonphosphorylative pathway for conversion of glucose to fructose which involves sorbitol as an intermediary metabolite and a sorbitol dehydrogenase as an intermediary enzyme. In addition to sorbitol dehydrogenase, the vesicular tissue also contains aldose reductase, which can reduce glucose to sorbitol in the presence of reduced form of NADP (NADPH). The pathway of this conversion is shown in Figure 13.4. The relative importance of two pathways for fructose secretory function in accessory glands remains unknown.

$$\text{Glucose} + \text{NADPH} + \text{H}^{+} \xrightarrow{\text{Aldose reductase}} \text{Sorbitol} + \text{NADP}^{+}$$

$$\text{Sorbitol} + \text{NAD}^{+} \xrightarrow{\text{Ketose reductase}} \text{Fructose} + \text{NADH} + \text{H}^{+}$$

$$\text{Glucose} + \text{NADPH} + \text{NAD}^{+} \longrightarrow \text{Fructose} + \text{NADH} + \text{NADP}^{+}$$

Figure 13.4: Formation of seminal fructose.

In species where fructose is a normal constituent of seminal plasma, anaerobic fructolysis is the metabolic process, which enables spermatozoa to survive without oxygen. Spermatozoa utilize and glycolyse fructose and glucose to lactic acid for energy needed for their motility.

Sorbitol and Inositol: Seminal plasma contains two polyols, sorbitol and inositol, both in sustainable quantities. The occurrence of sorbitol in seminal plasma was reported in ram, rabbit, bat, boar and human semen. The levels of sorbitol bear a definite relation not only to concentration of fructose in seminal plasma but also to activity of two-enzymes, aldose reductase and ketose reductase (sorbitol dehydrogenase) in the accessory organs.

Inositol is found in seminal vesicles of boar and also in many other species but its levels is 10-40 times lower than in boar. The experiments with rats indicate that content of inositol in the male accessory sex organs is regulated by androgens. Regarding the role of inositol there is evidence that inositol is metabolized directly by spermatozoa. In the boar, inositol is probably concerned with maintenance of the osmotic equilibrium of the seminal plasma. The medium where inositol is formed remains obscure, but several possible reaction routes are i) synthesized in a free form by breakdown of some of inositol lipids, ii) by hydrolysis of protein or peptide bound inositol phosphates, iii) it may arise from glucose or other sugars.

Citric Acid: Citric acid in the seminal plasma is derived from the male accessory organs of reproduction. In man, it is found in prostatic secretion. In boar and bull, it is found in seminal vesicular secretion while in rat, citric acid is present in seminal vesicles and ventral prostate. Just like fructose, there is a close relationship between the formation of citric acid in male accessory glands and the levels of testicular hormone, testosterone. In castrated rats it is found that a direct relationship exists between the dose of testosterone injected and response of seminal vesicles to produce citric acid. Therefore, this parameter is used as a sensitive and quantitative assay of androgen function. Removal of hypophysis (**hypophysectomy**) in rats and other mammals produces the same end-result as castration that is, it decreases the secretory activity of these glands.

Citric acid is one of the intermediate of TCA (Tricarboxylic acid) cycle. The rat seminal vesicle has remarkably little aconitase and therefore, it is possible that citric acid accumulates because its further breakdown is prevented due to absence of aconitase. On the other hand, rat ventral prostate, which also secretes citric acid, possesses the complete enzyme system for the oxidation of citrate via TCA cycles. The human prostate as well as seminal vesicle has high transaminase activity and free amino acid including glutamic acid. These points suggest the possibility of citric acid being formed from oxaloacetic acid, which arises from glutamic acid as a result of transamination. William Ashman (1958) pointed out that since both fructose and citric acid involve active participation of NAD, it is possible that their formation is dependent on balance between NADPH and NADH and that citrate would tend to accumulate whenever the ratio NADPH/NADP+ becomes unfavorable for isocitrate dehydrogenase activity. The absence of aldose reductase in ventral prostate and seminal vesicles also results in high rate of citric acid accumulation. In the absence of this enzyme, there is no reduction of glucose to sorbitol and consequently no oxidation of NADPH to NADP+, which is required by enzyme isocitrate dehydrogenase. Thus, the presence or absence of aldolase in a male accessory organ seems to be the decisive factor, which determines whether a given organ produces fructose or citric acid. The physiological role of citric acid is not clear. Perhaps citric acid in combination with potassium and sodium ions plays a part in maintaining osmotic equilibrium in semen.

Ascorbic Acid, Uric Acid, Lactic Acid and Pyruvic acid: Ascorbic acid is present in the vesicular secretions of guinea pig, man, bull, boar and is responsible for the reducing power of semen. Uric acid is a normal constituent of seminal plasma, not only in man but also in other mammals including bull, ram and boar. It is probably formed by enzymic oxidation of purines like xanthine and hypoxanthine in seminal vesicles. Lactic acid is also a normal constituent of seminal plasma. The lactic acid found in fresh semen comes from fluid produced by seminal vesicles. It may be an outcome of active glycolysis going in epithelial tissue of seminal vesicle. Fructolysis may also result in the formation of lactic acid and pyruvic acid in semen.

Nitrogen Bases: Among chemical characteristics, which distinguish seminal plasma from other body fluids are certain nitrogenous bases like spermine, spermidine, choline and ergothioneine.

In human semen, after ejaculation crystals of spermine are formed. It is in the form of phosphate ($C_{10}H_{26}N_4$-spermine). The oxidation of spermine gives rise to a volatile base associated with characteristic odor of semen. Spermidine is another base present in semen. Choline accumulates in semen only after ejaculation. This is formed as a result of hydrolysis from precursors like glyceryl phosphoryl choline and phosphoryl choline.

Choline, phosphoryl choline and glyceryl phosphoryl choline (GPC) are linked with metabolism of phospholipids in either male accessory organs or spermatozoa. GPC occurs in a significantly higher concentration in epididymis than in any other part of male reproductive system. This leads to the suggestion that mainly epididymis contributes to the seminal content of GPC.

Ergothioneine ensures sperm motility and fructose utilization by protecting essential sulphydryl group-binding substances and agents, which are capable of oxidizing the sulphydryl groups.

Lipids: Lipids are in the form of lipoprotein plasmalogens (phosphatidyl ethanolamine or phosphatidylcholine), and free cholesterol. Sperm phospholipids and plasmalogen play an important role in the metabolism of semen, mainly as substrates for spermatozoa for endogenous respiration. The lipids are also found in seminal plasma in the form of phosphorylated derivatives of choline. In human, they are derived from prostatic secretion. In bull, vesicular secretion contributes to the lipid present in seminal plasma.

Prostaglandins: The lipid soluble substances, which occur in seminal plasma, are called prostaglandins. The two main types are the prostaglandin E and prostaglandin F. Prostaglandin E_1 has been isolated in crystalline form from vesicular glands of ram and human seminal plasma. Prostaglandin F_1 has been isolated from seminal vesicles of ram. Other forms of prostaglandins, that is prostaglandin E_1 and prostaglandin F_1 have also been demonstrated in seminal plasma. The mechanism of their formation in male accessory sex organs and their full physiologic significance in reproduction are not fully understood.

Proteins, Proteases and Free Amino Acids: The seminal plasma also contains some extra-cellular proteins and proteases in human, ram, bull, boar and other species. Several assays for free amino acids show the presence of amino acids like glycine, threonine, alanine, valine etc. There is some evidence that amino acids and proteases present in semen play a role in sperm survival.

Mucoproteins and Sialic Acid: The mucoproteins of seminal plasma form a gelatinous mass. One distinct type of seminal mucoprotein in man as well as in other species is sialic acid (N-acetyl neuraminic acid). In boar, bulbo urethral glands secrete it. It also occurs in seminal plasma of other species like stallion (secreted by ampulla and epididymis). The physiological role of sialic acid in sperms remains to be investigated.

Proteolytic Enzymes: The seminal plasma and male accessory sex gland's secretions contain considerable proteolytic activity, which is implicated in proteolysis of seminal proteins to form free amino acids. There also exists a correlation between several proteolytic enzymes involved in coagulation and liquefaction of semen, two processes, which occur spontaneously in ejaculated semen of certain species like man, for example, presence of vesiculase in coagulating glands, and coagulase and fibrinolysin (plasmin) for liquefaction in prostate.

Phosphatase: Semen has powerful phosphatase activity. Among the most active and best known are acid phosphatase, alkaline phosphatase, 5-nucleotidases and several enzymes which split adenosine triphosphate. Acid phosphatase is secreted by prostate. The freshly ejaculated human semen contains phosphoryl choline, which on ejaculation is rapidly dephosphorylated by acid phosphatase to free choline and orthophosphate. Alkaline phosphatase is capable of hydrolyzing a number of phosphoric acid esters like 1-phospho fructose, 6-phospho fructose, 1-6 diphospho fructose. It has been suggested that rat's ventral prostate contains an alkaline phosphatase which is Zn^{++} dependent.

Hyaluronidase: Hyaluronidase is commonly associated with the sperm. It is a mucolytic enzyme, which depolymerises and hydrolyses hyaluronic acid. It facilitates fertilization by liquefying a passage for sperm through cumulus cells surrounding the ovum.

Other Substances: Other substances in semen include creatine, creatinine, epinephrine, and norepinephrine. Table 13 .2 compares the composition of the fluids taken from the ejaculated semen with those of the secretions of the epididymis and seminal vesicle in case of boar.

Table 13.2: Composition of ejaculated semen, epididymal semen and seminal vesicle secretion in Boar

Constituents ↓ Composition of fluid portion (mg/100ml)	**Ejaculated Semen**	**Epididymal Semen**	**Seminal Vesicle Secretion**
Total volume (ml)	375 (± 24)	12	174
Fructose	9 (± 0.5)	Trace	43
Ergothioneine	17 (± 1.1)	Trace	81
Citric acid	173 (± 9)	14	831
Lactic acid	21	19	21
Total dry weight	3970	6420	15020
Dry weight of non-dialyzable material	2745	4235	10615
Total phosphorus	39	227	34
Acid soluble phosphorus	32	224	31
Sodium	587	88	62
Potassium	197	188	212
Calcium	6	5	12
Hexosamine (after acid hydrolysis)		128	80

13.3 Coagulation of Semen

At coitus the semen in some species such as man, cow, sheep and rabbit is deposited directly into the vagina. But in few other species such as mare, sow and rodents, it may be forced through the cervix into the uterus. In different species, the semen coagulates to different degrees after ejaculation and this is very important in retaining the spermatozoa and preventing them from leaking through the vagina. The secretion from the coagulating glands (that is why called as the coagulating) forms what is known as the **vaginal plug** or '**copulation plug**' after copulation at the vaginal opening. In rodents such as mice, rat etc., the coagulum is especially large and tough and fills the vagina. It may persist for one or two days.

There exists a correlation between several of the proteolytic agents secreted by the male accessory organs. Semen coagulation and liquefaction are two processes, which occur, simultaneously in the ejaculated semen of certain species including man.

The mechanism of semen coagulation has been extensively studied in rat and guinea pig. It is believed to involve two enzyme reactions. The action of enzyme vesiculase secreted in coagulating glands on the protein procoagulase contributed by seminal vesicles with the formation of clotting enzyme proper or coagulase. The clotting of coagulinogen, a coagulable protein produced in seminal vesicle by the enzyme coagulase. The two reactions are shown in Figure 13.5.

In human semen the coagulation and liquefaction process is believed to involve three distinct stages.

1) The formation of a fibrin-like clot by the action of a clotting enzyme produced in the prostate on a fibrinogen like protein substance contributed by seminal vesicle.
2) Fibrinolysis that is splitting of the fibrin, a plasmin like enzyme of prostatic origin formed from an inactive precursor (plasminogen activator) and

3) Further proteolysis of the Iysed fibrin, leading to the formation of free amino acids and NH_3.

Procoagulase —*Vesiculase enzyme*→ Coagulase

Coagulinogen —*Coagulase enzyme*→ Coagulated protein

Figure 13.5: Coagulation of semen.

13.4 Physiological Significance of the Seminal Plasma

In addition to spermatozoa, seminal plasma is also a very important constituent of semen and plays many physiologically significant roles.

The seminal fluids or plasma acts as a normal diluent and vehicle for the thick mass of closely packed epididymal spermatozoa. Seminal plasma provides buffering capacity for transferring spermatozoa from the male to the female genital tract. This combats the acidic condition of the vagina. Seminal plasma is a composite mixture of secretions from the male accessory organs of reproduction. Some components of seminal plasma stimulate the activity and metabolism of the spermatozoa and others provide the necessary nutrients for energy production. Seminal plasma exerts a distinct stimulating effect on sperm motility. This may be due to dilution effect. However, the activation by seminal plasma is linked with the occurrence of specific substances secreted by the different accessory sex glands. Seminal plasma contains pharmacodynamically active substances such as prostaglandin, which elicit contraction of the smooth muscle of the female genital tract to aid in sperm transport. Also, the prostaglandins in semen decrease the viscosity of mucus guarding the entry (cervix) of the uterus. The presence of hormone relaxin and certain enzymes in semen enhance sperm motility. Semen also contains an antibiotic chemical called **seminal plasmin**, which destroys certain bacteria. Mixed semen from different bulls has been claimed to improve conception rate and yields better offspring. The coagulum/coagulation plug formed at the time of coitus in some animals like rats and mice from the secretion of accessory sex glands prevents leakage of spermatozoa from the vagina, thus ensuring fertilization.

Summary

Epididymis is a tightly coiled tube on the outside of the testis that conveys the spermatozoa into the vas deferens. It stores and nourishes immature spermatozoa and promotes their maturation.

Mammalian spermatozoa released from the testis undergo a series of morphological, physiological and biochemical changes during their transit through the epididymis. These are called maturational changes. These changes result in acquiring the spermatozoa of a characteristic motility and fertilizing ability. This process is androgen dependent and is affected by hypophysectomy, castration or treatment with androgen antagonist.

On completing their journey through the epididymis, spermatozoa are stored in the cauda epididymides and vas deferens till they are released to the outside during ejaculation. During sexual intercourse (coitus), semen is ejaculated into the vagina.

Semen is composed of a cellular component, the sperm cells and a fluid component, the seminal plasma.

The seminal plasma is a composite mixture of secretions of all the accessory sex glands, such as ampullary glands, seminal vesicles, prostate, coagulating glands, and bulbourethral glands.

Volume and sperm count of semen varies from species to species. In normal adult male, an ejaculate contains 2-5 ml of semen containing 50-130 million sperm per milliliter.

Semen is an alkaline fluid that dilutes and transports spermatozoa. Important constituents of seminal plasma are nutrients to provide energy, phosphates, electrolytes, enzymes, seminalplasmin, prostaglandins, hormones etc.

Semen activates sperm cells, but these sperm cells are coated with the decapacitation factor. This factor has to be removed in the female genital tract to enable the sperm to penetrate an egg for fertilization (capacitation).

Questions

1. What is maturation of spermatozoa? Where does it occur?
2. Describe the maturational changes in spermatozoa.
3. Describe the changes undergone by spermatozoa during their transit through the male tract.
4. What are the components of semen? Discuss their importance.
5. How does coagulation of semen takes place?
6. Discuss the physiological significance of seminal plasma.
7. Discuss the sources and functions of components of semen.
8. Discuss the role of accessory glands of reproduction in males.
9. What are the major constituents of seminal plasma and which glands secrete them? Comment on their functions.
10. Give a brief account of the biochemical constituents of semen and their functions.
11. Enumerate various biochemical components of semen. Discuss their importance in reproductive process.
12. Which of the following does not add a secretion that makes a major contribution to semen a) prostate, b) bulbourethral glands, c) testes, d) **vas deferens**.

Chapter 14

Female Reproductive System

The female reproductive tract is structurally and physiologically very malleable, serving to help attract the male during courtship, produce ova for fertilization and nourish the embryo. Organs of reproduction in females include the **ovaries**; the **uterine (fallopian) tubes**, or **oviducts**; the **uterus**; the **cervix**; the **vagina**; and the **external genital organs** that constitute the **vulva**, or **pudendum**. The **mammary glands** are also considered part of the female reproductive system. Figure 14.1 illustrates the structures of the female genital tract.

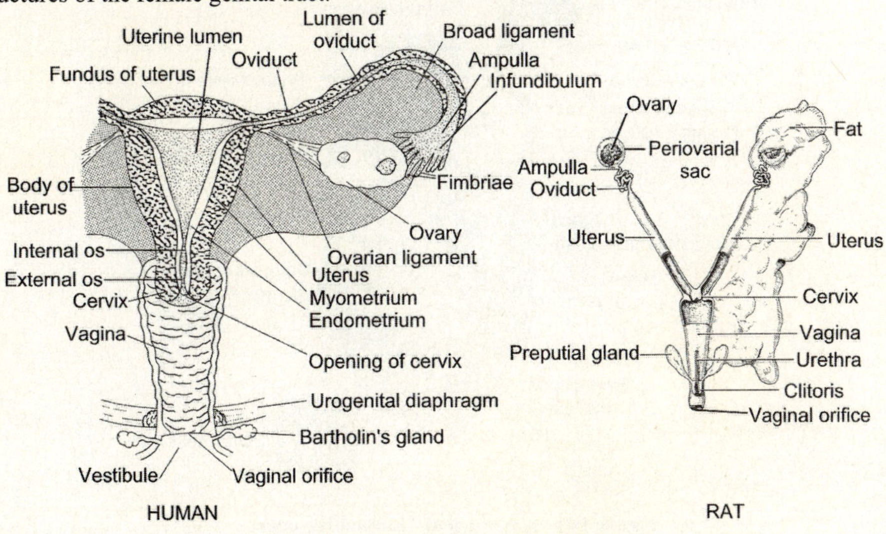

Figure 14.1: Female reproductive system of Human and Rat.

14.1 Ovary

The ovaries (= egg receptacles) are paired glands that resemble unshelled almonds in size and shape. They are homologous to testes as having the same embryonic origin. They are located in a shallow depression (ovarian fossa) one on either side in the lateral wall of the pelvic cavity.

Descent of the ovary: Ovary descends to the brim of the superior portion of the pelvic cavity during the third month of fetal development in humans and remains attached to the lateral pelvic wall.

Attachments of the Ovary: Each ovary is held in place within the peritoneal cavity by several ligaments. The **ovarian ligament** anchors the ovary medially to the uterus. The **suspensory ligament**

anchors it laterally to the pelvic wall and the **mesovarium** suspends it in between. Both the suspensory ligaments and the mesovarium are part of the **broad ligament**, which is a peritoneal fold, that " tents" over the uterus and supports the uterine tubes, uterus, and the vagina. The fibrous ovarian ligaments are enclosed within the broad ligament. The ovaries are served by the ovarian arteries, which are the branches of the abdominal aorta, and also by the ovarian branch of the uterine arteries.

Structure of the Ovary: Like the testis, the external surface of an ovary is surrounded by a fibrous **tunica albuginea.** A layer of polyhedral (columnar or cuboidal) epithelial cells known as the **'germinal' superficial epithelium** covers the tunica albuginea externally. The epithelium is continuous with the peritoneum of the mesovarium and is tenuously attached to the tunica albuginea. The term germinal epithelium is a misnomer here, as it does not give rise to ova. Generally the free surfaces of these cells are covered with a large number of microvilli, which can attain an average density of between 300-350 units per square millimeter of cell surface. These microvilli are uniform in appearance. Ovary consists of two distinct regions: an outer **cortex**, and an inner **medulla** (Figure 14.2). The cortex consists of dense connective tissue containing forming gametes while medulla consists of loose connective tissue, blood vessels, lymphatics, and nerves. The forming gametes are many tiny saclike structures in various stages of development and are called **ovarian follicles**.

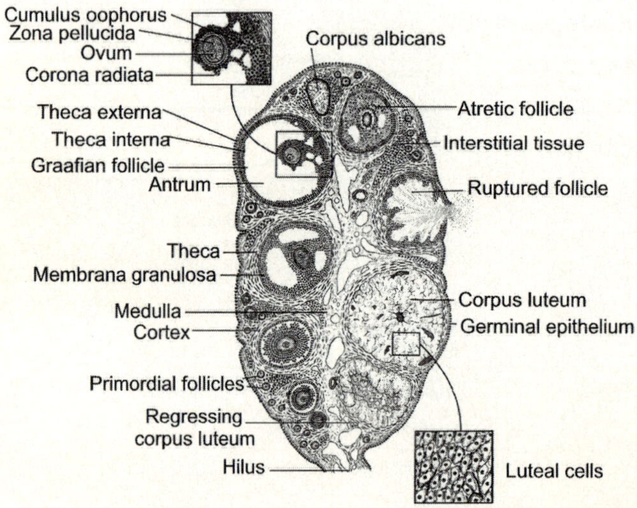

Figure 14.2: Structure of Mammalian ovary.

Follicular Development: At an outset of growth, ovarian follicles are approximately 40-50 μm in diameter and contain an oocyte of 15-30 μm in diameter surrounded by single layer of irregularly shaped flattened cells. These follicles are termed **primordial** or **unilaminar** or **primary follicles** and the oocyte is called a **primary** or **quiescent oocyte**. Small follicles are usually separated from the surrounding stroma by a thin basal lamina, which increases in thickness considerably during subsequent stages of follicular growth. Concomitant with the growth of the oocyte, the flattened granulosa cells of the primordial follicle begin to proliferate rapidly and in the process assume an irregular, polyhedral appearance and form multilayered, stratified epithelial-like structure called the **stratum granulosum** or simply **granulosa** which surrounds the oocyte. Such follicles are **secondary** or **multilayered** or **growing follicles**. Towards the end of proliferative phase, granulosa cell of secondary follicles under the influence of gonadotropins from the anterior pituitary, begin to secrete a fluid, called **liquor folliculi**, which accumulates in intercellular spaces. The continued secretion and accumulation of liquor folliculi result in the dissociation of granulosa cells, which subsequently leads to the formation of a large, fluid filled cavity called the **antrum**. When follicles possess a large antrum, they are referred to as **vesicular** or **tertiary follicles**, and finally these follicles attain maturity. The fully-grown follicles are called the **Graafian** or **pre-ovulatory follicles**. In the Graafian follicle, continuous accumulation of fluid separates granulosa cells closest to the oocyte from other cells in the follicle and also displaces the oocyte with its surrounding mass of follicle cells, called **cumulus oophorus** to an eccentric position within the antrum (Figure 14.2). During the course of oocyte development and follicle growth, an amorphous material rich in mucopolysaccharide is deposited in the space between the oocyte and the surrounding granulosa cells. This material is subsequently transformed into a continuous jelly-like coat, called the **zona pellucida**. Origin of the zona is still somewhat uncertain. It appears likely that the stratified nature of the zona pellucida in the mature follicle result from a discontinuous secretory process involving both oocyte and granulosa cells.

The innermost layer of granulosa cells becomes firmly attached to the zona pellucida and is called the **corona radiata**. The outermost granulosa cells rest on a basement membrane that separates them from the surrounding ovarian stroma. This outer region is called the **theca folliculi**. As primary follicle continues to grow, the theca differentiates into two layers, the **theca interna**, a vascularized internal layer of secretory cells, and the **theca externa**, an outer layer of spindle-shaped connective tissue cells. The cumulus is generally found on the wall of the antrum opposite the surface that ruptures at ovulation.

Each month in adult women, one of the ripening follicles ejects its oocyte from the ovary. This event is called **ovulation**. After ovulation, the ruptured follicle is transformed into a very different looking structure called the **corpus luteum** (= yellow body, plural is **corpora lutea**), which eventually degenerates. Degenerating corpus luteum is fibrous tissue called **corpus albicans** (=white body). Figure 14.2 illustrates the detailed structure of the mammalian ovary.

The initiation of the growth of the oocyte is most likely regulated within the ovary so that the number of oocyte that enters the growth phase is related to the size of the pool of nongrowing oocyte. Typically, both oocyte and follicle grow coordinately, and in a sequence of definable morphological stages so that at ovulation depending upon the species an oocyte may range between 100-150 μm in diameter, and follicle may attain a diameter of nearly 12 mm.

14.2 The Female Duct System

The female duct system consists of the uterine or fallopian tubes, the uterus, the cervix and the vagina.

The Uterine Tubes: The uterine tubes, also called **fallopian tubes** or **oviducts**, form the initial part of the female duct system (Figure 14.1). These are paired muscular ducts with **four** distinct regions (**infundibulum, ampulla, isthmus** and **intramural**) that extend from the immediate vicinity of the ovary and communicate directly with the uterus. Depending upon the species, the oviducts vary considerably in length and also in degree of convolution. Embryonically, the oviducts arise from the cranial part of the Mullerian ducts. During adult life, the oviducts provide, a) the channel through which spermatozoa and oocyte are transported, b) the site of egg fertilization, and c) the essential physical and nutritional milieu for the cleaving embryo during the early preimplantation stages of pregnancy. Thus, the fallopian tubes receive the ovulated oocyte, provide a site where fertilization can occur, and transport the fertilized eggs to the uterus.

Each uterine tube is about 10 cm long and extends medially from the region of an ovary to empty into the supero-lateral region of the uterus via a constricted region called the **isthmus**. The function of isthmus is to transport spermatozoa to the site of fertilization and also fertilized eggs to the uterus for implantation. The distal end of the uterine tube expands as it curves around the ovary, forming the **ampulla**. In human, it is the longest region. Fertilization usually occurs in this region. The ampulla ends in the **infundibulum,** an open, funnel-shaped structure bearing ciliated, finger-like projections called **fimbriae** that drape over the ovary thus ensuring close proximity to the ovarian surface (Figure 14.1). The fourth portion of uterine tube is the **intramural** region as it lies within the uterine wall. This region is much more developed in some species such as primates and much less developed in others as in rodents. The juncture of the fallopian tube and the uterus is called the **utero-tubal junction** and it is this region of the oviduct that crosses directly into the uterine cavity.

Histologically, the uterine tubes are composed of three layers (Figure 14.3). These layers from the duct lumen towards outside are **mucosa**, **muscularis** and **serosa**. Numerous tall, ramified mucosal folds give a highly irregular contour to the lumen of the uterine tube, and their extensions into the lumen form deep grooves between the folds. The internal **mucosa** contains simple ciliated columnar epithelial cells, which help move the fertilized ovum along the tube, and non-ciliated peg-shaped secretory cells, which have microvilli and may provide nutrition for the ovum. The lamina propria is well vascularised with loose connective tissue. The middle layer in the wall of the uterine tube is the **muscularis** and is composed of an inner thick circular ring of smooth muscle and an outer, thin region of longitudinal smooth muscle. A third layer of longitudinal fibers is usually present in the region of the isthmus, especially near the uterus. The thickness of the muscle layers generally increases from the infundibulum toward the uterus. Peristaltic contractions of the muscularis and the ciliary action of the mucosa help to move the oocyte or fertilized ovum toward the uterus. The outermost layer in the wall of the uterine tubes is a serous membrane called the **serosa**.

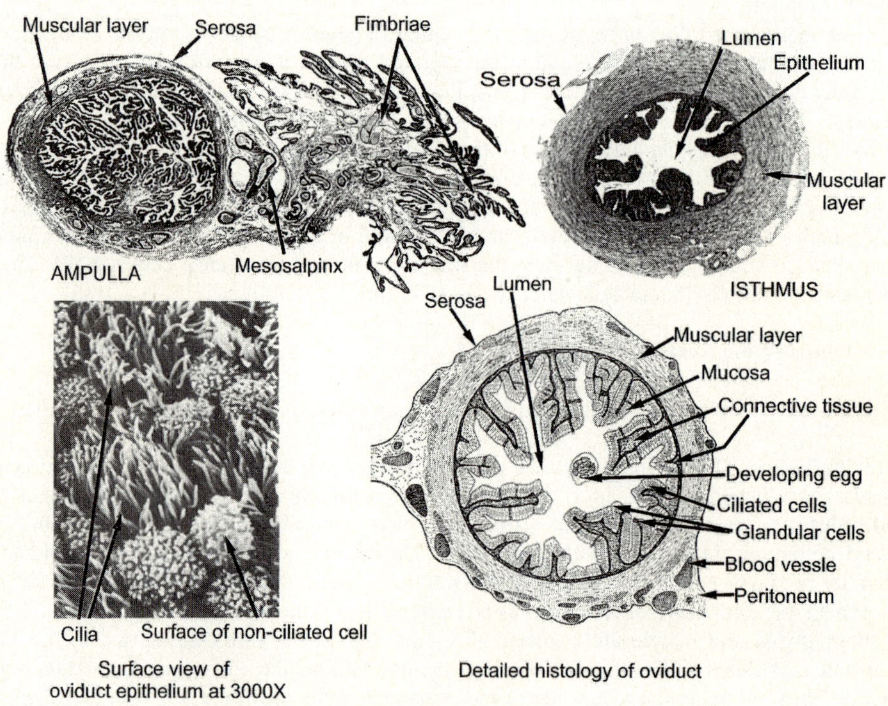

Figure 14.3: Transverse sections of Human oviduct.

The fimbriae and the infundibulum represent pre-ampulla region of the oviduct. Generally the wall of the pre-ampulla is quite thin and the cells of the epithelium are almost entirely ciliated since the function of this region is devoted to the transport of ovulated oocyte from the ovary to the site of fertilization, the ampulla. Wall of the ampulla is thicker than that of pre-ampullary region and its epithelium contains a comparatively reduced population of ciliated cells (Figure 14.3). Isthmus has a pronounced muscular coat and its epithelium is composed primarily of nonciliated secretory cells. These secretions fill the lumen of the tube. The muscle layers of the junctura are well developed, and the epithelium contains a larger number of ciliated cells than encountered in the isthmus. The lumen of the junctura is the narrowest of the entire oviduct. Except at estrus or when the eggs are passing into the uterus following their period of tubal transport, the utero-tubal junction is closed. In rat and mouse, the ovary is enclosed in a sac and is closely applied to the fimbriae. The fimbriae gather the shed ova or ovum, and with the help of ciliated cells, which beat towards the uterus, transport the ovum to the site of fertilization. Further, movement of the ovum is effected by peristaltic and segmental muscular contractions until in many species ovum transport is prevented by the constriction of the oviduct at the ampullary-isthmic-junction. The isthmic part of the oviduct undergoes contractions, which help the movement of sperm towards the ovum and later aid the movement of the fertilized ovum to the uterus. The utero-tubal junction may control sperm transport by providing sperm from the pocket-like diverticulae of the uterus. These diverticulae protrude into the uterine lumen in animals, which show uterine insemination such as rat, hamster, mouse, ferret, dog, mare, and pig. However, in woman, cow, and ewe, the junction is simple as in these, insemination is intra-vaginal. Externally, the uterine tubes are covered by visceral peritoneum and are supported along their length by a short mesentery (part of broad ligament) called the **mesosalpinx**.

Unlike the male duct system, which is continuous with the tubules of the testes, the uterine tubes have no actual contact with the ovaries. An ovulated oocyte is cast off into the peritoneal cavity, and many oocytes are lost there. However, the uterine tubes perform a complex sequence of movements to capture the oocytes. The infundibulum bends to cover the ovary while the fimbriae stiffen and sweep the ovarian surface, and the beating cilia on the fimbriae then create currents in the peritoneal fluid that act to carry the oocyte into the uterine tube, from where it begins its journey toward the uterus. The fact that the uterine tubes are not continuous with the ovary places the women at risk for **ectopic pregnancy** in which an ovum get fertilized in the peritoneal cavity and begins its development there itself. Such pregnancies are not normal and abort naturally often with substantial bleeding. Another problem with such a system of tubes in females is that of genital tract infection that easily spreads into the peritoneal cavity and this represents the **pelvic inflammatory diseases (PID)**.

The Uterus: The uterus (Latin word for "womb") is located in the pelvis, anterior to the rectum and postero-superior to the bladder. It is a hollow, thick walled organ that functions to receive, retain, and nourish fertilized ovum/ova.

Anatomically, uterus includes a dome-shaped portion superior to the uterine tubes (extend above the point of entry of the oviduct) called the **fundus**, the expanded central portion called **the body**, and an inferior narrow portion called the **cervix** that opens into the vagina (Figure 14.1) as the **portio vaginalis**. Between the body of the uterus and the cervix is the **isthmus**, a constricted region about 1 cm long. The interior of the body of the uterus is called the **uterine cavity**.

The shape of the uterus varies with species. For example, it may consist of two completely separated horns, two cervixes, and no uterine body. This is the **duplex** uterus of rodents; it may be **bicornuate** as in pig or **bipartite** as in ruminants; or **simplex** as in primates, while mare's uterus is in between bipartite and simplex, though more towards bipartite (Figure 14.4). Mammals that give birth to many young (**polytocous**) have primitive **duplex** uterus with least fusion between the embryonic Mullerian ducts (e.g. rodents and Lagomorphs). Slightly more fusion occurs in the ducts in the bicornuate condition, giving rise to the separate uterine horns, but a small uterine body and a single cervix, e.g. insectivores, pig, primitive primates, bats and popoises. Further fusion of the uterine horns give the bipartite condition with a moderate sized uterine body divided into two halves by a septum with long horns and a single cervical canal, e.g. carnivores and ruminants. Complete fusion of uterine horns and body result in simplex uterus of primates, usually associated with **monotocous species** (that give birth to single young).

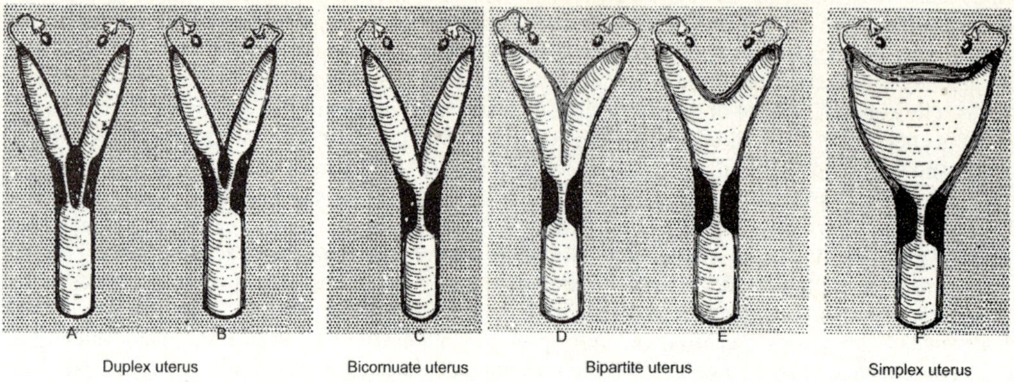

Figure 14.4: Four basic types of uterus in mammals, A (Rat, Mouse, Rabbit) and B (Guinea Pig) are duplex uterus, C (Pig, Insectivores) represent bicornuate uterus, D (Cat, Dog, Cow, Ewe with a septum separating the horns) and E (Mare with prominent uterine body) represent bipartite uterus and F (Primates) show simplex uterus with one cervix, prominent body but no horns.

The uterus is supported laterally by the **mesometrium** that is a portion of the broad ligament. More inferiorly, the **lateral cervical** or **cardinal ligaments** extend from the cervix and superior part of the vagina to the lateral walls of the pelvis, and the paired **uterosacral ligaments** secure the uterus to the sacrum posteriorly. The uterus is bound to the anterior body wall by the fibrous **round ligaments**, which run through the inguinal canals to anchor in the subcutaneous tissue of the labia majora. Despite the many anchoring ligaments, the muscles of the pelvic floor provide the principal support to the uterus.

Histologically, uterus also consists of three layers of tissues similar to those of the oviduct. These are the **serosa**, the **muscularis** (more commonly called **myometrium**), and the **mucosa** or the **endometrium** (Figure 14.5). The outer layer serosa is also known as perimetrium (*peri*= around, *metrium*= uterus). It is a part of visceral peritoneum and is composed of simple squamous epithelium and areolar connective tissue. The middle layer is the myometrium (*myo*=muscle), consisting of three layers of smooth muscle fibers. It is thickest in the fundus and thinnest in the cervix regions. The middle muscle layer is thicker and circular, whereas the inner and outer muscle layers are longitudinal or oblique. During the childbirth, coordinated contractions of the myometrium in response to oxytocin hormone from the posterior pituitary gland help to expel the fetus from the uterus. The inner layer of the uterus is the endometrium (*endo*= within). It is highly vascular and is composed of an innermost layer of simple columnar epithelium consisting of ciliated and secretory cells overlying a broad lamina propria. The epithelial layer lines the lumen. An underlying endometrial stroma is a very thick region of areolar connective tissue. Endometrial glands develop as invaginations of the luminal epithelium of endometrium and extend almost to the myometrium. The endometrium is divided into two layers, the **stratum functionalis** (functional layer) that lines the uterine cavity and is shed during menstruation, and a deeper layer, the **stratum basalis** (basal layer), which is permanent and gives rise to a new stratum functionalis after each menstruation (Figure 14.5).

To understand the cyclic changes of the uterine endometrium, discussed later in the chapter, it is essential to understand first the **vascular supply** of the uterus. The **uterine arteries** arise from the **internal iliac** in the pelvis, ascend along the sides of the uterine body, and send branches into the uterine wall. These branches break into several **arcuate arteries** within the myometrium. The arcuate arteries send **radial branches** into the endometrium, where they give off **straight arteries** to the lamina or stratum basalis and **spiral** or **coiled arteries** to the lamina or stratum functionalis (Figure 14.6). The spiral arteries undergo repeated degeneration and regeneration, and it is their spasms that actually cause shedding of the functionalis layer during menstruation. Veins in the endometrium are thin walled and form an extensive network with occasional sinusoidal enlargements. The extensive blood supply of the uterus is essential to support regrowth of a new stratum functionalis after menstruation for implantation of a fertilized ovum, and for the development of the placenta.

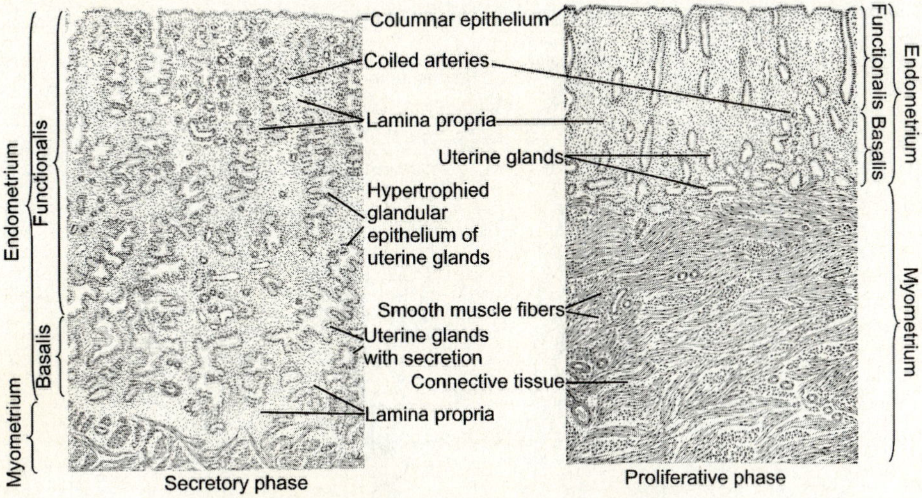

Figure 14.5: Histological structure of the Human uterus.

Cyclic Changes in the Endometrium: Both the structure and function of the endometrium, including the epithelium, lamina propria, glands and blood vessels are subjected to the influence of ovarian steroid hormones (Figure 14.7). Generally, three stages of cellular reorganization are observed during each menstrual cycle. These are 1) a **proliferative phase**, 2) a **secretory phase**, and 3) a **menstruation phase**. During the estrous cycle also, the uteri undergo progressive enlargement and become distended owing to the accumulation of luminal fluid (Chapter 15).

The endometrium of the uterus undergoes pronounced cyclical changes every month during a woman's reproductive years (Figure 14.8). These changes consist of a gradual building of tissue in preparation for receiving a fertilized egg followed by abrupt breakdown of this layer and a menstrual flow if pregnancy does not occur. The endometrial and superficial connective tissue layers of the uterine lining are at their maximum height (nearly 6-mm) during the fourteenth to twenty-sixth days of menstrual cycle. At this time, the endometrial glands are well developed and secrete a fluid that nourishes the embryo. Therefore, this period is referred to as the **secretory phase**. There are abundant blood vessels present in the superficial layer of endometrium at this stage. These are elongated and follow a spiral course as they extend from the basal portion to the surface epithelium. If no pregnancy occurs, drop in estrogen and progesterone levels makes the terminal portions of these vessels constrict. This deprives the superficial layers of the uterine lining of a supply of oxygen (**ischemia**) and results in their degeneration. About two days after the vasoconstriction takes place, the affected parts of the uterine lining begin to shed resulting in bleeding called the menstrual flow. This constitutes the **menstruation phase**. The menstrual fluid consists of epithelium, connective tissue, and blood. This blood normally clots in the uterus and the clots are broken up by enzyme action before flowing from the cervix. However, if menstruation at any given time is abnormally rapid, the blood may clot in the vagina. The normal blood loss during a menstrual period is variable, with an average of about 50 ml. Menstruation normally takes four days, with an average of three to six days. At this stage, the endometrium is only about 1 mm thick (Figure 14.8). It goes in to a three-day repair phase during which i) continuity of the epithelium is re-established, ii) the remaining blood vessels start to grow upward again, and iii) development of glands is initiated as invaginations of epithelium. Rapid growth of the epithelium, blood vessels, and connective tissue takes place during the next week. This is called the **proliferative phase**. It is followed by another **secretory phase**. All these changes are closely timed with those occurring in the maturing follicle of the ovary.

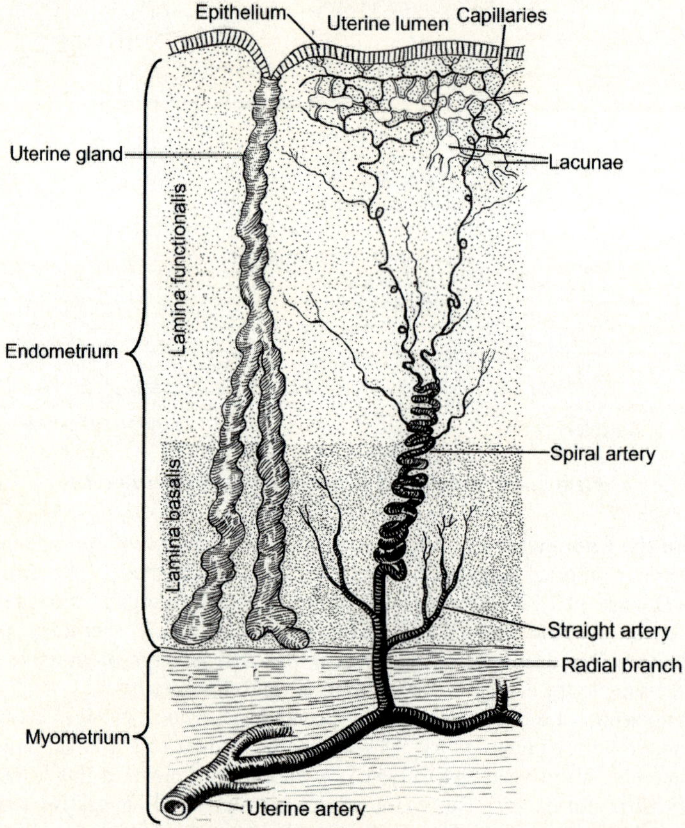

Figure 14.6: Vasculature of Human uterine endometrium.

Many other tissues of the reproductive tract of the female also undergo changes during the menstrual cycle, but to a much less extent. These changes are i) in motility of cilia of the oviduct (it is maximal at ovulation), ii) in the viscosity of the cervical mucus, and iii) in the cells of vaginal epithelium (see Chapter 15).

In general, the secretions that line the uterine mucosa during the progestational (secretory) phase are rich in carbohydrates, mucopolysaccharide, and proteins. Ionic composition of the uterus also undergoes marked alteration during the preimplantation stages of pregnancy. Also, in species in which capacitation of spermatozoa is a prerequisite for fertilization, the uterine secretions may be involved in an alteration of the plasma membrane overlying the spermatozoa acrosome, and change it to the fertilizable state. Unlike the oviduct, the uterus contains a reduced population of ciliated cells. Although the function of the ciliated cells of the uterus is not as apparent as that of the oviduct, it seems likely that these elements participate in the release and distribution of secretory material throughout the mucosa.

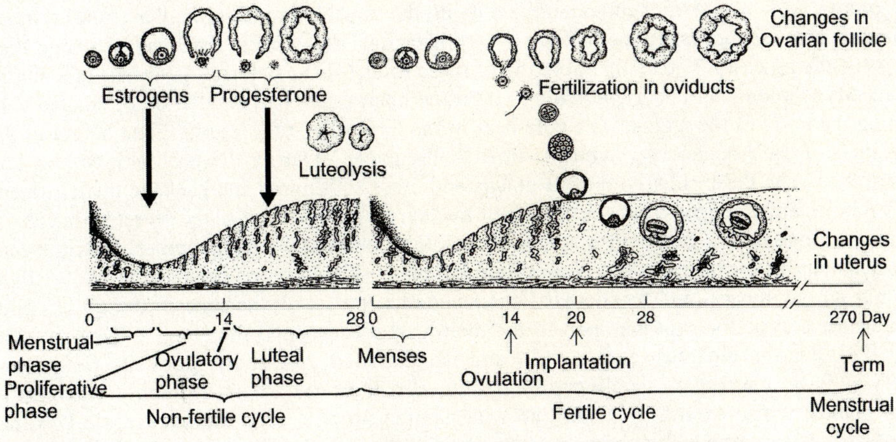

Figure 14.7: Correlation of pituitary and ovarian hormones with structural changes in ovary and uterus during menstrual cycle.

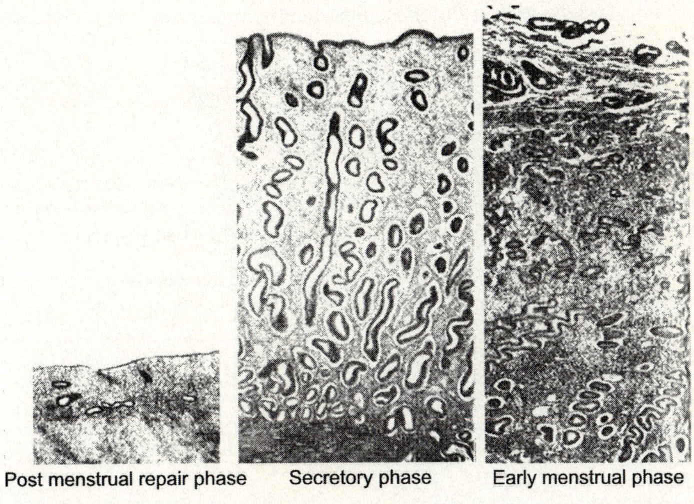

Figure 14.8: Changes in uterine endometrium during menstrual cycle of women.

The Cervix: The cervix is a neck-like region that extends from the uterus into the vagina. It is a sphincter-like fibrous organ, dilation of which allows passage of the fetus at birth. The interior of the narrow cervix is called the **cervical canal** and is nearly 3 cm long and slightly distended in the middle in human female. The cervical canal opens into the uterine cavity at the **internal os** and into the vagina at the **external os** (Figure 14.1).

Histologically wall of the cervix, like that of oviduct and uterus is also made up of three coats. These are **serosa** on the outside, **muscularis** in the middle and **mucosa** on the inner side (Figure 14.9). The mucosal lining of the cervix is called the **endocervix** and is continuous with that of the body of the uterus. However, both differ sharply in the epithelium as well as in the underlying stroma. In humans, the mucous membrane of cervix is 3-5 cm thick and forms very complex deep furrows known as the **plicae palmatae**. These are compound clefts in the mucous membrane that run in transverse, longitudinal and oblique directions to form a very irregular arrangement that may penetrate the entire thickness of the mucosa. The epithelial lining of these folds (plicae palmatae) consists of a single layer of tall mucus secreting columnar epithelium. It has comparatively less population of ciliated cells than that lining the body of the uterus. The cilia beat in the direction of the vagina. The height of the cells and position of their nuclei vary with the time of the cycle. During the proliferative and secretory phases of the cycle, these cells synthesize mucus and other substances and package them in membrane bound vacuoles and during active secretion, their nuclei rise to the center as the secreted mucus distends the lumina of the glands. Sometimes, a few of the plicae become occluded and dilate with secretions. Such occlusions or cysts are called **Nabothian follicles**. The cervical canal is normally filled with mucus but its biophysical and biochemical characteristics vary with the time of the cycle. However, mucosa of the cervix does not take part in the menstrual changes and therefore, it does not slough or rupture but after the menopause, it shrinks and its glandular epithelium gradually flattens and the secretory activity is arrested. Columnar epithelium also lines the numerous highly branched tubular cervical glands, which extend deep into the wide lamina propria. The lamina propria become more fibrous from cellular type in the cervix in comparison to the uterus. The mucosal columnar epithelium changes abruptly into squamous and stratified in the external os of the cervical canal as well as in the portion of the cervix that extends into the vagina (**portio vaginalis**), similar to that present in the vagina (Figure 14.9). The muscularis of cervix is not as compact as in the body of the uterus and more connective tissue is interspersed in it. Both muscularis and lamina propria are well vascularised.

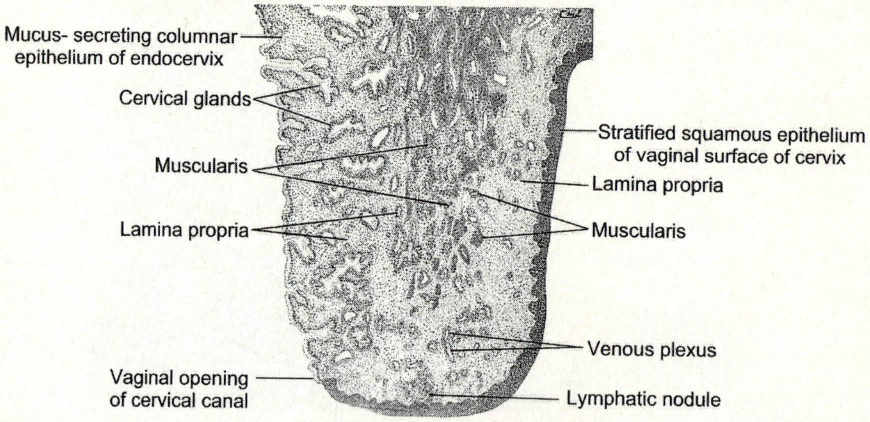

Figure 14.9: Longitudinal section of cervix in Women.

The maintenance of cervical cilia does not appear to require ovarian steroid hormones as is noted for the oviduct. However, synthesis and secretion of cervical mucus by nonciliated cells are under the influence of ovarian steroids since mucus production is found to increase significantly during steroid stimulation. The nonciliated cells of mucosa that line the cervical canal actively synthesize and secrete mucus. The cervical mucus changes both chemically and physically during the reproductive cycle so that a clinician can readily determine and correlate these changes_with the day of the menstrual cycle (Figure 14.10). The **cervical mucus** is a mixture of water, glycoprotein, serum-type proteins, lipids, enzymes, and inorganic salts. It is more hospitable to sperm at or near the time of ovulation because at this time, it is less viscous and more alkaline (pH 8-8.5). At other times or during pseudopregnancy, viscous cervical mucus forms a cervical plug that physically impedes sperm penetration. Cervical mucus supplements the energy needs of sperm and both the cervix and cervical mucus serve as a sperm reservoir. Cervical mucus protects sperm from the hostile environment of the vagina, and also from phagocytes. Further, it promotes sperm penetration and migration towards oviducts for fertilization. The cervix may also play a role in **capacitation**, which is a functional change that sperm undergoes in the female reproductive tract before it is able to fertilize a secondary oocyte.

Thus, in a typical menstrual cycle, two types of cervical mucus are met, each with its own cellular and chemical components. During late pre-ovulatory and ovulatory phase, 97 % mucus is type E, i.e. estrogenic. It is thin, watery with low viscosity, estrogenic, and voluminous. It forms bundles of long, parallel strands. The spaces between the strands are filled with cervical plasma. Sperm can pass through these spaces. By contrast, in early pre-ovulatory period and after ovulation, 90 % of the mucus is type G, i.e. gestogenic. It is thick, viscid, and opaque. Their macromolecules form a dense irregular network that does not allow sperm to enter.

In ruminants, the cervix acts as a sperm reservoir while in cow and rabbit, cervix has folded structures within the lumen that consists of mucus secreting crypts into which the sperm swim while traveling along the mucus fibrils, and are released slowly into the uterus. This delay in sperm transport has been suggested to be important for spontaneous ovulators where coitus may not be coincident with ovulation

Spinnbarkeit: It is the property that allows cervical mucus to be stretched or drawn into a thread. Thus, menstrual cycle time can be estimated by stretching a sample of cervical mucus between two glass slides and measuring the maximum length of the thread formed from the mucus before it breaks. At mid-cycle, spinnbarkeit usually exceeds 10 cm (Figure 14.10).

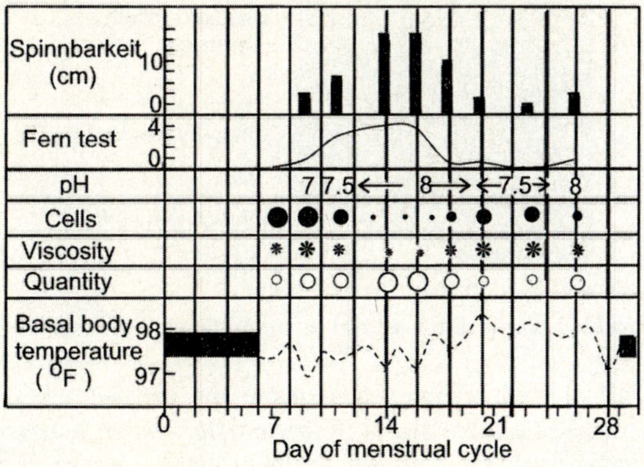

Figure 14.10: Changes in composition and properties of Human cervical mucus during a menstrual cycle.

Ferning or **Arborization**: Cervical mucus forms characteristic microscopic pattern when dried on glass slide (Figure 14.11). This is called ferning and it results from the crystallization of inorganic salts around small and optimal amounts of organic material present in cervical mucus. As estradiol increases in blood, the composition of cervical mucus changes so that dried mucus begins to show ferning in the latter part of follicular phase. Ferning is most prominent in the pre-ovulatory period when the estradiol levels are maximal and just prior to significant progesterone secretion. At this time, mucus is thin, watery and contains few cells. As the progesterone levels rise following ovulation, the quality of the mucus changes and ferning disappears. Persistent ferning throughout the menstrual cycle indicates anovulatory cycle or insufficient progesterone secretion.

The Vagina: The vagina is a thin walled 8-10 cm long fibro muscular tube, lying between the bladder and the rectum. It extends from the cervix to the body exterior (Figure14.12). The urethra is embedded in its anterior wall. Since it provides a passageway for delivery of an infant, it is often called as **birth canal**. Vagina is also a passage for menstrual flow and a female organ of copulation. In some species, such as armadillo, the urethral orifice opens into the urogenital sinus since a true vagina is absent. Sometimes, urethra opens into vagina at its distal end as in cow, mare, sow and rabbit or joining of urethra with the vagina as in elephant forms a long urogenital canal.

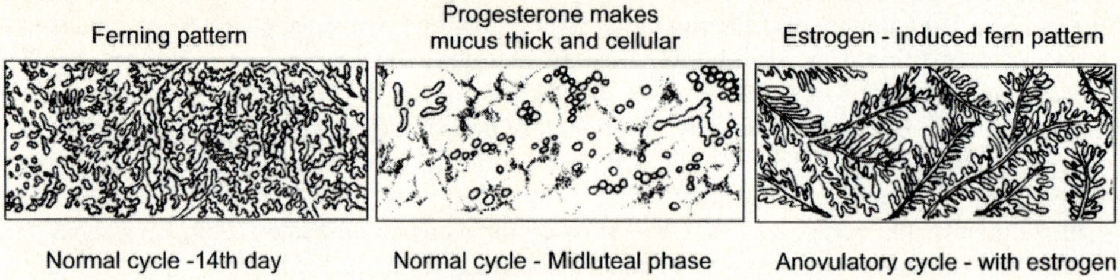

Figure 14.11: Smear of Human cervical mucus to check its ferning pattern.

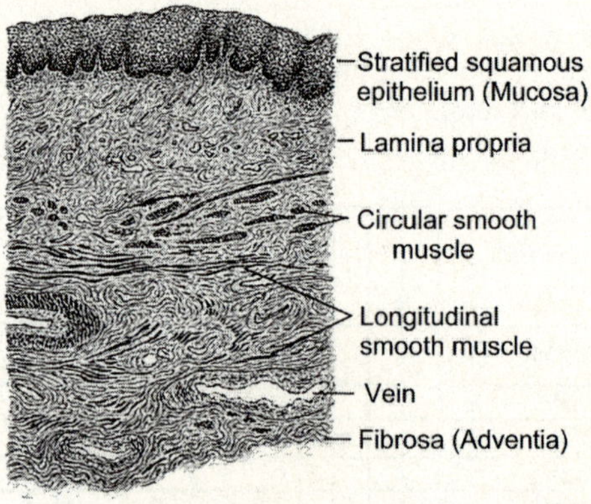

Figure 14.12: Longitudinal section through the wall of Human vagina.

Histologically, vaginal wall is highly distensible and consists of three coats, an outer fibro-elastic **adventitia**, a smooth muscle **muscularis** in the middle, and an innermost **mucosa**. Transverse ridges or folds called **rugae** mark the mucosa of the vagina. These stimulate the penis during intercourse (Figure 14.12). The mucosa of the vagina is continuous with that of the uterus and consists of non-keratinized stratified squamous epithelium adapted to stand up to friction. The cells of the vaginal epithelium are flattened. They accumulate mucus and glycogen during the secretory phase of the reproductive cycle. Certain mucosal cells are dendritic cells and act as antigen-presenting cells. These are thought to provide the route of HIV transmission from an infected male during sexual intercourse. The vaginal mucosa has no glands, and the cervical mucous glands lubricate it. Its epithelial cells release large amounts of glycogen, which is anaerobically metabolized to lactic acid by residual bacteria. Consequently, the pH of a woman's vagina is normally quite acidic and this helps the vagina to keep healthy and free from infection, but it is hostile to sperms. The broad lamina propria is moderately dense with irregular connective tissue having excessive elastic fibers. However, it is looser in the deeper area and extensions from it pass into the muscularis. Small blood vessels are numerous throughout the lamina propria. The muscularis is composed of less numerous inner layers of circular fibers and predominant outer layer of longitudinal and obliquely arranged bundles of muscle fibers. These layers of smooth muscles can stretch considerably to accommodate the penis during sexual intercourse and also a child during its birth. The adventitia anchors the vagina to adjacent organs such as the urethra and urinary bladder anteriorly and rectum and anal canal posteriorly. Numerous blood vessels are present in the adventitia.

In virgins, the mucosa near the distal **vaginal orifice** forms an incomplete partition called the **hymen**. This membrane or partition is very vascular and tends to bleed when it ruptures during **first coitus** (sexual intercourse). However, its durability varies and in some females it ruptures during sports activity.

In some rodents, the stages of the cycle can be detected by taking a vaginal smear and looking at the population of cornified epithelial cells, uncornified epithelial cells, and the leucocytes (leukocytes) coming from the vaginal wall (Figure 14.13). However, in humans, the cyclic changes of the vaginal epithelium are not as obvious as in most laboratory animals, but in all mammals these changes are strictly dependent upon the secretion of ovarian hormones.

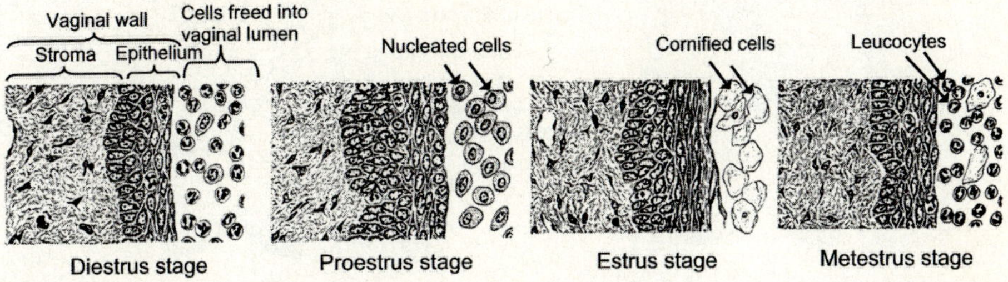

Figure 14.13: Section through wall of Rat vagina to show different types of cells in its lumen.

14.3 External Genitalia

The female reproductive structures that lie external to the vagina are called the **external genitalia**. (Figure14.14). The external genitalia, also called **vulva** or **pudendum** include the mons pubis, labia, clitoris and structures associated with the vestibule. Anterior to the vaginal and urethral openings is the **mons pubis**, an elevation of adipose tissue covered by skin and coarse pubic hair that cushions the pubic symphysis. From the mons pubis, two longitudinal folds of skin called the **labia majora** (*labia*=lips, *majora*=larger, singular is **labium majus**), extend inferiorly and posteriorly. The labia majora are covered by pubic hair and contain an abundance of adipose tissue, sebaceous glands and apocrine sudoriferous or sweat glands. These are homologous to scrotum of the males. Medial to labia majora are present two smaller folds of skin called the **labia minora** (*minora*=smaller, singular is **labium minus**). These are hair-free and are homologous to the penile urethra of the males and enclose a recess called the **vestibule**. The vestibule contains the external opening of the urethra (**external urethral orifice**) more anteriorly followed by that of the vagina. On either side of the external urethral orifice are the openings of the ducts of the **paraurethral (Skene's) glands**, which are embedded in the wall of the urethra and secrete mucus. These are homologous to the prostate gland while the vestibule is homologous to the membranous urethra of the males. Flanking the vaginal opening are the pea-size **greater vestibular (Bartholin's) glands** that are homologous to the bulbourethral glands of males. These glands release mucus into the vestibule and help to keep it moist and lubricated, thus facilitating intercourse. Several **lesser vestibular glands** also open into the vestibule. Just anterior to the vestibule is the **clitoris**, a small protruding structure, composed largely of erectile tissue. The exposed portion of the clitoris is the **glans** and is homologous to the glans penis of the male. A skin fold called the **prepuce** of the clitoris hoods it. The clitoris is richly innervated with sensory nerve endings, and is sensitive to touch contributing to a female's sexual arousal. The **bulb of the vestibule** consists of two elongated masses of erectile tissue just deep to the labia on either side of the vaginal orifice. It becomes engorged with blood during sexual arousal, thus narrowing the vaginal orifice to place pressure on the penis during intercourse. The bulb of vestibule is homologous to the corpus spongiosum penis and bulb of the penis of males. The **Perineum** is the diamond-shaped area medial to the thighs and buttocks of both males and females that contains the external genitalia and anus.

Surgical removal of ovaries is called **ovariectomy**. It results in loss of oviducal cilia, its secretion and muscular activity, uterus hypertrophies with reduction in blood supply. Hormone replacement (estrogen injections) restores all these structures to normalcy. Sexual behavior in females is also clearly dependent on hormones.

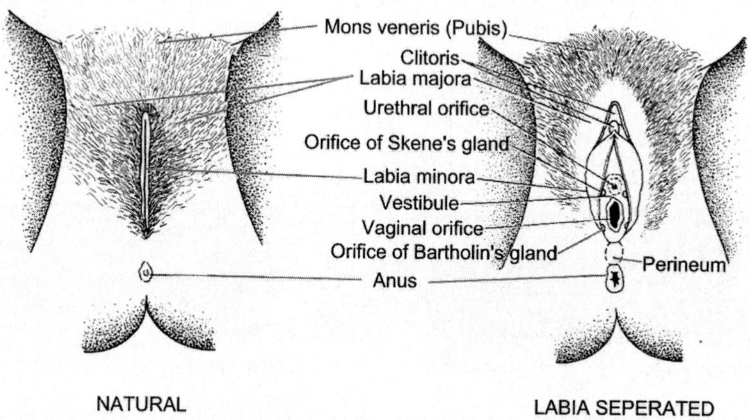

Figure 14.14: External genitalia of Women.

14.4 The Mammary Glands

The mammary glands are present in both sexes, but these normally function only in females. Since the biological role of the mammary glands is to produce milk to nourish a newborn, these are actually important only when reproduction has already been accomplished.

The **mammary** (*mamma*=breast) **glands** are modified sweat glands that produce milk. Their number varies in different mammals. In humans, there are two mammary glands. Each mammary gland in humans is contained within a rounded skin-covered breast anterior to the pectoral muscles of the thorax. Slightly below the center of each breast is a ring of pigmented skin, the **areola**, which surrounds a central protruding **nipple** (Figure 14.15). Large sebaceous glands in the areola make it slightly bumpy and produce sebum that reduces chapping and cracking of the skin of the nipple. Autonomic nervous system controls smooth muscle fibers in the areola and nipple of the mammary gland. It causes the nipple to become erect when stimulated by tactile or sexual stimuli and also when exposed to cold. Internally, each mammary gland consists of 15-25 **lobes** that radiate around and open at the nipple. The lobes are padded and separated from each other by fibrous connective tissue. The interlobular tissue forms **suspensory ligaments (Cooper's ligaments)** that attach the breasts to the underlying muscle fascia and to the overlying dermis. Within the lobes of each mammary gland are present smaller unit called **lobules,** which contain glandular **alveoli** that produce milk in lactating woman (Figure 14.15). Surrounding the alveoli are spindle-shaped cells called **myoepithelial cells**, the contraction of which helps propel milk toward the nipples. These compound alveolar glands pass the milk into the **lactiferous** or **mammary ducts**, which open to the outside at the nipple. Just deep to the areola, each lactiferous duct has a dilated region called a **lactiferous sinus**. Milk accumulates in these sinuses during nursing. In non-pregnant women, the glandular structure of the breast is largely underdeveloped and the duct system is rudimentary. The essential functions of the mammary glands are the synthesis, secretion and ejection of milk and these functions together constitute **lactation**. Lactation is associated with pregnancy and childbirth and is described in the Chapter 18.

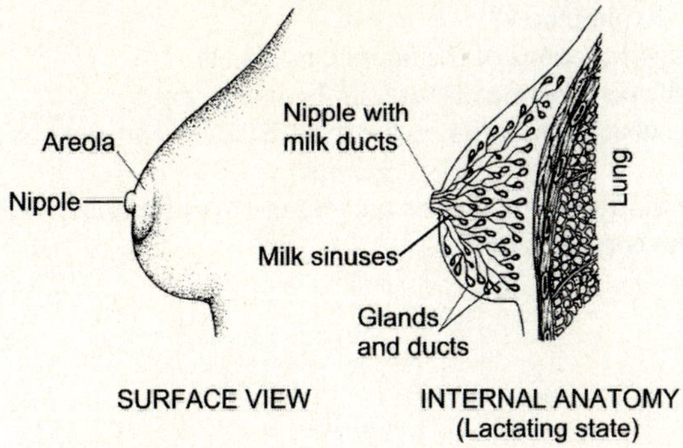

Figure 14.15: Structure of breast in Women.

Summary

The reproductive organs of the female have been summarized below in Table 14.1.

Table 14.1: Female reproductive organs

Organ	Location	Function
Ovary	Lateral wall of pelvic cavity	Produces egg cells and female sex hormones
Uterine Tubes	Close to ovary	Conveys egg cell toward uterus, site of fertilization, Conveys developing embryo to uterus
Uterus	Next to uterine tubes, Uterus lower ⅓ is cervix	Protects and sustains embryo during pregnancy
Vagina	Extends from uterus to the outside	Conveys uterine secretions to outside of body, Receives erect penis during sexual intercourse, Provides open channel for offspring during birth
Labia Minora	Either side of vestibule, between the labia majora	Form margins of vestibule, protect openings of vagina and urethra
Labia Majora	On the outside enclosing urethral and vaginal openings	Enclose and protect other reproductive organs
Clitoris	At the anterior end of vulva, between labia minora	It is richly supplied with sensory nerve endings associated with feelings of pleasure during sexual stimulation
Vestibule	A space enclosed by labia minora	Space between labia minora that includes vaginal and urethral openings
Vestibular Glands	Either side of vaginal Opening	Secrete fluid that moistens and lubricates vestibule
Mammary Glands	Subcutaneous tissue of anterior thorax	Accessory organs specialized to secrete milk following child birth during lactation

Questions

1. What are the sex organs of the female?
2. Describe the structure of the ovary.
3. What changes occur in a follicle during its maturation?
4. Where are the fallopian tubes located? What is their function?
5. Describe the structure of the uterus.
6. Discuss the blood supply to the uterus. Why is an abundant blood supply important?
7. Describe the structure of cervix and vagina.
8. Both the epithelium of vagina and the cervical glands of uterus help to prevent invasion and spread of vaginal pathogens. Explain how?
9. Discuss the structure and functions of the mammary glands.
10. Hormone that makes the cervical mucus viscous-**Progesterone**.
11. In females, it exerts feedback inhibition on the hypothalamus and anterior pituitary-**Estrogen** and **Progesterone**.
12. Spermatozoa are to seminiferous tubules as oocytes are to a) fimbriae, b) corpus albicans, **c) ovarian follicles** and d) corpora lutea.

Chapter 15

Reproductive Cycles

Neither gametogenic, nor the endocrine functions are continuous processes in the females. These fluctuate rhythmically during the life of an individual. Hormones from the anterior pituitary-gonadal axis regulate the periodic changes of the female reproductive system. The hypothalamus appears to be the source of factors that pass through the portal veins to the adenohypophysis where they act to promote the differential release of hormone. These variations follow a cyclic pattern to result in what is known as **reproductive cycles**. The duration of each reproductive cycle varies from species to species with fluctuations significant between cycle length and life expectancy of any one species. Mating may occur either anytime or it may be confined to a specific period of the reproductive cycle.

Most mammals have a distinct mating or breeding season and in most cases their breeding occurs with respect to the seasons in order to take advantage of favorable temperature and food supply. Short cycles promote quick breeding and facilitate production of multiple litters during one breeding season. Probably the shortest breeding season is that of the arctic ground squirrel, which emerges from hibernation in late May and copulates only during the first two weeks of June. In contrast, tropical mammals, such as the hippopotamus, can conceive in every month of the year. Many marine forms have their reproductive cycles tuned to the tides and to definite phases of the moon. The reproductive cycles of mammalian species thus present a plethora of information regarding rhythms of hormone secretion, their pulsatile patterns imposed on circadian rhythms, which in turn influence not only continuous reproductive cycles of finite duration but also the photoperiod control of seasonal breeding.

15.1 Components of the Cycling System

The reproductive cycles are considered to be the expression of the cyclic function of the **hypothalamo-hypophyseal-ovarian (H-H-O) complex** operating on the female reproductive tract. Their operating system can be divided into two general elements. These are i) the **controlling element** (the H-H-O complex), and ii) the **controlled** or **target element (the reproductive tract)**. The functions of the three components (H-H-O) of the controller are closely interrelated. The integrity of the ovary is dependent on the pituitary; the pituitary functions are completely dependent on the hypothalamus; and the function of the hypothalamus and pituitary are modulated by the feedback signals from the ovary. The ovary inherently is a cyclic organ with two endocrine structures, the follicle and the corpus luteum. These two ovarian structures have sequential life spans. The ovarian hormones not only provide feedback signals to the hypothalamo-pituitary complex, but through local or short-loop feedback also perform critical control functions within the ovary itself. In addition, presence of a hormone 'inhibin' recently demonstrated in follicular fluid provides a preferential control of secretion of follicle stimulating hormone (FSH) from anterior pituitary. The genital tract (oviducts, uterus, cervix and vagina) is the target of the H-H-O system. It responds to cyclic H-H-O input during the reproductive years of female life and undergoes cyclic changes, which are seen in the form of cycles.

15.2 Types of Reproductive Cycles

The cyclic nature of adult ovarian secretion imposes cyclicity on both phenotype and behavior in females. The external manifestations of internal ovarian cycle were first noticed in many mammals in terms of behavioral characteristics. It was seen that female mammals of most species are receptive to males and are willing to mate only around the time of ovulation. Such females are said to be 'in heat' and this period of heat is hormonally conditioned and is accompanied by some changes in behavioral characteristics. The frisky (playful and lively) state observed in some mammals, example horse, was given the name oestrus (attacked by gadflies). However, in primates, external manifestation of ovarian cyclicity is observed as shedding of bloody uterine endometrial tissue via the vagina and this hormonally conditioned event is called menstruation (monthly event). In both cases, these events repeated at definite intervals of time, which was specific for a particular species and therefore, were referred to as reproductive cycles.

There can be numerous ways of defining and classifying the types of sexual or reproductive cyclicity in females. Basically, two types of reproductive cycles are met in mammals, based on the response of the uterine epithelium to the stimulation of hormones. These are called i) **estrous cycle**, and ii) **menstrual cycle**. The series of events associated with the maturation of an egg in a cycle is called **ovarian** cycle. Concurrent series of changes occur in the endometrium of the uterus to prepare it for the arrival of a fertilized ovum. These constitute the **uterine cycle**. The events that occur in ovary and uterus follow a set rhythmic pattern and repeat in every cycle. For example, in certain rodents uterine epithelium undergoes mild stimulation followed by a resorptive process. Such a cycle is called an **estrous cycle** and is seen in **nonprimate mammals**. In contrast, in the **menstrual cycle**, which occurs in **primates**, the progesterone stimulates the uterine epithelium so that the sudden changes in hormonal levels cause a sloughing of uterine lining and is associated with hemorrhage. This is called **menstruation**. However, estrus mammals do not menstruate.

Cycles can also be defined according to the number occurring during a given calendar year. Animals with single estrous cycle annually fall in the category of **monestrous** and example is elephant. They show a long **anestrous** (no cycle) period separating the heats (periods of sexual excitement). **Diestrous** animals complete two cycles in a year, example, dog. **Polyestrous** forms repeat their cycles throughout the year if not interrupted by pregnancy, and examples are rat, mice, hamster and guinea pig. Polyestrous animals do not exhibit a seasonal effect on cyclicity due to the lack of seasonal clues in laboratory. Further, on the basis of type of ovulation, reproductive cycles may be **spontaneous ovulatory cycle** and **reflex** or **induced ovulatory cycle** (see Chapter 16).

15.3 Duration of Reproductive Cycle

The duration of the reproductive cycle varies in different mammalian species (Table 15.1). For example, the reproductive rhythm or cycle of female rats and mice repeats at intervals of four to five days, the guinea pig every fifteen days, the mare, sow and cow every three weeks, the monkey and human every four weeks, the chimpanzee every five weeks, and of dog and cat twice or thrice a year.

Table 15.1: Length and duration of estrous cycles in different species

Species	Duration of cycle	Duration of Estrus
Rat	4-6 days	9-20 hours
Mouse	4-5 days	9-20 hours
Hamster	4 days	4-23 hours
Guinea Pig	16-19 days	6-15 hours
Dog	22 days	7-13 days

15.4 The Estrous Cycle

Among mammals, other than primates, the recurring periods of sexual excitement in the adult female are known as '**heat**' or biologically as '**estrus**'. The period of one estrus to the next make up an **estrous cycle**. However, length and duration of the estrous cycle varies with species (Table 15.1). During heat or estrus, the female is physiologically and psychologically conditioned to receive the male. Structural changes occur in the female genital ducts according to the different phases of the estrous cycle.

Phases of Estrous Cycle: The estrous cycle is completed in a sequence of **four phases** or **stages**. These are **proestrus, estrus**, **metestrus**, and **diestrus**. In rodents such as rat or mouse, the estrous cycle is completed in 4-5 days, and the four stages of this cycle can easily be recognized and studied in the laboratory with the help of a compound microscope from the vaginal smears (Figure 15.1).

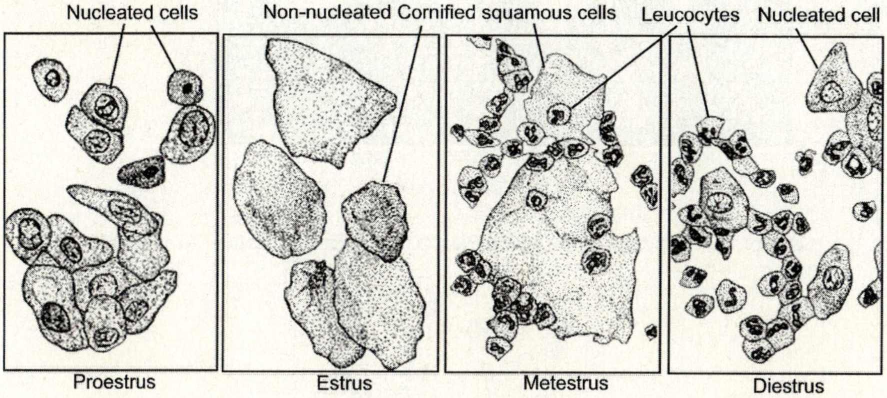

Figure 15.1: Vaginal smears at different stages of estrous cycle in Rat.

Proestrus: Proestrus lasts for about 10 hours. It is a proliferative phase, which precedes the heat period. The functional involution of corpora lutea and pre-ovulatory swelling of the follicles characterize ovary. During proestrus, estrogens from the ovarian follicles condition the endometrium, and so this stage constitutes the follicular phase. Fluid collects in the uteri and they become contractile. Endometrial vascularity increases, the surface epithelium becomes low columnar in height, and the endometrial glands undergo some growth although they remain straight and only slightly branched. The vaginal smear shows mainly **nucleated epithelial cells** that occur singly or in sheets (Figure 15.1). Vaginal smear of early proestrus stage shows few leucocytes with many nucleated epithelial cells, whereas of late proestrus shows a few cornified cells along with the nucleated cells. The female does not permit copulation during early proestrus but become receptive towards late proestrus..

Estrus: It lasts for 12 hours and is the period of heat. Estrus is characterized by a period of sexual receptivity when the females allow copulation. During this period, certain behavioral changes are observed such as increased running activity (Figure 15.2), quivering of ears and **lordosis** (arching of back) in the presence of a male. Under the influence of FSH, dozen or more follicles grow rapidly. Estrus is thus a period of increased estrogen secretion. The uteri undergo progressive enlargement and become distended owing to accumulation of luminal fluid during late proestrus or early estrus phase (Figure 15.3). Much mitosis occurs in vaginal mucosa and as new cells are added, superficial layer of cells become **squamous**, **nonnucleated** and **cornified** (Figure 15.1). These cornified cells are exfoliated into the vaginal lumen and their presence in the vaginal smear is indicative of estrus.

Ovulation occurs during estrus and is preceded by histological changes in the follicle suggestive of early luteinization.

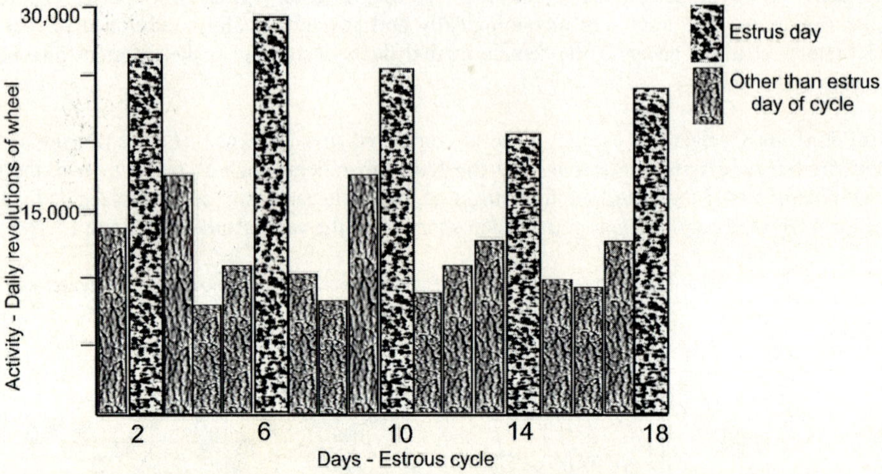

Figure 15.2: Changes in the activity levels of female Rat during estrous cycle.

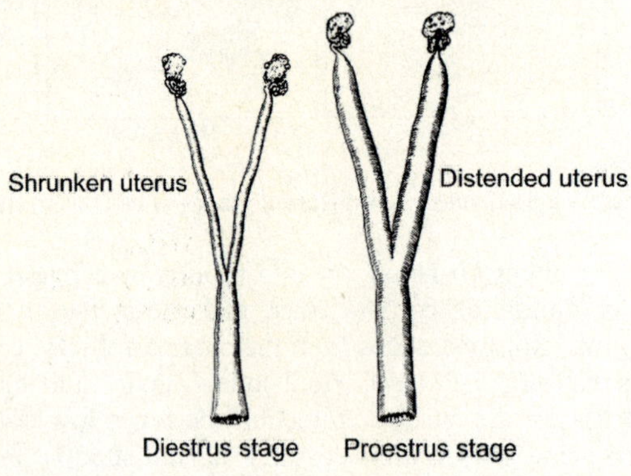

Figure 15.3: Female genitalia of Rat during two phases of estrous cycle.

Metestrus: Metestrus occurs shortly after ovulation, that is in between estrus and diestrus. It lasts for 10-14 hours. Mating is not permitted during metestrus. The ovaries contain corpora lutea and small follicles. Uteri diminish in vascularity and contractility. The exfoliated vaginal cytology (or vaginal smear) shows many leucocytes (leukocytes) and only a few cornified cells (Figure 15.1).

During the period between estrus to early diestrus (constituting the luteal phase), the progesterone from the corpus luteum controls the structure of the endometrium. The endometrium thickens and its surface epithelium becomes high columnar type. The uterine glands grow to their maximal size. These are larger, more coiled and more highly branched than at other phases of the cycle. The glands are actively secretory.

Diestrus: Diestrus is the longest phase and lasts for 60-70 hours. In the ovary, functional regression of corpora lutea occurs. The uteri are small, anemic, and only slightly contractile. The endometrium shrinks and its glands lose size and cease to secrete. It is characterized by thin vaginal mucosa and the vaginal smear consists of **leucocytes (leukocytes)**. There is no acceptance of male during diestrus.

These cyclic changes occur whether fertilization takes place or not. In most estrous mammals, excepting the mouse and rat, the uterus thickens appreciably under the influence of ovarian hormones, and deterioration and sloughing of the uterine lining occur at the end of the cycle. However, the periodic sloughing of the endometrial surface during the estrous cycle does not cause bleeding, which occurs during the menstruation cycle of primates, as substantial portion of the endometrium is lost during menstruation.

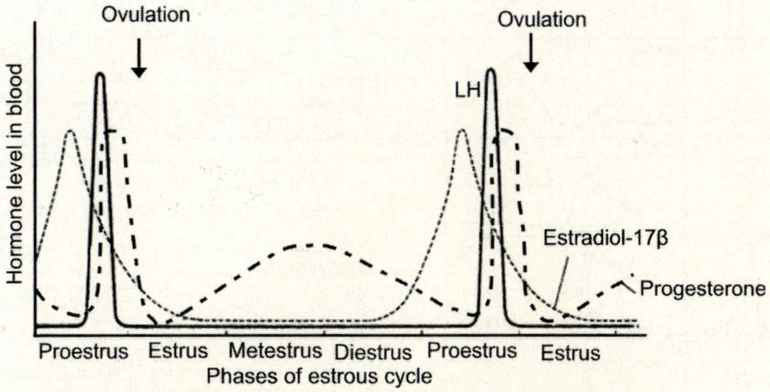

Figure 15.4: Hormonal regulation of estrous cycle (Rat).

Hormonal Regulation of the Estrous Cycle: The reproductive cycles are governed by interplay of pituitary and gonadal hormones. According to current concepts, a feedback mechanism operates in which gonadotropin (FSH and LH) released from the anterior pituitary is controlled by the levels of estrogen and progesterone in circulation (Figure 15.4). It is not known what factors are originally responsible for activation of pituitary-ovarian axis, but it has been postulated that very low levels of estrogens coming from the premature follicles may stimulate the pituitary to augment the release of FSH. The significant production of estrogens by the follicles apparently requires both FSH and LH. When the estrogen level goes high in the blood, indicating the full growth of ovarian follicles, it acts to prevent a greater release of FSH by pituitary but simultaneously promotes an augmented release of LH. Pre-ovulatory swelling and definite lutein changes occur in the walls of the mature follicles under the rising levels of LH. The pre-ovulatory follicles undoubtedly secrete small amounts of progesterone as well as large amounts of estrogen (Figures 15.4 and 15.5). This accelerating process peaks late in the light phase of the day of proestrus when the high levels of estradiol cease inhibiting LH via negative feedback activity and actively promotes the ovulatory surge of this hormone. The estradiol titer determines the day of this surge, but a circadian clock regulates the time of the day. These two processes interact to produce an ovulatory release of LH late in the afternoon of proestrus and ovulation occurs in a few hours. Sexual receptivity is programmed steroidally to occur at about the time of ovulation (Figure 15.5). Estradiol is the primary hormone responsible for promoting sexual receptivity in the rats, but progesterone may enhance this effect. Estradiol may also be important in terminating receptivity, as there is a fall in the circulating estrogen levels after ovulation. The ovulated follicles are then transformed into corpus luteum, which becomes functional under the influence of LH and prolactin. The release of LH from anterior pituitary seems to be inhibited by rise in progesterone level. The source of the progesterone peak that occurs late in proestrus is partly adrenal in origin. Circulating levels of prolactin also peak at this time and play a major role in producing the rat's short-lived corpus luteum (Figure 15.5). The corpora lutea secrete modest amounts of progesterone for a day or two, as they remain functional only for a short period, unless pregnancy or pseudopregnancy occurs. The ovaries of cyclic rats always contain several sets of corpora lutea of several past estrous cycles in different stages of disintegration. Various environmental factors such as photoperiod, temperature, stress, nutrition, humidity, pheromones, copulation and suckling also affect the estrous cycles.

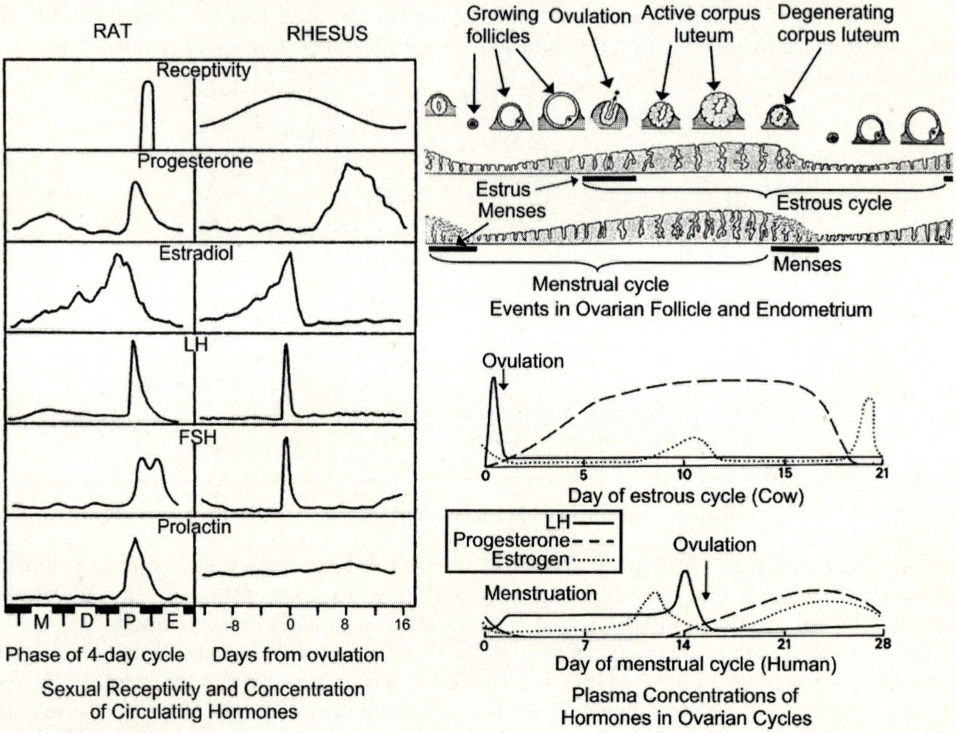

Figure 15.5: Correlation of events of estrous (Rat) and menstrual (Rhesus) cycles, M-metestrus, D-diestrus, P-proestrus and E-estrus phases of 4-day cycle.

15.5 The Menstrual Cycle

One of the dramatic changes that occur at puberty in human females is the onset of menstruation and is called **menarche** (the first menstruation at puberty). Menstruation normally occurs at fixed intervals throughout reproductive life span of the female. The period between two successive menstrual flows constitutes the **menstrual cycle**. The menstrual cycle, is characteristic of primates and it does not occur in other vertebrates, including mammals.

Menstrual cycle is fundamentally comparable to the estrous cycle (Figure 15.5) but there are two important differences. Firstly, there are no unequivocal peaks of heightened sexual receptivity in menstrual cycle and secondly, the breakdown of the endometrium at the end of the cycle is accompanied by a loss of blood called **menstruation**. Also, menstrual cycle is of longer duration in comparison to estrous cycle and only one egg is ovulated in each menstrual cycle. The cycle is characterized by more obvious and prolonged follicular and luteal phases, with estradiol being the dominant steroid secreted during the former and progesterone secretion dominating the later phase (Figure 15.6).

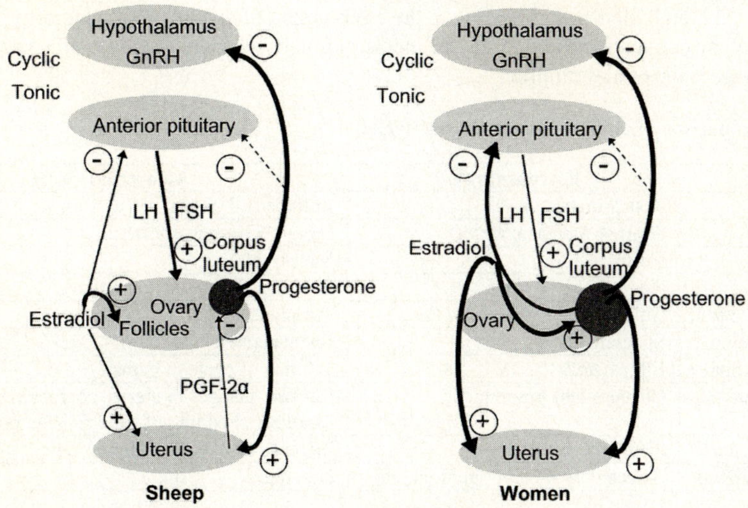

Figure 15.6: Hypothalamic-pituitary-ovarian relationships in the luteal phase of ovarian cycles in Sheep and Women.

However, both rat showing estrous cycle and monkey showing menstrual cycle are **spontaneous ovulators** that is, they ovulate in every cycle whether or not copulation occurs. Therefore, the cyclic changes in the ovary, uterus, vagina and hormones at the hypothalamic-pituitary-gonad axis in these are very distinct. In contrast, in some other mammals, such as cat, ovulation is **induced** by copulation and accordingly in the ovaries of these animals, one crop of eggs is always mature and ready for ovulation, at least during the breeding season. In them estradiol levels are always relatively high along with the sexual receptivity and the tactile stimulation in them during copulation elicits a neurogenic signal that reflexively elicits the ovulatory release of LH followed by ovulation.

Table 15.2 compares the estrous and menstrual reproductive cycles. Basically, both estrous and menstrual cycles are regulated by the same interplay of pituitary and ovarian hormones, and the effects of the ovarian hormones on the reproductive tract are also comparable in most respects (Figure 15.6). The secretion of progesterone from the corpus luteum inhibits the positive feedback effect of estradiol in both estrous and menstrual cycles. However, in menstrual cycle as seen in women, the corpus luteum controls the basal secretion of gonadotropins through the negative feedback of estradiol at tonic center while in estrous cycle as exemplified by ewe, the corpus luteum does not secrete estradiol and secretion of gonadotropins is controlled by the negative feedback of estradiol secreted by the follicles, which continue to develop throughout the luteal phase. Thus, in estrous cycle as shown in Figure 15.6 in sheep, reduction in the activity of corpus luteum at the end of luteal phase depends on an additional negative feedback that involves the production of prostaglandin from the uterus.

The median menstrual cycle length in women is 28 days (24-35 days) during the major reproductive years. It is somewhat longer at the two ends of the reproductive life of an individual. The prolonged cycles are expression of the frequent occurrence of anovulation, common in adolescence and in the transition to menopause. The cycle in chimpanzee requires about 35-37 days and rhesus monkey, 23-33 days.

Phases of the Menstrual Cycle: The menstrual cycle can also be functionally divided into four phases: the **menstrual phase**, the **proliferative** or **follicular phase**, **ovulatory phase**, and the **postovulatory** or **luteal** or **progestational phase** (Figures 15.7). The circulating levels of gonadotropins, estrogens, androgens and progestins exhibit cyclic patterns in synchrony with the phases of the menstrual cycle

(Figure 15.8). Although menstrual bleeding is the culmination of cyclic hypothalamo-hypophyseal-ovarian activity, by convention the first day of menstruation is accepted as Day 1 of a menstrual cycle, and the mid cycle is the ovulation time.

Table 15.2: Comparison of estrous and menstrual cycles

Feature	Estrous Cycle	Menstrual Cycle
Example	Non-primate	Primate and human
Duration	Short, 4-5 days in rat	Long, 28 days in human
Phase	Estrus	Menstrual
Bleeding	No bleeding	Bleeding during menstruation
Sexual receptivity	Only during estrus phase (heat)	Throughout
Type of Ovulation	Spontaneous	Spontaneous
Time of Ovulation	Early estrus	14th day of cycle in human
Uterine mucosa	Changes less pronounced	Marked changes in uterus, characterized by bleeding, shedding of superficial endometrium
Body Temperature	No noticeable change	Increase of 2^0 C at ovulation time
Environment effects	Affected by factors like light, etc.	No effect

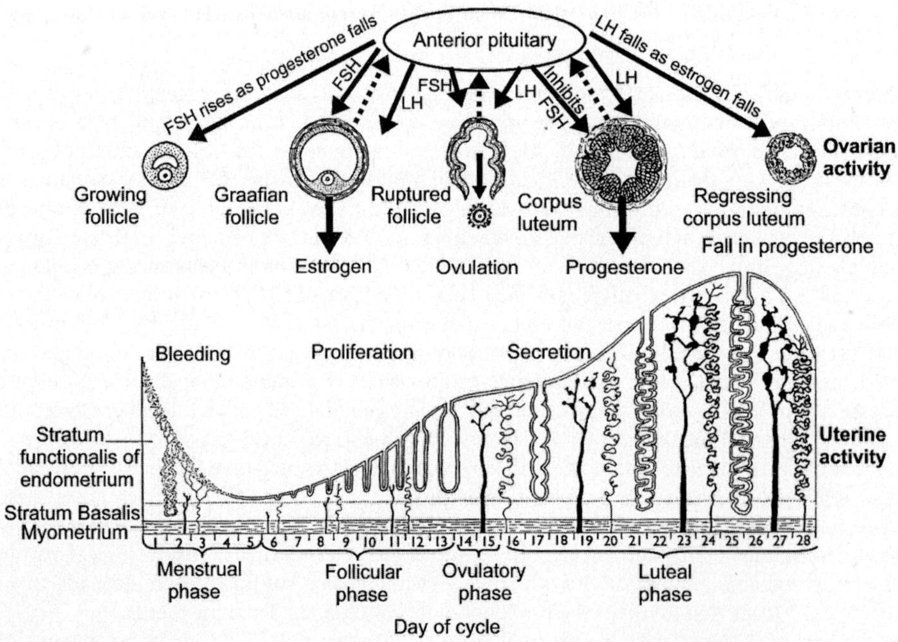

Figure 15.7: Changes in ovary and uterus during menstrual cycle in Women, FSH-follicle stimulating hormone (causes follicle to mature and secrete estrogen), LH-luteinizing hormone (causes ovulation and corpus luteum to develop and secrete progesterone).

Menstrual Phase: Also called **menstruation** or **menses** (=month), lasts for roughly first five days. The first day of menstruation marks the first day of a new cycle. Following the peak of luteal activity on about Day 22, the corpus luteum begins to regress so that by Day 1 of the ensuing cycle, its hormonal production is markedly reduced. This rapid estrogen and progesterone withdrawal induces dramatic morphologic changes in the endometrium including its vasculature. Events in ovaries include enlargement of nearly 20 secondary follicles with accumulation of fluid in antrum while those in uterus are mainly discharge of menstrual flow of blood, tissue fluid, mucus, and epithelial cells derived from endometrium. This discharge occurs because of the declining level of ovarian hormones, especially progesterone, which stimulates release of prostaglandin. This causes the spiral arterioles of uterus to constrict and as a result, the cells they supply oxygen die. Eventually, the entire stratum functionalis sloughs off. Thus, if uterus alone is considered, menstrual phase represents the terminal event with the regression of the corpus luteum. The uterine endometrium is very thin at the end of this phase as only stratum basalis remains (Figure 15.9). The menstrual flow passes from uterine cavity to cervix, vagina, and to the exterior. The human vaginal smear from the 5th day of menstrual cycle shows predominance of intermediate cells (Figure 15.10). A few superficial acidophils and superficial basophils and a few leucocytes are also present.

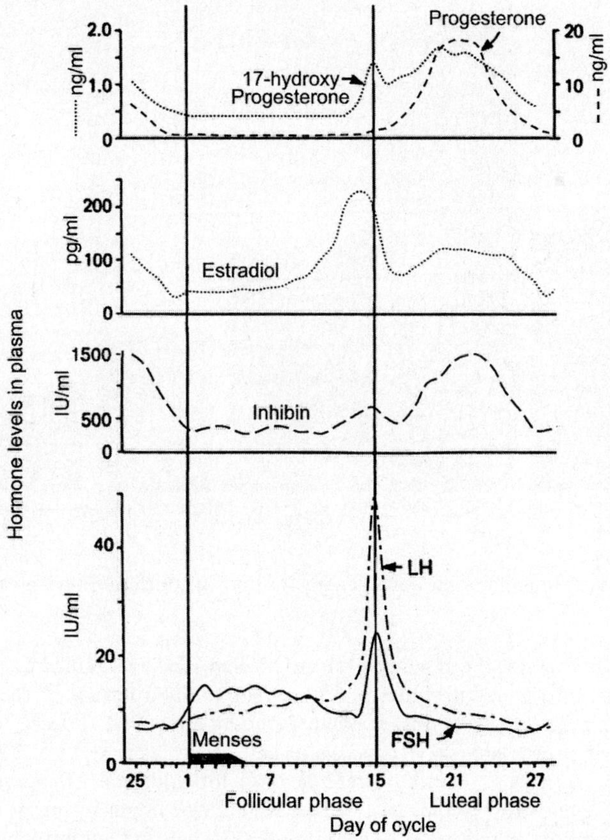

Figure 15.8: Hormonal changes during a typical Human menstrual cycle.

Proliferative or follicular Phase: This phase is more variable in length than other phases of the cycle and lasts from day 6-13 in 28 day cycle. This phase is characterized by a rise in serum levels of FSH (Figure 15.8), and under the influence of FSH, the secondary follicles grow and begin to secrete estrogens and inhibin. By the later half of this phase, one of the follicle grows fully and become mature or Graafian follicle. This follicle forms a blister-like bulge on the surface of the ovary. Estradiol increases slowly at first and then rapidly reaches a maximum on the day of the peak of the LH surge (Figures 15.7 and 15.8). The maturing follicle continues its estrogen production under the influence of increasing level of LH. The rise in plasma estrogen levels is accompanied by a decrease in FSH level. This divergence in the pattern of FSH and LH secretion is probably related to-i) a preferential inhibitory action of estrogen on FSH release (negative feedback), and ii) secretion by the maturing follicle of "inhibin", which selectively inhibits FSH secretion. Small amounts of progesterone are also produced a day or two before ovulation by the mature follicle. The estrogen simultaneously repairs the endometrium (Figure 15.9) and as the estrogen titters rise, it acts on thin, poorly vascularized uterus to restore its glandular and vascular patterns, and prepares it for implantation. Similar changes occur in vagina, and the vaginal mucosa becomes thicker. The vaginal smear is composed of squamous, stratified epithelium, which undergoes cornification. The cervical mucous becomes copious and watery.

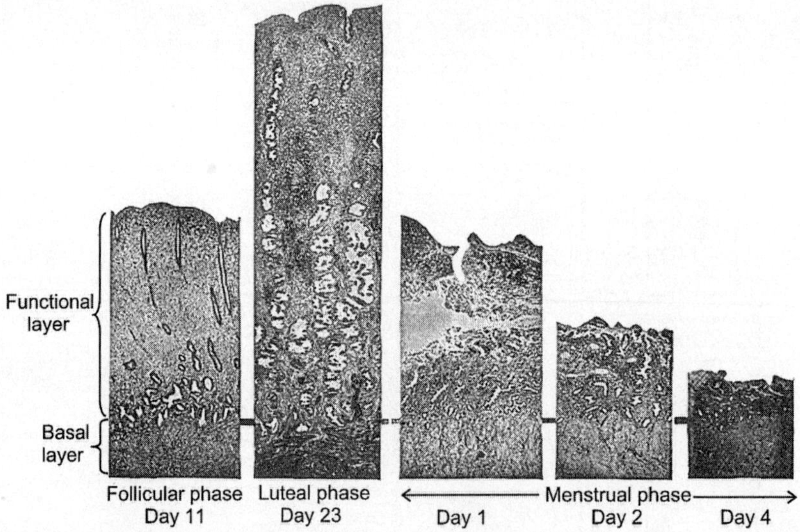

Figure 15.9: Vertical sections of Human uterine endometrium to show its thickness during various phases of menstrual cycle.

Ovulatory phase: On about Day 13, the rapid rise in the plasma LH level, known as the LH surge leads to the final maturation of a Graafian follicle. Follicle rupture and release of secondary oocyte usually occurs on day 14 in a 28-day cycle, that is about 24 hours after the LH peak. This process is known as ovulation. Ovulation is a precisely timed event and occurs as a result of LH surge that is triggered by high levels of estrogens. Shortly after the onset of midcycle LH surge and prior to ovulation, plasma estradiol levels drop precipitously and a further rise in plasma progesterone occurs. LH surge stimulates continuation of reduction division of the oocyte, the leutinization of granulosa cells and synthesis of progesterone and prostaglandin within the follicle. No conspicuous changes occur in the endometrium during the ovulatory phase (Figure 15.9). A vaginal smear from the 14th day of human menstrual cycle is characterized by the predominance of large superficial acidophils, reduction in superficial basophils and intermediate cells and absence of leucocytes (Figure 15.10). This is due to the high estrogenic level achieved by the time of ovulation and therefore, the smear is called the 'follicular type'. The superficial cells mature with increase in estrogen and become acidophilic. Cyclic variations in the body temperature of the human female correlate with the hormonal changes occurring during a menstrual cycle. A distinct rise in basal body temperature occurs at ovulation and remains high until the onset of the next menstrual period. The changing titers of hormones during the menstrual cycle seem to be responsible for the basal body temperature fluctuations.

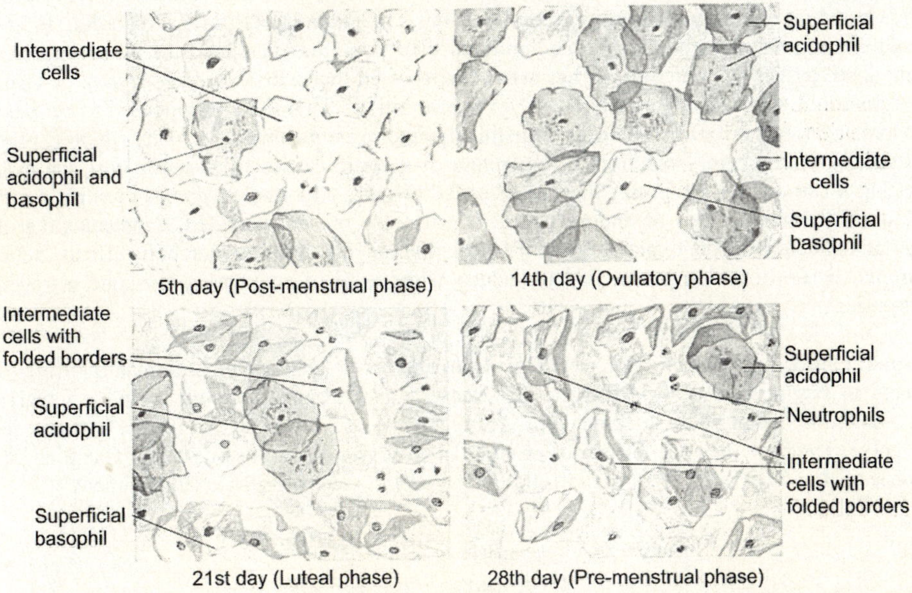

Figure 15.10: Vaginal smears of Human female during various phases of menstrual cycle.

Postovulatory or **Luteal** or **Progestational phase:** This phase of the cycle is the most constant in duration and lasts for 14 days, from days 15 to 28. It represents the time between ovulation and the onset of next menses. Following ovulation, LH stimulates the remnants of ovulated follicle to develop into **corpus luteum**, which secretes progesterone and some estrogen. The corpus luteum has a life span of two weeks. If fertilization occurs, the corpus luteum persists and is maintained by hCG, a hormone produced by the chorion of the embryo to continue secretion of progesterone to maintain pregnancy. Progesterone and estrogen produced by the corpus luteum promote growth and coiling of endometrial glands that begin to secrete glycogen, vascularization of the superficial endometrium, thickening of endometrium (Figure 15.9) and increase in amount of tissue fluid. These changes reach at peak one week after ovulation, corresponding to the time when a fertilized ovum might reach the uterus for implantation. In vagina, there is secretion of thick mucous and the epithelium is profusely infiltrated with leucocytes. Thus, the vaginal smear from 21st day of human menstrual cycle due to high levels of progesterone and diminished estrogens shows the predominance of large intermediate cells (precornified superficial cells) with folded borders which aggregate into groups. Superficial acidophils, superficial basophils and leucocytes are scarce. By 28th day of cycle, great predominance of intermediate cells with folded borders occurs and these tend to be in groups. Also, there is an increase in neutrophils and a scarcity of superficial cells (Figure 15.10). The cervical mucous becomes thicker, viscous and opaque inhibiting migrating sperms. If the oocyte is not fertilized, corpus luteum activity declines, and it degenerates into **corpus albicans**. With the decrease in ovarian hormones, release of GnRH, FSH, and LH occurs due to loss of negative feedback suppression by the ovarian hormones. This resumes follicular growth. But uterine epithelium undergoes degenerative changes. Leucocytes invade it and necrotic changes occur in its stroma. The spiral arteries first constrict and then dilate and rupture producing hemorrhage or bleeding (Figures 15.7 and 15.9). This is accompanied by sloughing of the uterine mucosa and a new cycle begins. Immediate cause of mechanism of menstruation has continued to be the topic of special interest for many years and the most frequently discussed hypothesis regarding its mechanism is the one proposed by Marllee (1946), which is based on direct observation of vascular changes in endometrial grafts. According to him, the immediate cause of menstruation is the injurious effects of anoxia upon tissues of endometrium brought about by vasoconstriction. It has also been reported that a toxic substance may be formed in the endometrium, which may be responsible for menstruation. This toxin is supposed to be present in the endometrium just prior to and during menstruation and resembles with necrosin, which is produced as a result of inflammatory reactions. Regardless of specific causes of menstruation, the evidence shows that it can occur even in the absence of coiled arteries, endometrial glands or surface mucosa, and is unrelated to thickness of endometrium. Further, the present knowledge indicates that it is a stromal phenomenon and an explanation of menstruation may be found in metabolic effects induced in the stromal tissue of endometrium due to sudden withdrawal of supporting hormone estrogen and progesterone.

Hormonal Control of Menstrual Cycle: Hormonal changes during a typical human menstrual cycle are given in Figure 15.8. The hypothalamus releases gonadotropin-releasing hormone GnRH) into portal circulation in a pulsatile manner. This is necessary to support the cyclic female hormone pattern that involves feedback between hormones produced in ovary and anterior pituitary. The gonadotropic hormones FSH and LH are both needed to stimulate ovarian cycles of follicle development.

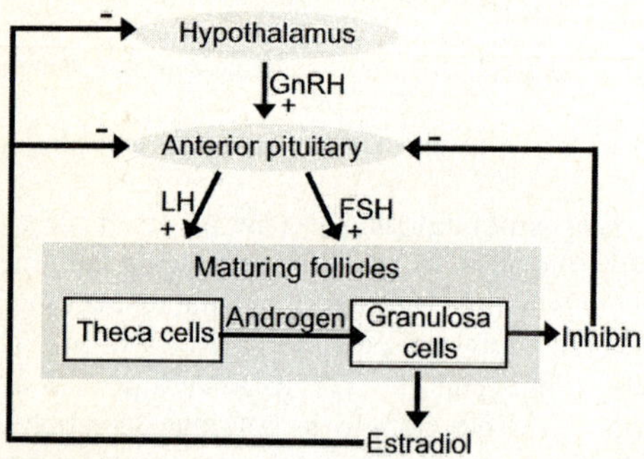

Figure 15.11: Regulation of gonadotropin secretion through negative feedback loops of estradiol and inhibin secreted by ovaries during a menstrual cycle in Women.

On day 1 of cycle, rising levels of GnRH from the hypothalamus stimulates increased production of and release of FSH and LH by the anterior pituitary. FSH with synergistic effect of a little LH stimulates the growth of young follicles. During early follicular phase, FSH exerts its main effects on the follicle cells, whereas, LH more specifically targets the thecal cells. As the follicles enlarge, estrogen secretion begins. LH prods the thecal cells to synthesize androgen. The androgens diffuse through the basement membrane, where they are converted to estrogens by the FSH-primed granulosa cells (Figure 15.11). FSH stimulates the granulosa cells to make the enzyme necessary for converting androgen to estrogens. FSH also stimulates production of inhibin by granulosa cells. The rising estrogen levels in plasma exert negative feedback on the anterior pituitary, inhibiting its release of FSH and LH (Figure 15.12), while simultaneously prodding it to synthesize and accumulate these gonadotropins. Within the ovary, estrogen increases estrogen output by intensifying the effect of FSH on follicle maturation. Inhibin, released by granulosa cells, also exerts negative feedback controls on FSH release during this period. However, when the levels of estrogen reach a critical concentration in blood, a strange reversal occurs. The negative feedback is converted to a positive feedback on the brain and anterior pituitary. They increase their output of gonadotropins even more steeply than rate of rise of estrogen. The increase of LH in response to rapidly rising estrogen is called **LH surge,** which is the hormonal trigger for ovulation (Figure 15.12). The sudden flush of LH stimulates the primary oocyte of the dominant follicle to complete the first meiotic division. The secondary oocyte that results after first meiotic division continues on to metaphase II of second meiotic division. LH surge results in ovulation at or around day 14. Perhaps LH induces the synthesis of proteolytic enzymes too, but whatever the mechanism, the blood stops flowing through the protruding part of the follicle wall. Within 5 minutes, that region of the follicle wall bulges out, thins and oozes fluid, and then abruptly ruptures to result in ovulation. The role of FSH in this process is unknown. Shortly after ovulation, estrogen levels decline, probably reflecting the damage to the dominant estrogen-secreting follicle during ovulation. The LH surge also transforms the ruptured follicle into a corpus luteum, hence the name "luteinizing" hormone and it also stimulates the newly formed endocrine gland (corpus luteum) to produce progesterone and estrogen almost immediately after it is formed. Rising levels of progesterone, estradiol, and inhibin during luteal phase exerts a powerful negative feedback effect on anterior pituitary release of LH and FSH (Figure 15.12). Presence of effective numbers of receptor sites for estrogen and progesterone on the endometrium during the course of the menstrual cycle correlates well with the changing levels of these hormones (Figure 15.13). As gonadotropins decline after ovulation, development of new follicles is inhibited and additional LH surges that might cause additional oocyte to be ovulated are prevented. As LH blood levels decline, the stimulus for corpus luteum activity also ends, and the corpus luteum begins degenerating. During late luteal phase, deterioration of the corpus luteum leads to a decrease in estrogen, progesterone and inhibin production. However, if implantation of an embryo occurs, the activity of the corpus luteum is maintained by LH-like hormone released by the developing embryo. A marked decline in ovarian hormones at the end of cycle (days 26-28) induces positive feedback on pituitary and thus level of gonadotropins begins to rise with a start of a new cycle.

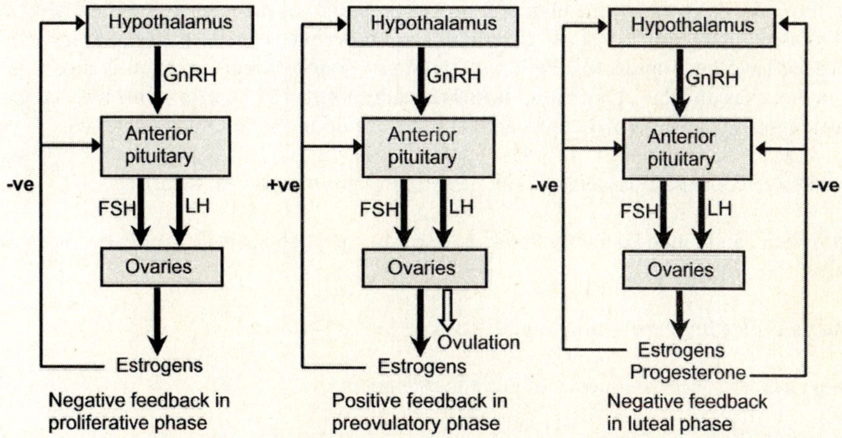

Figure 15.12: Estrogen and progesterone feedback on hypothalamus-pituitary axis in a menstrual cycle.

Current evidence indicates that the functional life span of the corpus luteum in primates is 'preprogrammed'. Although the capacity of luteal tissue to synthesize progesterone can be extended by exogenous LH or chorionic gonadotropin, its effect is transient. The hCG-LH receptors eventually become refractory and the corpus luteum regresses in spite of continued **luteotropic** (factors that contribute to corpus luteum survival and function) stimulation. Although the precise mechanism for the obligatory regression is unknown, both estrogen and prostaglandin produced by the luteal tissue are known to be **luteolytic** (factors that contribute to the demise of corpus luteum) and may represent a 'self-destruct' mechanism that limits the life span of the corpus luteum.

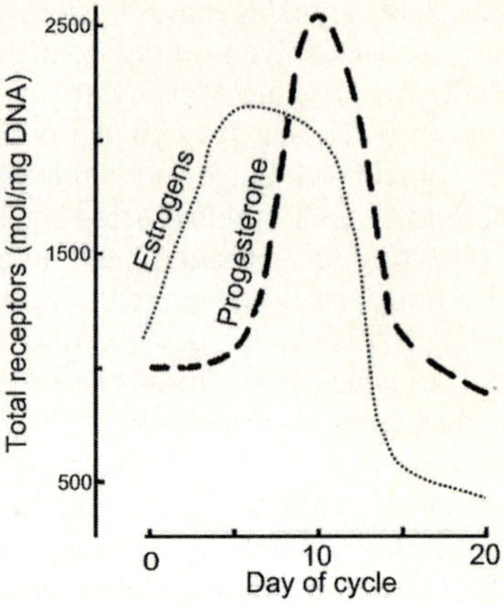

Figure 15.13: Receptor sites for estrogen and progesterone on uterine endometrium in a menstrual cycle.

Abnormalities occurring during Menstrual Cycle: Given below are some of the common abnormalities associated with menstrual cycle in women.

Amenorrhea is an absence of the monthly menstrual flow. It may be due to a deficiency in estrogen production and thus a failure in the monthly proliferative growth of the endometrium resulting in the absence of monthly sloughing of the uterine lining. The failure of the menses to be initiated at puberty is referred to as **primary amenorrhea**. **Secondary amenorrhea** refers to a failure to menstruate after regular menses have been initiated. Failure of pituitary gonadotropin secretion is also a defect that results in amenorrhea and this abnormality is known as **hyperprolactinemia**. However, pregnancy and menopause are examples of normal physiological bases for failure to resume the menses.

Dysmenorrhea refers to pain associated with menstruation or it is painful menstruation.

Hypomenorrhea and **menorrhagia** refer to scanty and abnormally profuse menstrual flow respectively.

Metrorrhagia is bleeding from the uterus between periods or menses.

Oligomenorrhea is reduced frequency of periods or menses.

Premenstrual Syndrome refers to symptoms such as irritability, bloating, edema, emotional liability, decreased ability to concentrate, depression, headache, and constipation during the last 7-10 days of the menstrual cycle.

Around the age of 50, a woman's menstrual periods become less regular and ultimately disappear. This is called **menopause**. The cause of menopause is a decrease in number of follicles and their hypo responsiveness to gonadotropins and is a normal physiological process in women's life. Symptoms of menopause are due to marked decrease in plasma estrogen (see Chapter 11).

Summary

Female mammals show cyclic variations in their reproductive pattern and behavior. These are depicted in the form of reproductive cycles.

Two types of reproductive cycles are seen in mammals. These are **estrous** and **menstrual** cycles. Basically, these are similar showing ovarian and uterine cyclic changes, characterized by cyclic variations in the vaginal epithelium also. These changes are expression of the cyclic function of the hypothalamic-pituitary-ovarian hormone complex.

Changes during **estrous cycle** can easily be recognized and studied in the laboratory in rats or mice in vaginal smears using compound microscope.

Four phases of estrous cycle are proestrus, estrus, metestrus and diestrus. Each phase has nearly fixed duration. Table 15.3 summaries the cytological and behavioral characteristics of the four phases of rat estrous cycle.

Table 15.3: Changes in reproductive organs, vaginal cytology and behavior during estrous cycle in Rat

Cycle Phase (Duration)	Ovary	Uterus	Vaginal Mucosa	VaginalSmear (cell type)	Behavior
Proestrus (12 hrs.)	Follicles grow rapidly, degenerating corpora lutea of previous cycle	Uterus distended with increasing fluid	Slightly dry	Mainly round, nucleated cells	Sign of acceptance of male towards end of this phase
Estrus (12 hrs.)	Follicles largest, become mature, ready for ovulation	Uterus reaches greatest distension, epithelium thins	Dry, lusterness	Predominantly cornified, few nucleated	Lordosis, acceptance of male
Metestrus (21 hrs.)	In early metestrus, ovulation occurs, in late stage follicles smallest, young corpora lutea, ovulated eggs in oviducts,	Uterine epithelium undergoes vacuolar degeneration, at late stage regeneration also begins	Slightly moist	Cornified and few leucocytes	No acceptance of male
Diestrus (57 hrs.)	Follicles of different sizes, corpora lutea continue to grow	Uterine epithelium undergoes regeneration	Moist	Mainly leukocytes, few leucocytes	No acceptance of male

Menstrual cycle is characterized by a period of bleeding called menstruation and is characteristic of primates. A typical menstrual cycle in human is of 28 days. Events occurring during Menstrual Cycle are summarized in Table 15.4.

Day 1-5: Estrogen and progesterone are low because the previous corpus luteum has completely regressed. Endometrial lining is sloughed off resulting in menstruation. Secretion of FSH and LH is released from inhibition and their plasma concentration rises, therefore, several follicles are stimulated to grow.

Day 6: Dominant follicle is selected.

Day 7-12: Plasma estrogen rises because of secretion by the dominant follicle and endometrium is stimulated to proliferate.

Day 12-13: High plasma estrogens induce LH surge, therefore, oocyte is induced to complete first maturational division. Follicle is stimulated to secrete certain lytic enzymes and prostaglandins resulting in ovulation.

Day 14: Ovulation occurs.

Day 15-25: Corpus luteum forms under the influence of LH. It secretes progesterone and estrogen. Secretory endometrium develops. Secretion of FSH and LH is inhibited, lowering their plasma concentrations. No new follicles develop.

Day 26-28: Corpus luteum degenerates. Therefore, plasma progesterone concentration declines. Endometrium begins to slough by day 28 and a new cycle begins with menstruation.

Table 15.4: Summary of events during a menstrual cycle

Days	Ovary	Uterus	Hormones
1-4	Follicular phase begin, corpus luteum degenerates, several follicles begin to mature	Menstrual phase, outer layer of endometrium sheds after estrogen and progesterone levels fall	FSH, LH, estrogen and progesterone levels all low
5-13	Follicular phase continues, FSH stimulates follicle Maturation	Proliferative phase, endometrium regrows	Estrogen rising Progesterone low, FSH and LH low
14	Ovulatory phase, LH surge causes ovulation	Cervical mucus becomes thin and watery	LH and FSH sharp rise, estrogen falls after follicle ovulates
15-28	Luteal phase, corpus luteum secretes estrogen and progesterone	Secretory phase, endometrium secretes uterine milk	Estrogen and Progesterone high, FSH and LH low

Questions

1. What are reproductive cycles? How many types of these are met in mammals?
2. Define estrous and menstrual cycles. How do they differ from each other?
3. Describe estrous cycle along with the hormonal changes during each phase.
4. Trace the events of the menstrual cycle. What effect does progesterone have on the endometrium?
5. Discuss the hormonal regulation of the menstrual cycle.
6. Compare the principal events of the ovarian and uterine cycles in human.
7. What causes menstrual flow?
8. Explain the hormonal and physical factors responsible for the shedding of stratum functionalis in menstruation.
9. Hormones that directly regulate the ovarian cycle-**FSH and LH**.
10. The sequence of phases in menstrual cycle starting from the first day of cycle is **a) menstrual, proliferative, secretory** b) menstrual, secretory, proliferative c) secretory, menstrual, proliferative d) proliferative, menstrual, secretory e) secretory, proliferative, menstrual.

Chapter 16

Ovulation and Fertilization

In the ovaries of adult females, there are always several follicles at different stages of maturation. As a rule, one follicle outstrips the others to become a dominant follicle. How this follicle is selected is still not clear. This dominated follicle matures, becomes Graafian follicle and undergoes ovulation.

16.1 Ovulation

Rupturing of the mature follicle to release an ovum is called ovulation. **Ovulation** thus can be defined as a physiological event, which results in the expulsion of the mature ovum from the Graafian follicle to the fronds of the fallopian tube. It releases the **egg** from the ovary at the right time for its fertilization and further development. The term egg generally refers to a single cell that is released from the ovarian follicle at the time of ovulation, though what is ovulated in most animals is a secondary oocyte with the first polar body emitted and the chromosomes arranged on the spindle for the second meiotic division

The process of ovulation: When an ovarian follicle reaches the Graafian stage of development, it is prepared for ovulation (Figure 16.1). The initial event associated with the development of a follicle to the pre-ovulatory stage is the rapid increase in the secretion and accumulation of liquor folliculi. Accompanying this secretion is a marked swelling of the antrum and a series of successive morphological changes that occur in the oocyte, in each of the cellular layers of the follicle and in the apex portion of the follicle related to the ovarian surface. Thinning of the granulosa layer occur simultaneous to these changes. In most mammals, these changes take place roughly 10-15 hours prior to the rupture of the follicle. At this time, the liquor folliculi is markedly less viscous than previously and is composed of both the secretion of granulosa cells and plasma proteins that enter the follicle by transudation. The leakage of plasma proteins into the antrum is probably a consequence of both the increased vascularization of the pre-ovulatory follicle and increased permeability of thecal capillaries. As a consequence numerous granulosa cells, originating primarily from the stratum granulosum and also from the cumulus oophorus become dissociated from each other. They lose their intercellular contacts, or remain connected by thin strands of cytoplasm in which small junctional complexes are still evident. Further contact between granulosa cells is also maintained by means of processes that invaginate into the cytoplasm of adjacent cells, forming gap junctions at the interface of the two plasma membranes. The dissociation of granulosa cells is most pronounced in the region of the cumulus oophorus that is nearest to the apex of the follicle. Fluids that likely originate from surrounding capillaries also distend the intercellular spaces within the theca interna. The dissociation of the granulosa layer in the pre-ovulatory follicle seems to be caused by components of the plasma that enter the granulosa through large gaps in the basal lamina and become mixed with liquor folliculi initially secreted by granulosa cells.

The infiltration of fluids into the pre-ovulatory follicle is usually restricted to the apical portion of the follicle. Just prior to ovulation, the appearance of these fluids seems to be correlated with the dissociation of granulosa cells to the distension and disorganization of other cellular layers such as the theca, tunica albuginea, and the superficial epithelium. It is likely that the disorganization of these structures contribute to the characteristic distended appearance of a pre-ovulatory follicle. Most of the granulosa cells in the area corresponding to the anticipated site of follicle rupture are flattened, lose their intercellular contacts, and become detached from the granulosa layer. Within a few hours or even moments before ovulation, the cumulus oophorus is detached from the stratum granulosum and float freely in the antrum. Detachment of the oocyte from the granulosa layer probably involves the mechanical dissociation of cells as a result of the passive infiltration of fluid into the antrum. In addition, the amoeboid contractions of granulosa cells, which contain extensive microfilamentous networks, composed of the contractile protein actin and myosin, may contribute to the detachment of the cumulus oophorus. Just prior to ovulation, the processes of coronal cells that traverse the zona pellucida and contact the surface of the oocyte are withdrawn. Pre-ovulatory follicles are generally blister-like structures that protrude markedly from the ovarian surface. At the apices of some pre-ovulatory follicles, irregular, fluid-like drops are seen either free on the surface of cell or in the process of being extruded from the cytoplasm and/ or intercellular spaces among the superficial cells. This fluid-like material, which permeates the intercellular spaces of the theca, tunica albuginea and superficial epithelium, seems to be correlated with the disruption of collagen fibrils. A number of enzymes have been found in follicular fluid that probably brings necrotic changes in the membrana granulose. Follicular cells in which relevant proteins can be detected histochemically produce apparently proteolytic enzymes. It seems that the enzymes have only a local effect. All this leads to marked weakening of the apical wall. In addition, a reduction in blood flow (**ischaemia**) to a circumscribed region on the external surface of the follicle probably contributes to lysis of the thecal and granulosa cells in that area. Finally, just prior to ovulation, antral fluid is observed to mix with this amorphous material as a direct consequence of the disorganization of the basal lamina, which separates the granulosa and theca layers.

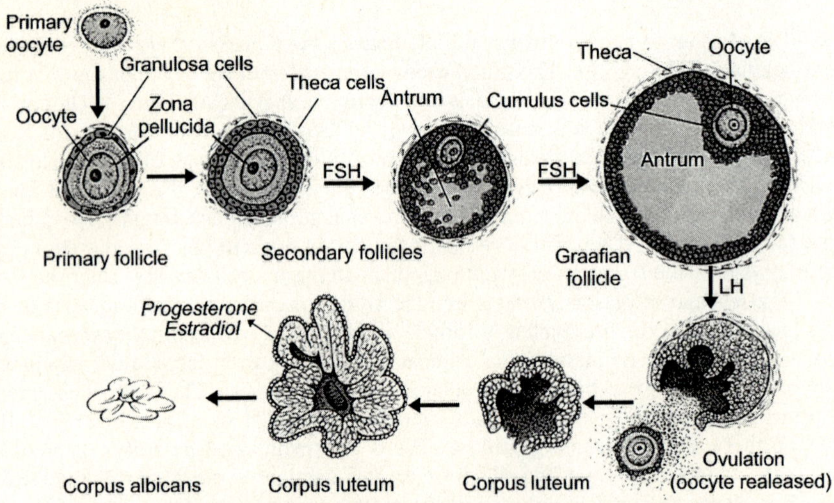

Figure 16.1: Life cycle of an ovarian follicle showing ovulation and formation of corpus luteum.

At the moment of ovulation, large, irregular areas of the apex of a follicle are ruptured (Figure 16.1). It is rather difficult to view the oocyte and corona radiata during the process of ovulation directly by scanning electron microscopy (SEM) since an ovulating or recently ovulated follicle is usually covered by a large quantity of a viscous material and cellular debris as large amount of follicular fluid is expelled along with the oocyte.

Many theories have been put forth to define what "causes" a follicle to ovulate. These are, i) an increase in intrafollicular pressure prior to ovulation, ii) the contraction or 'squeezing' of the follicle by smooth muscle cells, iii) the enzymatic digestion of the follicular apex, iv) vascular changes within the follicle, and v) nervous control of pre-ovulatory events. However, at present, no single theory is widely accepted as being the actual cause of ovulation. It appears that ovulation occurs only if a follicle is in the process of transforming into a corpus luteum during the pre-ovulatory stage and is in a superficial position in the ovarian cortex with enough of the weakened follicular wall exposed to allow rupture. If such a follicle is located in a more interior region of the stroma, the oocyte may not be expelled. Such follicle develops into a corpus luteum, termed **false corpus luteum** or **atretic** or **arctic follicle**, and the oocyte rapidly degenerates. Thus, ovulation seems to be a gradual process in which the oocyte, immersed in a gel-like material (antral fluid) escapes from the fractured surface of the ovary.

Entry of egg into the oviduct is a highly efficient process and a number of theories have been put forth to explain how egg enters the fallopian tube at ovulation. The most accepted view is that the vigorous actions of the cilia on the fimbriae create a fluid flow towards the tubal ostium and the muscular activity of the tube and even of the ovary itself also contribute to this action. Movements of all these structures increase at the time of ovulation and this is presumably due to raised circulating levels of ovarian hormones. The released ovum is then transported to the ampullary region of the fallopian tube where it meets the spermatozoa introduced into the vagina or uterus during copulation to result in fertilization. The timing of the two events, estrus and ovulation, in non-primates is crucial because both egg and spermatozoa have very short lives. Table 16.1 gives the ovulation time in the reproductive cycle of some mammals.

Table 16.1: Time of ovulation in reproductive cycles of some Mammals

Species	Length of Cycle(Days)	Duration of Estrus (hours)	Ovulation	
			Time	Type
Rat	4-5	13-15	8-10 hrs. after start of estrus	Spontaneous
Hamster	4	10	8-12 hrs. after start of estrus	
Mouse	4	10	2-3 hrs. after start of estrus	
Guinea pig	16	20	10 hrs. after start of estrus	
Cow	21	13-14	12-16 hrs. after end of estrus	
Goat	20-21	1-3 days	30-36hrs. after onset of estrus	
Sheep	16	20-48	12-24 hrs. before end of estrus	
Pig	21	2-3 days	35 hrs. after onset of estrus	
Horse	19-23	4-7 days	1-2 days before end of estrus	
Dog	60	7-9	1-3 days after start of estrus	
Monkey	28*	None	14 days prior to onset of menses	
Human	28*	None	14 days prior to onset of menses	
Fox	90	1-5	1-2 days after onset of estrus	
Squirrel	16	6-11	8-12 hrs. after mating	Induced
Cat	-	4days with male da	20-30 hrs. after mating	
Ferret	-	Continuous	30 hrs. after mating	
Mink	8-9	2 days	40-50 hrs. after mating	
Rabbit	No cycles	Continuous	10 hrs. after mating	

- Menstrual Cycle

Basically the reproductive cycle of the female is linked with ovulation and it occurs more or less at the same time in each cycle. For example in rat, the cycle is 4-5 days and estrus takes about 14 hours, ovulation occurs 8-11 hours after the start of estrus. Ovulation in sheep occurs 18-24 hours after the beginning of estrus. The timing of ovulation is extremely variable in primates. For example in rhesus monkey, it can occur anywhere between 9-20 days (generally 13 days) after menstruation, and in human beings from 9th to 17th day (generally 13-14 days) after the start of menstruation. The detection of ovulation is of great importance in artificial insemination (Chapter 25) and in human contraceptive practice (Chapter 23). Some women experience a twinge of pain in the lower abdomen at the time of ovulation. This episode is called **mittelschmerz** (German word meaning "middle pain") and is caused by the intense stretching of the ovarian wall during ovulation.

In 1-2% of all ovulations, more than one oocyte is ovulated. This can result in multiple births. This phenomenon increases with age. Since different sperms fertilize different oocytes, the siblings produced are **fraternal** or **non-identical twins**. However, **identical twins** result from the fertilization of a single oocyte by a single sperm followed by separation of two daughter cells in early development.

Types of Ovulation: Ovulation is of two types. It can occur either spontaneously at regular intervals as it happens in animals exhibiting estrous cycles such as rat, hamster, guinea pig, mouse etc. and menstrual cycle, example primates including humans or by induction with a stimulus as in rabbit, cat, ferret etc. Accordingly, ovulation is known as **Spontaneous Ovulation**, and **Reflex** or **Induced Ovulation** (Table 16.1). This results in spontaneous ovulatory cycles and reflex ovulatory cycles. The chains of events in both types of ovulation are basically similar (Figure 16.2). Further, precocious ovulation can be induced experimentally in the rat by the administration of LH-RH, PMSG (pregnant mare serum gonadotropin), estradiol and 5α-androstane-3β, 17β-diol.

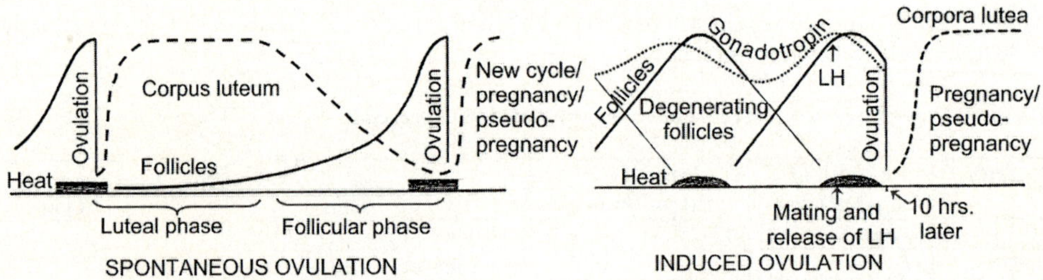

Figure 16.2: Comparison of events occurring in the ovary of spontaneous and induced ovulating females.

Spontaneous Ovulation: In this, ovulation recurs at regular intervals and is basically independent of external environment. Species with the intrinsic rhythm of LH release are spontaneous ovulators.

Reflex or Induced Ovulation: In reflex or induced ovulators, ovulation is dependent upon stimulus of mating or some nervous stimulus as seen in cat, rabbit, ferret, mink. Control of follicular growth and cycles and control of ovulation are dissociated from each other in these animals.

Hormonal control of ovulation: Ovulation is a dynamic phenomenon controlled by the hormones. It occurs due to the release of LH surge in both types of ovulators but the trigger for this release differs in two cases.

Spontaneous ovulators: The increase of LH in response to rapidly rising estradiol called **LH surge** is the hormonal trigger for ovulation (Figures 16.3 and 16.4) in spontaneous ovulators. The recurrent reproductive cycles of mature animals depend on the rhythmic secretion of hormones of the anterior lobe of the pituitary gland and the ovary. The rhythm is imposed by the hypothalamus and the related structures of the brain and begins to function with the onset of puberty. The gonads and the pituitary gland of prepuberal animals are not insensitive to the stimulus of tropic hormones. However, the stimulus from the hypothalamus is missing before puberty. Females with regular estrous cycles have the cyclic pattern of gonadotropin secretion. Anestrous females and male animals have an acyclic pattern of gonadotropin secretion. The type of gonadotropin secretion depends on the sexual differentiation of the hypothalamic functions. The inherent pattern of sexual differentiation of the hypothalamus is to develop into cyclic type or the female type.

Periodic increase of FSH and LH release is required for the induction of estrus and ovulation. The tonic release of FSH and LH is controlled by the neural centers in the anterior hypothalamus. The release of FSH-RF is regulated in the area of the anterior hypothalamic nucleus (FSH-control centers), and release of LH-RF, in the area of the preoptic and suprachiasmatic nuclei (preoptic LH-trigger). However, recent studies in primates indicate that the ovaries and pituitary can carry out the entire cycle of positive feedback that leads to ovulation. A constant pattern of pulsatile release but no coordinated signal from the hypothalamus is required to drive the female cycle. However, the pattern of GnRH secretion in males and females is not significantly different. These results show that that a timing signal from the hypothalamus is not necessary for triggering the LH surge. But the cycle cannot be carried out if GnRH is totally absent, or if the timing of the pulses is abnormal. Estrogens and progesterone also exert a positive feedback effect on the secretion of FSH and LH. Figure 16.3 illustrates the stepwise pathways that provide a positive feedback to LH secretion during follicular phase to result in a LH surge at the end of this phase and it brings about rupturing of follicle or ovulation. After ovulation, the remnants of the follicle become a corpus luteum and if pregnancy does not occur, it degenerates leaving a scar like corpus albicans and a new cycle begins. Cyclic changes in gonadotropins and ovarian hormones during a menstrual cycle are shown in 16.4. In estrous cycle, progesterone in synergism with estrogens secreted during the pre-ovulatory period facilitates ovulation. Rats in persistent estrus do not ovulate spontaneously and have large follicles, but treatment with progesterone restores ovulation in them. Progesterone may also interrupt the anovulatory cycle of the rhesus monkey and induce ovulation.

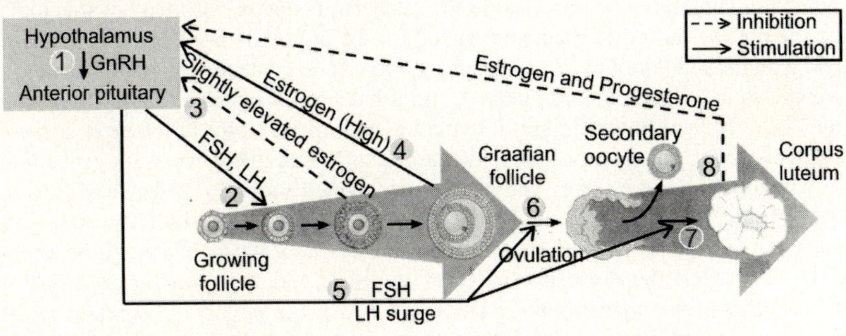

Figure 16.3: Pathways that provide positive feedback to LH secretion in follicular phase of menstrual cycle, number in circles indicate the sequence of events.

Reflex or **Induced Ovulators:** The secretion of FSH is either continuous, as in rabbit, or occurs during the breeding season, as in mink. Estrous cycles are characterized by waves of growing follicles (Figure 16.2). In seasonal breeders, length of day and temperature play an important role in inducing hypothalamic centers to stimulate gonadotropin secretion. Induced ovulators generally mate during estrus. After mating, LH, also called ovulating hormone, is normally released in large amounts by neural mechanism acting via the hypothalamus. Reflex pathways from the spinal cord and connections from the higher centers including the cerebral cortex all play a part in the pre-ovulatory release of LH. In rabbit, release of LH is also partly due to psychic excitation of the brain. In reflex ovulators, the pre-ovulatory release of LH is brief, in rabbit it lasts for nearly 2 hours and the hormone remains in the circulation for an additional 4 hours. In these animals, estrogens and progesterone facilitate the ovulation just as in the cyclic mammals. Administration of progesterone less than four hours before mating or before the mechanical stimulation of the vagina facilitates ovulation in rabbit. Inhibition of ovulation occurs if progesterone is given 24 hours before each stimulus.

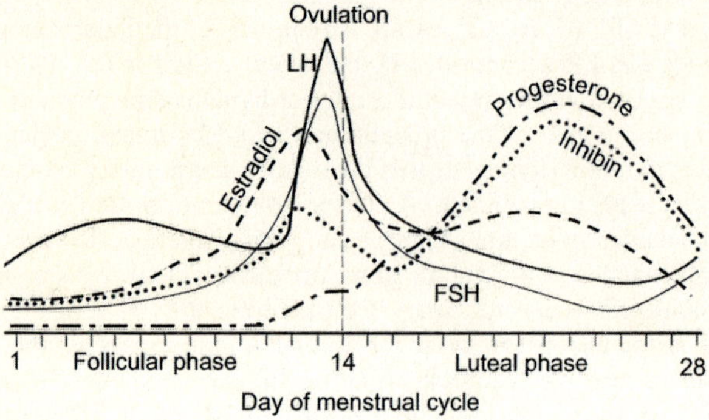

Figure 16.4: Cyclic changes in gonadotropins and ovarian hormones during a menstrual cycle.

Thus, a relationship exists between the circadian system and reproductive system-firstly in those species, which have ovulatory cycles throughout the year and secondly in mammals who are seasonal breeders and whose onset of estrus is determined by the changing length of day. In "non-seasonal breeders" a neural signal generated at circadian intervals determines the timing of ovulation. Some animals when maintained in constant light either cease to cycle or have lengthened estrous cycles. Also timing of ovulation can be shifted by twelve hours by reversing the light/dark cycle. Light-entrained LH surges can be observed in the estrogen treated or "primed" ovariectomized rat and hamster and the precise timing of the neural signal for the pre-ovulatory LH surge in these animals is tightly linked with the light/dark cycle. Conversely, there is no evidence for a circadian organization of reproductive cycles in guinea pig and monkey, and it has been suggested that in these species steroid feedback may be sufficient to the timing of ovulation and organization of the estrous cycle. It seems that in rats and hamsters, the anterior hypothalamus/preoptic area is important for generating the neural trigger for ovulation while in monkey and guinea pigs, which show no evidence of internal circadian oscillators governing the timing of ovulation the basal hypothalamic-pituitary axis is required for ovulation. The circadian pacemaker in rats and hamsters appears to reside in the suprachiasmatic nuclei (SCN). However, the close proximity of the SCN and the preoptic area may have led to conflicting conclusions in suggesting the relationship between a circadian oscillator in the SCN, the preoptic area and the neural timing of ovulation

Apart from SCN, the pineal gland also plays a role as a circadian pacemaker in determining the timing of ovulation. Thus, the timing of ovulation in some non-seasonal breeders is entrained to light/dark cycles and circadian rhythms and this involves the SCN, while estrous cycle in some mammals appear to be independent of autonomous circadian pacemakers and ovulation is determined solely by the feedback of gonadal steroids. On the other hand, the seasonal patterns of reproduction are controlled by the environmental photoperiod and the onset of the breeding season is normally connected with changes in the day length. In many species, females only show cyclic ovarian activity for limited periods of the year while the males of the species only develop active testis at this corresponding period. Animals whose breeding season is stimulated when the days shorten, e.g. sheep, deer, are termed **short day breeders** while other mammals such as horse, come into season with the lengthening days and are referred to as **long day breeders**. The onset of breeding season is brought about by activation of the hypothalamic-pituitary axis by photic stimuli. The onset of reproductive activity is marked by a gradual increase in the frequency and amplitude of LH pulses and a slow but delayed rise in FSH levels. The increased gonadotropin secretion consequently stimulates the gonads and the synthesis of testosterone and estrogen. When the testis become fully active as in ram, secreting high concentrations of testosterone, the amplitude of the pulsatile LH secretions is decreased. This change may be attributed to the frequency of GnRH pulses reaching the pituitary coupled with the feedback effects of steroids on the gland. The evolutionary significance of seasonal breeders is apparent in that the process of natural selection would favor those species whose offspring are born at a time of the year, which favors the growth, and development of the young.

16.2 Formation of Corpus Luteum

Transformation of a follicle into corpus luteum usually begins before ovulation and is initiated under the influence of pituitary gonadotropins, particularly luteinizing hormone (LH), which is abundant in the circulating blood at this time. After ovulation, when the corpus luteum is fully differentiated, its structure and function are those of a typical endocrine gland and it secretes progesterone and some estrogen. This secretion of steroid hormones by the corpus luteum, i) prepares the endometrium for implantation, ii) enables the blastocyst to implant, and iii) maintains pregnancy after implantation. The functional life span of a corpus luteum is completely dependent upon the fate of the embryo. If implantation takes place, the corpus luteum undergoes extensive enlargement and continues to synthesize and secrete steroid hormones and becomes corpus luteum of pregnancy. If an embryo fails to implant or if the oocyte is not fertilized, the corpus luteum undergoes atrophy and eventually degenerates. It is known as the **corpus luteum of menstruation** in humans. In both situations, the developmental changes leading to the formation of corpus luteum are similar, as are the subsequent regressive events. Regressing corpus luteum leads to the formation of small white nodule called the **corpus albicans** (Figure 16.1). Luteal regression is called **luteolysis**. Life span of a corpus luteum varies greatly with the species, for example, it persists for nearly 28 days in a pregnant rabbit and about 2-3 months in a pregnant woman. However, if implantation does not take place, it remains functional only for 14 days in both cases.

Structure of Corpus Luteum: During the initial stages of transformation into a corpus luteum, granulosa cells mixed together with thin strands of connective tissue and numerous small vessels hypertrophy become polyhedral and rapidly accumulate lipid or lutein droplets. These modified cells are termed **granulosa-lutein** cells or simply **luteal cells**. Another putative cell type present in the early corpus luteum is the "**K**" cell, so called because of the high Ketosteroids content of the cytoplasm. These cells appear to migrate from the theca interne to the granulosa layer of a recently ovulated follicle. At present it is not clear whether "K" cells or Momigliano's cells (after the investigator who first described them in 1937), or "paraluteal" or "theca-lutein" cells are distinct individual cell types or simply represent transitional forms during the differentiation from a single, initial cell type. Luteal cells have lipid droplets, mitochondria and endoplasmic reticulum, characteristic of other steroidogenic cells. The termination of secretory activity by the luteal cells involves both the atrophy and degeneration of these elements and involution of entire luteal mass. Regressing luteal cells contain autophagic vacuoles, heterogenous lysosomes, large lipid inclusions and myelin figures. Formation of a hyaline or fibrous body, the corpus albicans or fibrosus is the final result of complex degeneration and regression of the corpus luteum. While the corpora albicantia of a reproductive cycle in which pregnancy has not taken place generally shrink and disperse into the ovarian stroma rather rapidly, the complete regression of corpora lutea of pregnancy in some species may require several years before finally disappearing into the stroma.

16.3 Sperm Transport through the Male Ducts during Ejaculation

Spermatozoa leave the male genital tract at ejaculation. This may be provoked by copulation or masturbation (stimulation by hand etc.) or in spontaneous emissions or failing these events, sperm pass out in a slow steady discharge that is carried away by the urine. In ejaculation, spermatozoa from vas deferens and from the tail of the epididymis are rapidly forced into the urethra by muscular contractions of the duct walls and get mixed with the secretions of the accessory glands whose ducts lead into the urethra. During sexual intercourse, the male deposits semen-containing sperm in the vagina near the cervix. To reach the site of fertilization, the sperm move upward through the uterus and uterine tube.

16.4 Sperm Transport in the Female Genital Tract

The mechanical factors responsible for propelling the semen into the female tract include i) muscular contractions in the wall of the urethra, ii) the piston-like action of the penis during coitus, and iii) the orgasmal contractions of the female tract. Spermatozoa do not appear to depend solely upon their own swimming movements to reach their destination. They generally swim in wide circles and there is no sound evidence of anything in the female tract that would give them a sense of direction. Also, the passage to the site of fertilization is not an easy task for spermatozoa because of the pressure of two difficult points in the female genital tract (the utero-tubal junction and the uterine-cervix junction, when semen is deposited in the vagina). In addition, spermatozoa are subject to considerable dilution in the secretions of the female genital tract. Thus, migration of sperm through the female genital tract is accomplished by contractions of the uterus and oviduct and partially by motility of the sperm. The contractions of the female genital tract play a fairly prolonged role provoked by the hormone oxytocin from the posterior pituitary gland. Also, semen contains prostaglandins, which are capable of stimulating strongly the muscles in the walls of the female tract. Thus, the spermatozoa accompanied by differing amounts of seminal plasma reach near the utero-tubal junction. This junction in many species has a narrow bore and the region represents a partial barrier to sperm transport. Spermatozoa that do manage to negotiate the utero-tubal junction are carried along the oviduct chiefly by the irregular contractions of the wall of the organ, which cause a mixing of the contents. In addition, there are bands of cilia on the walls of the female genital tract. They beat in the direction of the ovaries and consequently there is to some extent a current of fluid favoring passage of spermatozoa to the site of fertilization.

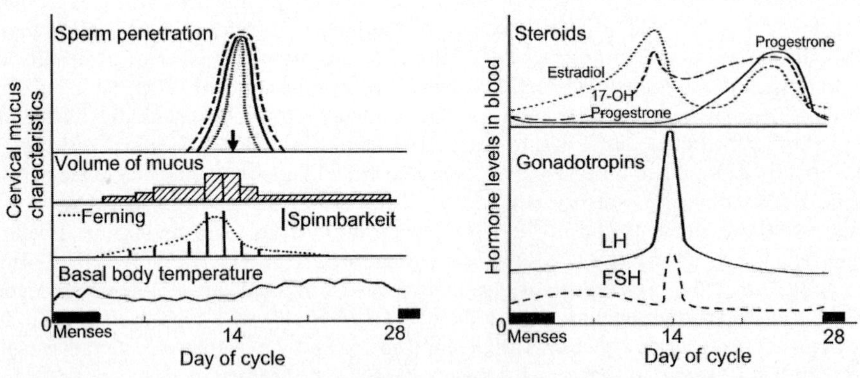

Figure 16.5: Characteristics of cervical mucus, basal body temperature and endocrine profile and its correlation with sperm penetration through cervical mucus during a menstrual cycle of Human female.

Passive transport of spermatozoa through the female genital tract is also affected by the phase of the menstrual cycle (Figure 16.5). Penetration of sperm through the cervical mucus reduces drastically during the luteal phase and post menstruation and early follicular phase of menstrual cycle as shown in Figure 16.5, correlating well with the other characteristics of cervical mucus and also with the endocrine profile during a menstrual cycle. Sperm penetration also reduces during metestrus and diestrus phases of estrous cycle, and is almost nil during pseudopregnancy or under the influence of progesterone. This is because cervical mucus becomes very viscous and impermeable to spermatozoa under the influence of progesterone. In mammals, it takes less than fifteen minutes for the sperm to reach the site of fertilization in the ampulla of the oviduct. Millions of sperm are deposited at coitus but only a few hundred reach the site of fertilization. During copulation, **300** to **500 million sperm** are deposited in the vagina by a single ejaculation, but only a few hundred reach a secondary oocyte in the ampulla of the oviduct, a distance of nearly 5 inches. Millions of them leak from the vagina almost immediately after being deposited there. Of those that remain, millions more are destroyed by the vagina's acidic environment and unless the thick "curtain" of cervical mucus has been made fluid by estrogens, additional millions fail to make it through the cervix. Those that do manage to enter the uterus are subjected to forceful uterine contractions, where thousands more are destroyed by resident phagocytic leukocytes. Therefore, only a few thousand and sometimes fewer than 200 sperm, out of the millions in the male ejaculate, finally reach the uterine tubes for fertilization.

Like the eggs, spermatozoa also have a short fertile life span in the female genital tract. A Secondary oocyte may survive for 12-24 hours following ovulation, whereas sperm may live up to a day or two within the female reproductive tract in most mammals. Table 16. 2 give the estimated fertile life of spermatozoa (following coitus) and eggs (following ovulation) in some mammals assessed on the basis of successful pregnancies. Motile spermatozoa have been found in the human oviduct up to 85 hours after coitus; however, fertilizing capacity of spermatozoa is usually lost before their motility. Thus, sexual intercourse must occur no later than 72 hours before ovulation or within 24 hours following ovulation for fertilization to take place. Sperm reach the upper portions of the uterine tube within an hour following sexual intercourse. Although many sperm may reach a secondary oocyte, but only one sperm actually fertilizes it and the remaining gets phagocytized.

Several layers of follicle cells, radially arranged near the egg surface, surround the egg at ovulation and this arrangement of cells probably orient the sperm head towards the egg. Once the egg reaches the site of fertilization, its outer layer of cells is rapidly lost due to the mechanical action of cilia and muscular movements of the uterine tube and also through the presence of an enzyme **hyaluronidase**, released from the sperm acrosome during acrosome reaction.

Table 16.2: Estimates of fertile life of spermatozoa and eggs in some Mammals

Species	Duration of fertile life of spermatozoa (Hrs.)	Duration of fertile life of ovulated egg (Hrs.)
Cow	28-50	22-24
Ferret	36-126	Approximately 36
Guinea Pig	21-22	Not more than 20
Hamster	-	5-12
Horse/Mare	144	Nearly 24
Man	28-48	Not more than 24
Mouse	6	8-12
Pig	-	Approximately 20
Rabbit	30-32	6-8
Rat	14	12-14
Sheep	30-48	15-24

16.5 Pre-fertilization Changes in Sperm

Although spermatozoa that have passed through the epididymis are fully fertile, yet these must undergo some further changes before they can actually engage in fertilization. These changes normally take place in the female genital tract in order to gain the capacity to penetrate and fertilize the egg. These changes are referred to as **capacitation** and **acrosome reaction**.

Capacitation: Freshly deposited sperm in the vagina are incapable of penetrating the oocyte. They must be **capacitated**, that is, the membranes of spermatozoa must become fragile so that the hydrolytic enzymes in their acrosomes are released. The exact mechanism of capacitation is still a mystery, but it is clear that as sperm swim through the cervical mucus, uterus, and uterine tubes, the cholesterol that keeps their acrosomal membranes "tough" and stable is depleted, and the sperm undergoes a gradual capacitation over the next 6-8 hours. Also, capacitation is an elaborate mechanism for preventing the spilling of acrosomal enzymes. If sperm had fragile acrosomal membranes while still within the male reproductive tract, they could rupture prematurely, causing some degree of autolysis of the male reproductive system. Thus, capacitation seems to be a process in which sperm undergoes certain morphological changes while residing in the female genital tract in order to obtain the capacity to fertilize the egg. Some feel that maturation of spermatozoa does not stop at the moment of ejaculation but continues in the female genital tract as part of the capacitation process that finally leads to the acquisition of full fertilizing capacity.

In 1951, Austin and Chang observed that the mammalian spermatozoa require a period of time in the female reproductive tract before becoming capable of penetrating the cellular and noncellular investments of an ovulated oocyte. This phenomenon was later termed "**capacitation**" by Austin in 1952.

Capacitation process thus, can be defined as a conditioning of spermatozoa within the female tract, which when completed, permits the acrosome reaction to occur, usually in the immediate vicinity of the oocyte or within the cumulus cell mass. The time required for capacitation ranges from one and half-hours in sheep to six hours in rabbits. The end result is to improve the chance of establishing contact between the sperm and egg and to enable the sperm to penetrate the zona pellucida.

During capacitation, both a glycoprotein coat and seminal plasma proteins are removed from the acrosomal region of spermatozoa. These surface elements are deposited on spermatozoa in the epididymis to stabilize the plasma membrane that overlies the acrosome. Capacitation process seems to involve at least two specific changes in the spermatozoa. I) Removal of polysaccharide from the surface of sperm, and is called the decapacitation factor (D.F.) of the seminal plasma. And 2) loosening of the acrosome, which release enzyme hyaluronidase for sperm passage through the cumulus and a lipoprotein, which is a lytic agent active on the zona pellucida. Hormones influence the capacitating ability of the female genital tract. Estrogen enhances the process while progesterone inhibits it. An important physiological correlate of capacitation is a marked increase in respiratory activity and intensity of motility of spermatozoa. Although capacitation has been shown to be a pre-requisite for the fertilization of rabbit, rat, hamster, ferret, sheep, and pig oocyte (Austin 1969), it may not be necessary for the fertilization of mouse, cow, monkey, and human oocyte (Austin 1969).

Acrosome Reaction and **Sperm Penetration**: The corona radiata and deep to that, the zona pellucida encapsulates the ovulated oocyte. Both of these must be breached before sperm can penetrate the oocyte itself. This is done with the help of **acrosome reaction**. During acrosomal reaction, acrosomal enzymes such as **hyaluronidase, acrosin, protease**, and others are released in the immediate vicinity of the oocyte. Hundreds of acrosome must rupture to break down the intercellular cement, rich in hyaluronic acid, that holds the granulosa cells together and to digest holes in the zona pellucida. Calcium ions (Ca^{2+}) appear to promote the acrosome reaction in capacitated spermatozoa and it is noticed that this reaction fails to occur in motile spermatozoa in the absence of calcium. Also, calmodulin, a calcium-dependent enzyme activator appears to be located in the acrosomal region of spermatozoa and may have a functional link through which action of calcium is mediated within the membranes of the acrosome.

The mammalian sperm acrosome is a cap-like membrane-limited organelle, which is located in the anterior two-thirds of the sperm head (Figure 16.6). It contains hydrolytic enzymes that are important in fertilization. This organelle has various sizes and shapes in different animals, but always consists of a continuous limiting membrane composed of an outer region, an inner region, the equatorial segment or acrosomal collar, the subacrosomal space (the perforatorium), and the soluble contents of the acrosome. When a mammalian spermatozoon is in the immediate vicinity of the cumulus oophorus, a series of morphological alterations occur on the surface of the acrosomal region. These alterations, known collectively as '**acrosomal reaction**' takes place subsequent to the completion of capacitation in species that require this process for fertilization. The occurrence of the acrosome reaction in mammals was first recognized by Austin and Bishop (1958) and later defined by Austin in 1963. It is an essential precondition of successful fertilization.

Acrosome reaction consists of multiple point fusion by vesiculation and/or vacuolations of the outer acrosomal membrane with the overlying plasma membrane. The resultant formation of vesicles or membranous discontinuities is presumably required for the activation and/or release of the acrosomal contents. Normally, the process of vesiculation extends only to the limits of the acrosomal cap, with the outer acrosomal and plasma membranes fused at the equatorial region in order to ensure the continuity of the posterior plasma membrane and maintenance of sperm motility. The acrosome reaction is completed during the passage of spermatozoa through the cumulus and coronal cells and must be accomplished during this passage in order to expose the inner acrosomal membrane, which is necessary for spermatozoa to traverse the zona pellucida. Acrosome reaction liberates and activates acrosomal contents, permitting spermatozoa to first penetrate the cumulus mass by degrading bonds in the extracellular matrix formed primarily between glycoprotein and hyaluronic acid and then to traverse the zona pellucida by breaking protein-carbohydrate linkages (Figure 16.7). Mammalian acrosome shows the presence of both hyaluronidase and hydrolytic enzymes. Hyaluronidase facilitates the passage of spermatozoa through the zona pellucida by cleaving zona polysaccharides. When removal of the acrosome or acrosome reaction is completed, the inner acrosomal membrane is exposed (Figure 16.6) and the proteolytic enzymes bound to this membrane and capable of digestion to create a narrow path through the zona pellucida are released. Once a path is cleared, a single sperm makes contact with the oocyte's membrane receptors (Figure 16.7), and its nucleus is pulled into the oocyte cytoplasm (Figure 16.8). Each sperm carries a special two-part binding apparatus on its surface. The **beta protein** part acts first and binds to a receptor on oocyte membrane (identified as glycoprotein **ZP3**). This event engages the **alpha protein** part, causing it to insert into the membrane. This somehow causes the membranes of sperm and egg to open and then fuse together. This process is known as **syngamy** and it results in the formation of **zygote**.

16.6 Cortical Reaction and Zona Reaction

The presence of a gradient, polarity, or mosaicism in the structural organization of the cortex and the spatial distribution of macromolecules in the vitelline membrane are relatively new concepts as applied to mammalian oocyte and ova. Such polarities are common in the oocyte of amphibian and insects where the entrance and/or penetration of a spermatozoon are limited to a specific region of the plasma membrane of egg.

Austin first described the existence of cortical granules in mammalian oocyte and their behavior during fertilization in 1956 from light microscopic observations of golden hamster oocyte. Recent investigations have shown that either fusion of the gametes or parthenogenetic activation of oocyte is required for cortical granule release. The discharge of cortical granules and the release of cortical contents into the perivitelline space of oocyte appear to occur by a process of exocytosis. This process is known as **cortical reaction**. Cortical reaction results in the release of "factors" that I) render the oocyte membrane impermeable to accessory spermatozoa, and ii) alter the structure and/or molecular composition of the zona pellucida possibly through the inactivation or removal of species-specific receptor sites for spermatozoa. This later process is termed **zona reaction** and is observed in many, but not all, fertilized mammalian eggs.

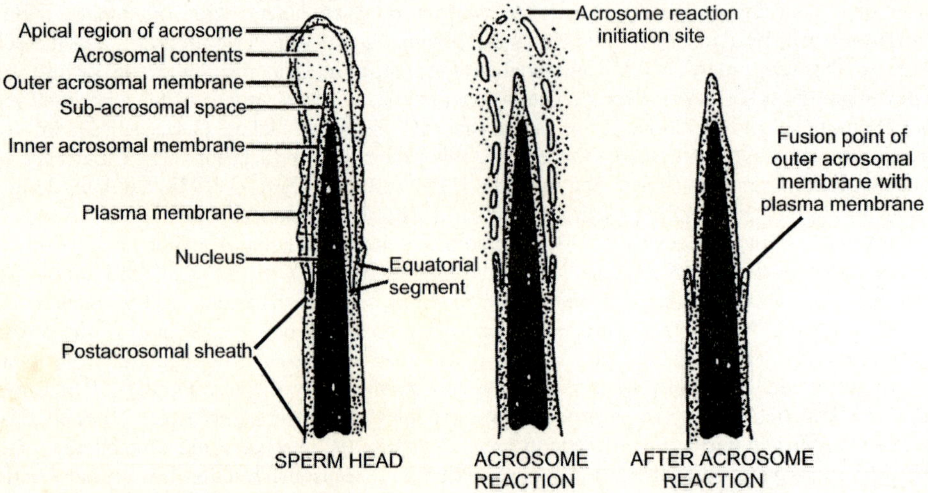

Figure 16.6: Changes in acrosome during acrosome reaction in Rabbit.

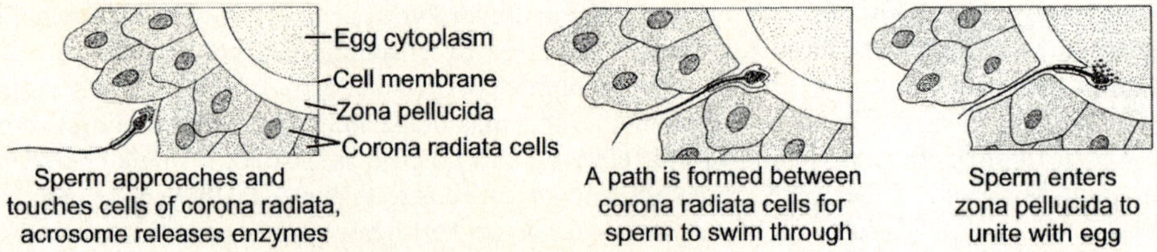

Figure 16.7: Sperm penetration through corona radiata and zona pellucida during the process of fertilization of egg in a laboratory Mammal.

Once the sperm enters the oocyte membrane, ionic calcium (Ca++) is released into the oocyte cytoplasm. Rise in intracellular Ca++ activates the oocyte to prepare it for cell division and also causes cortical reaction. The **cortical granules** located just deep to the plasma membrane spill their contents into the extracellular space beneath the zona pellucida. The spilled material binds water, and as it swells, it detaches all sperm still in contact with receptors on the oocyte membrane, accomplishing the permanent **slow block to polyspermy**.

16.7 Polyspermy

Polyspermy is the entry of several (accessory or supernumerary) spermatozoa into an egg or oocyte and it occurs in some animals, but in humans and as a rule only a single sperm is allowed to penetrate the oocyte. Both the fusion of the gametes and the block (s) to polyspermy involve cellular, molecular and physiological modifications in the cortex of the oocyte and in the oocyte membrane. Two mechanisms ensure **monospermy** (entry of one sperm into an egg). One is opening of the sodium channels as soon as the plasma membrane of one sperm contacts the oocyte membrane, and then diffusion of sodium into the oocyte from the extracellular space, causing its membrane to depolarize. This electrical event, known as the **fast block to polyspermy** prevents other sperm from fusing with the oocyte membrane. Polyspermy if at all it occurs in rare cases, results into nonviable embryos due to too much of genetic material.

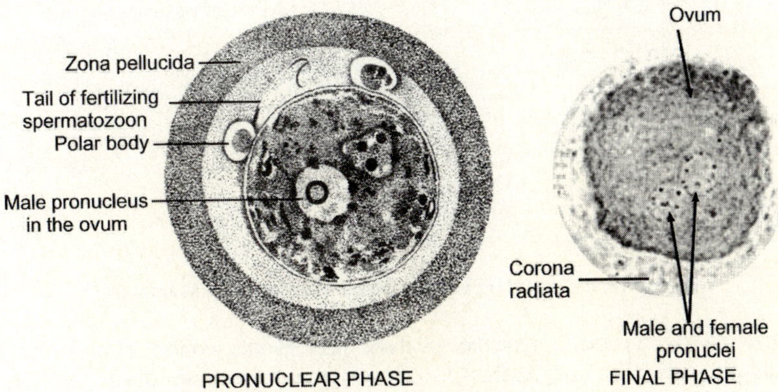

Figure 16.8: Fertilization in a Mammalian egg.

16.8 Fertilization

New life begins at fertilization, with the union of two gametes, the egg and the spermatozoon (Figure 16.8). Site of fertilization in nearly all mammals is the ampulla, a wide part of the fallopian tube or oviduct (Figure 16.9). After fertilization in the ampulla, the egg, or more correctly called as zygote and later the embryo, passes through the rest of the oviduct, and then into the uterus where it attaches to the wall of the uterus so that development can takes place as illustrated in Figure 16.9.

Events taking place during Fertilization: The secondary oocyte, activated by the ionic calcium signal, now completes meiosis II to form the ovum nucleus and ejects the second polar body. The ovum and sperm nuclei swell, becoming **female** and **male pronuclei**, and approach each other (Figure 16.8). The pronuclei membranes rupture, releasing their chromosomes and the true movement of fertilization occurs as the maternal and paternal chromosome combine. Fertilization not only establishes the diploid state for the embryo but is also the time at which the sex of the embryo is decided.

Mammalian oocyte is ovulated with chromosomal maturation "arrested" at the second metaphase of meiosis. The first polar body extruded at the first meiotic division, is still present in the perivitelline space and is often connected to the oocyte by means of a cytoplasmic bridge containing microtubules. Major features of the period immediately preceding fertilization are the disruption of tight and gap junctions between coronal cell processes through the zona pellucida. Prior to ovulation, the continued contact of coronal cells and the oocyte appears to be essential for the normal growth and meiotic maturation of the mouse, pig, and rabbit oocyte. Coronal cell processes are withdrawn from the surface of the oocyte either during the first or second meiotic metaphases. At the intracellular level, the formation of electron-dense granules from elements of the peripheral Golgi complexes and the distribution of these granules within the cortical cytoplasm are major features of the pre-fertilization periods (Cortical reaction). Fusion of gametes rarely occurs in the region of the vitelline membrane devoid of cortical granules and microvilli.

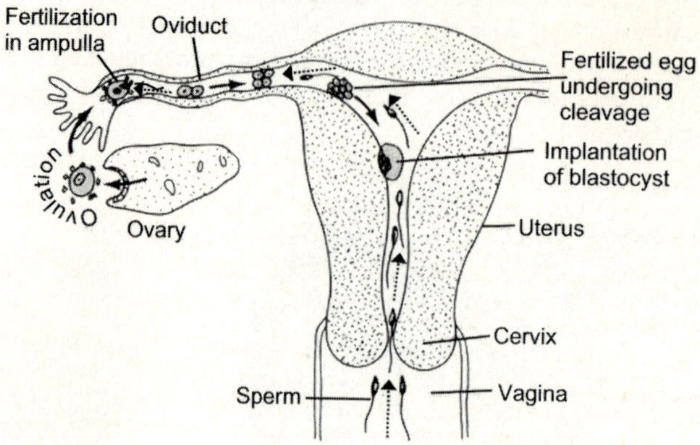

Figure 16.9: Site of fertilization and implantation in Mammals.

Fertilization encompasses a sequence of three basic events: contact of spermatozoon with an oocyte at the investments of an oocyte; fusion of the external membranes of the gametes; and finally the actual mixing of the maternal and paternal genomes (i.e. syngamy) at the metaphase of the first mitotic division. Fertilization of a mammalian oocyte involves: i) passage of a spermatozoon through the cellular layers of an oocyte, ii) attachment of the spermatozoon to the surface of the zona pellucida- a process that for some species is apparently mediated by species-specific receptors for spermatozoa, iii) passage through the zona pellucida, iv) fusion of the spermatozoa and oocyte plasma membranes, and v) the actual penetration of the fertilizing spermatozoon into the oocyte with the resultant decondensation and dispersion of chromatin. Fine structural aspects of each of these events have been studied by scanning and transmission electron microscopy (Austin 1968) and Gwatikin 1977). Mammalian fertilization involves the fusion of the limiting membrane of the gametes, thus producing a single cell with a diploid complement of chromosomes and bounded by a membrane that, at least initially is a composite or mosaic of the two-gamete membranes. Additional correlates of fertilization process are the cortical and zona reactions.

After traversing the zona pellucida, an acrosome-reacted mammalian spermatozoon reaches the vitelline membrane rather rapidly, although the duration of residence in the perivitelline space prior to contact varies among and within species. Only acrosome-reacted spermatozoa are capable of undergoing fusion with the vitelline membrane. The inner acrosomal membrane of mammalian spermatozoa does not fuse with the oocyte plasma membrane; rather, fusion is usually accomplished between the vitelline membrane and the portion of the spermatozoal plasma membrane that covers the posterior region of the head. The mechanics of fusion appear to involve a two-step process: i) fusion of the vitelline membrane with the portion of the spermatozoal plasma membrane extending from the posterior margin of the acrosome to the tip of the tail, and ii) engulfment of the anterior two thirds of the head within a cytoplasmic vacuole formed from the portions of the oocyte cytoplasm that surround the anterior region of the head. It appears likely that receptor molecules present on the surface of an oocyte are capable of interacting only with a specific population of spermatozoal macromolecules located in the posterior plasma membrane, and this interaction provides for species-specific binding. It is only upon fusion of the gametes, a series of morphogenetic events occurs in the cortex of egg cytoplasm that prevents additional spermatozoa from undergoing fusion (cortical and zona reaction).

The zona and cortical reactions are the resumption of meiotic maturation and the "activation" of the egg accompanying fusion of the gametes. Shortly after the incorporation of a fertilizing spermatozoon into the oocyte cytoplasm, the nuclear membrane of the spermatozoon disintegrates by means of a lytic process and its chromatin begins to swell and decondense into filamentous strands, which then diffuse into the cytoplasm. Spermatozoal chromatin is both exceptionally stable and rich in disulfide bonds and exposure of the chromatin to the hydrating conditions of the oocyte cytoplasm is insufficient to cause decondensation. However, presence of a factor or a set of factors possibly enzymes that reduce disulfide bonds in the oocyte cytoplasm may be responsible for the decondensation of the chromatin. These postulated factors, termed "male pronucleus growth factors" by Thibault and Gerard (1973) and Thibault (1973, 77), and "sperm-nucleus decondensing factors" by Yanagimachi (1977) are probably synthesized in the pre-ovulatory oocyte following the breakdown of the germinal vesicle. At present, the existence of these factors is still only hypothetical. After decondensation, spermatozoal chromatin usually lies in a subcortical location over which the plasma membrane generally devoid of microvilli, protrudes markedly. Then a nuclear envelope develops to enclose the chromatin, thus forming the **male pronucleus**. Concomitant with the fusion of the gamete plasma membranes is the resumption of meiotic maturation, culminating in the abstraction of the second polar body. The more internal set of chromosomes quickly become surrounded by a double membrane envelop resulting in the formation of **female pronucleus**. After the enclosure of the chromosomes, the two pronuclei enlarge significantly, move toward the central portion of the ovum, and come to lie in juxtaposition (Figure 16.8). Depending upon the species as many as 30 or more nucleoli are present in the pronuclei, but each pronucleus appears to be nearly identical in size and structure. In mammals, the association of the maternally and paternally derived genomes, a process termed "**syngamy**" occurs in the absence of the fusion of the pronuclear membranes. During the growth and movement of pronuclei, DNA synthesis is initiated resulting in the duplication of chromosomes. The actual association of the maternal and paternal genomes is affected when breakdown of two pronuclear envelopes occurs and numerous nucleoli also disappear. Then the two groups of chromosomes assume positions on the first cleavage spindle for the first mitotic division of the egg. Following the mixing of the maternal and paternal genomes and the first mitotic or cleavage division, the **zygote** enters the period of **post-fertilization development**, which includes cleavage, and blastocyst formation, and is termed the **preimplantation period**. However, successful attainment of two haploid sets of chromosomes (maternal and paternal) within the ovum cytoplasm is critical for the formation of future embryo. Abnormal number of chromosomes (condition is known as **aneuploidy**) results in embryonic abnormality and usually its death. This is due to normal block to polyspermy and also failure in normal reactivation of second meiotic metaphase with polar body extrusion. Such failures are common in ageing eggs.

Most mammalian eggs are ovulated at metaphase of meiosis II and only these eggs complete second meiosis if activated by appropriate stimuli. Under normal conditions *in vivo*, the fertilizing spermatozoon provides the activation stimulus. But it seems likely that a wide range of stimuli can induce a series of biochemical events, which closely resemble this type of activation.

Errors of Fertilization: Occasionally errors of fertilization occur and these bring about abnormal chromosome numbers in the egg. These are the following:

Polyspermy is fertilization by more than one spermatozoon. It occurs naturally in few cases and can be enhanced by ageing of the egg before fertilization.

Polygyny occurs due to a failure to extrude the second polar body and thus results in an extra set of female chromosomes in the zygote. However, it is a rare error.

Gynogenesis is a type of sexual reproduction in which spermatozoa activate oocytes but do not contribute genetic components to the embryo. It is nearly same as parthenogenesis.

Androgenesis is the development of a haploid embryo whose genome is exclusively contributed by the spermatozoon or parental chromosomes, accomplished when the maternal nucleus of a fertilized ovum degenerates. This form of development occurs in a few species, but is not possible in mammals.

Summary

An ovary contains many growing follicles but only one of them advances to mature follicular stage per menstrual cycle. Under the influence of FSH, it reaches the Graafian stage.

A surge of LH at the mid-cycle causes the Graafian follicle to rupture and release an ovum. This process is called ovulation.

Ovulation is of two types: spontaneous and induced or reflex type. Spontaneous ovulation occurs at regular intervals independent of mating or external environment as seen in rat, hamster, mouse, cow, goat, sheep human, monkey etc. Induced or reflex ovulation is dependent upon stimulus of mating as seen in cat, rabbit and mink. The chains of events are basically similar in both types of ovulation.

The ovulated follicle is entrapped in the fimbriae of the oviduct and it moves to the ampullary region, which is the site of fertilization.

An oocyte is fertilizable for up to 24 hours and the sperm are viable within the female reproductive tract for up to 72 hours.

Lashing of sperm tails and muscular contractions within the walls of the uterus and uterine tube, stimulated by prostaglandins in the semen, aid the sperm journey in the female genital tract. Also, under the influence of high estrogen concentrations during the first part of the menstrual cycle, uterus and cervix contain a thin, watery secretion that promotes sperm transport and survival in these ducts. Conversely, during the later part of the cycle, when the progesterone concentration is high, the female reproductive tract secretes a viscous fluid that hampers sperm transport and survival in it.

Many millions of spermatozoa are deposited in the vagina but the numbers reaching the site of fertilization rarely exceed a hundred in the small animals, and a few hundred to a few thousand in the larger animals. The magnitude of sperm numbers at the site of fertilization may still appear well in excess of needs. Still, the population is very sparse when one takes into account the minute size of the spermatozoa, in comparison to the enormous volume of space within this region of the oviduct.

For successful fertilization, availability of capacitated sperm to mature oocyte is essential. Therefore, sperm must survive the hostile environment of the vagina and become capacitated. Hundreds of sperm release their acrosomal enzymes in acrosome reaction to break down the egg's corona radiata and zona pellucida. A path is formed between corona cells for sperm to swim through. When one sperm penetrates the egg, it triggers first the fast block to polyspermy and then cortical reaction occurs with the release of cortical granules. This occurs in the isthmus of oviducts. Following sperm penetration, the secondary oocyte completes meiosis II. Then the ovum and sperm pronuclei fuse resulting in fertilization and formation of a zygote.

Pre-embryonic development results in the formation of blastocyst, which consists of the trophoblast and an inner cell mass.

The trophoblast adheres to, digests, and implants in the endometrium about 14 days after ovulation.

Questions

1. Define ovulation. What causes ovulation and what happens to an oocyte following this process?
2. How does an egg move into the infundibulum following ovulation?
3. Discuss the hormonal control of ovulation.
4. What factors aid the movements of the egg and sperm cells through the female reproductive tract?

5. Where in the female reproductive tract does fertilization normally takes place? List the events of fertilization.
6. Write a note on corpus luteum, acrosome reaction, capacitation, cortical reaction and polyspermy.
7. The structures that draw an ovulated oocyte into the female duct system are **a) cilia, b) fimbriae,** c) microvilli, d) stereocilia
8. The corpus luteum is formed in a) fertilization, **b) ovulation**, c) menstruation, d) implantation..
9. The zygote contains chromosomes from a) the mother only, b) the father only, **c) both the mother and father, but half from each**, d) from each parent.
10. Identical twins result from the fertilization of **a) one ovum by one sperm** b) one ovum by two sperm, c) two ova and two sperm, d) two ova by one sperm.

Chapter 17

Implantation and Pregnancy

Fertilization results in the formation of zygote that remains in the oviduct for a further few days and is then transported through the isthmus of the oviduct or uterine tube into the uterus. In some marsupials, such as opossum and rat kangaroo, this may take 24 hours or less while in some carnivores, fertilized egg may stay in the fallopian tubes for up to a week. However, in most mammals the journey of the fertilized egg from ampulla to the uterus takes 2-4 days (Table 17.1). And this delay in reaching the uterus is essential for the survival of the embryo as the estrus uterus is distended and provides a favorable environment for the spermatozoa but a very unfavorable one for the embryo.

Table 17.1 Implantation time and duration of pregnancy in various Mammals

Species	Type of Implantation	Entry of embryo into uterus(days)	Time of implantation (days)	Luteal regression if mating infertile (days)	Duration of Pregnancy (days)
Rat	Invasive	3	4.5-5.5	10-12	22
Mouse		3	4.5	10-21	21
Rabbit		3.5	7-8	12	28-30
Dog		4-6 (?)	14-21	61	61
Man		3.5	6(?)	12-14	270
Sheep	Non-Invasive	2-4	16	16-18	145-150
Pig		2-4	18	16-18	114
Cow		3-4	30-45	18-20	282
Horse		4-5	30-40	20-21	340

Cilia of the genital tract are the primary active transporters of the embryo. Also, transfer may be facilitated by the changing endocrine milieu of the female genital ducts during this early luteal phase with its rising ratio of progesterone to estrogens. This hormonal change affects the musculature of oviducts and uterus and also relaxes the isthmus sphincter. On reaching the uterus, embryo engages in an elaborate interaction with the mother during which several messages are transmitted in both directions. Because of these, embryo makes the maternal pituitary-ovarian axis aware of its presence, and establishes physical and nutritional contact with the maternal uterine endometrium. This results in implantation of the embryo in the mother's uterus. In the absence of these events, regression of corpus luteum occurs followed by menstruation and beginning of a new cycle.

The first formal description of preimplantation of rabbit conceptus was by de Graaf in 1672. However, Von Baer in 1827-28 published the first descriptive reports of the early stages of pre-implantation development and the conformation of the actual existence of the mammalian ovum in the uterus. With the application of the electron microscope and elegant biochemical techniques to the study of early embryonic development, it has become possible to define more clearly the sequence of cellular and macromolecular steps that prepare the conceptus for implantation.

17.1 Pre-implantation Processes-Blastocyst Formation

After fertilization in the oviduct, rapid mitotic cell divisions (called **cleavage)** of the fertilized egg or **zygote** occur (Figure 17.1). Cleavages eventually produce a solid sphere of **blastomeres** called **morula**. This is still surrounded by the zona pellucida. It shows a marked quantitative increase in its biosynthetic capacity so that net synthesis of RNA and protein increases, transport of amino acids and nucleotides into cells rises and changes in the synthetic patterns of phospholipids and cholesterol occur. Morula continues to move through the uterine tube toward the uterine cavity (Figure 17.1). At 5th day after fertilization, a dense cluster of cells develops into the hollow ball of cells. This transforms morula to next embryonic stage in development called **blastocyst**. The blastocyst has an outer covering of cells called the **trophoblast or trophectoderm** surrounding a fluid filled cavity called the **blastocoel**. In the blastocyst, a cluster of cells is placed eccentrically against one pole of the cavity. This is called the **inner cell mass** (Figure 17.2). The trophoblast and part of the inner cell mass ultimately form the membranes composing the fetal portion of the placenta. Rest of the inner cell mass develops into an embryo. It is during the transition from a morula to a blastocyst stage that the embryo enters the uterus and attaches to its wall and this occurs around 7th day from fertilization.

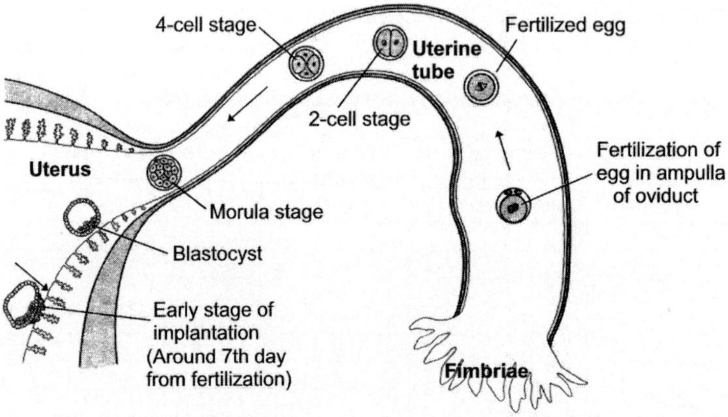

Figure 17.1:Transport and implantation of Human embryo after fertilization.

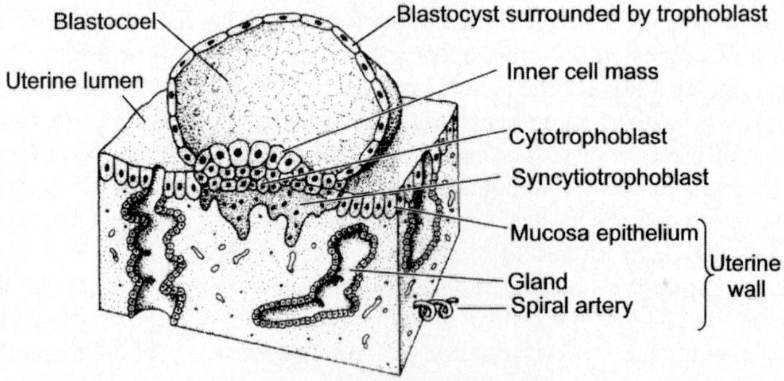

Figure 17.2: Structure of implanting blastocyst within the uterus of a Mammal.

17.2 Implantation

The blastocyst remains free within the cavity of the uterus for about 2 days before it attaches to the uterine wall. The free-living blastocyst is bathed in the secretions of the uterus and draws the oxygen and metabolic substrates that it requires for its continued growth and survival from these secretions. It actively accumulates organic molecules and ions by specific, cellular transport mechanism. However, exchange of oxygen and carbon dioxide occurs by diffusion. During this phase of the cycle, the endometrium is in its secretory phase, and the blastocyst receives nourishment from the glycogen-rich secretions of the endometrial glands. This secretion is also called as uterine milk. However, there is a limit to the size that a free-living conceptus can attain before such exchanges become inadequate. Therefore, before this critical stage is reached, the conceptus develops its own blood vascular system that supplies the essential metabolites etc. to the growing embryo. The conceptus also develops a distinct and highly vascularised region on its extra-embryonic surface through which interchange of materials with maternal tissues takes place. To achieve this, the blastocyst and the uterine endometrium interact locally with one another. During this time, the zona pellucida disintegrates and the blastocyst attaches itself to the uterine wall. This is called **implantation** (also called **nidation**) and it occurs about 6-7 days after fertilization. With the successful conclusion of implantation, a corresponding specialized and vascularised region develops in the maternal endometrial tissue. This zone of adjacent and highly vascularised contact between mother and conceptus is called the **placenta.** The placenta is the ultimate outcome of the primary interactions between mother and conceptus that occur at implantation.

Implantation Sites: On entering the uterus, the embryo is positioned for implantation. The location of implantation site within the uterus tends to be characteristic for each species. Generally, the blastocyst implants in either the posterior portion of the fundus or the body of the uterus. It is oriented such that the inner cell mass is toward the endometrium (Figure 17.2). But, little is known of the mechanisms by which the implantation site is determined. There seems to be two major factors involved in the orientation of the blastocyst to the endometrium. One is the shape of the blastocyst and its response to the contraction of the uterus, and second is specific adhesiveness of the trophoblast as in the first stage of implantation; only certain regions of the blastocyst are adhesive. However, insufficient evidences do not generalize the role of these two factors in implantation of the blastocyst in most species. Further, in ruminants, a distinct area of projecting aglandular uterine mucosa known as **caruncles** is the only site at which close attachment of conceptus tissue occurs. In polytocous species (those having several embryos) a 'spacing mechanism' also operates to ensure that blastocysts are distributed along the whole uterine axis rather than clustering at one site.

Within a few hours of the initiation of implantation in the region of contact between the blastocyst and the endometrium, the trophoblast develops two layers. These are **syntiotrophoblast** and a **cytotrophoblast**. The syntiotrophoblast contains no cell boundaries (sycytium) and is formed by the fusion of some trophectodermal cells. The cytotrophoblast lies between the inner cell mass and syntiotrophoblast and has distinct cells that may serve as a proliferative source for generating more trophoblastic cells (Figure 17.2). These layers of trophoblast as they grow further become part of the **chorion**, that is one of the fetal membrane. During implantation, the syntiotrophoblast secretes enzymes that enables the blastocyst to penetrate the uterine lining by digesting and liquefying the endometrial cells. The endometrial secretions further nourish the burrowing blastocyst for about a week after implantation. Eventually, the blastocyst becomes buried in the endometrium and derives the nutrients through the placenta.

The events subsequent to attachment vary with species and accordingly implantation may be classified into two categories:

Invasive Implantation: In invasive implantation, the conceptus ultimately breaks through the surface epithelium and invades extensively the underlying stroma of the uterus as seen in primates, cat, dog, mouse, rabbit. The blastocyst of these species is nurtured at first by uterine secretions but this free-living phase is relatively short-lived (Table 17.1). As a result, invasive embryos tend to be smaller at attachment. When intimate contact is made with the maternal epithelium, only relatively few trophectodermal cells are involved in developing this contact. The tissues of the conceptus erode not just the epithelium but also stromal cells, connective tissue and, in man, even the walls of the blood vessel. Thus, a primary signal from the conceptus is effectively transferred through the epithelium to the stroma and is then amplified. The stromal response to invasive implantation seems to anticipate the event by developing protective devices, which limit and control the depth of invasion. One of the earliest visible response to this event is an increased vascular permeability in the stromal tissue underlying the conceptus, followed by edema and compositional changes in the intercellular matrix, changes in the morphology of stromal cells and a progressive sprouting and ingrowth of capillaries. This is called **decidualization,** and can easily be observed in man and rodents. The major endometrial component of placenta involved in decidualization is called **decidua**. It is clear that the rapid progression of changes in the endometrium underlying the attachment site is organized and stimulated by a message derived from the blastocyst. The nature of the message could be a low molecular weight secretory product of the blastocyst or more likely the blastocyst stimulates the adjacent uterine tissue to secrete a 'decidualizing molecule', which then spreads through the stroma. Both histamine and prostaglandins have been suggested as the decidualizing molecule (s) since both of these are present in the progestational endometrium and induce decidualization if injected locally. However, in rat and probably also in human, maximal decidual response is elicited by the conceptus if endometrial epithelium and stroma are primed with progesterone and then exposed to elevated levels of estrogen. The depth to which the conceptus invades maternal tissues varies with species.

Non-invasive Implantation: In non-invasive implantation, epithelial integrity is more or less retained and the epithelium becomes incorporated within the placenta. Therefore, it is the uterine epithelium in non-invasive implantation and not the underlying stroma, which limits and controls the invasion of the conceptus. Non-invasive implantation is seen in pig, cow, horse and sheep (Table 17.1). Attachment of non-invasive conceptuses is initiated relatively late than that of invasive ones. During the prolonged interval prior to attachment, the free-living conceptuses continue to draw on richer and more copious secretions from uterine glands called the uterine 'milk'. This secretion is a rich source of ions, amino acids, sugars and lipid precursors and the conceptus utilizes these resources and grows to a much greater preimplantation size than the embryos of invasive implantation such as of human or rodent. Also, no proper decidual response is induced in the underlying uterine stroma but limited stromal changes provide evidence of the recognition of embryonic presence. These include increase in vascularity and distinct changes in cellular morphology. All these changes result in the implantation of the blastocyst and formation of placenta in non-invasive implantation.

The relation of the chorionic sac to the uterine wall also varies among placental mammals and accordingly three types of implantation are seen. These are, 1) **Superficial** or **Central**, in which growth of chorionic sac brings it into contact with the lining of main uterine cavity, e.g. ungulates, carnivores, monkey; 2) **Eccentric** in which chorionic sac lies in a fold or pocket that closes off from the main cavity, e.g. rat, squirrel, dog, cat, rhesus monkey and 3) **Interstitial** in which chorionic sac penetrates into the substance of uterine lining, e.g. guinea pig, ape, man.

Delayed Implantation: In a number of species, after the blastocyst stage is reached, there is a prolongation of the time before implantation occurs. The blastocyst development during this period becomes relatively quiescent. This extension of the pre-implantation period is referred to as **delayed implantation**. It is primarily due to the conditions in the maternal reproductive tract. The phenomenon of delayed implantation is widespread and is found in such diverse groups as seals, armadillos, European roe deer, mink, mice, rat, gerbils etc. Delay of implantation may be natural due to suckling large litters and this type is called **facultative delayed implantation**. It occurs due to natural suppression of endogenous estrogen secretion in females, which are suckling young of the previous litter and it helps to prevent too great a metabolic drain on the lactating mothers. Thus, in these animals if the litters are removed or if exogenous estrogen is given to the mother, implantation proceeds within 24 hours. In contrast, there are many species such as elephant, seal, mink, fruit bat, brown bear, roe-deer and wolverine in which an **obligate delayed implantation,** also called **diapause** is an essential and normal part of the pregnancy. In these species, a prolonged period of weeks or months is spent with blastocysts of their pregnancy, in delay. Diapause confers distinct biological advantages. For example, roe deer mates in July and August when the adults are well fed and are in their prime, ensuring effective competition for mates. The embryo remains as a blastocyst until January and then it reactivates for delivery of young in May and June when the nutritional conditions become optimal for the new offspring.

Hormonal Control Of Implantation: The blastocyst provokes a response of considerable magnitude in the uterus for implantation and the uterus can only take part in these interactions if suitably primed by steroid hormones. The uterus must be prepared for receiving the blastocyst in order to support implantation in most species. Estrogen-dominated uterus is rather hostile to the conceptus. Under estrogen domination, the uterus cannot accommodate an implanting embryo and thus, premature entry of an embryo into the uterus results in its death. In the normal course of events, progesterone titers are comparatively high at the time of implantation. Progesterone increases rapidly from the pre-ovulatory period during which there was a relatively high estrogen titer and continues so during implantation and pregnancy. Under progesterone domination, the uterus is appropriately primed to engage in conversation with the blastocyst. In addition, the luteal phase of the cycle is characterized by distinctive patterns of uterine secretions rich in sugars and proteins. Elaboration of these secretory products is dependent upon progesterone action and their release requires the presence of estrogens in luteal phase. For optimal uterine sensitization, a high level of estrogens at the time of estrus seems to be necessary, followed by a period of several days when progesterone, produced by the developing corpora lutea, is the dominant hormone. It appears that estrogen stimulates the epithelium of the uterus in two ways. First, it stimulates the release of a glandular secretion of a characteristic composition, including specific macromolecules, such as the zona proteolytic enzyme, and also glucose, amino acids and ions, which cause embryonic activation. Second, the estrogen also acts on the epithelial cells to make them responsive or sensitive to a blastocyst signal so that they acquire the capacity to transmit effective evidence of the blastocyst's presence at attachment to the underlying stromal cells, and thereby instruct them to commence decidualization. Thus, it appears that the embryo first produce estrogens needed for implantation to stimulate the progesterone-primed uterus, the uterine epithelium may then respond by secreting embryotrophic factors indicating increased sensitivity to embryo attachment. Finally, the embryo may co-respond by the initiation of implantation and attachment Therefore, synchronous timing of embryonic and uterine development is vital for implantation to be successful. Another secretion of the trophoblast is the human chorionic gonadotropin (hCG), which has actions similar to LH. Human chorionic gonadotropin rescues the corpus luteum from disintegration and sustains its secretion of progesterone and estrogens. These hormones maintain the uterine lining in a secretory state and thus prevent menstruation.

17.3 Placenta

The placenta is an organ jointly formed by maternal and fetal tissues. Elaboration of placenta is associated with **viviparity** (giving birth to living young). So, when embryos develop within body of the mother, instead of within laid eggs, it has to establish functional relationships with the maternal tissues and also reduce the supply of yolk stored in the egg as the developing embryo derives its nutrients from the body of the mother. This is accomplished with the help of extra-embryonic membranes and formation of placenta.

Mammals like reptiles and birds have the same basic extra-embryonic membranes. These are **amnion**, **chorion**, **allantois** and **yolk sac**. The amnion surrounds the embryo proper; chorion is an outer layer of ectoderm (the trophoblast) that is vascularised by the mesoderm layer of either the yolk sac or the allantois and the allantois is an endodermal sac to store waste of the embryo. The yolk sac does not surround the yolk as the mammalian egg is almost yolkless but is in the same general position and is the first area to develop hemopoietic centers. In most marsupials, the allantois remains relatively simple sac and only the yolk sac vascularises the chorion. This region is closely apposed to the maternal endometrium and therefore, the placenta formed in these mammals is known as **chorio-vitelline**. Transportation of materials from maternal to fetal blood stream occurs through the endothelium, the connective tissue, the epithelium of the uterine endometrium, and then through the trophoblast, the connective tissue, and the endothelium of the mesoderm of the apposed yolk sac. In higher (eutherian) mammals, on the other hand, the vessels of the allantois, instead of yolk sac, vascularise the trophoblast (chorion) and such a placenta is known as **chorio-allantoic**.

The shape of the placenta and its size relative to the whole chorionic sac is governed by the distribution-pattern of the villi. On this basis, placenta may be classified into four categories (Figure 17.3). These are 1) **diffuse** (villi are retained over the entire chorion, e.g. lemurs, and some ungulates such as sow, mare), 2) **cotyledonary** (villi are grouped in well-spaced, prominent rosettes, known as **cotyledons** separated by stretches of smooth chorion, e.g. cattle, sheep and deer), 3) **zonary** (villi occupy a girdle-like band about the middle of the chorionic sac, e.g. carnivores) and 4) **discoid** (villi are limited to one or two disc-shaped areas, e.g. insectivores, bats, rodents and primates).

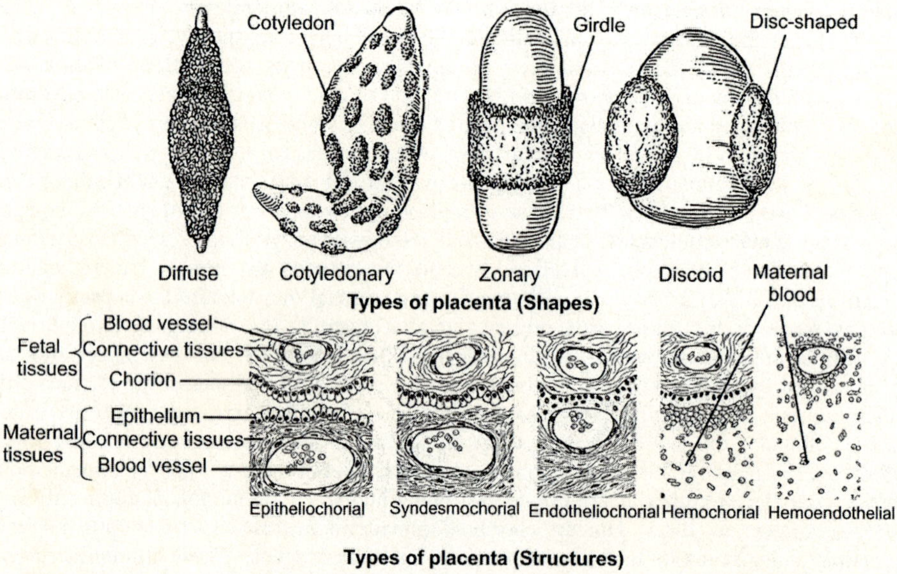

Figure 17.3: Types of placenta in Mammals on the basis of their shape and structure.

Further, if the chorionic villi lie in apposition with the uterine lining and do not fuse with it, the association is described as **semi placenta**. At the time of parturition, the villi are drawn out without much damage to the uterine wall and without much bleeding in such associations and therefore, this type of placentations are called **nondeciduate**. On the other hand, in case of **true placenta** (also called

placenta vera), the chorionic villi fuse with the eroded uterine mucosa in such a manner that at the time of birth, uterine lining also tears away with extensive hemorrhage. This type of placentation is called **deciduate**. The depth to which the conceptus invades maternal tissues and develops intimacy with it varies with species and accordingly on this structural basis, placenta can be divided into number of types. Therefore, **depending upon the progressive elimination of barriers between the maternal and fetal circulations**, placenta can be of five types (Figure 17.3).

A. Epithelio-choriol: The chorio-allantoic composite membrane comes in direct relation with the uterine lining and the simple chorionic villi fit into the corresponding pits in the mucosa of the uterus. Therefore, all the three tissues of the mother and fetus (epithelium, connective tissue and endothelium of blood vessels) lie opposite to each other as seen in Figure 17.3. Examples are sow, mare and lemurs and marsupials.

B. Syndesmo-choriol: In this type of placenta, local destruction of uterine epithelium allows the chorionic ectoderm to come into direct contact with the vascular maternal connective tissue. Examples are ruminants. Once gestation period is over, the chorionic villi are withdrawn and maternal tissue is not torn, and therefore, there is no bleeding.

C. Endothelio-choriol: In carnivores, the fetal-maternal union in the region of placenta shows a marked advance in intimacy. Therefore, in this type of placenta, erosion of the uterine mucosa practically bares the endothelium of its blood vessels and the syncytial chorionic epithelium then packs around these maternal vessels.

D. Hemo-choriol: A still more intimate placental relation occurs in lower rodents, insectivores, bats and anthropoids. In this type of placenta more thorough erosion of the superficial uterine mucosa occurs so that maternal blood circulates in channels within the fetal syncytium.

E. Hemo-endothelial: In higher rodents, such as rat, guinea pig, and rabbit actual intermingling, of the blood of the two circulations (fetal and maternal) occur. Thus, in this type of placenta, the chorionic villi lose their layers to such a degree that in most places, the bare endothelial lining of their vessels alone separates the fetal blood from the maternal sinuses.

Physiology of placenta: The primary function attributed to placenta is the interchange of materials present in the blood streams of the mother and embryo. The main functions of placenta are to pass nutrition from mother's blood to fetus, and to bring about respiration and excretion. Smaller molecules such as monosaccharides, hormones, vitamins, water, oxygen, carbon dioxide, soluble inorganic materials, certain antibodies and drugs pass through the placenta by simple diffusion. Physiologically, placenta acts as a selective barrier or like an ultra filter or semi permeable membrane thus allowing certain substances to pass through and some not. It is impermeable to some particulate matter such as bacteria and larger molecules. Many drugs used medically may penetrate the placental barrier and sometimes cause adverse effects on the embryo.

17.4 Parthenogenesis

The term parthenogenesis means literally virgin birth. It is applied to development that begins without the participation of a spermatozoon, that is without prior sexual intercourse and therefore without fertilization. However, it is different from **gynogenesis** in which spermatozoon induces activation of oocyte but takes no further part in the development of an embryo. Parthenogenesis is a regular method of reproduction in some insects and can be induced experimentally in some animals, such as frog.

However, it does not seem to occur naturally in any mammal, though it is a normal process in several non-mammalian groups, especially common among insects.

17.5 Pregnancy

The ovulated egg has two possible fates. It may fail to fertilize and if this happens during a typical menstrual cycle, the corpus luteum degenerates about two weeks after ovulation. Consequently, estrogen and progesterone concentrations decline rapidly, the uterine lining is no longer maintained, and the endometrium sloughs off as menstrual flow. However, if this occurs following implantation, the embryo is lost and this is called **spontaneous abortion**. On the other hand, if the ovum is fertilized, the resultant **conceptus** grows into **blastocyst** and implants in the uterus and grows further, it becomes **fetus** ("the young in the womb"). This results in pregnancy. The term **pregnancy** refers to events that occur from the time of fertilization (**conception**) until the **infant** is born. The pregnant women's developing offspring is called the **conceptus** (that which is conceived) and at birth, it is an **infant**. The time period during which development of the conceptus occurs is referred to as the **gestation period** (*gestare*= to carry). It extends from the last menstrual period to until birth of an infant and is approximately 280 days in human (Table 17.1).

The size of the uterine myometrium increases significantly during pregnancy and on this basis, the uterus may be categorized as **parous** and **nulliparous** (Figure 17.4). Parous uterus is the one that has borne one or more children. On the other hand, uterus of a woman who has never borne a child is called nulliparous.

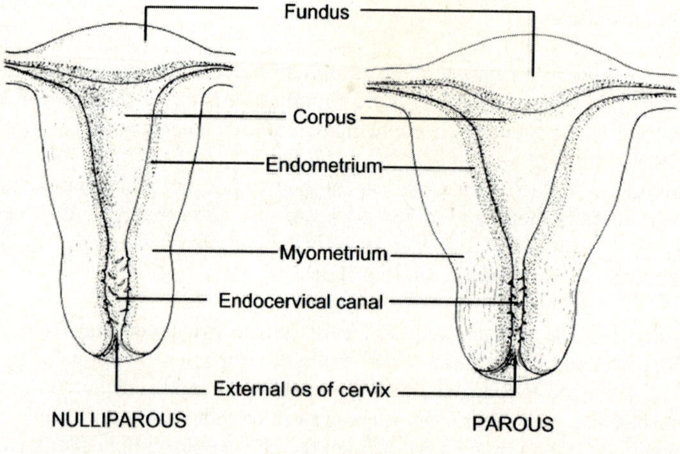

Figure 17.4: Changes in the size of uterine myometrium during pregnancy in Women.

Ectopic Pregnancy or Extra Uterine Pregnancy: Normally a fetus develops in the endometrium but rarely the fetus may be found located at various situations such as ovary, fallopian tube, mesentery, interstitial tissues, uterus, vagina etc. Such pregnancies are known as **ectopic** or **extra-uterine pregnancies**. Normally such pregnancies do not last long.

Hormonal Regulation Of Pregnancy: In all mammals, the corpus luteum formed after ovulation in the ovary persists for some time. If fertilization occurs, it does not regress and instead enlarges in response to stimulation by gonadotropic hormones secreted by the placenta. The placental gonadotropin in humans is called human chorionic gonadotropin (hCG). The enlarged corpus luteum of pregnancy secretes estrogen, progesterone and relaxin (Figure 17.5). The relaxin helps to maintain pregnancy by inhibiting contractions of the uterine myometrium. In most species, removal of ovaries at any time during pregnancy results in abortion, but in humans, the placenta produces sufficient estrogen and progesterone from maternal and fetal precursors to take over the function of the corpus luteum after 6th week of pregnancy. Therefore, ovariectomy before 6th week of gestation period leads to abortion but thereafter has no effect on pregnancy. The function of the corpus luteum in humans begins to decline after eight weeks of pregnancy but it persists throughout pregnancy.

Human Chorionic Gonadotropin (hCG): LH-like hormone known as **human chorionic gonadotropin (hCG)** maintains the viability of the corpus luteum once implantation occurs. hCG is a glycoprotein and is secreted by the trophoblast cells of the blastocyst. By the eighth day after fertilization or third week of gestation, hCG can be detected in the blood of a pregnant woman to confirm pregnancy. Main function of hCG is to maintain the corpus luteum of pregnancy beyond the period of menstrual cycle. It stimulates the corpus luteum to continue production of estrogens and progesterone, which are essential for the maintenance of the endometrium and also for the suppression of menstruation. hCG also causes the fetal testes to produce small amounts of testosterone, which stimulate the development of male sex organs and the descent of the testicles into the scrotum. Peak levels of hCG are reached at about ninth week of pregnancy but afterwards, it declines sharply during the 4th-5th month and is then maintained at a lower level until the end of pregnancy (Figure 17.5).

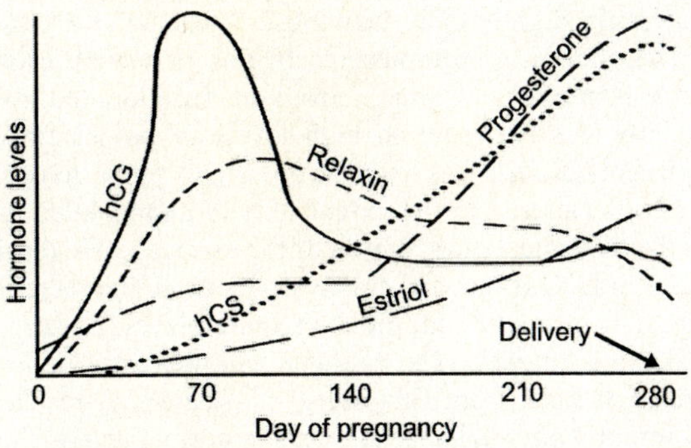

Figure 17.5: Hormone levels during normal pregnancy in Women, hCG-human chorionic gonadotropin, hCS-human chorionic somatomammotropin.

Progesterone: Progesterone is produced by the corpus luteum in early pregnancy and in much larger amounts by the placenta. From about 8th week onwards, the production of progesterone is taken over by the placenta. Progesterone secretion reaches a peak value at the end of pregnancy when it is nearly ten times the levels of early pregnancy (Figure 17.5).

Progesterone plays multiple roles in the maintenance of gestation. It delays ovulation by the suppression of LH secretion. It acts on the endometrium to prepare it for the reception of the embryo. It renders the contractile myometrium quiescent so that implantation proceeds normally and the expulsion of embryos is prevented. **Arpad Csapo** has called this property of uterus as the **'progesterone-block'** of myometrial activity.

Progesterone increases the endometrial nutrient stores in early pregnancy. This provides the developing embryo with an important source of nourishment. High levels of progesterone stimulate and maintain the uterine lining. During pregnancy, progesterone inhibits uterine contractions by decreasing the contractility of the myometrium. A high level of progesterone ensures that the uterine myometrium is relaxed and that the cervix is tightly closed. Together with estrogens, progesterone prepares the breast for lactation. Progesterone causes development of the duct system of mammary glands and prepares them to secrete milk. Placental estrogen and progesterone also inhibits secretion of FSH and LH from anterior pituitary gland. Placental progesterone has an important role to play as a precursor for fetal steroid synthesis. Therefore, progesterone of the placenta is converted to dehydroepiandrosterone (DHEA) by the fetal adrenal cortex and DHEA is then converted to estriol by the placental enzymes. Thus, the production of placental estrogens depends on both, the fetus and the placenta, which together constitutes the **feto-placental unit**.

Estrogens: The placenta secretes large amounts of estrogens, mainly in the form of estriol (Figure 17.5), in contrast to ovaries, which produce mainly estradiol, a more potent estrogen. The precursors for placental estrogens come from the fetal adrenal. Therefore, maintenance of secretion of placental estrogens depends on a living fetus. Intrauterine fetal death results in a sharp fall in maternal plasma estrogen levels.

Placental estrogens enlarge the reproductive organs. They promote the growth and enlargement of the uterus to accommodate the developing embryo and then fetus. Estrogens also promote the growth of the glandular tissues of the breast. By the end of pregnancy, both the duct and the glandular systems of the mammary glands are developed and become ready to produce milk. The external genitalia also enlarge and the pelvic ligaments and joints relax. These changes help the passage of the fetus through the pelvis during labor.

During the first 3-4 months of pregnancy, the corpus luteum continues to secrete progesterone and estrogens that maintain the lining of the uterus during pregnancy. The amounts secreted by the corpus luteum, however, are only slightly more than those produced after ovulation (luteal phase) in a normal menstrual cycle. The chorion of the placenta begins to secrete estrogens after the first 3-4 weeks of pregnancy and progesterone by 6th week. From the third month through the remainder of the pregnancy, placenta itself provides the required high levels of progesterone and estrogens (Figure 17.5). It is estimated that placenta produces as much as one gm of progesterone per day towards the end of pregnancy. Levels of estriol increase to the extent of a thousand folds in the latter stages of the pregnancy compared with the mid-luteal phase levels of the estrogen. By the 4th month, when placenta is fully established, secretion of hCG is reduced drastically because the secretions of the corpus luteum are no longer essential. Thus, the placenta supplies the required levels of estrogens and progesterone to maintain pregnancy from 3rd to 9th month. The estrogen and progesterone levels also show a gradual increase in urine of pregnant women from first week of pregnancy, reaches a peak shortly before parturition and then drops abruptly after delivery to return to normal levels (Figure 17.6).

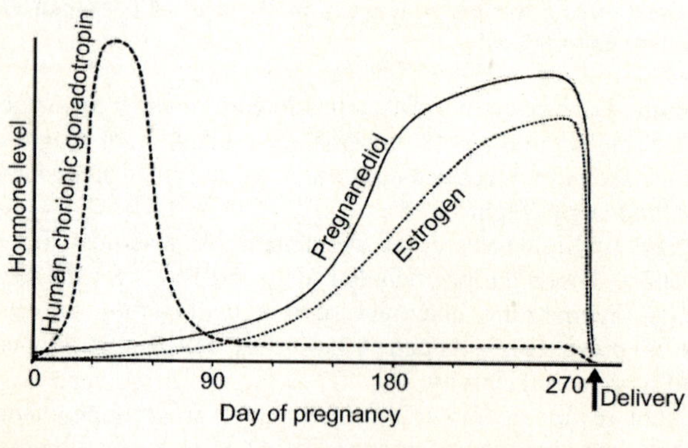

Figure 17.6: Urinary excretion of human chorionic gonadotropin, estrogen and pregnanediol during pregnancy and at parturition in women.

Relaxin: Relaxin is produced first by the corpus luteum of the ovary and later by the placenta (Figure 17.5). Relaxin from corpus luteum like placental progesterone also inhibits uterine contractions. Relaxin increases the flexibility of the pubic symphysis and ligaments of the sacro-iliac and sacro-coccygeal joints and helps to dilate the uterine cervix during labor to ease delivery of the baby.

Human chorionic somatomammotropin (hCS) or Human placental lactogen (hPL): Chorion of placenta produces another hormone called human chorionic somatomammotropin (hCS), also known as human placental lactogen (hPL). It is a protein hormone and is first detected in the maternal circulation around the 5th week of pregnancy. The rate of secretion of this hormone increases in proportion to placental mass, reaching maximum levels after 32 weeks and remains relatively constant after that (Figure 17.5). It is believed to help to prepare the mammary glands for lactation, enhance maternal growth by increasing protein synthesis, and regulate certain aspects of metabolism in mother and fetus alike, such as decreased use of glucose by mother, thus making it more available for fetus. In addition, hCS promotes the release of fatty acids from adipose tissue, providing an alternative to glucose for the mother's ATP production.

Recently, placenta is found to produce another hormone called **corticotropin-releasing hormone (CRH)**. In non-pregnant females, only neurosecretory cells in the hypothalamus secrete CRH. CRH is now thought to be the "clock" that establishes the timing of birth. Secretion of CRH by placenta begins at about 12 weeks and increases enormously toward the end of pregnancy. It has been noticed that women who have higher levels of CRH earlier in pregnancy are more likely to deliver prematurely, whereas those who have low levels deliver after their due date. CRH from placenta also increases secretion of cortisol, which is needed for maturation of the fetal lungs and the production of surfactant.

Aldosterone from the adrenal cortex promotes reabsorption of sodium and **parathyroid hormone** from the parathyroid glands helps to maintain a high concentration of maternal blood calcium during pregnancy.

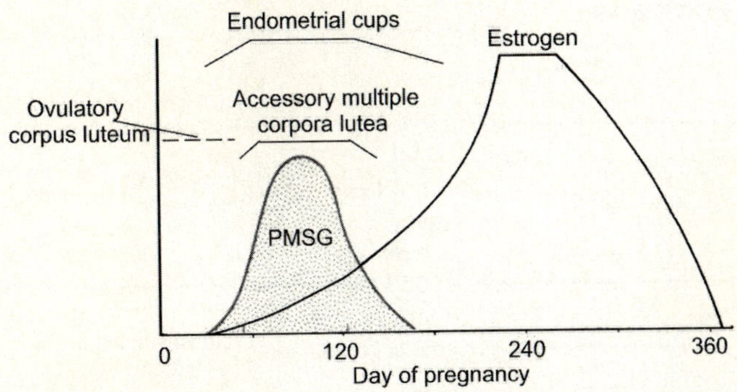

Figure 17.7: Sequence of events during gestation in Mare- with increase in serum gonadotropin (PMSG- pregnant mare serum gonadotropin), ovulatory corpus luteum wanes and accessory corpora lutea are formed, development and regression of fetal gonads correlate with rise and fall of maternal estrogens, urinary estrogens reach a peak at about 220 days and fall before parturition.

Equine Gonadotropin: The blood serum of pregnant mares contains a gonadotropin called **pregnant mare serum gonadotropin (PMSG)**. It is a glycoprotein and resembles FSH in its biological properties. Unlike hCG and pituitary FSH and LH, PMSG remains in blood and lymph and is practically absent from the urine. PMSG appears in the blood of the mare on about the 40th day of pregnancy and remain high until about day 120. Then it drops and is absent after day 180 (Figure 17.7). Whereas the placenta, (specifically the **Langhans cells** of the fetal chorion) produces hCG, PMSG appears to be formed in the **endometrial cups** and hence is **uterine in origin**. Under the influence of PMSG, the mare's ovaries form large vesicular follicles. Some of these follicles ovulate and produce corpora lutea, whereas others undergo luteinization without ovulating. In this manner a crop of accessory corpora lutea is normally formed during pregnancy.

17.6 Feto-placental Unit

With the demise of corpus luteum in primates, function of production of estrogen and progesterone is taken over by the placenta. However, the placenta is not capable of producing these steroid hormones without a supply of precursors from both the fetus and the maternal compartments. Thus, fetus and placenta form a joint functional unit called **feto-placental unit** to carry out synthesis of these steroids (Figure 17.8).

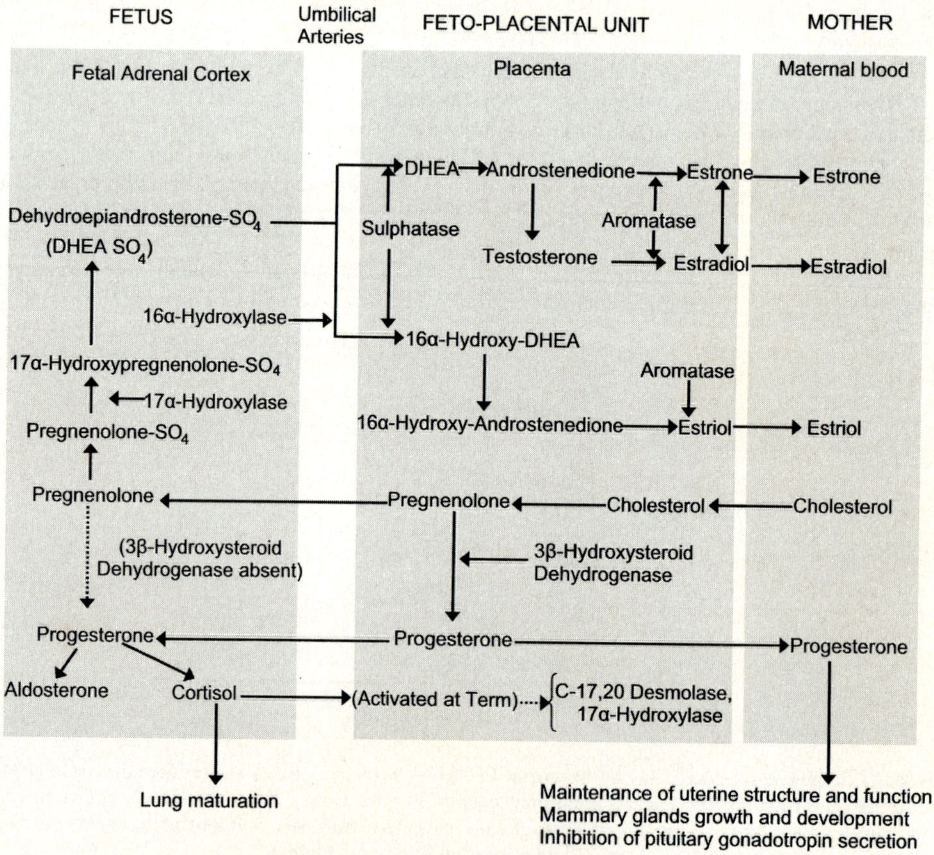

Figure 17.8: The feto-placental unit.

Although the placenta can synthesize progesterone from cholesterol, yet it is dependent on the supply of cholesterol derived from the maternal blood supply for the de novo biosynthesis of progesterone. Besides serving its own functions, placental progesterone is also used as a substrate for corticoid such as aldosterone and cortisol production by the fetal adrenals that lack an active 3β-hydroxysteroid-dehydrogenase. Pregnenolone of placental origin is used by the fetal adrenals for the production of precursors for estrogen production within the placenta. The placenta itself has only a limited capability for estrogen synthesis due to minimal 17α-hydroxylase activity. However, this enzyme within the fetal adrenal cortex is responsible for production of dehydroepiandrosterone sulphate (DHEA-SO_4). This steroid metabolite serves as a precursor substrate for the synthesis of estrone and estradiol by the placenta. However, much of this substrate is converted by the fetal adrenal 16α-hydroxylase to precursors that result in the production of large amounts of estriol. Figure 17.8 shows the pathways of steroid biosynthesis and metabolism and their interdependence within the maternal-fetal-placental unit.

17.7 Pseudopregnancy

Pseudopregnancy is a kind of false pregnancy seen in few mammals. In some mammals, such as rat, mouse and dog estrous cycles cease during condition of **pseudopregnancy** as seen in normal pregnancy in which the estrous cycles always cease and hormones modify accordingly to act on the female genital tract for the protection and nourishment of the developing embryo. Pseudopregnancy can be induced in many laboratory mammals by procedures that prolong the secretory function of the corpora lutea, thus holding in the onset of the next estrus. In mammals, such as rat and mice, which have short estrous cycles, the luteal phase of the ovary is so abbreviated that the uteri do not undergo the extensive progestational changes generally associated with progesterone action. Thus, in these animals pseudopregnancy may be induced easily by stimulating the cervix of the estrus animal with a glass rod or other mechanical means, or by electrical stimulation, or by mating with a sterile male. The onset of next estrus is delayed by about 13 days. Thus in pseudopregnancy, except for the fact that there are no developing young in the uteri, the endocrine balance is very similar to true pregnancy. In most species, pseudopregnancy lasts for about half the length of time required for a normal pregnancy. The pseudopregnancy state may be prolonged by administering estrogens or by traumatizing the uterus to produce deciduoma. The corpora lutea of pseudopregnancy maintain the uterus in a state capable of receiving blastocysts and conspicuous proliferation of mammary glands also occur. Pseudopregnancy occurs in wild rabbit but rarely in other wild mammals.

17.8 Pregnancy Tests

Since chorionic gonadotropin is secreted by placental tissue, its presence in blood or urine forms the basis of many tests for pregnancy. All pregnancy tests used today are **antibody tests that detect hCG** in a woman's blood or urine. Early pregnancy tests detect tiny amounts of hCG in the urine that begins to be excreted about 8 days after fertilization.

Immunological Techniques: The test kits can detect pregnancy as early as the first day of a missed menstrual period that is about 14 days after fertilization. Color change in the chemicals of the kit indicates a positive reaction between hCG in the test urine and hCG antibodies included in the kit, thus indicating a positive test for pregnancy. Several of the test kits available at pharmacies are as sensitive and accurate as test methods used in many hospitals. However, false-negative and false-positive results can occur. A false-negative result may be due to ectopic pregnancy while false-positive result may be due to excess protein or blood in urine or to hCG production due to a rare type of uterine cancer.

Ascheim-Zondek test depends on the capacity of pregnancy urine, when injected into female mice and rats, to induce ovulation within 96 hours of treatment.

In **Friedman Test,** pregnancy urine causes ovulation in immature rabbits within 24 hours of treatment.

Xenopus test involves female frogs and toads, which ovulate within 6-8 hours after injection of pregnancy urine into dorsal lymph sacs.

Summary

Once fertilization occurs, zygote is formed.

It is transported through the isthmus of the oviduct into the uterus.

Cilia of the genital tract are the primary transporters of the embryo. Also, it is facilitated by the changing endocrine milieu of the female genital ducts during this early luteal phase.

During the period in the oviduct, fertilized egg undergoes rapid mitotic cell divisions and becomes morula, and by the time it reaches into the uterus, morula is transformed into next embryonic stage called blastocyst.

The blastocyst remains free within the cavity of the uterus for about two days and then attaches to the wall of the uterus. This is called implantation.

Implantation can be invasive or non-invasive. Also, it may be superficial, eccentric and interstitial.

Attachment of the blastocyst to the wall of the uterus is done with the help of an organ or tissue jointly formed by the maternal and fetal structures called placenta.

Placenta may be non-deciduous or deciduous and also chorio-vitteline and chorio-allantoic in lower and higher mammals respectively.

Shape of the placenta and the depth to which conceptus invades maternal tissues for the formation of placenta varies with species.

Main function of placenta is to transport nutrients from mother's blood to fetal blood and bring about exchange of gases etc. It also acts as a selective barrier.

Hormonal control of implantation involves both estrogen and progesterone. Implantation results in pregnancy.

The corpus luteum of pregnancy is maintained by placental hCG, and the corpus luteum and later the placenta secrete progesterone, and estrogen to support pregnancy and breast development for lactation.

Hormonal changes during pregnancy are- following implantation, cells of trophoblast secrete hCG, which maintains the corpus luteum, thus it continues secreting estrogen and progesterone. As placenta develops, it secretes large quantities of estrogen and progesterone to stimulate the uterine lining to continue development, and maintain the uterine lining, inhibit secretion of FSH and LH from anterior pituitary, and stimulate development of the mammary glands. Placental progesterone inhibits uterine contraction while its estrogen enlarges the reproductive organs. Relaxin from corpus luteum also inhibits uterine contractions and relaxes the pubic ligaments. The placenta secretes placental lactogen that stimulates development of breast.

With the demise of the corpus luteum in the primates, estrogen and progesterone production is taken over by the placenta. However, the placenta is not capable of producing these steroids without a supply of precursors from both the fetus and maternal compartments. Thus, fetus and placenta form a joint functional unit called feto-placental unit to carry out synthesis of these steroids.

Pregnancy can be detected and confirmed by a number of tests.

Questions

1. Define implantation. How does an embryo implant in the uterine formation wall?
2. Discuss the hormonal control of implantation.
3. What mechanism maintains the uterine wall during pregnancy?
4. What is the source of hCG during the first few months of pregnancy?
5. Discuss the hormonal changes during pregnancy.

6. What is parthenogenesis and pseudopregnancy?
7. Write a note on fetal-placental unit.
8. The usual site of embryo implantation is a) the uterine tube, b) the peritoneal cavity, c) the vagina and d) **the uterus**.
9. The outer layer of blastocyst which later attaches to the uterus is the a) decidua, **b) trophoblast**, c) amnion and d) inner cell mass.
10. The fetal membrane that forms the basis of the umbilical cord is the **a) allantois**, b) amnion, c) chorion and d) yolk sac.
11. Which of the following cannot pass through the placental barriers? **a) blood cells**, b) glucose, c) amino acids and d) antibodies.

Chapter 18

Parturition and Lactation

In the previous chapters we have learnt how various process in reproductive organs occur to result in initiation and maintenance of pregnancy. Pregnancy is suspected when a female in case of humans and primates misses an otherwise regular menstrual period or if a new cycle does not start after diestrus phase in rodents. As early as 5-6 weeks after the last menstrual period or 14 days after conception, a hormone known as human chorionic gonadotropin can be detected in the urine of pregnant woman. Role of hormones in the maintenance of pregnancy became more prominent with the evolution of viviparity, when a series of innovations first appeared. These have been i) reduction in the contents of yolk sac, ii) formation of the placenta, iii) retention of the young within the female genital tract (uterus) and iv) parental care of offspring. All this resulted in the birth of a living young one (viviparity) from an egg laying condition as seen in oviparous animals.

18.1 Parturition

The fetus lies within its fetal membranes in the uterus during pregnancy and is retained there by the cervix. The duration of normal pregnancy is called **gestation period**. It is about 40 weeks from the first day of the last menstruation in human, following which birth of the infant occurs. The sequence of events involving birth of an infant is called **labor** or **parturition** or **eutokia**. Thus, parturition is the process by which the uterus expels the products of conception at a time when the newborn child called infant can exist semi-independently of the mother. The mechanism and timing of onset of parturition is probably the same in all species such as goat, sheep, human etc. The act of parturition is termed as labor or delivery in human; calving in cow, buffalo, camel and elephant; foaling in mare; kidding in goat; lambing in ewe; farrowing in sow; whelping or puppying in bitch; and kittening in cat.

During most of the normal gestation period, the uterine smooth muscle is relatively quiet, but as the fetus grows, the muscle is stretched. The stretching increases the contractility of the muscle called **stress activation**. This results in some uncoordinated, irregular, painless uterine contractions during pregnancy. These are known as **Braxton-Hicks contractions**. However, onset of labor is marked by regular uterine contractions, initially widely spaced but gradually increasing in frequency and strength.

18.2 Onset of Parturition

It is difficult to predict the exact day and time of parturition. However, symptoms associated with the onset of parturition help to predict the exact time of parturition in certain animals. The symptoms of the onset of parturition are changes in the size of birth canal, its progressive extensibility to permit safe passage of the fetus, and hypertrophy of the mammary glands. During labor, the uterine smooth muscles characteristically contract and retract or shorten. This phenomenon is important as it ensures gradual descent of the infant. The initiation of labor is probably due to several factors, and is accompanied by pain, uneasiness, general disturbances and violent efforts, generally termed as "labor pains".

18.3 The Stages of Labor

The labor and delivery process is divided into three stages. The first stage is marked by the dilation of the cervix. The second stage is the delivery of the infant. And the third stage is the delivery of the placenta (Figure 18.1). A series of interactions between the fetal adrenal and pituitary glands, along with an increased synthesis of prostaglandins by the uterus may trigger the initiation of labor (Figure 18.2). When the time of delivery is near, the cervix, already softened by the action of estrogen is gradually taken up and shortened in response to relaxin. It is promoted by uterine contractions. This process is known as **cervical effacement**. Softening of cervix is called **ripening of cervix**.

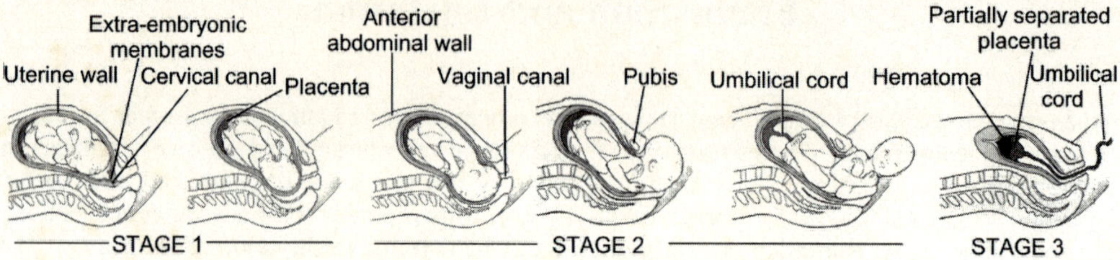

Figure 18.1: Stages of labor in the delivery of an infant.

The opening of the cervical canal before labor is small normally obliterated and plugged with mucus. **Stage one of labor (Dilation of cervix)** is marked by the onset of regular uterine contractions that **open** or **dilate** the cervix from 0-2 cm to 7-10 cm to push the baby's head against the opening of the cervix and progressively dilate it. The average duration of this stage is 12 hours in a first pregnancy and 7 hours in successive ones, but it may be as short as 2-3 hours.

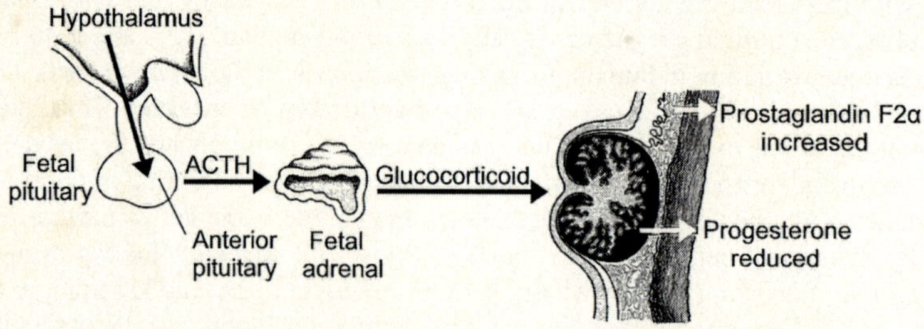

Figure 18.2: Diagrammatic representation of pathways involved in onset of labor in fetal lamb.

Stage two (Expulsion of fetus) begins when the baby begins to move through the cervix and ends when the **baby is delivered** (Figure 18.1). This stage may last for several hours in first delivery, but may be as brief as a few minutes in women who have previously delivered. During second stage of labor and when the cervix is fully dilated, the character of the uterine contractions changes. They begin to move the baby down the birth canal ("**bearing down**") instead of merely causing the head to impinge against the cervix. Most women are aware of this change and spontaneously begin to assist the uterus by voluntarily holding their breath and increasing abdominal pressure with each contraction as it is an important part of this stage and it helps to shorten its duration.

In **stage three** of labor **(Expulsion of placenta membrane)**, the **placenta is delivered** after the childbirth and this stage may last only for few minutes (Figure 18.1). The placenta usually becomes detached right after the baby is born as the uterus continues to contract. These contractions expel the placenta. Further contractions help to clamp down on uterine blood vessels to minimize blood loss.

The total time required for parturition varies between the species and individuals. The contractions of the uterine myometrial cells depends on the movement of calcium ions (Ca^{2+}), which may be liberated from intracellular binding sites or enter the muscle cell from the extra cellular fluid. Calcium ions bind to regulatory sites on the contractile protein actin and myosin. This allows expression of ATPase activity resulting in uterine contraction. The term **Dystokia** (*Dys* = difficult, *tokos* = birth) is used to indicate various types of obstructions in the process of parturition. Normal birth is called **Eutokia**. Dystokia generally occurs when first and second stage in parturition is prolonged and when artificial aid becomes necessary for the extraction of fetus.

18.4 Ferguson's reflex

During parturition, in the second stage of labor, the head of the fetus tends to dilate the cervix by its rhythmic movements. The head of the fetus brings about a neuroendocrine reflex that travels through brain stem to the hypothalamus and is responsible for production of large amounts of oxytocin. This oxytocin produce dilation of the cervix to the size equal to the fetal head and it also stimulates production of more prostaglandins by fetus by the positive feedback mechanism on the secretions of PGF 2α (Figure 18.2). The reflex produced by the rhythmic movement of the fetal head in the uterus (**neuroendocrine reflex**) that brings about large secretions of oxytocin from the adenohypophysis is called **Ferguson's reflex**. It is observed in the labor stage (stage two) of parturition and oxytocin brings about the final parturition of the fetus from the uterus. Several factors such as physical, neural, biochemical and hormonal are involved in the act of parturition. As the fetus enlarges, it distends the uterine musculature and stimulates the sensory nerve endings of the uterus. This stimulation causes increased secretion of certain hormones, which are involved in parturition.

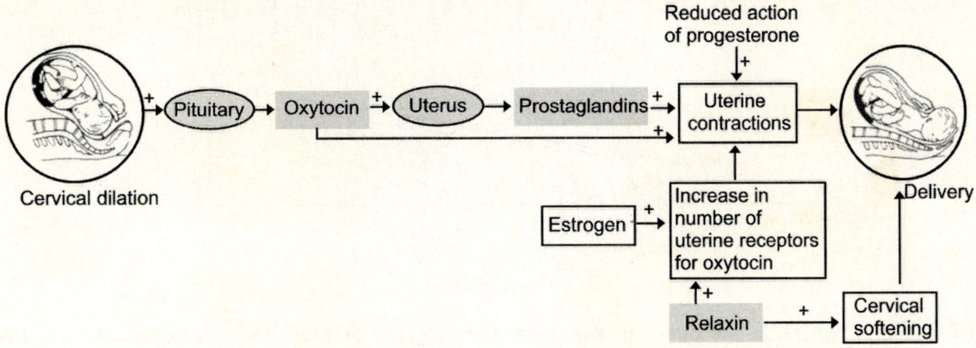

Figure 18.3: Hormonal factors involved at the onset of parturition in Human.

18.5 Hormonal Control of Parturition

The hormonal factors involved in the onset of labor are illustrated in the Figure 18.3. One of the factors that initiate and maintain labor is the rising sensitivity of the uterine muscle to oxytocin. During early pregnancy, there are few oxytocin receptors, but as pregnancy progresses these appear in increasing numbers on the uterine myometrium and decidua cells. Maternal estrogen increases and progesterone decreases near term in humans (Figure 18.4). The increase in myometrial activity in late pregnancy corresponds with the time when the concentration of estrogens in blood reaches its highest levels as seen in rat, guinea pig, goat, sheep and human female. This is also the time when spontaneous uterine activity and reactivity to oxytocin show a dramatic increase. It appears that the removal of the 'progesterone-block' of myometrial activity towards the end of gestation may be related not only to a reduction in the local concentration of progesterone, but also to the antagonism of a raised estrogen level. These hormonal changes increase the sensitivity of the uterus to oxytocin. Binding of oxytocin to its receptors has two effects. First, it causes uterine smooth muscle contraction. Second, it stimulates the uterus to make prostaglandins ($PGF_{2\alpha}$ and PGE_2) that also activate uterine smooth muscle. At parturition, prostaglandins act mainly by liberating Ca^{2+} from intracellular binding sites. During labor, oxytocin has a direct action on the rate of Ca^{2+} influx and also lowers the excitation threshold of the muscle cell. Prostaglandin is found in high concentration in the amniotic fluid and placenta at term or parturition. It has strong stimulating action on the uterus. Because of this action, prostaglandins are used artificially to induce labor or to assist in delivery. The cells in the endometrial-derived portion of the placenta that are responsible for the large increase in prostaglandin release are macrophages. These cells are highly responsive to a range of stimuli, including steroid hormones, oxytocin, and factors associated with infections and inflammation. Despite increasing levels of oxytocin and prostaglandins, progesterone directly inhibits uterine smooth muscle and blocks its response to oxytocin and prostaglandin. Yet maternal progesterone levels do not fall abruptly before labor and also a drop in progesterone does not precipitate labor. However, the propagation of contractile activity in the myometrium certainly increases after progesterone withdrawal.

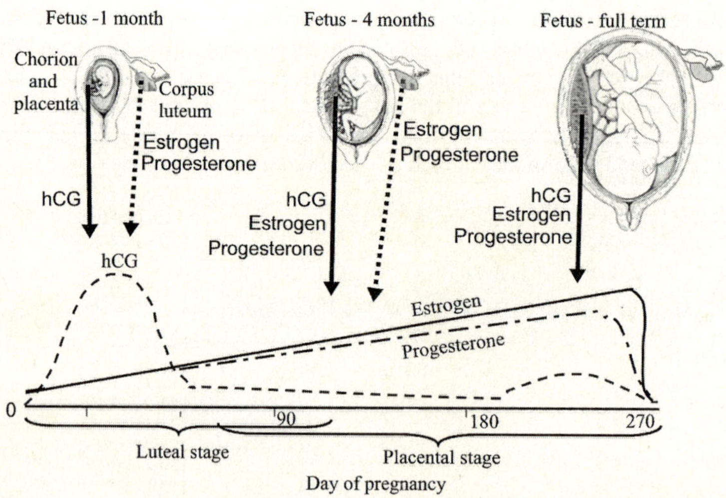

Figure 18.4: Changes in hormones during pregnancy and at term in huma; hCG-human chorionic gonadotropin, in third trimester-placenta is the major source of estrogen and progesterone.

Thus, the contractile activity of the uterus expels the fetus at parturition as at this time, the inhibitory action of progesterone is withdrawn. This allows uterine contractions to develop to the point where the cervix of the uterus dilates and labor progresses to delivery. In early pregnancy, the source of progesterone is always the corpus luteum of the ovary. But during late pregnancy, this function of the corpus luteum is taken over by the placenta in some mammals. Mammals accordingly may thus be divided into two groups. One in which maintenance of pregnancy is dependent on corpus luteum function. And the other in which dependence on the corpus luteum ceases at some point during pregnancy. In general, species having short gestation period belong to the first group, and those with long gestation period belong to the second with few exceptions. Does this mean that different mechanism control parturition in these two groups? The mechanism of one group is concerned with control of corpus luteum function while in the other with the placental function. However, a common mechanism appears to apply to most mammals, and it is the conceptus or the fetus itself and not the mother, that controls the onset of parturition.

Much of the studies on the control of parturition in **placenta-dependent mammals** are based on sheep. These show that the chain of events leading to parturition at term begins in the fetal hypothalamus. Fetal pituitary responds to hypothalamic activity by releasing ACTH-adrenocorticotropic hormone (Figure 18.2). The fetal adrenal, in turn, is stimulated to secrete more corticosteroids. The fetal mechanisms are so potent that premature labor could be induced at any time in the second half of pregnancy by artificial means. Withdrawal of the inhibitory effects of progesterone on the uterine musculature and increase in prostaglandin concentration control the onset of labor.

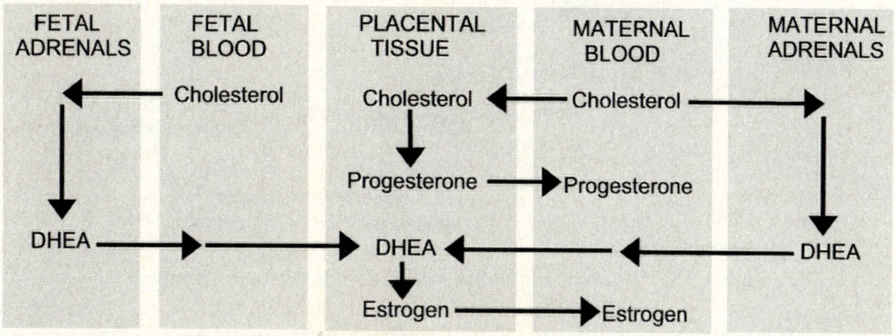

Figure 18.5: Cooperation of mother and fetus adrenals in conversion of cholesterol to progesterone and estrogen in placenta; DHEA- Dehydroepiandrosterone.

In humans, maternal plasma progesterone concentrations do not fall at parturition (Figure 18.4). Instead, fetal adrenal influences synthesis of placental estrogens by providing androgen precursors. These androgens are secreted from the specialized fetal zone of the adrenal gland and constitute 80-90 % of substrate for placental estrogen synthesis, late in pregnancy (Figure 18.5). Thus, factors that may be involved in initiation of labor in humans are as follows. Secretion of ACTH by the fetal pituitary near term causes an increase in cortisol secretion by fetal adrenals. Increased secretion of fetal adrenals inhibits progesterone synthesis by the placenta. This causes estrogen levels to rise relative to progesterone levels. Also increasing synthesis of prostaglandins stimulates excitability of myometrium. Once contractions of uterus become strong enough, they trigger oxytocin secretion. Oxytocin derived from the fetus may provide the stimulus for the increased production of prostaglandins at the onset of labor. This sets in a positive feedback loop of strong, coordinated waves of contraction that continues until delivery is complete. At the onset of labor, the pressure of the head of the fetus against the cervix initiates a hormonal reflex (Figure 18.6) that increases oxytocin secretion. Oxytocin greatly potentiates uterine contractions, setting up a positive feedback loop of strong, coordinated waves of contraction until baby is delivered. During this stage, the strong uterine contractions result in poor circulation to the placenta. Therefore, rapid progress in these processes is vital for a safe delivery. Parturition ends with the complete delivery of the placenta and membranes.

Parturition in corpus luteum-dependent mammals is preceded by regression of the corpora lutea and a fall in the concentration of progesterone in the blood. Factors controlling the luteal regression are responsible for determining the time of onset of labor. Maternal pituitary gonadotropins are responsible for regulating the function of corpus luteum. In goat (although a close relative of sheep, but is a corpus luteum-dependent mammal), abortion occurs after maternal hypophysectomy or ovariectomy at any stage of pregnancy. In these mammals, it is the ovarian and, not the placenta, secretion of progesterone that is affected by the activity of fetal adrenal gland.

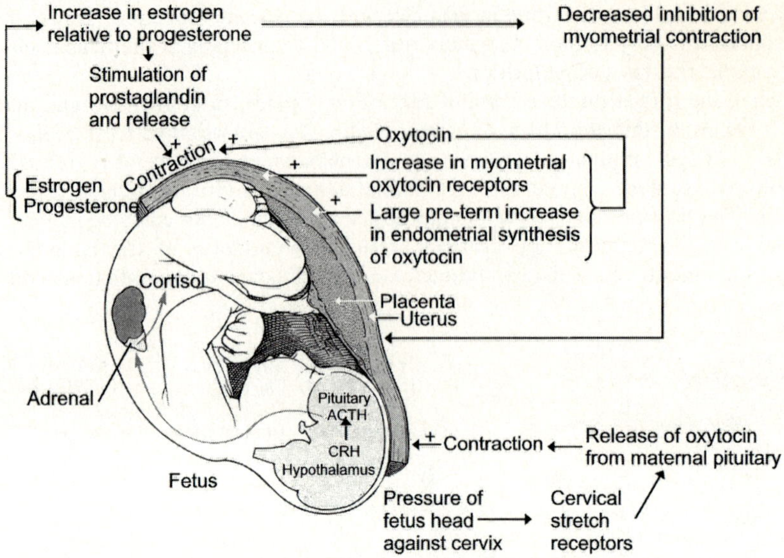

Figure 18.6: Factors controlling initiation of labor in Human.

Role of Relaxin in Parturition: Another possible contributing factor in timing of labor is **relaxin** that promotes an increase in the number of oxytocin receptors on uterine muscle (Figure 18.7). Relaxin is one of the most recently recognized hormones. In 1926, Hisaw reported that an aqueous extract of the corpora lutea of pregnant sow relaxes the pubic symphysis of the guinea pig. This biologically active substance was purified and named 'relaxin'. Structurally relaxin is a peptide, similar to insulin with about 40 % homology between the residues. Corpus luteum is the source of relaxin in most mammals including humans. But later in pregnancy, most relaxin probably comes from the uterine muscle and placenta. Relaxin may also be produced and stored within granulocytes localized in the endometrium of rhesus monkey and adult human females. The amount of relaxin in maternal blood peaks just before delivery, and then drops off rapidly to remove its relaxing effects on uterine muscle. In humans, relaxin concentrations are four times higher in the ovarian vein draining the ovary containing the corpus luteum of pregnancy than in either peripheral plasma or the contra lateral ovarian vein.

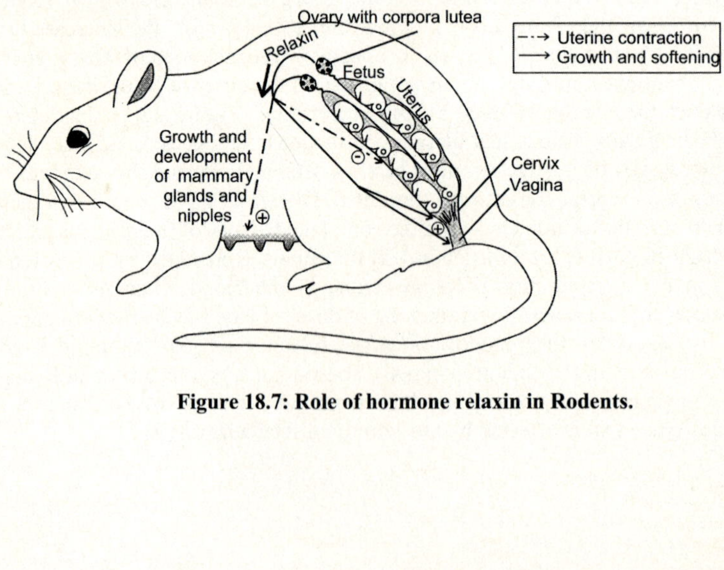

Figure 18.7: Role of hormone relaxin in Rodents.

The biological effects of relaxin are associated with pregnancy and parturition. Relaxin acts on pubic symphysis and transforms the connective tissue from cartilaginous type to more flexible structure. Thus, relaxin softens connective tissue between the bones of the pelvic girdle, so that the pelvic aperture is enlarged and the baby passes through more easily at the time of birth. Relaxin withdrawal just before delivery may contribute to the uterine muscle responsiveness to contraction-producing agents present in labor.

18.6 Carbohydrate and Fat Reserves in Fetus and Infant

During the latter part of gestation, the fetus of many species accumulates large amounts of glycogen, particularly in the liver. As long as adequate supplies of glucose can reach the fetus from the mother, the total amount of carbohydrate stored in the various tissues depends mainly on the fetal adrenal activity. As preparation to birth, probably related in part to accentuate adrenal activity near term, enhanced rate of storage normally occurs. The pronounced tolerance of newborn animals to severe oxygen deficiency (hypoxia) is attributed, in addition to other factors, to the high concentration of glycogen present in cardiac muscle. And this glycogen reserve allows the heart to continue its contractile activity in the absence of oxygen, by anaerobic glycolysis. The brain has no glycogen reserves and has to rely on circulating blood glucose. Neonatal hypoglycemia is commonly seen in babies who show signs of intra-uterine growth retardation.

Storage of fat is regulated by insulin rather than by corticosteroids. When nutrition is good and blood glucose is maintained at relatively high levels, the action of insulin ensures that glucose available after the requirements of growth are fully met, is then diverted to fat reserves. In addition to the usual **white fat**, fetuses have substantial deposits of a peculiar form of adipose tissue, called the **brown fat** (Figure 18.8). The usual white fat on oxidation liberates fatty acids and glycerol into circulation to be metabolized in tissue elsewhere. In contrast, the brown fat is oxidized and releases its energy in the form of heat largely within itself. This plays an important part in maintaining body temperature after birth when the newly born is no longer within the neutral thermal environment of the mother.

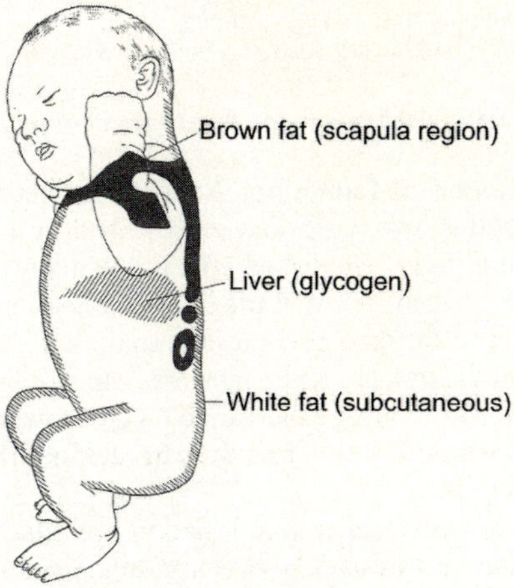

Figure 18.8: Sites of energy stores in Human fetus- glycogen is for immediate needs of newborn but may get exhausted rapidly, then white fat is metabolized until feeding is established, brown fat is the source of heat for the newborn.

18.7 Cesarean Section

It is a procedure by which the baby is delivered through surgical incisions made in the abdominal wall and uterus. The name was derived from a belief that Julius Caesar was born this way. Cesarean section is done in various situations. i) The pelvic outlet is too small for normal delivery. ii) The uterus fails to function normally or properly. iii) The baby's orientation is not correct, for example a breech presentation. iv) Certain emergency situations that may lead to a threat to survival either of baby or of mother.

18.8 Lactation

Lactation is production of milk by the hormone-prepared mammary glands. The evolution of mammary glands from sweat glands was a defining step in mammalian evolution. At the onset of puberty, the mammary gland starts to develop and breast become prominent due to deposition of more fat than glandular tissue. Breast development at puberty is stimulated mainly by estradiol although growth hormone, insulin, thyroid hormones, and cortisol have permissive effects (Figure 18.9). Progesterone results in proliferation of the sinuses and ducts and in breast enlargement so that the size of the breast varies even during the menstrual cycle. The presence of normal pituitary function is essential for the effects of the sex hormones on mammary glands.

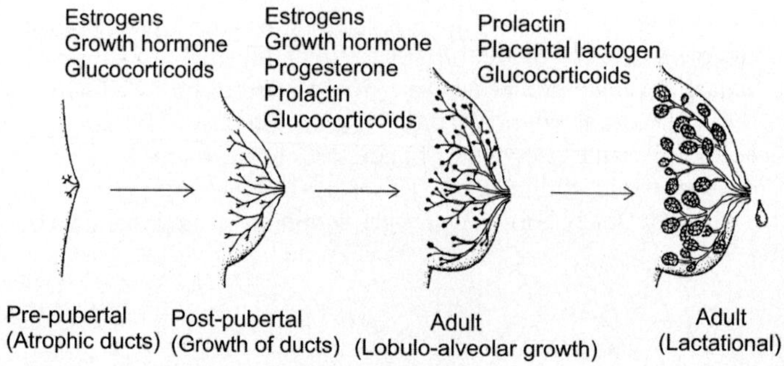

Figure 18.9: Hormonal regulation of growth and development of mammary glands in Human.

Preparation for Birth and Initiation of Lactation: At birth, separation from the placenta suddenly deprives the newborn of the supplies of oxygen and glucose and in normal circumstances breathing starts within seconds of birth and is fully established after a few minutes. Glucose is rapidly released from carbohydrate reserves, i.e. glycogen stored in the liver and heart muscle. This source of glucose is exhausted within a few hours and fat then becomes the main metabolic fuel, supplying both fatty acids and glycerol for oxidation in the tissues. Even fat stores can sustain life only for a limited period. But this period is more than sufficient to bridge the variable gap between the birth time and beginning of suckling. Successful transition from intra-uterine to extra-uterine life is thus dependent on events that have preceded birth of a young one.

In most mammals, man being an exception, lactation precedes labor by a variable number of days. This enables the young animal to obtain substantial quantities of food soon after birth. The mechanisms controlling the initiation of milk secretion (called **lactogenesis**) and maintenance of milk secretion (called **galactopoiesis**) emanate from the fetus and placenta. This exhibits an example of preparation by the fetus for its birth.

18.9 Hormonal Control of Lactation

During pregnancy, estrogen and progesterone levels increase much beyond the levels of the luteal phase of the menstrual cycle. This results in the considerable proliferation of the alveoli and alveolar ducts (Figure 18.9). In addition, two other hormones, **prolactin (PRL)** and **placental lactogen (hPL)** also play important role in preparing the breasts for milk production. Withdrawal of estrogen and progesterone at birth is critical and it removes the block to prolactin-induced milk secretion (Figure 18.10). Withdrawal of human placental lactogen (hPL) also has a similar effect.

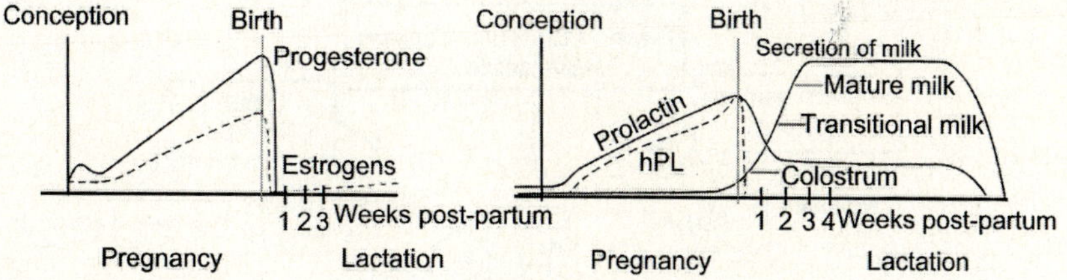

Figure 18.10: Hormonal changes in maternal circulation during pregnancy and at the onset of lactation in Women-withdrawal of estrogen and progesterone at birth removes a block to prolactin-induced milk secretion, hPL-human placental lactogen has the similar effect.

Prolactin (*pro* = for, *lact* = milk) is produced by anterior pituitary. It causes development of alveoli of breasts and stimulates milk production. Release of prolactin from the adenohypophysis is under a tonic inhibitory control as illustrated by the fact that hypothalamic lesions elevate circulating levels of prolactin. Hypothalamus controls prolactin secretion through prolactin inhibiting and releasing factors (PIFs and PRFs). A major inhibitory factor that alters prolactin release is the neurotransmitter, dopamine, whereas the nature of a specific prolactin releasing factor remains to be defined, but it is thought to be serotonin. In males, the influence of PIF predominates, but in women, prolactin levels rise and fall in rhythm with estrogen blood levels. Low estrogen stimulates PIF release, while high estrogen promotes release of PRF and thus of prolactin. Control of prolactin secretion is very complex and many other factors seem to be involved in neural control of its secretion (Figures 18.11 and 18.12). For example, Thyrotropin releasing hormone (TRH) and vasoactive intestinal peptide (VIP) are known to have powerful stimulatory effect on prolactin secretion. A brief rise in prolactin levels just before menstruation partially accounts for the breast swelling and tenderness some women experience at that time. But since this PRL stimulation is so brief, the breast do not produce milk.

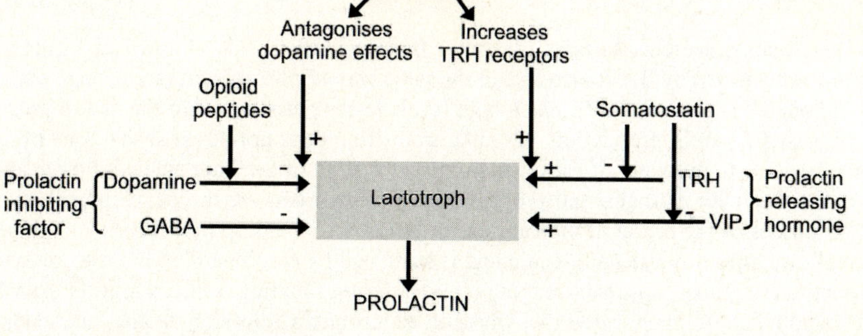

Figure 18.11: Possible factors that interact at pituitary lactotroph to control prolactin secretion.

Prolactin is secreted in small amounts from puberty; its secretion is greatly enhanced during pregnancy, and further increases during lactation. Prolactin stimulates growth and secretory activity of the mammary alveoli (Figure 18.9). Prolactin levels in blood rise dramatically toward the end of pregnancy, and milk production by the breasts becomes possible (Figure 18.10). After birth, suckling by the infant stimulates PRF release in the mother (Figure 18.12). This results in continued milk production and availability. Hypersecretion of prolactin is more common than its hyposecretion and is known as **hyperprolactinemia**. It results in inappropriate lactation (**galactorrhea**), lack of menses, infertility in females and impotence in males.

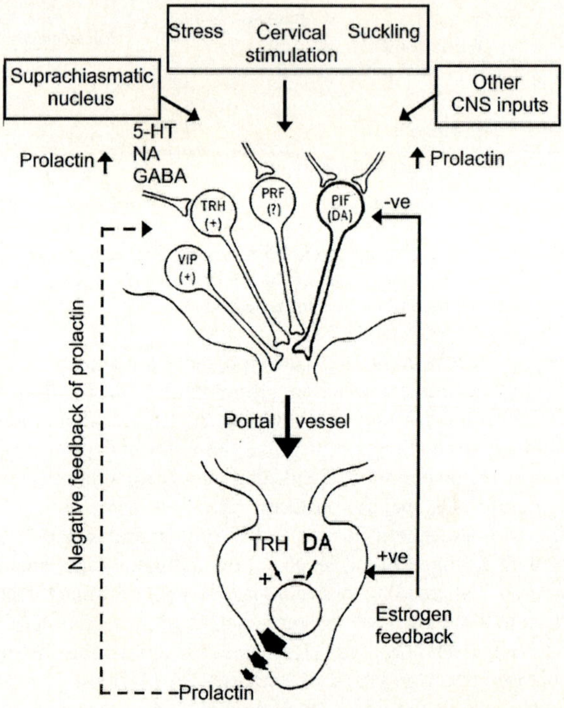

Figure 18.12: Neural control of prolactin secretion, 5-HT-5 hydroxytryptamine, NA-noradrenaline, GABA-γ amino butyric acid, TRH-thyrotropin releasing hormone, VIP-vasoactive intestinal polypeptide, PRF-prolactin releasing factor, PIF-prolactin inhibiting factor, DA-dopamine.

The placenta secretes **human placental lactogen** (**hPL**), also known as **human chorionic somatomammotrophin** (**hCS**). It also acts in the same way as pituitary prolactin, augmenting alveolar growth. Although prolactin and hPL reach high levels in the plasma toward the end of pregnancy, and breasts are primed for milk production, yet milk production does not begin at that time because of the inhibitory effects of high levels of estrogen and progesterone in the later stages of pregnancy. These hormones, together with estrogen and progesterone are important for the development of the lobules and alveolar tissues of the breast in preparation for lactation. The drop in estrogen and progesterone at parturition allows milk production to begin and is sustained by continued prolactin secretion as long as suckling continues. According to current hypothesis, during suckling, sensory signals from the nipples cause the hypothalamus to increase the secretion of prolactin releasing factor, maintaining plasma prolactin levels and resulting in milk production. Increase in the frequency or duration of suckling stimulates prolactin release to match the needs of the growing baby. If a mother does not feed her infant, prolactin levels fall and milk production stops after a few days.

The movement of milk from the alveoli into ducts is called **milk letdown**. Milk production and milk letdown are two distinct processes. Milk letdown involves a reflex in which stimulation of the nipple by an infant's suckling causes release of oxytocin from posterior pituitary which causes contraction of smooth muscle cells around the alveoli and delivers milk to the nipples (Figure 18.13). The reflex becomes conditioned after a short time and movement of milk from alveoli into ducts begins with sound or sight of the infant. Oxytocin also stimulates uterine contraction, which is important after delivery, as it reduces blood loss and speeds the recovery of the stretched uterus to return to its original shape.

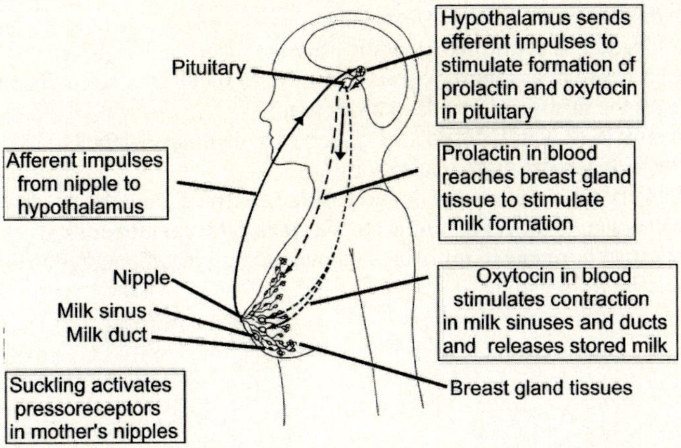

Figure18.13: Positive feedback mechanism of milk letdown reflex (suckling reflex) in Women.

After delivery, milk production does not begin for a day or so. The initial breast secretion is known as **colostrums**. It is a yellow, watery fluid having a high protein content, almost no fat but large quantities of maternal antibodies (IgA) produced by lymphocytes in mammary gland. The antibodies help to protect the new–born against infections (**passive immunization**), in particular, those affecting the gastrointestinal tract. Antibody secretion continues after milk production begins and by the fourth month of lactation, it may amount to as much as 0.5 g/day.

Summary

The sequence of events that result in the birth of an infant is called labor or parturition.

There are three stages of labor. Stage one of labor open or dilate the cervix. In stage two, baby begins to move through the cervix and ends when the baby is delivered. In stage three, the placenta is delivered.

Initiation of labor occurs when estrogen levels are sufficiently high. These stimulate oxytocin receptors on the myometrial cells and inhibit progesterone's quieting effect on uterine muscle. With this, weak, irregular contractions begin. Fetal cells produce oxytocin, which stimulates prostaglandin production by the placenta. Both hormones stimulate contraction of uterine muscle. Increasing stress activates the hypothalamus, causing oxytocin release from the posterior pituitary. This sets up a positive feedback loop resulting in true labor.

The breasts are prepared for lactation during pregnancy by high blood levels of estrogen, progesterone, prolactin and placental lactogen. Milk is produced around day 3 after labor in response to suckling, which stimulates the hypothalamus to prompt anterior pituitary release of prolactin and posterior pituitary release of oxytocin. Prolactin stimulates milk production, and oxytocin triggers milk letdown. Continued breast-feeding is required for continued milk production. Colostrums, a premilk fluid, are rich in protein and poor in fat and contain antibodies from mother's body to provide passive immunization to the infant.

Questions

1. Describe the stages of labor.
2. Describe the role of progesterone in initiating labor.
3. Discuss the hormonal regulation of parturition.
4. Explain how dilation of the cervix affects labor.
5. Explain how bleeding is controlled naturally after the placenta is expelled.
6. Describe the structure of a mammary gland. How does pregnancy affect the mammary glands?
7. What stimulates the mammary glands to produce milk?
8. What causes milk to flow into the ductile system of a mammary gland?
9. Discuss the hormonal regulation of lactation.
10. Following delivery of the infant, the delivery of the afterbirth includes a) placenta only, b) placenta and decidua, **c) placenta and attached, torn fetal membranes**, d) chorionic villi.
11. The most important hormone in initiating and maintaining lactation after birth is a) estrogen, b) FSH, **c) prolactin**, d) oxytocin.

Part III

Reproductive Health and Human Welfare

- AIDS
- Cancer and Hormones
- Infertility
- Assisted Reproductive Technologies
- Family Planning
- Demography

Chapter 19

AIDS

AIDS is one of the most serious health problems that mankind has ever faced. The impact of this disease is much more severe in developing countries such as India. Millions of people have died already, and more than 12 million young people are living with HIV/AIDS. Today's young people are the AIDS generation. Epidemic among youth remains largely invisible to adults and to youth people themselves. Of the over 60 million people who have been infected with HIV in the past 20 years, about half became infected between the ages of 15 and 24. Young women are several times more likely to be infected with HIV than young men.

19.1 What is AIDS?

AIDS stands for **Acquired Immunodeficiency Syndrome** (sometimes called "slim disease"). It is a viral disease, caused by the AIDS virus. AIDS is a condition in which a person experiences a telltale assortment of infections as a result of the progressive destruction of immune system, leaving the victim vulnerable to a host of life-threatening opportunistic infections, neurological disorders, or unusual malignancies. By 1983, researchers linked HIV to AIDS. HIV targets lymphocytes in lymph nodes, and CD4 helper T cells.

19.2 The Causative Agent

AIDS is due to an infection by the **Human Immunodeficiency Virus**, commonly known as **HIV**, and AIDS represents the end stage of infection by HIV. The special feature of HIV infection is that once infected, it is probable that a person will be infected for life. A person who is infected with HIV may be free of symptoms for many years and may spread the virus unknowingly. However, HIV infection is serious, and is usually fatal as the virus attacks the body's immune system. It takes control of and destroys the very cells that the body deploys to attack the virus. AIDS kills everyone by destroying the cells of the body, which fight against diseases thus making the person vulnerable to infections and certain cancers that healthy persons can otherwise resist. Approximately 50 % of adults die within 1-1½years after AIDS symptoms appear, and the death rate in children is still higher.

How does this infection occur: HIV infection may occur from unprotected sex, infected blood or infected pregnant mother to her child. Thus, it can be caused by the exchange of semen, vaginal secretions, blood or milk, which is infected by the virus. The virus can enter the body through the vagina, penis, rectum, or mouth. Anal intercourse, with or without a condom, is risky, as the rectum can easily be injured during intercourse. HIV spreads fastest and farthest in conditions of poverty, powerless, and lack of information.

Incubation period for HIV infection to the development of AIDS is uncertain, varying from a few months to 6 years or more. The virus may be silent in the body for many years. It has been estimated that 75 % of those infected with HIV develop AIDS by the end of 10 years.

19.3 Transmission of the infection

The transmission for HIV (**Epidemiology**) occurs through practices that involve the exchange of blood or body fluids between people since HIV is present in blood and some body fluids. i) It may be transmitted in semen or vaginal fluid during anal or vaginal unprotected intercourse or oral sex, however, the infection with HIV is higher with anal than with vaginal intercourse. ii) It is also transmitted through "needle sharing" from an infected person to a healthy person in cases of intravenous drug abusers (IVDA) by direct blood-to-blood contact. iii) HIV is also transmitted through infected blood or blood products (coagulation factors for disease hemophilia) from one individual to another during blood transfusion, and iv) It can also be transmitted from an infected mother to her fetus during pregnancy, birth or through breastfeeding to her infant. Hugging or sharing household items does not transmit by insect bite or by casual contact the infection with an HIV-infected person, such as.

Adolescent women are at even greater risk than adult women since their vagina and cervix are less mature and less resistant to HIV and other STIs (sexually transmitted infections). Changes in the reproductive tract during puberty make the tissue more susceptible to penetration by HIV. Also, hormonal changes associated with the menstrual cycle often are accompanied by a thinning of the mucus plug, the protective sealant covering the cervix. Such thinning can allow HIV to pass more easily. Also, young women produce only scant vaginal secretions, providing little barrier to HIV transmission.

According to epidemiological and ecological studies, male circumcision is associated with lower rates of HIV acquisition. Male circumcision is the surgical removal of the foreskin (prepuce) of the penis. Uncircumcised men are 2-8 times more likely to have HIV infection. In addition, male circumcision also protects against other STDs, and reduces the risk of penile carcinoma and urinary tract infections. It is believed that the foreskin provides a ready portal of entry to HIV and other pathogens. The inner surface of the foreskin is rich in special cells called Langerhans cells, which are particularly vulnerable to HIV. It appears to be the primary means through which HIV enters into the penis. Further, foreskin is more susceptible to trauma during intercourse, which can make it vulnerable to HIV. However, the age at which a person undergoes circumcision is important to HIV. For example, circumcision before the age of 12 years is associated with decreased risk of HIV, but not if performed at 13 years or more, HIV prevalence is 7 % for men who are circumcised at the age of 12 years or less, 15 % for men circumcised at 13 years or more, and 14 % for uncircumcised men.

It is important to remember that AIDS is sexually transmitted, and the AIDS virus is not the only infection that is passed through intimate sexual contact. Other sexually transmitted diseases (STDs), such as gonorrhea, syphilis, herpes, and chlamydia can also be contracted through oral, anal, and vaginal intercourse. However, chances of getting AIDS are increased in a person who is infected with any one of the STDs and is also engaged in risky behavior. These can be sharing drug needles and syringes, anal sex, with or without a condom, vaginal or oral sex with someone who use intravenous drugs or engages in anal sex or having sex with someone you do not know well or with someone you know has several sex partners, or unprotected sex (without a condom) with an infected person.

Who suffers with the disease: The disease occurs among homosexuals, contaminated bisexuals, promiscuous heterosexuals, drug abusers, people receiving blood transfusion, and babies born to or taking milk of HIV positive mothers. Of the 40 million people infected with HIV worldwide in the year 2000, about half are women and one quarter are children.

19.4 HIV

HIV belongs to a group of "**retroviruses**", which have an RNA genome and transcribe a DNA copy of the RNA genome after penetration in the host cell. They are called retrovirus because the genetic information is carried in RNA instead of DNA. To replicate, a virus must enter a host cell, where it uses the cell enzymes, ribosome, and nutrients to reproduce copies of its genetic information.

HIV consists of a single strand of **genetic material** or **RNA genome** surrounded by a **protective protein coat**. The coat is wrapped by an **envelop** with **high lipid content** rendering it sensitive to organic compounds. The envelope is composed of a **lipid bilayer** penetrated by a distinctive assortment of **glycoproteins**, and one of the glycoprotein is **GP 120**. The protein is composed of many molecules in the coat, and is termed **P24**. GP120 functions as the docking protein that binds to CD4 molecules on T cells, macrophages, and dendritic cells. In addition, HIV must simultaneously attach to a co-receptor in the host cell's plasma membrane (a molecule designated CCR5 in antigen presenting cells and CXCR4 in T cells) before it can gain entry into the cell. The other glycoprotein is called **GP 41**, and it helps the viral lipid bilayer to fuse with the host cell's lipid bilayer. Binding of HIV's docking proteins with the receptors and co-receptors in the host cell's plasma membrane causes receptor-mediated endocytosis. This brings the virus into the cell's cytoplasm. Using the invaded cell's machinery, HIV replicates, filling the cell with its RNA and protein.

Once inside the cell, HIV sheds its protein coat. A viral enzyme called **reverse transcriptase** reads the viral RNA strand and makes a DNA copy of the viral RNA. Then the viral DNA copy becomes integrated into the cell's DNA, and the viral DNA is duplicated along with the host cell's DNA during normal cell division. In addition, the viral DNA can cause the infected cell to begin producing millions of copies of viral RNA, and assemble new protein coats for each copy. These new HIV copies bud off from the plasma membrane and circulate in the blood and infect other cells. HIV damages principally CD4 helper T-lymphocytes (T4) cells and even can infect and impair the function of many other cell types mainly cells of the monocytes, dendritic cells and B-lymphocytes. Over 100 billion viral copies may be synthesized each day and the viruses bud so rapidly from an infected plasma membrane that cells lyses eventually occurs. In most HIV-infected individuals, the body is able to replace HIV infected T4 cells at about the same rate that they are destroyed. This process continues for many years. However, the body's ability to replaceT4 cells is slowly exhausted, and the population of T4 cell in circulation slowly declines at an estimated rate of approximately 20 million cells per day.

19.5 Signs and Symptoms of HIV Infection

Most people experience a brief flu-like illness immediately following infection with HIV. Common signs and symptoms include fever, rash, headache, joint pain, sore throat, swollen lymph nodes and fatigue. Approximately 50% of infected people have night sweats. After 3-4 weeks, plasma cells begin secreting antibodies to components of HIV protein coat and these antibodies are detectable in blood plasma and form the basis for some of the screening tests for HIV. If antibody test is negative even when acute HIV infection is suspected, laboratory tests based on detection of HIV's RNA or P24 of coat protein in blood plasma can confirm the presence of HIV.

19.6 Diagnosis of HIV infection

HIV infection can be confirmed by detecting the presence of antibodies to HIV in the patient's serum. These antibodies are detected by **ELISA (Enzyme-Linked Immune Sorbent Assay) test**, which is simple and cheap, with very low false negative rate, and becomes the routine screening test for the "same day" testing service. However, all positive results are normally confirmed by the more precise

western blot test. Following infection, detection of antibodies to HIV may not occur for three months and sometimes even longer.

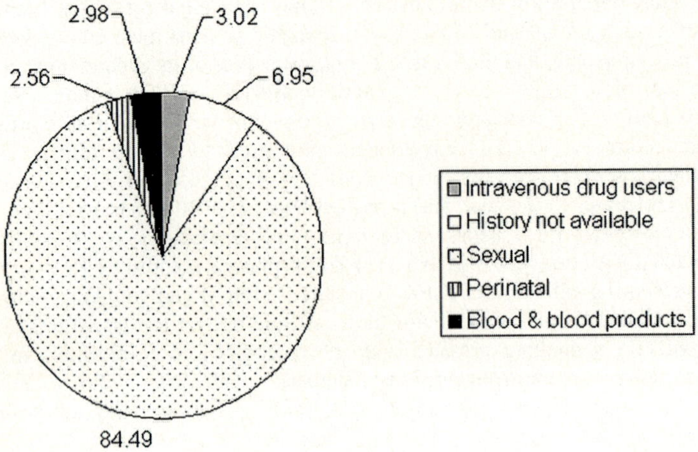

Figure 19.1: Probable source of AIDS infection (%) in India from May 1986 to August 2002 (total reported cases = 39742).

Estimation of HIV infection among adult population: Applying the following formula makes HIV infection estimates:

$$V = (P/T)\ (R),$$

where V is the total estimate, P is the number of HIV positive, T is the number of samples tested, and R is the estimated size of population. Distribution of likely source of infection is mapped in Figure 19.1 while the age distribution of cumulative AIDS cases in India are given in Table 19.1. High prevalence states of HIV infection in India are Maharashtra, Karnatka, Tamil Nadu, Andhra Pradesh, Manipur and Nagaland.

19.7 Protection and preventive Measures

Stopping HIV/AIDS requires comprehensive strategies that focus on youth. Recent declines in incidence of HIV/AIDS infection cases have been reported in a few countries. Signs that young people are changing their risk-taking behavior gives some hope for future in protecting and preventing people from getting HIV/AID. AIDS today is widely seen as a social crisis. Therefore, a combination of approaches may succeed in finding solutions to AIDS epidemic.

AIDS may be controlled through four basic approaches and these are prevention through a) education and awareness programs, b) primary health programs, c) anti-retroviral treatment, and d) specific prophylaxis to treat the manifestations of AIDS.

HIV can be eliminated from personal care items and medical equipment's by exposing them to heat at 135^{0}F for 10 minutes or by cleaning them with disinfectants such as Lysol, rubbing alcohol, hydrogen peroxide, household bleach, or germicidal cleansers such as Hibiclens or Betadine. Routine clothes washing and dishwashing also kills HIV. The disease can also be prevented from spreading by taking care of those actions or practices, which help it to spread. The chance of transmitting or getting infected by HIV during vaginal or anal intercourse can be minimized by the use of latex condoms. Health programs may be aimed in encouraging intravenous drug users not to share needles, and also to check the blood for HIV positive test before transfusion. Further, prophylactic administration of certain drugs such as AZT (3-azido-3' deoxythymidine) to pregnant HIV-infected women has proved remarkably effective in minimizing the transmission of the virus to their newborn babies.

Table 19.1: Age distribution of AIDS infected cases in India up to 31st August 2002

Age Group in years	Female	Male	Total
0 – 14	583	938	1521
15 – 29	4556	9756	14312
30 – 44	4087	16789	20876
> 45	609	2424	3033
Total	9835	29907	39742

19.8 Treatment

At present, **AIDS cannot be cured,** and despite of intensive research, no effective vaccine is yet available to provide immunity against HIV. Several antiviral agents have been tried without satisfactory results. Drug therapy is also not effective for prevention, progression or spread of the disease. Counseling and preventive measures are the important and valuable in the AIDS treatment and control. However, two lines of treatment have proved successful in extending life to AIDS patients.

The first category of drugs recommended for AIDS for regular clinical use are **reverse transcriptase inhibitors** that inhibit the spread of infectious virus into uninfected cells. But these do not affect replication of the HIV genome once it is integrated into host cell. Drugs of this category are **zidovudine**, commonly called **AZT**, **didanosine (dideoxyinosine, DDI)**, **zalcitaline (dedeoxycytidine, DDC)**, and **stavudine (D4T)**. However, these drugs have side effects also, for example. AZT causes nausea, vomiting, anemia, headache, neutropenia, and sometimes leucopenia and thrombocytopenia. Macrocytosis also develops in most patients.

The second and more recently discovered category is the **protease inhibitors** that interfere with the action of **protease**. Protease is a viral enzyme, which cuts proteins into pieces that are assembled into the coat of newly produced HIV particles. Drugs in this category are **nelfinavir**, **saquinavir**, **indinavir**, and **ritonavir**.

Triple therapy (a combination of two differently acting reverse transcriptase inhibitors and one protease inhibitor) has been found useful in late 1995 in treatment of most HIV-infected individuals. This therapy results in a drastic reduction in viral load (the number of copies of HIVRNA in a milliliter of plasma), and an increase in the number of T4 cells in whole blood, and thus delays the progression of HIV infection to AIDS. Also, many individuals with AIDS experience disappearance of opportunistic infections. But, triple therapy is very expensive and also all people cannot tolerate the harsh side effects of these drugs. However, people who can afford it and find the drugs helpful must keep taking them for a long time may be for life. Better understanding of the biology of HIV infection, plus new drug weapons, and clues from survivors, is providing what has long been lacking in the global fight against AIDS.

National AIDS Control Program: WHO (World Health Organization) has launched a "Global Program on AIDS" on February 1, 1987 to provide global leadership and to support the development of national AIDS programs.

Summary

AIDS is Acquired Immune Deficiency Syndrome. It is not one disease, but a set of diseases, and not all people who develop AIDS suffer from the same disease. Because of this, it is called a "syndrome".

AIDS is caused by a retrovirus, called Human Immunodeficiency Virus (HIV). It affects the body's immune system, making it liable to infections and cancers to which it would normally be resistant. It is possible to get infected with HIV from someone who appears fit and healthy, or to carry the virus oneself without being aware of it. Once infected, a person carries the virus for life, and can transmit the virus to others.

HIV multiplies in the body, and takes away the power of the body to combat the infections. The most common opportunistic infections are pneumonia, a variety of gastro-intestinal infections resulting in diarrhea and weight loss, a skin cancer (Kaposi's sarcoma), and disorders of nervous system.

HIV is found in most body fluids, but is only infectious in blood, semen and vaginal secretions. HIV can be transmitted by infected blood and blood products in blood transfusion, unsterilized hypodermic needles or other medical implements, needle-sharing in drug users, having sex-oral, anal, or vaginal with someone who is infected with AIDS virus, and from an infected mother to her baby in the womb or during birth.

AIDS is not transmitted through every day's casual contact such as saliva, kissing, telephone, utensils, sweat, urine, clothes, toilet seat, traveling in a bus or train, tears, and insect bite etc.

HIV attacks progressively inactivate CD4 helper T cells, which are vital in controlling the body's defense to many diseases. HIV infection may live in human body for years before actual symptoms appear. It primarily affects by making an individual unable to fight other diseases, which can prove fatal. Using the invaded cell's protein synthetic machinery, HIV replicates, filling the cell with its RNA and proteins. The dying T cell no longer release cytokines or stimulate B cells to manufacture antibodies, instead it bursts, unleashing many new HIV particles.

HIV replicates at an astounding rate, producing 3 billion new particles a day, from the start of the infection. The immune system cells can remove only 100 million to a billion per day, and therefore, the coordination of the immune response collapses, and opportunistic infections set in the body.

The diagnosis of AIDS is given when certain unusual opportunistic infections and tumors develop, and antibodies to HIV are found in the bloodstream, called the viral load.

HIV can be detected by ELISA test (Enzyme-Linked Immuno Sorbent Assay) and confirmed by western blot test.

There is no cure for AIDS. Treatment of AIDS can be done through two categories of drugs. These are reverse transcriptase inhibitors, and protease inhibitors. A triple therapy has also been introduced in 1995. Combining drugs can keep viral load low and delay symptoms onset and progression of HIV infection to AIDS. Goal is to enable infected people to live normal life spans in relatively good health.

Questions

1. What is AIDS? How the disease is transmitted.
2. What is HIV? What are its signs and symptoms?

Chapter 20

Cancer and Hormones

Control of cell reproduction is absolutely crucial for maintenance of proper health. Though frequent mitosis is an important phenomenon in the development of an embryo, or in the growth of a child, or in the healing of a wound, yet it may produce an abnormal and unwanted growth (neoplasm) in the body. This growth may develop into a disorganized mass called a tumor.

20.1 Tumor

A **tumor** is defined as an abnormal mass of tissue. The study of tumors is known as **oncology** (*onco* = swelling or mass).

Types of Tumor: Tumors are of two types: I) When the developed mass remains well recognized like a lump and does not invade other tissues, it is called a **benign tumor**. It may be harmless, or if it interferes with a normal body function or become disfiguring it can be surgically removed. 2) On the other hand, a type of tumor that spreads by invading other tissues is called a **malignant tumor** or **malignancy** or **cancerous tumor**. This is much more dangerous and is commonly referred as **Cancer**.

20.2 Cancer

Cancer is a collection of disorders characterized by uncontrolled cell proliferation, and can be distinguished by their site of origin and the affected cell type. The name "Cancer" comes from its resemblance with a crab with outreaching claws, since the cancerous tumor is invasive, extending into surrounding tissue. By simple physical examination, it may be impossible to determine whether a tumor is benign or malignant (cancerous) but microscopic examination of the small piece of tumor, surgically removed from the site, provides a definitive diagnosis and this test is called a **biopsy**.

Types of Cancer: After cardiovascular disease, cancer is the second most common disease resulting in death. Humans of all ages can develop cancer. It can affect a wide variety of organs. Most human cancers are **carcinomas** (*carcin* = cancer, *-omas* = tumors) or malignant tumors that arise from epithelial cells. The name of the cancer is generally derived from the type of tissue in which it develops. For example, **Leukemia** is a cancer of blood-forming organs characterized by rapid growth of abnormal leukocytes or white blood cells; **Sarcoma** is any cancer arising from muscle or mesodermal cells or connective tissue; **Lymphoma** is the cancer of the lymphatic tissue such as lymph nodes; **Prostatic Cancer** is that of prostates; **Breast Cancer** of breasts, and so on.

Cancer associated with Male and Female Reproductive Organs: Many portions of the male reproductive tract can develop cancer, and the most common site is the prostate gland. Nearly 16 percent of all cancers in men are prostatic and its occurrence is second to lung cancer (21 %).

However, prostatic cancer has a very low death rate as it occurs primarily in older men and is slow growing. Cancer of penis and testicles are relatively rare.

Cancer is common in generative organs in females. 22 percent of all malignant tumors in women occur in the breasts, 5 percent in the ovaries, and 17 percent in the uterus. However, direct inspection, palpation or cytological tests such as Pap smear can easily detect them. The female reproductive tract can develop both benign as well as malignant tumors. A common form of benign tumor that develops in the female reproductive tract is the uterine tumor, which develops in the myometrium, and is commonly known as **fibroid tumor**. This is a hard mass of smooth muscle, that is usually innocuous and it decreases in size after menopause. However, numerous fibroids or a large one when present in the uterus prevent pregnancy. Or it may cause excessive menstrual flow. In the latter case, surgical removal of the uterus (called **hysterectomy**) becomes essential for correction of the disease.

Characteristics of Cancer Cells: Cancerous cells have the ability to spread or **metastasize**. They lose cell cycle control, contact inhibition, as well as specialized characteristics, such as dedifferentiation. Thus, a cancer cell multiplies to form more cancer cells. It also has transplant ability that is if a cancer cell is implanted into another individual, it will cause cancer to develop. Cancer cell is invasive in nature. It has the ability to induce local blood vessel formation (**angiogenesis**).

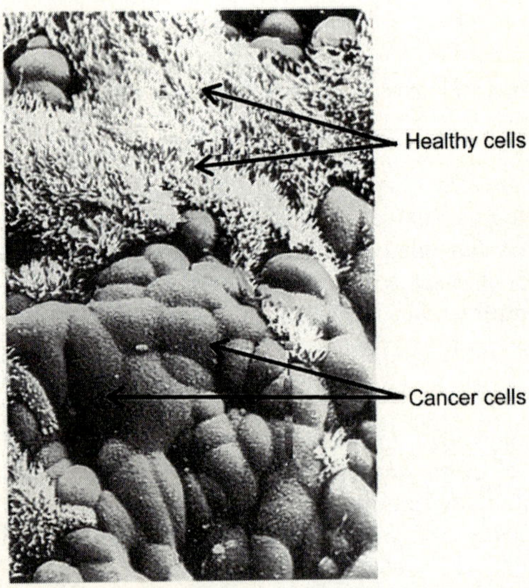

Figure 20.1: Cancer cells and the healthy cells-a cancer cell is rounded and less specialized than healthy cell.

Growth and Spread of Cancer: Once a cell becomes a tumor cell, its composition and behavior do not remain static. Cancerous cells duplicate rapidly and continuously, and invade surrounding tissue (Figure 20.1). This is manifested by increasingly abnormal karyotypes, increasing rates of growth, and an increasing tendency to invade and metastasize. They also trigger the growth of new networks of blood vessels or **angiogenesis** (Figure 20.2). The proteins that trigger angiogenesis in tumors are called **tumor angiogenesis factors (TAFs)**. The important phenomenon of progression appears to reflect a fundamental instability of the genome of tumor cells. It seems likely that mutations in DNA repair genes are involved in this phenomenon, creating a mutator phenotype. The activation of additional oncogenes may be involved. Cells with faster rates of growth have a selective advantage.

These fast growing cells tend to maximize the anabolic processes involved in growth, cut down on catabolic functions and dispense with the differentiation functions shown by their normal ancestors.

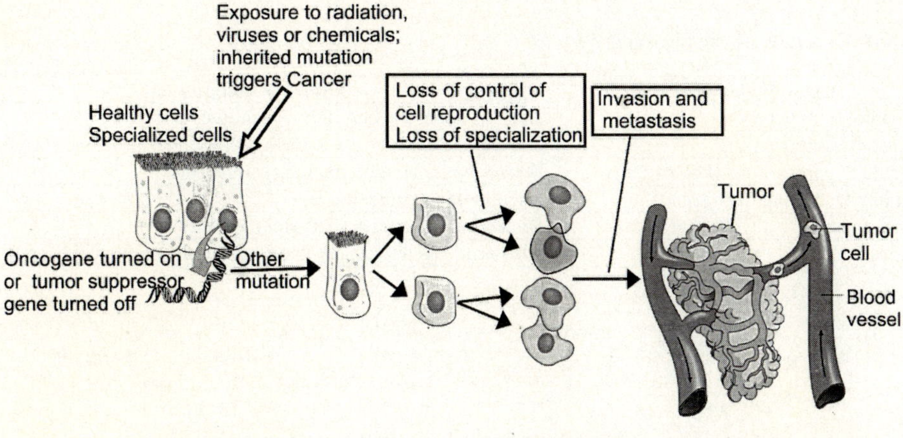

Figure 20.2: Invasion, metastasis and angiogenesis by cancer cells.

As cancer grows, it starts competing with surrounding normal tissue for space and nutrients. The normal tissue slowly decreases in size and dies. Some of the cancerous cells may detach from the **primary tumor** and enter circulation to invade other body tissues (Figure 20.2). **Metastasis** is the spread of cancer cells from a primary site of origin to other tissues. There, they grow as **secondary tumors**. When the tumor presses on nerves or blocks a passageway in an organ due to its growth, it causes pain.

Causes of Cancer: Several factors or agents are responsible to trigger a normal cell to lose controls and become cancerous. Broadly, these can be classified into three groups: i) **Radiant energy**, ii) **Chemical compounds**, and iii) **Viruses**. A chemical agent or radiation that produces cancer is called a **carcinogen**. Common carcinogens are hydrocarbons found in cigarette tar, ultraviolet or UV radiation in sunlight, radon gas from earth, and many environmental agents (considered as its pollutant) we breath in through air, the water we drink, and food we eat. In general, cancerous agents induce **mutations**. Mutations are permanent structural change in DNA base sequence of a gene.

i) Radiant Energy: Ultraviolet rays, x-rays, and γ-rays are mutagenic and carcinogenic, and damage DNA in several ways. Ultraviolet radiation may result in the formation of pyrimidine dimers, thus creating apurinic or apyrimidinic sites by eliminating corresponding bases. Single- and double-strand breaks or cross-linking of strands may occur, causing damage to DNA. Apart from direct effects on DNA, x-rays and γ-rays cause free radicals to form in tissues, and the resultant OH, super oxide, and other radicals interact with DNA and other macromolecules, leading to molecular damage and producing carcinogenic effects.

ii) Chemical Compounds: Many compound as shown in Table 20.1 and Figure 20.3 are carcinogenic. Many of these compounds have been tested in the laboratory by administering them to rodents and other animals. It has been found that many environmental chemicals are carcinogenic, and these substances enter the human body through air or water or food and cause approximately 80 % of human cancers. World Health Organization estimates that carcinogens may be associated with 60-90% of all human cancers. Benzene, asbestos, cigarette smoke, certain therapeutic drugs are some of the known chemical carcinogens. Both organic and inorganic molecules may be carcinogenic (Table 20. 1). However, great diversity of these compounds indicates that they do not possess one common structural feature that confers to their carcinogenicity.

Table 20.1: Examples of chemical carcinogens

Class of chemical	Nature of compound
Inorganic Compounds	Arsenic, asbestos, beryllium, cadmium, chromium
Aromatic Amines	2-Acetylaminofluorene,N-methyl-4-aminoazobenzene (MAB)
Aromatic Hydrocarbons (Polycyclic)	Benzo[a]pyrene, dimethylbenzanthracene
Naturally Occurring Compounds	Dactinomycin, aflatoxin B_1
Nitrosamines	Dimethylnitrosamine, diethylnitrosamine
Various Drugs	Alkylating agents (e.g. cyclophosphamide), diethylstilbestrol

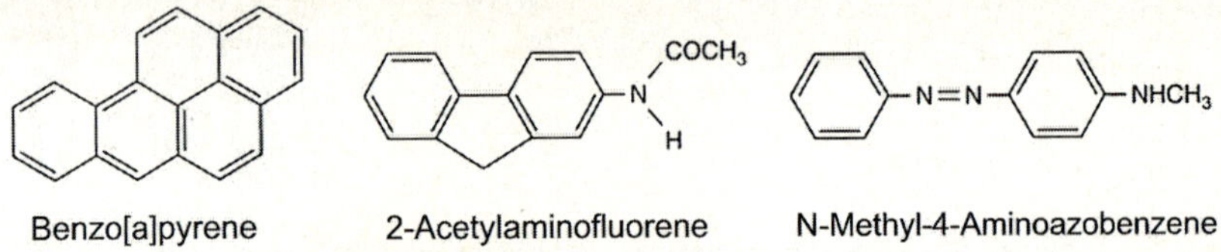

Figure 20.3: Structures of few important experimentally used carcinogens in case of Human.

Some chemical carcinogens interact directly with target molecules to cause cancer and are called **direct carcinogen** (e.g. mechlorethamine and β-propiolactone), while others require prior metabolism (metabolic activation) to become carcinogenic and are known as **procarcinogen**. The intermediate compounds formed are called **proximate carcinogens**, and the final compound that reacts with DNA is the **ultimate carcinogen**. A possible sequence of action of procarcinogen may be as follows.

Procarcinogen → proximate carcinogen → Ultimate carcinogen

It is believed that ultimate carcinogens are **electrophiles**, the molecules deficient in electrons, which readily attack nucleophilic groups in DNA, RNA, and proteins. The enzymes responsible for metabolic activation of procarcinogens are principally species of cytochrome p450, located in the endoplasmic reticulum. The activities of the enzymes metabolizing chemical carcinogens are affected by a number of factors, such as species, age, sex, or genetic considerations, and this explains the appreciable differences often seen in the carcinogenicity of these chemicals among different species etc. The ultimate carcinogen has been found to interact with the purine, pyrimidine, or phosphodiester groups of DNA, and the most common site of attack is guanine. The covalent interaction of direct or ultimate carcinogens with DNA result in several types of damage, which can be repaired, yet certain modifications of DNA caused by these chemical carcinogens persist for long periods. It is likely that these **persistent unrepaired lesions** cause mutations critical to carcinogenesis.

Ames assay has proved useful in screening for potential carcinogens. It identifies approximately 90% of known carcinogens, and is becoming a routine test for detecting mutagenicity in the newly synthesized chemicals, which are to be introduced commercially for wide use in the industry.

iii) Viruses: Viruses are tiny packages of nucleic acids, either DNA or RNA, that are capable of infecting cells, and converting them to virus-producers. Although link between viruses and cancer is strongly established for animal cancers, yet in cases of human cancers, it is less clear. Evidences suggest that chronic viral infections are associated with up to one-fifth of all cancers in human. Table 20. 2 lists the major viruses associated with tumors in humans.

Table 20.2: Major viruses associated with tumors in Humans

Class of Virus	Type of Virus	Members
DNA Viruses	Adenovirus	Adenoviruses 12,18, and 31
	Hepadnavirus	Hepatitis B virus
	Herpesvirus	Epstein-Barr virus
	Papovavirus	Polyomavirus, SV40 virus, human papillomaviruses
RNA Viruses	Retrovirus type B	Murine sarcoma and leukemia viruses, avian sarcoma and leukemia viruses,
	Retrovirus type C	human T cell leukemia viruses and II, Mouse mammary tumor virus

20.3 Mechanism of action of Oncogenes

Cancer causing genes are called **oncogenes**, and the process by which cancer develops is called **carcinogenesis**. Oncogenes are aberrant forms of normal genes (proto-oncogenes) that control growth and differentiation.

Carcinogenesis is a multi-step process in which as many as ten distinct mutations may have to accumulate in a cell before it becomes cancerous. Carcinogenic mutation, chromosomal rearrangement, and gene amplification are several of the known genetic mechanisms that can activate normal proto-oncogenesis. Several factors may trigger a normal cell to lose control on cell cycle, and become cancerous in a stepwise genetic changes resulting in the activation of proto-oncogenes, and the inactivation of so-called anti-oncogenes or tumor suppressor genes necessary for progression to the fully formed malignant phenotype (Figure 20.4). Hormones probably contribute to this process, since many natural and synthetic steroids and steroid-like compounds are known to be carcinogenic.

Many human tumors appear to produce mitogenic polypeptides that are called **cellular** or **transforming growth factors (TGF)**. Tumor cells also synthesize membrane-binding proteins for these same growth factors, and these growth factor receptors commonly possess protein kinase activity that transduces the mitogenic signal from cytoplasm to nucleus (Figure 20.4). Evidences suggest that the cyclins, the cyclin-dependent kinases (cdks), and cdk inhibitors are affected in cancer, either by mutation or secondarily. Inhibitors of cdk include members of the kinase inhibitory protein (KIP) family (example-p21, p27, and p57) and members of the inhibitors of cdk4 (INK4) family (example-p16) of proteins. Elevations of various cyclins (example D and E) and members of the INK4 family of proteins have been documented. The protein products of tumor suppressor genes, such as pRB, p53, and p16 (an inhibitor of cyclin kinases), which are frequently mutated in cancer cells, play important roles also in regulating the cell cycles. The products of oncogenes (example the sis oncogene) may also imitate the action of a polypeptide growth factor or imitate an occupied receptor for a growth factor (example the erb-B oncogene). Chronic exposure to increased amounts of a growth factor or to decreased amounts of a growth inhibitory factor could alter the balance of cellular growth. The effects of growth factor may be **endocrine**, **paracrine**, or **autocrine**. Growth factors, like polypeptide hormones, must transmit a message across the plasma membrane to the interior of the cell (**transmembrane signal transduction**). In the case of growth factors, the message will ultimately affect one or more processes involved in the cell cycle and mitosis (Figure 20.4). Most growth factors have high-affinity protein receptors on the plasma membrane of target cells. It seems likely that gene activation, whether of normal genes or proto-oncogenes, is involved in the action of most growth factors. The products of certain oncogenes such as *sis* (encoding the B chain of PDGF-platelet-derived growth factor), *erb*-B (encoding a truncated form of receptor for EGF-epidermal growth factor), *ras* (encoding a G type protein), *src* (encoding a protein-tyrosine kinase) and C-MYC (alter gene expression) may ultimately alter cellular metabolism and thereby stimulate growth. Cyclic AMP can affect a number of cellular processes by activating cAMP-dependent protein kinases, which affects the activities of a number of target proteins. Also, polypeptide growth factors are known to be mitogenic. However, control of cell growth is complex, and both positive and negative regulatory factors seem to be involved. Further, certain types of cancer, for example of breast show an increased familial incidence and by now considerable progress has been made in isolating genes that increase susceptibility to cancer, example gene BRCA1influencessusceptility to early-onset of breast and ovarian cancer. Genetic factor contribute to nearly 5 % of all cases of breast cancer. Once a cell becomes a tumor cell, composition and behavior of its progeny do not remain static and its tendency to become malignant increases with increasing abnormal karyotype, rate of growth and tendency to invade and metastasize, thus reflecting a fundamental instability of genome of tumor cell.

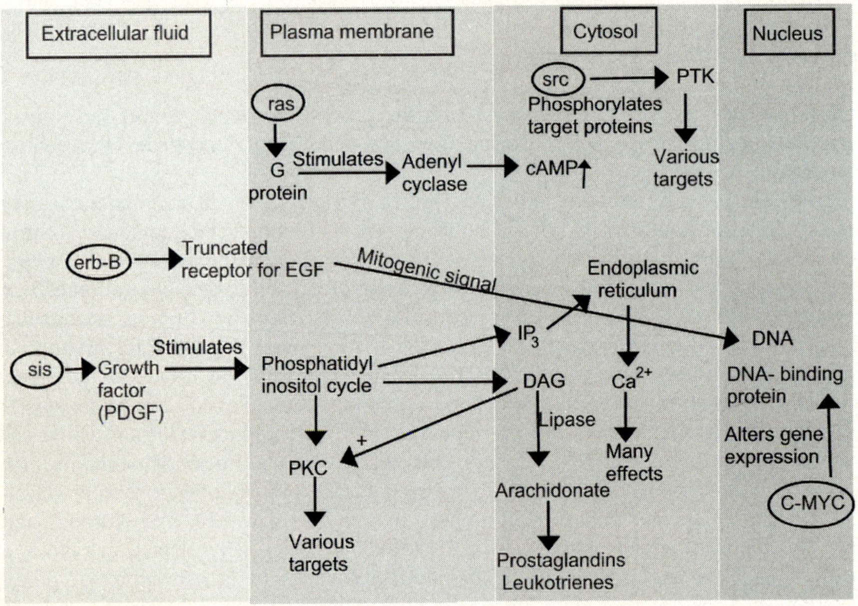

Figure 20.4: Mechanisms by which products of five oncogenes alter cellular metabolism to stimulate growth, PDGF-platelet-derived growth factor, EGF-epidermal growth factor, PKC-protein kinase C, PTK-protein tyrosine kinase, DAG-diacyl glycerol.

20.4 Hormones and Cancer

The cancers frequently promoted by **sex steroids** include those common tumors arising from **breast** (male and female), **endometrial**, and **prostatic tissue**. Studies demonstrate associations between sex steroids, especially estrogens and vaginal, ovarian, and laryngeal carcinomas. It has been suggested that sex steroids alone may play a pathogenic role in almost 30% of all cancer cases in USA. Thyroid, testicular, and ovarian tumors occur in glands under the tropic influences of TSH, FSH, and LH. Estradiol enhances breast cancer cell production by auto stimulating mitogens (agents that promote cell proliferation) such as TGFα, EGF, IGF-1, and IGF-2, and by paracrine factors, such as PGDF, and PGFs. Additionally, estradiol can depress synthesis of the bi-functional growth factor TGFβ, which normally inhibits proliferation of breast cancer epithelial cells while paradoxically stimulating growth of mesenchymal cells.

Nonsecretory primary or metastatic tumors may invade and replace normal glandular tissue and thereby cause loss of endocrine function. The most common syndrome in this is hypopituitarism due to pressure necrosis that occurs gradually during tumor growth or that occurs abruptly from tumor infarction (a necrotic area formed following interruption of the blood supply to the region) and bleeding. On the other hand, several types of benign and malignant tumors secrete hormones or hormone-like substances. Tumors can cause endocrine syndromes by secreting hormones inappropriately. This was, first proposed by Fuller Albright. He suggested in 1941 that the cause of hypercalcemia and hypophosphatemia in patients with renal carcinoma might be due to production of parathyroid hormone (PTH) by the tumor. To describe such situations, Liddle then coined the term "ectopic hormonal syndrome".

Secretion of hormones by tumors often differs qualitatively from glandular secretion of hormones. Firstly, secretion by tumors is rarely suppressible, and secondly, tumors lack the ability to process peptide hormones normally, and they secrete larger precursor forms whose biologic activity is reduced. Thirdly, tumor-associated syndrome may involve secretion of hormone homologues rather than hormones themselves.

20.5 Laboratory Tests For Cancer

Laboratory tests help in the management of cancer patients. The molecules used in the tests are known as **tumor markers**, and their application in diagnosis and early management of some types of cancers is of great importance. Table 20.3 gives a list of few of the commonly used tumor markers in cancer diagnosis.

Table 20.3: Commonly used tumor markers in cancer diagnosis

Tumor Marker	Associated Cancer
Alpha-fetoprotein (AFP)	Liver, Germ Cell
Calcitonin (CT)	Thyroid (medullary carcinoma)
Carcinoembryonic antigen (CEA)	Colon, Lung, Breast, Pancreas
Human chorionic gonadotropin (hCG)	Trophoblast, Germ Cell
Prostatic acid phosphatase (PAP)[2]	Prostate

20.6 Treatment of Cancer

The lethal effects of cancer may be best prevented by its early diagnosis, and treatment. The treatment of cancer is the surgical removal of the growth, followed by radiation therapy, or chemotherapy, or some combination of both. However, in cases where cancer is widely distributed throughout the body or in organs such as brain, surgery is not possible and only radiation therapy and chemotherapy are used. Radiation therapy destroys the chromosomes of cancerous cells with the help of radiation, while chemotherapy involves administration of drugs (anticancer chemicals) that poison the cancerous cells. Radiation and chemotherapy kill cells that are dividing through mitosis, and prevent them from increasing. Since cancerous cells divide rapidly, they are more vulnerable to the destructive effects of radiation and chemotherapy than the normal cells, nevertheless, both therapies can kill or disrupt the functions of some of the normal cells as well. Some compounds that have been used in the treatment of cancer are listed in Table 20.4. Many of these compounds are used because they inhibit DNA synthesis, but because of this reason, they also damage normal tissues whose cells divide continuously such as gut and bone marrow. Further, a major problem in cancer chemotherapy is development of resistance during the course of treatment to the agents used. To overcome this, combination chemotherapy has been tried. Combination chemotherapy i.e. combining three or four agents, have proved successful in some cancers as the drugs may act synergistically, the onset of resistance is delayed, and toxicity also is often less.

Table 20.4: Names of some compounds used in cancer treatment

Compound	Example	Site of Action	Treatment
Alkylating agents	Melphalan	Alkylates DNA and other molecules	Myeloma
Antimetabolites: Folate antagonists Purine antagonists Pyrimidine antagonists	 Methotrexate Mercapto-purine Fluorouracil	 Inhibits dihydrofolate reductase Converted to'fraudulent'nucleotide & inhibits purine synthesis Converted to'fraudulent'nucleotide & inhibits thymidylate synthetase	 Choriocarcinoma Acute myelo-cytic leukemia Colorectal cancer
Antitumor antibiotics	Doxorubicin	Intercalates in DNA & stabilizes the DNA-topoisomerase II complex	Hodgkin's disease
Corticosteroids	Prednisone	Inhibits proliferation of lymphocytes	Myeloma
Sex hormone	Estrogens	Block effects of androgen in prostatic tumors	Cancer of the prostate
Other agents	Cisplatin Hydroxyurea	Causes strand breakage in DNA Inhibits ribonucleotide reductase	Carcinoma lung Chronic myelo-cytic leukemia
Plant compounds	Vinblastine	Binds tubulin, and inhibits microtubule formation	Kaposi's sarcoma

Another difficulty encountered by blood-borne anticancer drugs is the physical barrier developed by solid tumors, such as those arises in the breasts, lungs, colon, and other organs. The high-pressure areas deep within such tumors collapse blood vessels in the tumors. This makes it difficult for blood borne anticancer agents to penetrate the tumor.

Table 20.5: Response of tumors known to contain estrogen receptors to endocrine therapy

Type of Tumor	Percentage Positive for ER	Response Rate to Endocrine Therapy
Breast Carcinoma	50-60 %	30 %
Endometrial Carcinoma	40-50%	30 %
Ovarian Carcinoma	30-40 %	< 20 %

Table 20.6: Antitumor endocrine agents

Endocrine Agent (s)	Mechanism	Tumor Targets
Anandrone, casodex	Androgen antagonists	Prostate
CGS-16949A, 4-hydroxy-androstenedione (4-OHA)	Aromatase inhibitors	Breast, endometrium, ovary
Finasteride, 4-OHA	5α-Reductase inhibitors	Prostate
Flutamide	Androgen antagonist	Prostate
Goserelin, buserelin	GnRH analogues	Prostate, breast, endometrium, ovary
ICI-164384	Estrogen antagonist	Breast
Mifepristone (RU-486)	Progestin antagonists	Breast, endometrium
Octreotide acetate	Somatostatin antagonist	Breast, ovary, prostate

At present, endocrine treatment is also of therapeutic value in cases of breast, endometrial, and prostatic cancers (Table 20.5) and (Table 20.6). This treatment is based on the response of steroid receptors (estrogen receptors-ER, and progesterone receptors-PgR) to endocrine therapy (antiestrogen or progestins). The therapeutic importance of receptors depends on both, a functioning receptor mechanism and a growth-regulating receptor response. Receptors (ER positive) can be assayed by monoclonal antibody. Steroid agonists and antagonists are now being combined with ablative therapies to try to increase endocrine response rates. For example, combining medroxyprogesterone acetate with aminoglutethimide brings into play at least two mechanisms of interaction that could result in enhanced inhibition of ER-positive tumors.

Summary

Cancer or malignant cells are characterized by loss of growth control, invasiveness, and metastasis, while benign tumor cells, though has lost growth control, yet they do not metastasize.

Physical, chemical, and biological agents such as radiation, chemicals, and environmental pollution can cause Cancer. These agents damage or alter DNA.

Normal cells contain potential precursors of oncogenes, called proto-oncogenes. Activation of these genes to oncogenes is achieved by at least five mechanisms. These are: promotor and enhancer insertion, chromosomal translocation, gene amplification, and point mutation.

Activated oncogenes influence cellular growth by perturbing normal cellular mechanisms of growth control, by acting as growth factors or receptors.

Growth factors act in endocrine, paracrine, or autocrine manners. They affect cell division.

Tumor suppressor genes are now recognized as key players in the genesis of cancer. They affect the transcription of genes involved in regulating events in cell cycle.

The phenomenon of metastasis may involve changes in surface glycoconjugates, altered activities of proteases, and alterations of cell adhesive molecules.

Treatment of cancer involves surgery, radiation therapy and chemotherapy.

Laboratory tests involving use of tumor markers are also available now, and are of great importance in the management of cancer patients.

Questions

1. Discuss various types of tumors. How tumor is different from cancer?
2. What are the characteristics of cancer cells?
3. What are the causes of cancer and how does it spread?
4. Describe the treatment of cancer.

Chapter 21

Infertility

Successful pregnancy requires fertilization of a mature ovum by a sperm and its subsequent implantation in a prepared endometrium. This process can be disturbed at several stages resulting in infertility. Physicians define **infertility** as the inability to conceive by a couple after a year of trying through unprotected intercourse. Demographic studies define a couple as infertile if woman reports no pregnancies or live births within a certain number of years of unprotected intercourse-usually the past one, two, or five years. World Health Organization (WHO) defines infertility as the inability to achieve conception within two years. In medical literature, the term **infecundity** often is synchronous with infertility since infecundity is defined as the inability to conceive or to impregnate. Both male as well as female factors are responsible for infertility.

Infertility can inflict a great amount of trauma on the minds of a barren couple. About 10-20 % of the couples find difficulty in having children. Incidents of infertility not only vary with countries but also within different population groups. Living conditions, nutrition, availability of health care, education, inheritance, and drugs are some of the factors, which may influence reproduction and result in infertility. It is a must for both the husband and wife to get tested for infertility. Treatment for infertility must be taken in specialized hospitals by a team of doctors consisting of medical specialists, physicians, psychologists, sexual workers and nurses. Also, in Family Planning clinics, simple interview and investigations may detect the cause of infertility.

In most of the infertile couples, a single factor in either partner (female or male) is responsible for infertility while in minority instances multiple factors resulting in infertility are involved. In poor population, sexual and unhygienic conditions such as inflammatory diseases predominate to cause infertility whereas in healthier environment, developmental and endocrinological factors predominate in causing infertility. In many regions pelvic inflammatory disease in women, due to sexually transmitted disease (STD) and other infections, accounts for nearly more than half of all female infertility. Although the woman is usually blamed when a couple cannot have children, yet male factors explain about one-third of all infertility. Low sperm count, often the result of infection, is the most important male factor in causing infertility.

Many of these factors cause **primary infertility** that is they are present before the occurrence of any pregnancy. **Secondary infertility** appears after the birth of one or more infant following which the couple is not able to achieve pregnancy. Some couples have no children as a result of **pregnancy wastage** (failure to carry a pregnancy to term) due to habitual abortion, and/or premature or stillbirth. However, pregnancy wastage is not classified as infertility though end result for the couple is the same. **Sterility** implies complete and permanent inability to conceive or impregnate even after treatment. **Childlessness** is a common measure of infertility and it means that a couple has not produced any children, whether due to infecundity, pregnancy wastage, contraception, or induced abortion.

21.1 Causes of infertility in a couple

Following causes may result in infertility in a couple:

- Sexual dysfunction,
- Mental or psychological factor,
- Immunological incapability,
- Genetic abnormality,
- Infectious diseases,
- Nutritional factor,
- Trauma or shock,
- Radiation (X-rays),
- Drug use,
- Endocrine factors,
- Bad habits and addiction,
- Environmental pollutants or Industrial hazards

Sexual dysfunction: It may be due to lack of basic understanding of reproductive physiology.

Mental or psychological factors include impotency, premature ejaculation, ejaculatory failure, and ovulation failure. Psychological factors may be produced by undefined and by indefinite pathways, hypothalamic and pituitary dysfunction, and sex with different partners. Either partner in a couple may prove otherwise fertile.

Immunological abnormalities may produce antibodies to sperm in both female and male and result in infertility.

Genetic factors to result in infertility may include Klinefelter's Syndrome or Turner's syndrome, and such infertility is not preventable. For instance, men with Klinefelter's syndrome, a genetic disorder found in 0.2 % of men, have low testosterone levels and thus are azoospermic. Some may also experience breast development and atrophied testes. In Kallman's syndrome, another genetic disorder, the hypothalamus fails to secrete gonadotropin-releasing hormone and thus the pituitary does not produce FSH or LH. Since these gonadotropins are necessary to stimulate the testes to develop and release testosterone, puberty never takes place.

Infectious diseases may cause pelvic inflammation in women or destruction of testicular or epididymal duct in men and result in infertility. Other infections may result in poor quality of genital secretion. Such infections include mumps, T.B. and sexually transmitted diseases (STD). Obstruction of vas deferens or tubes causes anatomical abnormalities interfering with sexual function or childbirth.

Malnutrition may affect hormone secretion or supporting function of genital organs. Males as well as females both experience reproductive problems in response to severe malnutrition, rapid loss of weight, vitamin deficiency, especially A, E, C, and B complex.

Trauma or **shock** may destroy or damage genital organs.

Radiation destroys ova and sperm. Excessive heat applied to the scrotum destroys sperm.

Drugs: Women treated with progesterone for menstrual pain or take tranquilizers may show lower fecundity. Habitual use of barbiturates or narcotics inhibits regular ovulation.

Endocrine factors: Diabetes, hypopituitarism, hypogonadism, hypo and hyper secretion of thyroid or adrenal glands can cause infertility. Hormonal imbalance that causes infertility is less common in males than in females.

Bad habits and addictions: Alcohol, drugs and tobacco can cause a range of fertility problems both in females and males.

Environmental Pollutants or Industrial Hazards: Various environmental pollutants or substances used in industry and agriculture may affect fecundity in both sexes. For example, exposure to lead can reduce sex drive and sperm count in males and reduces the ability to conceive and increases pregnancy wastage in females.

Relationships of some factors directly and indirectly involved with infertility in females and males are given in Tables 21.1 and 21.2 respectively.

Table 21.1: Some causes of infertility in Human female

<table>
<tr><th colspan="2">Direct and Indirect Cause of Infertility</th><th colspan="2">Resultant Infertility</th></tr>
<tr><td rowspan="2">STDs
Certain non-sexually transmitted organisms
Postpartum infection
Post abortion infection</td><td>Pelvic inflammatory disease (PID)</td><td rowspan="2">Tubal inflammation, damage, or distortion
Mild endometriosis</td><td rowspan="3">Inability to conceive</td></tr>
<tr><td>Endometriosis
Tuberculosis</td></tr>
<tr><td rowspan="3">Pituitary tumor
Stress</td><td>Hyperprolactinemia
Polycystic ovarian disease
Thyroid / adrenal disorders</td><td>Ovulation disorders</td></tr>
<tr><td>Complications of childbirth and illegal abortion</td><td>STDs
Certain systemic diseases
Uterine defects
Cervical incompetence</td><td rowspan="2">Pregnancy wastage</td></tr>
<tr><td>Some other causes</td><td>Hormonal disorders
Environmental factors
Alcohol, certain drugs and tobacco</td></tr>
</table>

Table 21.2: Some causes of infertility in Human male

<table>
<tr><th colspan="2">Direct and Indirect Cause of Infertility</th><th colspan="2">Resultant Infertility</th></tr>
<tr><td>STDs
Certain non-sexually transmitted organisms</td><td>Epididymitis
Other complications</td><td rowspan="2">Blocked sperm ducts</td><td rowspan="4">Poor semen quality</td></tr>
<tr><td rowspan="3">Genetic factors
Certain hormonal disorders
Complications of mumps</td><td>Certain systemic diseases
Congenital disorders</td></tr>
<tr><td rowspan="2">Lack of testicular function
Varicocele
Hormonal imbalance
Environmental factors
Alcohol, certain drugs, tobacco</td><td>Sperm production disorders</td></tr>
<tr><td>Sperm antibodies</td></tr>
<tr><td colspan="2">Some other causes</td><td>Psychological factors
Certain systemic diseases</td><td>Sexual malfunction</td></tr>
</table>

In addition to the above factors, there are some more factors that are responsible for causing infertility in females and male. The factors that may **cause infertility in women** are: ovulatory failure, tubal dysfunction-obstruction or blockage in oviduct, uterine factors, such as pH, endometriosis (growth of endometrial tissue outside the uterus), unfavorable cervical or vaginal secretions and inadequate body fat. Additional factors to cause infertility **in men** are impaired spermatogenesis, defective seminal secretions, obstructed seminal ducts, faulty delivery of semen, sexual dysfunction, antibody formation to sperm or seminal plasma, systemic illness and endocrine disorders such as of hypothalamus-pituitary axis or testis or androgen action or hypogonadism and adrenal insufficiency.

21.2 Causes of infertility in women

In 60 % of the time, abnormality to induce infertility lies in the female's reproductive system. In women, the reproductive parts consist of ovaries, fallopian tubes, uterus, cervix and vagina. Any abnormality in any of these structures can cause infertility (Figure 21.1). Generally, investigation of female infertility begins with an evaluation to determine if the woman ovulates. If the woman appears to ovulate and the hormonal system is adequate to support pregnancy, then the possibility of a physical obstruction in the genital ducts is evaluated, followed by evaluation of other possibilities.

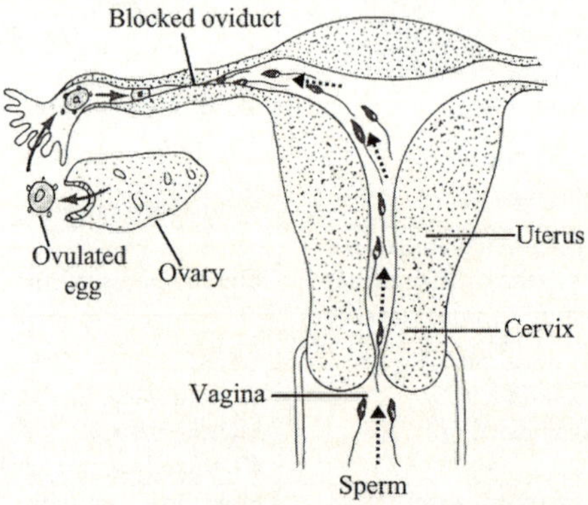

Figure 21.1: Infertility due to blocked oviducts in Women.

Ovulatory failure: One of the common causes of female infertility is hyposecretion of gonadotropic hormones from the anterior pituitary followed by failure to ovulate (anovulatory cycle). In addition to hypothalamic pituitary dysfunction, it may be due to hypoplasia and other developmental abnormalities of the ovaries. Ovulation disorders may also occur due to hyperprolactinemia, polycystic ovarian disease, and thyroid gland disorders. Ovarian diseases may also result from the use of oral contraceptives or other drugs. Since the concentration of progesterone normally rises following ovulation, no increase in pregnanediol in the urine during the later part of the menstrual cycle suggest lack of ovulation, thus can easily be detected. Stress may disrupt ovulation by affecting the autonomic nervous system, which in turn affects the endocrine system

Adolescent infertility in some girls lasts 12-18 months after menarche, and regular ovulation is not established until several years after menstruation has begun. Post-menarchial infertility may be due to anovulatory cycles, or may be caused by incomplete maturation of the uterus. However, the period of adolescent infertility enables the girls to attain greater maturity before reproduction and this is very advantageous as behavioral maturity lag behind physical development. Both dieting and intensive exercise may reduce body fat below the minimum amount and this may lead to infertility. However, this is reversible, if weight gain or reduction of intensive exercises, or both is taken care of properly. Studies of very obese women indicate that they, like very lean ones, experience problems with amenorrhea and infertility.

Tubal dysfunction: This may be caused by infection, developmental abnormalities or tumors including fibroids, endometriosis (damage of endometrium by chemical, mechanical and infectious factors) and drugs. Approximately 25 % of female infertility can be attributed to blocked tubes (Figure 21.1), scar tissue from infections in peritoneal cavity and endometriosis. Endometriosis is an important cause of female infertility. It is characterized by the growth of endometrial tissue on the fallopian tubes, ovaries, and other pelvic organs. It may occur when some endometrial tissue passes through the fallopian tubes during menstruation and implants on other organs. Under the influence of hormones during each subsequent menstrual cycle, this tissue grows and may shed, resulting in more implants. The implants eventually cause scarring and adhesions, both of which may distort the tubes and ovaries, interrupting ovum transport and causing infertility. Infection such as gonorrhea can inflame and obstruct the uterine tubes, or stimulate production of viscous mucous that can plug the cervix and prevent entry of sperm.

Cervical, uterine, and vaginal factors: Some congenital uterine and cervical abnormalities cause infertility. Techniques, such as **Laparoscopy** and **Hysteroscopy** are used to identify the cause of infertility due to structural abnormality in female genital tract. **Laparoscopy** is the visual examination of inside structures with the help of a long flexible rope-like instrument called **endoscope** passed through a tiny hole made on the abdominal wall, below the naval while **Hysteroscopy** is the visual examination of the uterus. **Cervical stenosis** (a small cervical canal) and **septate uterus** (a uterus divided into two chambers) are two examples of such abnormalities. Some factors, such as, unfavorable cervical and vaginal secretions inhibit sperm migration and cause infertility. Infertility may also occur due to metabolic and immunological changes or infections and chemical damage of cervical canals, vagina and accessory glands.

Pregnancy wastage: In addition to the causes of infertility in women, many women are unable to give birth to normal term baby for various reasons though they can become pregnant. Syphilitic disease is an increasing cause of pregnancy wastage, or spontaneous abortion.

Female Circumcision: It is practiced chiefly in certain African and Middle Eastern Countries. The operation varies from excision of the tip of the clitoris to removal of the clitoris, labia minora, and labia majora-termed **Pharanoic Circumcision**. It is performed on girls between ages of 4-10 years. All female circumcisions cause short-term risk of infection, hemorrhage, shock, and urine retention. Clinicians believe that Pharaonic Circumcision predisposes women to ascending infections and infertility. This is because the closure of the external genitalia prevents proper drainage of urine and menstrual blood and because tearing, which facilitates infection, is likely to occur at childbirth. However, infertility occurs in most cases because the circumcision makes penetration of full penis impossible.

Table 21.3: Relationship of increasing age with infertility in Women

Age (Years)	% Infertile
20-24	4.0
25-29	5.5
30-34	9.4
35-39	20.0

Age and female infertility: A woman's natural fecundity (fertility) varies considerably over the years between menarche and menopause. It is low immediately after menarche and before menopause, when hormonal patterns are quite irregular and peaks between ages 18 and 30. However, a marked drop in fertility has been found at ages 35-39 years through World Fertility Survey data than at any younger age (Table 21.3) suggesting that the risk of infertility increases with age.

21.3 Causes of infertility in men

Male infertility can be attributed to the inability of sperm cells to fertilize an egg cell. Approximately 40 % of the infertility cases are attributable to male factors and most of these are easy to detect. Several methods have been utilized to identify the causes of male infertility as indicated in Figures 21.2 and 21.3.

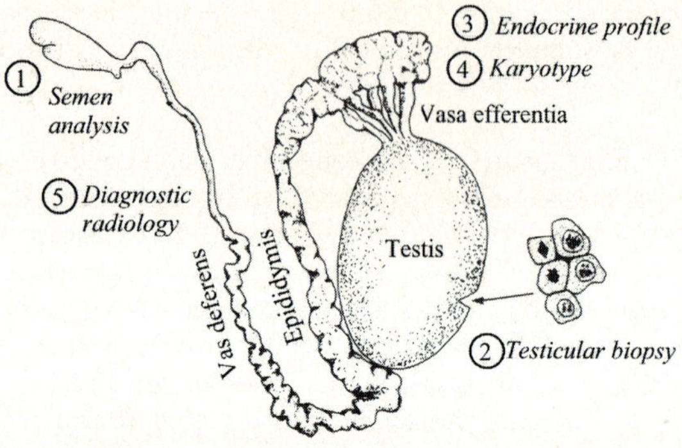

Figure 21.2: Methodologies used to identify causes of infertility in Men.

Male infertility is most often caused by one of the two conditions, either blockage of sperm ducts or disorders in sperm production. Both result in poor semen quality i.e. semen that contains too few sperm and/or abnormal sperm. On the basis of sperm count, men can be classified as either **azoospermic** (having no sperm in semen), or more likely, **oligospermic** (having a low concentration of sperm in semen) or **normospermic** (normal number of sperm in semen). **Infertility** occurs due to azoospermic conditions while **sub fertility** occurs due to oligospermia and is represented by sperm count below 20 million sperm per milliliter of semen. "**Idiopathic Oligospermia**" is oligospermia without apparent causes. The presence of large numbers of motile spermatozoa in mucus obtained from the internal os of the cervix rules out the male factors as a cause of infertility. But, if a post-coital test reveals **necrospermia** (dead sperm) or **asthenospermia** (slow moving sperm) or **sperm agglutination**, examination of the female partner for the presence of sperm-immobilizing antibodies or abnormalities in cervical mucus must be carried out.. A less common condition of male infertility is sexual malfunction that prevents ejaculation of semen.

Abnormal Spermatogenesis may be due to hypothalamic-pituitary dysfunction, testicular diseases (**orchitis**), undescended testes or **cryptochidism**, the higher temperature of the abdominal cavity or inguinal canal, other congenital testicular abnormalities, such as, **Sertoli cells syndrome** are the causes of infertility in males. Varicose veins of the scrotum can reduce fertility by increasing the temperature of the testes. **Varicocele**, a defective testicular vein or veins that cause abnormal blood flow to the testes may cause oligospermia. Incomplete valves in one or more testicular veins, allowing excess venous blood to flow around the testis, cause varicocele. This excess blood flow interferes with sperm production by raising the temperature or by increasing serum levels of toxic metabolites in the testes. Externally induced oligospermia may occur due to wearing tight underpants, excessive smoking, alcohol abuse, malnutrition, and undernourishment. In addition, high temperature, radiation, trauma or shock, testicular torsion, epididymitis, endocrine diseases, exposure to environmental pollutants, certain diseases such as mumps, viral infections, tuberculosis, syphilis, leprosy and stress etc. can induce infertility. Defective seminal secretions resulting from metabolic disease or genital infection affecting composition of the secretion of prostate gland and seminal vesicle may cause infertility. Obstructed (blocked) seminal ducts thus preventing free passage of sperm from testes to urethra reduce sperm count and result in infertility. Developmental abnormalities, faulty delivery of semen resulting from retrograde ejaculation (secretion into urinary bladder) is some more factors responsible for infertility in men. Severe malnutrition and weight loss in men results in less production of prostatic fluid and reduced numbers of sperm having decreased motility.

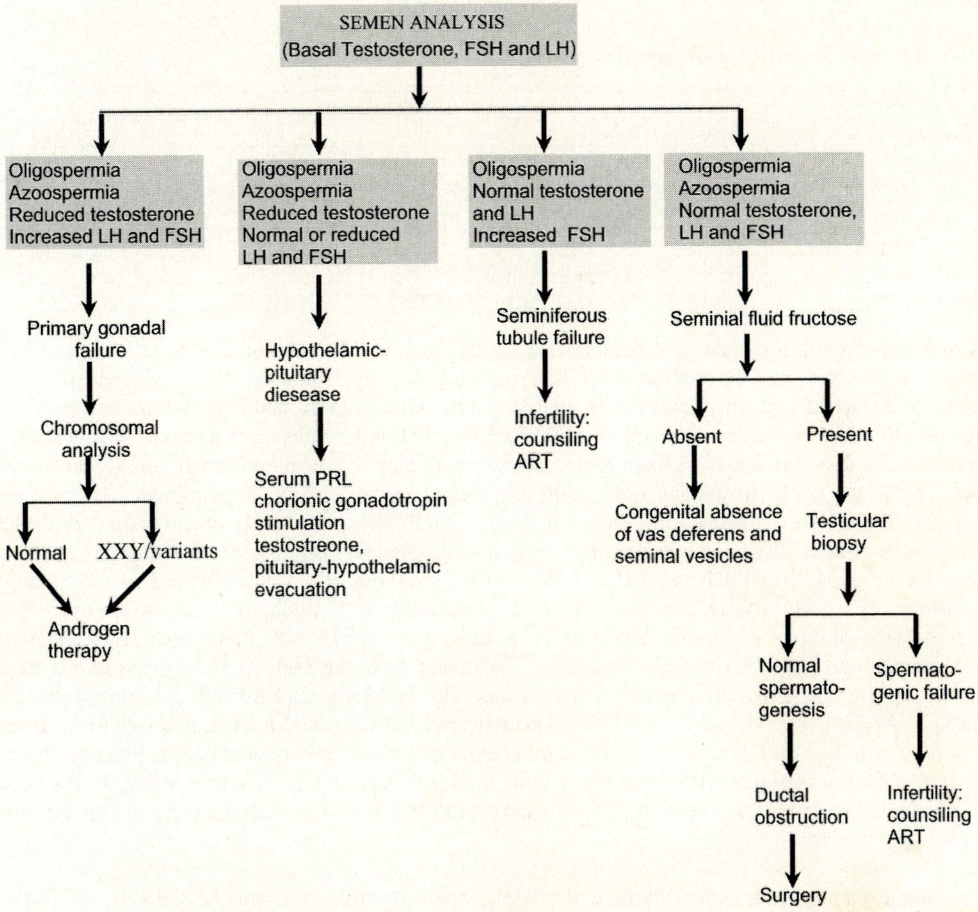

Figure 21.3: Semen analysis to identify the cause of infertility, its management and treatment in Men.

Impotence: Impotence implies to erectile dysfunction with or without associated disturbances of libido or ejaculatory ability. The overall prevalence of impotence in the general population is unknown, though it is probable that most men experience occasional episodes of impotence at some time during their lives.

21.4 Treatment and management of infertility in female

Simple methods should be tried to treat infertility in women. The first step in finding the right treatment for a particular patient is to determine the cause of infertility. Further, it is necessary to give reassurance to both the partners because there are many families where there is social pressure on couples that have failed to conceive following a period of living together. Emotional stress affects menstrual cycle. There are many cases of amenorrhea (no menstrual cycle), in which emotions upset the menstrual cycle and may inhibit ovulation. Table 21.4 gives various tests to assess female infertility.

Table 21.4: Assessment of female infertility in Women

Parameter	Assessment
Hormone levels	If ovulation occurs
Ultrasound	Placement, appearance, and structure of reproductive organs
Postcoital test	Cervix examined for thin mucus, immediately after intercourse
Endometrial biopsy	Samples of uterine lining viewed under microscope to see if it can support an embryo
Hysterosalpingogram	Dye injected into uterine tube, followed with scanner to see if tube is clear or blocked
Laparoscopy	Small optical device inserted near naval to detect scar tissue
Laparotomy	Scar tissue removed through incision made for laparoscopy

Treatment of ovulatory failures: Treatment depends on cause of ovulation failure. If amenorrhea is present, its causes may be studied before commencing any infertility treatment. Several forms of hormone therapy are given in cases of ovulation failure. One of them involves clomiphene treatment that elicits a rise in the serum levels of both FSH and LH and results in ovulation. An alternative treatment involves the use of gonadotropins, which maintains the development of oocyte, but in this form of therapy, it is difficult to control the number of oocyte, which is permitted to mature and ovulate. Failure to ovulate during lactation is associated with high levels of circulating prolactin. Many cases of infertility in women are likewise due to elevated levels of prolactin resulting in impaired response of gonads to FSH and LH. Treatment of such infertile women with Bromocriptine, a derivative of ergot, lowers prolactin levels accompanied with ovulation. It is useless where hypothalamic-pituitary function is absent or where there is no ovarian activity (premature menopause). It is given by mouth, 50 mg per day for 5 days. Treatment may be expensive and success rate is 50 %. Bromocriptine and gonadotropin may be used carefully blocking dangerous hyper-stimulation and multiple pregnancies. Gonadotropin treatment involves LH (hCG) and FSH in two sets of injection. Aim is to stimulate follicle formation, and to induce ovulation and formation of corpus luteum. Human menopausal gonadotropin (HMG) contains both FSH and LH and is available as single injection. Estrogen may be given for several days before and during ovulation to render the cervical mucous more penetrable to sperm.

Treatment of tubal blockage: Blockage of fallopian tubes towards the uterus is treated by removal of the blocked part of fallopian tube or oviduct and reconstruction. If endometriosis is the cause of blockage, progesterone treatment for 6-9 months can be tried. If tubes are irremediably blocked, fertilization can be carried out *in vitro* and blastocysts can be implanted in the uterus (**test tube babies**). The embryologist obstetrician team of **R.G. Edwards** and P.C. Steptoe of Cambridge, England pioneered the application of these techniques to human eggs and to women with blocked oviducts. Several decades of research by his team finally led, in 1978, to the first successful birth of a "test tube baby".

Anatomical defects or the obstruction of fallopian tubes can be examined by introducing an X-ray-opaque dye into the uterus. By using what may be the smallest telescope around, it is now possible to inspect and repair oviducts. In **falloposcopy**, a 0.5-mm telescope is threaded through the cervix into the fallopian tubes and connected to a video camera to provide a high-resolution color image of the sites of blockage or scar tissue, and as per requirement, video-aided fallopian surgery is performed. **Trans-cervical balloon tuboplasty (TBT)** applies a technique developed to open partially blocked coronary blood vessels to the opening of obstructed fallopian tubes. In TBT, a catheter with a deflated balloon is inserted through the vagina into the uterine cavity and up into the fallopian tube while a fluoroscope projects a x-ray image onto a television screen. The balloon is inflated and deflated several times to reopen the tube. By providing relief for one or more ovarian cycles, this procedure may be effective for thousands of infertile women whose fallopian tubes are blocked or if they close down again.

Besides tubal block, endometriosis can also be diagnosed by laparoscopy. Infertility associated with endometriosis can be cured either by surgery or by suppressing the activity of gonadotropin. This is done by danazol, a gonadotropin-suppressant or using continuous low dose oral contraceptive pill, which block the production of gonadotropin. Treatment by any of the drugs is accompanied with accurate monitoring and continuous evaluation of the menstrual cycle.

21.5 Treatment and management of infertility in male

Both the quantity and quality of sperm cells are essential factors in the ability of a man to father a child. Parameters normally used to analyze the quality of semen are given in Table 21.5. If a sperm head is misshapen, or it cannot swim, or there are too few sperm cells, or its entry in to an egg is unsuccessful, it will result in infertility (Figure 21.4).

Table 21.5: Parameters used in the analysis of semen

Parameter	Normal Value In Semen
Volume	2-6 ml/ejaculate
Sperm density	120 million/ml
Percent motile	More than 40 %
Motile sperm density	More than 8 million/ml
Average velocity	More than 20 micrometers/second
Motility	More than 8 micrometers/second
Percent abnormal morphology	More than 40 %
White blood cells	More than 5 million/ml

Treatment of azoospermia: If chromosome analysis shows abnormal genotype, then there is no treatment. Testicular biopsy is useful in cases of azoospermia to differentiate between obstructive and non-obstructive azoospermia, and in the later case, to determine the type and extent of disturbed function. In Sertoli cell syndrome, Klinefelter syndrome, and testicular atrophy, there is no use of any treatment since it represents permanent infertility. In hypogonadism, treatment with HMG with or without hCG may be beneficial. In obstructed azoospermia (blocked vas deferens) or some kind of infection in vas deferens, a course of antibiotics and anti-inflammatory drugs may be tried for infections. Surgical removal of vaso-vasal or vaso-epididymis anastomosis must be tried.

Treatment of oligospermia: In oligospermia, number of sperm is very low indicating shortage of FSH and LH. However, it is uncertain whether hypo-gonadotropinsm with oligospermia really exists. Testicular biopsy is also of diagnostic and prognostic value in cases of severe oligospermia. It is useful to evaluate the outcome of andrologic surgery, e.g. orchidopexy, varicocelectomy, epididymovasostomy, etc. Artificial insemination of husband's semen (AIH) is advantageous in cases of ejaculates with a small volume and ejaculates with large volume (first portion of the split ejaculate).

Treatment of oligospermia with FSH and LH or clomiphene with or without mestranol usually fails. It is due to shortage of androgens. Mestranol may be tried in cases of post tubular Leydig cells insufficiency. This is a syndrome where fructose contents are low and is the cause of oligospermia. Lack of liquefaction of semen as a result of an-enzymatic defect can be corrected in most cases by adding drops of seminal plasma from a normal donor and the use of AIH. Structural defects such as of varicose, varicocele, tubal blockage etc. can be treated by surgery. Oligospermia can be treated by artificial insemination of husband's semen into the cervix of the partner. Artificial insemination of husband's semen (AIH) can be done in cases of premature ejaculate, retrograde ejaculation, incomplete erection of the penis. Infertility due to azoospermia can be taken care by artificial insemination by donor (AID) who is anonymous, healthy male matching as far as possible with the infertile male.

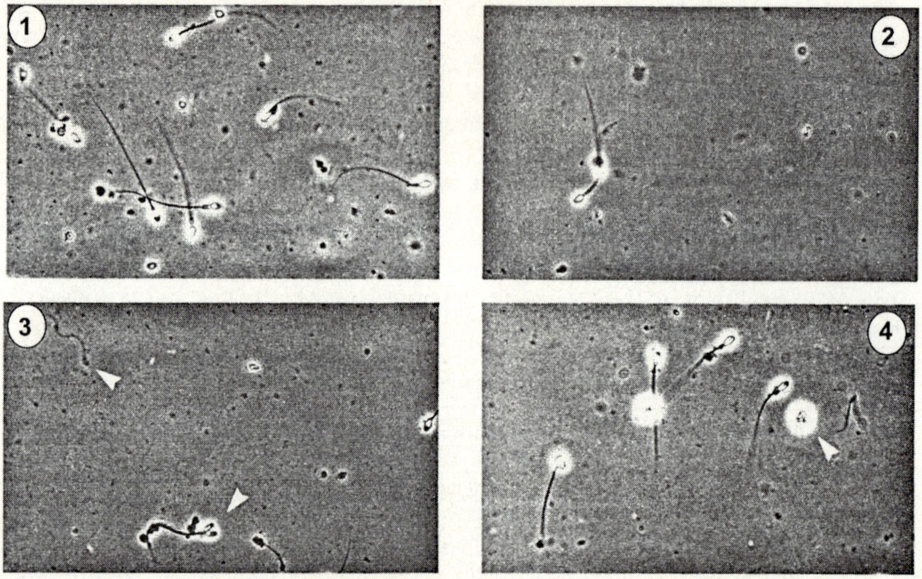

Figure 21.4: Phase micrographs of semen samples of Men, 1- normal sperm count containing nearly 200 million/ml of semen (20 million/ml is considered normal), 2-oligospermia with nearly 3 million/ml, 3-oligospermia with a high percentage of abnormal sperm, including 2-headed sperm, and sperm with small heads, 4-normal sperm count, but semen also shows leucocytes suggesting genital infection.

Until recently, sperm analysis was rather subjective, as it was based on a person's viewing the cells under a microscope. Now, **computer aided sperm analysis (CASA)** is standardizing and expanding criteria for assessing normalcy in human male seminal fluid and sperm cells it contains. Hundreds of CASA systems are now in use, mostly at fertility clinics helping the couple to know the cause of infertility through semen analysis. Figure 21.5 gives a CASA of normal sperm showing how the swimming pattern alters as they travel through the woman's body. The devices are also helpful in using sperm as "biomarkers" of exposure to toxins, such as solvent perchloroethylene used in dry cleaning industry and are believed to damage sperm.

Some cases of infertility result from male-female incompatibility. The mucous secretions of the cervix of some women never become penetrable to spermatozoa while in others, vaginal secretions are too acidic or contain antibodies that lead to the destruction of the spermatozoa. This problem of infertility can be solved **by artificial insemination**, which deposits a fresh sample of the husband's semen directly into the uterus (AIH). Also, a process known as **sperm washing** which removes the surface molecules that the female antibodies recognize on the sperm or **zona drilling**, also called "**zona blasting**" in which the outer surface of the zona pellucida is chemically stripped of to present less barrier to a sperm. This provides an easy excess for a limited number of sperm in to egg, and thus may be used to treat infertility. All these are **assisted reproductive technologies**, details of which are given in next chapter. With the help of these, even an individual sperm can be injected into an ovum. A last resort for infertile couples is placing gametes or a zygote into the fallopian tube (GIFT and ZIFT). If still all this is a failure, then adoption is the only measure.

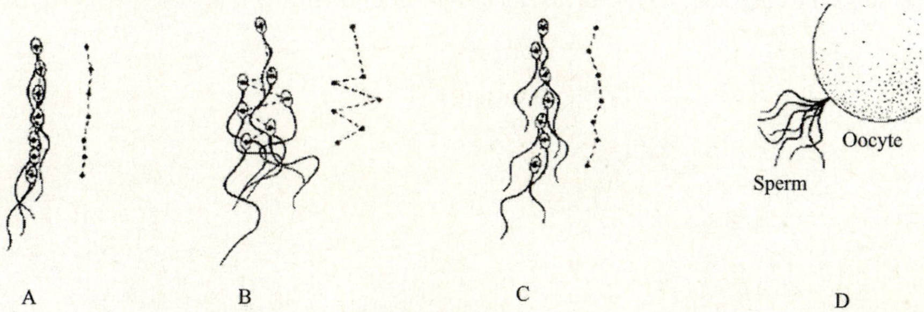

Figure 21.5: Computer-aided sperm analysis (CASA) of normal sperm of Men showing how their swimming pattern changes as they travel, A-sperm swim in straight line in semen, B-sperm trajectories widen in the woman's body, C-sperm in the mucus of a Woman's cervix, and D-sperm are attempting to penetrate the structure surrounding an oocyte.

Summary

Fifteen to twenty percent of married couples are unable to produce offspring, thus resulting in infertility.

Infertility is usually defined as a failure of conception by a couple that have been having intercourse for one year or more without using any contraceptive method. It may be caused due to male factors (40 %) and female factors (50-60 %) or both, i.e. couple factors (10 %).

Female infertility may be due to anovulation (15 %), tubal disease (20 %), cervical factors (5 %), abnormal body fat, immunological abnormalities, hormonal disorders and some unknown factors.

Male infertility is caused by abnormalities in semen (of both sperm as well as seminal plasma), high scrotal temperature, radiation exposure, use of drugs, smoking, use of alcohol, endocrine disorders and immunological abnormalities.

Genetic abnormalities, infectious diseases, psychological factors and nutrition may also result in infertility.

Infertility can be treated and managed both in males and females. However, treatment of infertility depends on its cause and manifestations.

Anatomical defects may be corrected with the help of surgery, while gonadal dysfunction with the help of hormones and/or drug therapy.

Infertility due to chromosomal abnormalities is generally permanent and cannot be corrected easily. Assisted reproductive technologies may be used in severe cases of infertility or sterility.

Questions

1. Differentiate between sterility and infertility.

2. What are the major causes of male and female sterility? Describe various methods to treat male sterility.
3. What are the causes of female infertility? Describe the methods to treat female infertility.
4. What are the main causes of male infertility? Describe various methods to treat male sterility.
5. Define infertility, and give various causes of infertility in human males.
6. Evaluate the procedures of male infertility. Indicate the role of sexually transmitted diseases therein.
7. Discuss the diagnosis, treatment and management of infertility in male.
8. Discuss the diagnosis, treatment and management of infertility in female.

Chapter 22

Assisted Reproductive Technologies

World over, infertility can be a source of suffering to both women as well as men. Enormous amount of money is spent and millions of visits to physicians are made every year for the complaints of infertility.

Several methods have been used to modify or stimulate the normal process of human reproduction to help the infertile and sterile males and females. **Assisted Reproductive Technologies (ART)** are new techniques that make babies outside the privacy of the bedroom to help such couples. These techniques overcome the hurdles that prevent spermatozoon and oocyte fusion and therefore, are developed to provide childless couples with offspring. Though these scientific breakthroughs are boons for childless couples, yet, they have raised the fear of a "brave new world" where babies will gestate in laboratory bottles and only those with the right gender or selected genetic traits will be chosen to live. Still recent focus on advanced technologies has overshadowed what appeared impossible few years back and with the rapid advances in the development and use of assisted reproductive techniques, there is a significant increase in the cure rate and management in almost every category of infertility. For many couples that have exhausted traditional clinical and surgical treatments for infertility, these technologies may offer the best hope for pregnancy. Women with otherwise untreatable infertility problems, through these procedures have given birth to healthy babies. However, successful reproduction through assisted reproductive technologies involves a careful coordination of both a medical and a scientific approach to each couple who undertake such a treatment cycle.

Some of the commonly performed assisted reproductive technologies are artificial insemination (AI) with fresh or frozen semen, *in vitro* fertilization (IVF), and embryo transfer (ET), also written as IVF-ET, gamete intrafallopian transfer GIFT), zygote intrafallopian transfer (ZIFT), pronuclear stage tubal transfer (PROST), tubal embryo stage transfer (TEST), intracytoplasmic sperm injection (ICSI), and microinjection fallopian transfer (MIF). Initially, some of these techniques were used when the woman had blocked or damaged or no fallopian tubes (tubal factor), but these are now used in patients with long-standing infertility not responding to conventional treatment, endometriosis, immunological problems, unexplained infertility, and male factor infertility, such as less sperm count. These technologies are described below.

22.1 Artificial Insemination (AI)

The major cause of infertility in man is a low concentration of healthy sperm in the ejaculate. Semen (ejaculate) always contains a fair number of immobile and abnormal sperm, but fertility problems can be expected when the concentration of healthy sperm cell dips below 50 percent. However, this cannot be detected always from a simple sperm count. Various pathological conditions of infertility associated with sperm number are a low count of viable sperm (**oligospermia**) or no sperm in the semen (**azoospermia**) or dead sperm in the semen (**necrospermia**), or slow-moving sperm in the semen (**asthenospermia**). There are several procedures that can be tried to treat cases of sub fertility or infertility in men occurring due to a low sperm count of viable sperm or due to slow-moving sperm. One method is to avoid intercourse for a full week before the woman's estimated ovulation time. This results in the natural increase in concentration of sperm and these are delivered to the female genital tract at the time of optimal fertility. Another technique is to inject the ejaculate directly into the uterus at the estimated ovulation time to avoid the dilution of viable sperm that normally occurs in the hostile vaginal environment. This procedure is called **artificial insemination** (**AI**). Thus artificial insemination can be defined as the intra-vaginal or intra-cervical injection/transfer of spermatozoa to achieve fertilization. It can be **intra-uterine insemination** (**IUI**), **sperm intrafallopian transfer** (**Sift**), and **direct intra-peritoneal insemination** (**Dipi**). For artificial insemination, either husband's sperm or donor's sperm depending upon the degree of infertility in the male partner may be used and accordingly, the technique is known as **AIH** (**artificial insemination using husband's semen**) or **AID** (**artificial insemination using donor's semen**) respectively.

Artificial insemination using the **husband's semen** (**AIH**) is performed when there is low sperm count or there are anatomic defects in male reproductive ducts that prevent sperm deposition in the cervix. Several methods have been used to treat the semen of infertile men for artificial insemination. In cases when sperm production is below optimal fertility level **(oligospermia)**, spermatozoa from husband's semen are concentrated either by **centrifugation**, or by **accumulation** using **deep freeze storage** technique over several months, and then used for AIH. Another technique known as the **split-ejaculate method** is also used in oligospermic men to get the optimal number of spermatozoa required for fertilizing an ovum. This technique is based on the fact that during ejaculation, semen comes in two or three fractions and the first half of ejaculate contains the majority of spermatozoa, while the later fraction of ejaculate contains mainly the secretions of all the accessory glands of reproduction. In split ejaculate method first part of the ejaculate is used for artificial insemination (AIH) when the husband's semen is either oligospermic or when the semen volume is too large due to which the number of sperm become low in the ejaculate. The split-ejaculate technique therefore, provides another method of concentrating the husband's semen spermatozoa required for artificial insemination in oligospermic condition to achieve successful fertilization. In addition to the number of spermatozoa, motility and morphology of spermatozoa are also better in the first half portion or fraction of ejaculate in comparison to the later part of ejaculate. Attempts have been made to separate motile sperm from nonmotile sperm. Certain substances, such as kalikrein, arginine, or albumin have also been used to improve motility of spermatozoa in split ejaculates. In addition, ejaculates of sub fertile men have also been cleaned to obtain large number of live and motile sperm and "Cleaned up" ejaculates are also used for artificial insemination.

A donor's semen is also used for insemination in cases where husband is severely oligospermic or azoospermic or necrospermic or asthenospermic and when there is no possibility of getting fertilizable sperm from husband's semen. However, donor insemination has complex emotional and legal issues associated with it, but it is very much in practice now. **Artificial insemination by donor (AID)** mainly focuses on couples where male is nearly or fully sterile. With the development of this facility, several **sperm banks** that collect, freeze, and store sperm from anonymous donors began to spring up and today there are several sperm banks all over the world with frozen ejaculates for sale. Artificial insemination technique is simple and requires only sperm, a syringe and a fertile woman. The detection of ovulation is of high importance in artificial insemination. The sperm are deposited with the help of syringe in the woman's vagina or cervix at the appropriate time of the menstrual cycle and then nature is allowed to take its course. However, strict guidelines and high regulatory standards are needed in donor selection, cryopreservation methods of semen, semen banking, and shipping, microbiologic contamination of semen, and confidentiality of donor-recipient relationships. Sometimes a mixture of semen from several donors is used so that actual father of the baby cannot be known. The couple is also encouraged to have frequent intercourses around the insemination time to raise the possibility that, in case pregnancy occurs, the child might be their natural one. With artificial insemination by donor, at least the mother's genes are transmitted to the embryo, and therefore, she gets the experience and emotional satisfaction of giving birth to a child.

22.2 In Vitro Fertilization (IVF)

In vitro fertilization is the fertilization of oocytes outside the female body, in the laboratory dish and because of this, young ones born with the use of this technology are commonly referred to as **test-tube babies**. In vitro fertilization technique was initially used for the woman who had blocked or damaged or no fallopian tubes (tubal factor). But now in addition to tubal factor infertility, this technique is also widely used in-patients with long-standing infertility not responding to conventional treatment, endometriosis, immunological problems, unexplained infertility and male factor infertility. Young embryos can also be nurtured in surrogate mothers in cases when a woman who donates the oocytes cannot support a pregnancy. In vitro fertilization is also used to acquire zygotes with desired genetic characteristics for experimental purposes, and also to study early embryonic development. *In vitro* fertilization is commonly used to increase the populations of rare and endangered species and expensive animal breeds (to get better milk yield or stronger breeds for fieldwork).

External fertilization as seen in several marine invertebrates and in some amphibians led people to believe that the same trick could also be applied to mammalian gametes as well for fertilization in the external environment. First attempts were made around 1880 and the efforts continued until it was realized that the spermatozoa are required to undergo capacitation before fertilizing an ovum. Therefore, spermatozoa were recovered from the female tract some hours after mating and then were used for *in vitro* fertilization, adding them to the eggs held in a suitable medium. Charles Thibault and Louis Dauzier made the first successful experiments on *in vitro* fertilization using rabbit sperm. A few years later, M.C. Chang showed that the embryos of rabbit obtained through *in vitro* fertilization were normal. In addition, when these embryos were transferred to the genital tracts of foster mothers, birth of healthy young rabbits occurred. Since 1960, *in vitro* fertilization in culture medium and subsequent introduction of the embryo into the uterus via cervix is being performed in pigs and cows.

The hamster and mouse spermatozoa were also used for *in vitro* fertilization as they readily undergo capacitation in comparison to rabbit spermatozoa that must reside for some hours in the female genital tract. Human spermatozoa evidently resemble those of mouse and hamster, and not those of rabbit, as they can complete their capacitation *in vitro* in a medium. Human eggs recovered after maturation from the ovary and then fertilized *in vitro* were able to develop normally in culture up to the stage of blastocyst. After this, further development required its transfer to a human recipient. The birth of Louise Joy Brown on July 12, 1978, in England was the first recorded case of the successful IVF procedure in humans by R.G. Edwards and P.C. Steptoe. In India, the first ever scientifically documented baby conceived by IVF was born in August 1986.

IVF is a method of assisted reproduction ("test tube baby") in which the man's sperm and the woman's egg are combined in a laboratory dish where fertilization occurs and the resulting embryo is transferred to the woman's uterus. Therefore, it requires appropriate patient selection, ovarian stimulation, monitoring and timing of oocyte retrieval, and *in vitro* fertilization with viable gametes capable of producing healthy embryos. Both men and women need to be investigated thoroughly as regards the cause of infertility before performing IVF technique. Most medical personals that perform *in vitro* fertilization first use hormonal therapy to stimulate ovarian activity followed by the induction of ripening of ovarian follicles that release the ova. Thus, the basic steps of IVF are **super ovulation**, **oocyte aspiration**, **insemination**, and **fertilization** and **embryo culture**. To obtain the oocytes for *in vitro* fertilization, the woman is primed with natural or synthetic gonadotropins to induce the development and maturation of several follicles (super-ovulation) in her ovaries in a single cycle rather than a single oocyte that normally develops each month. Ultra-sonographic screening of the ovaries monitors growth and maturation of the follicles. When several follicles are judged to be close to maturity, they are then sucked from the ovary through a small incision in the abdomen into which a viewing instrument, known as **laparoscope** is inserted. Several oocytes are collected in this way. On the day the eggs are harvested, the husband provides a semen sample. A few of these oocytes are fertilized with her partner's sperm in a glass receptacle, following which zygotes are formed (Figure 22.1). After a few days of growth of zygote, pre-embryo with normal early development (32-cell stage) is placed back into the uterus for implantation and subsequent growth. The other oocytes are also fertilized and frozen (**frozen embryos**) "for spares" in case the first implantation is not successful-hence, the catchy term **Popsicle babies** is used for such young ones. Since most IVF programs super-ovulate patients to grow many eggs, many patients are left with spare embryos.

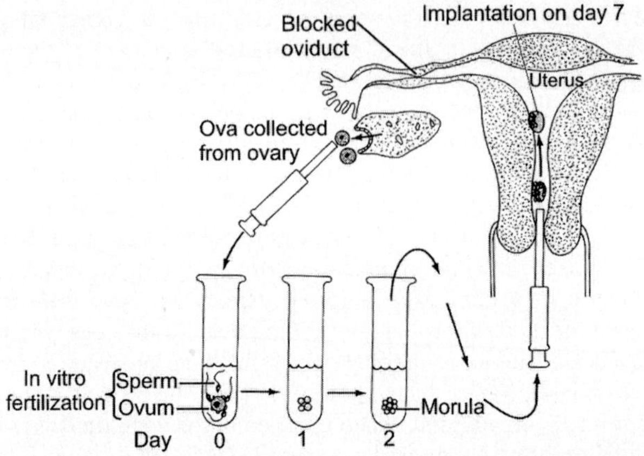

Figure 22.1: ***In Vitro*** **fertilization, culture and implantation of embryo in Women's uterus (IVF-ET).**

It is now possible to freeze the spare embryos after IVF and store them in liquid nitrogen. These embryos can be used later for the same patient if she does not get pregnant on the first cycle or wants another baby in the future without having to go through super-ovulation. Once stored, embryos thus can be used by the couple during a later treatment cycle or donated to another couple or removed from storage. Embryo freezing provides an avenue for successful pregnancy in the patients with hypergonadotrophic hypogonadism or inheritable genetic disorder.

In vitro fertilization is now a therapeutic option to women to achieve pregnancy. Although expensive but it is highly beneficial to many infertile couples. This technique has an added benefit for the couples whose families carry genes for genetic abnormalities. During **pre-implantation diagnosis** of the *in vitro* fertilized embryo, presence of the deleterious genes is tested and accordingly decision for implantation can be taken.

In vitro fertilization technology is improving very fast and many exciting advances have taken place recently. These technologies are now available in India. These include **zona pellucida drilling** by lasers or chemicals. Improved success in implantation is achieved by the thinning of the egg's outer surface done in zona pellucida drilling. The abraded surface of the ovum is the "sticky" site at which the initial attachment to the endometrium occurs. A still newer procedure extracts immature oocytes from the ovary and these isolated eggs are then matured *in vitro* by bathing with gonadotropins. This technique spares the woman from daily hormone injections and also substantially reduces the time and cost of IVF procedure.

22.3 Embryo Transfer (ET)

Embryo transfer is the artificial insertion of one or more young embryos into the uterus. It is a procedure used along with IVF in women to overcome some causes of infertility (IVF-ET). This technique involves placing of a fertilized ovum (zygote) directly into the uterus so that the first days of existence that normally occur in the oviducts and uterus are spent outside the body and the infertility caused by tubal factors is bypassed. Embryo transfer technique is also used to accomplish development in surrogate mothers, in cases where a normal fertile woman cannot bear a child and give birth. This is done by collecting the fertilized embryos from the fallopian tubes of mothers who are incapable of sustaining a pregnancy, and transferring them to the recipients uterus called the surrogate mother, capable of carrying the pregnancy to giving birth of a child. Surrogate animal mothers are also used to get quickly larger progeny of special highly valuable breeds, disease-resistant cattle et c. (see chapter 25) and to nurture endangered species when the natural mothers are scarce. They are also used for experimental purposes to investigate some aspects of reproduction in laboratory animals. The embryo transfer technology has been used extensively in laboratory and farm animals and also in man.

Walter Heape in Cambridge using rabbit in 1890 carried out the first successful embryo transfer but the potentialities of the technique as practical aid to animal breeding were realized only in the twentieth century. The importance of synchrony between the developmental stages of two uteri (that is of donor's and recipient's) was demonstrated in rabbits. This was through experiments involving surgical transfer of embryos following *in vitro* fertilization from a donor female at one stage of pregnancy to the uterus of a recipient female at a different stage. It was realized that embryo transfer gives a high success rate when donor and recipient females are at the same stage of uterine developments or better if the donor is somewhat more advanced in development than the recipient. In contrast, if the embryo is "younger" than the recipient's uterus and is not ready for implantation at that moment when the uterine endometrium is ready for implantation, the success rate becomes low. Synchronization has also been shown to be necessary for embryo transfer in mice, rats, rabbits, sheep and cows (see chapter 25).

Since R.G. Edwards and P.C. Steptoe announced the birth of the first "**test tube baby**" in 1978, treatment for infertility through *in vitro* fertilization and embryo transfer techniques (IVF-ET) gained much popularity, although it is generally used as a last resort for carefully selected patients. To maximize chances of implantation, the patient must remain stationary following introduction of the *in vitro* fertilized embryo into the uterus for four hours or more, followed by about 36 hours of bed rest. Progesterone is administered daily for 10 days during this period to decrease the chances of abortion.

In human, embryo transfer technology is used along with IVF technique in cases of infertility due to tubal factor, or using fertile secondary oocyte of the donor woman in case of infertile mother, or using surrogate mothers for women who cannot support pregnancy. Depending upon the cause of infertility, fertilization may be done *in vitro* or *in vivo* along with artificial insemination using a donor and a recipient for both a male and a female. Thus, it is possible to treat women without ovaries and make them pregnant with embryo transfer technology using a donor oocyte fertilized with the husband's spermatozoon, or eggs and sperm from a healthy donor. Spare eggs from IVF cases can be donated to couples that lack the capacity to produce these gametes. In addition, it is also possible from a woman who has ovaries but no uterus to contribute to the birth of a baby by fertilizing her oocyte with her husband's spermatozoon and transferring the resultant embryo to a surrogate mother. After in vitro fertilization, the morula (32-cell stage) or blastocyst is transferred to the fallopian tube or uterus of the natural or surrogate mother. The transfer of morula or blastocyst into the fallopian tube is called **intra fallopian transfer (IFT)** and into the uterus is called **intra uterine transfer (IUT)**. With embryo transfer technology an infertile recipient (natural mother) or a surrogate mother then carries the fetus to term (Figure 22.2). Harvesting procedure of the fertilized embryos for transfer in case of *in vivo* fertilization involves flushing of the donor's uterus out during the first week of pregnancy through a soft catheter or plastic tube. For IVF-ET, the gametes (ova and spermatozoa) are collected by micro aspiration.

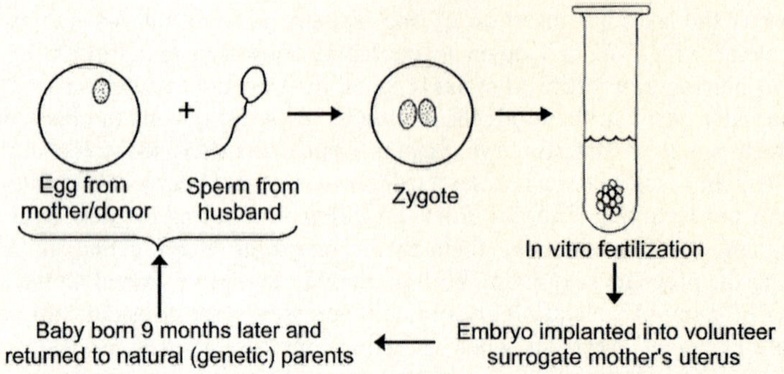

Figure 22.2: ***In Vitro* fertilization followed by surrogate motherhood procedure for successful pregnancy.**

Embryo transfer is a great boon for those women who are infertile or who suffer from serious genetic disorders and would not like to pass on their own genes to the offspring but will get the emotional satisfaction of delivering the baby or of having a baby born using the husband's sperm. However, this procedure is more complicated than ***in vitro*** fertilization, but still the first successful embryo transfer was done in early 1984 and this led to the birth of a healthy baby boy.

Embryo transfer technique is also used to investigate many problems. These are effect of crowding of embryos on embryonic and placental growth, on embryonic mortality, the effect of transferring relatively advanced embryos on the development of their younger foster sibling and the effect of young of varying conceptual age on the timing of parturition, and to analyze genetically the phenomenon of maternal inheritance. Embryo transfer technique has shown that the uterine environment and not the egg cytoplasm influence the growth of the fetus. Potential practical uses of embryo transfer are similar to those of artificial insemination. The number of various animal breeds can be increased with the help of embryo transfer technique using surrogate mothers for pregnancy purposes and high quality breeds as donors for gametes. Reproduction at a distance is also facilitated with the help of embryo transfer technology.

22.4 Gamete Intrafallopian Transfer (GIFT)

The gametes, that is eggs and sperm are reproductive cells. Therefore, the initials in **GIFT** stand for **gamete intrafallopian transfer** or **gamete intrafallopian tube transfer**. GIFT is a byproduct of IVF research and the procedure is suitable for women who have normal fallopian tubes, but suffering with unexplained (idiopathic) infertility. It is generally attempted when the ability of the sperm to fertilize the egg is proven but pregnancy does not result. GIFT is performed in IVF units and the patients who qualify for IVF can be accepted for GIFT. However, the most significant difference between these two techniques is that recipients of GIFT must have at least one healthy fallopian tube. On the other hand, IVF is appropriate treatment for women with tubal disease, or even those with no fallopian tubes at all. GIFT requires laparoscopy for transfer of gametes while an IVF treatment cycles can be completed without laparoscopy. In the case of GIFT, fertilization occurs unobserved inside the body, whereas in IVF, fertilization takes place in a laboratory dish and can be confirmed visually under the microscope.

The initial steps of two techniques, IVF and GIFT are the same. For example, as with *in vitro* fertilization technique, woman is given FSH or a preparation that contains it to stimulate maturation of several ovarian follicles. Ovulatory stimulant drugs such as LH or hCG is then administered to promote ovulation and secondary oocytes are collected by vacuum aspiration. But instead of attempting fertilization in a laboratory dish, the gametes (both, the egg and sperm) are placed in a fallopian tube with a hope that they will mate "naturally". In GIFT, the transfer of gametes in the fallopian tubes takes place within minutes of the egg extraction from the ovaries, it obviates the need for a second surgical procedure. After extraction, the eggs are examined under a microscope and the best are selected and in most units, a maximum of two eggs is used at any one time to reduce the possibility of multiple pregnancies. Also top-grade sperm from the partner's ejaculate are chosen for placement in the fallopian tube. While performing the GIFT technique, the eggs are drawn up into a catheter and a tiny air bubble is inserted to keep the two gametes (egg and sperm) apart from each other, and then sperm is drawn into the same catheter. Sometimes, the sperm are divided into two portions, with the first half being placed in the catheter before the eggs, an air bubble added, followed by the eggs, another air bubble, and then the rest of the sperm. The air bubbles are to ensure that an over-eager sperm does not penetrate one of the eggs before the gametes have been placed in a fallopian tube. The catheter is introduced directly into a fallopian tube through the abdominal incision and the gametes are deposited there for fertilization.

Vaginal GIFT: A major disadvantage with conventional GIFT is that a surgical procedure (laparoscopy) is needed to transfer the eggs and sperm into the fallopian tube. Recently, Dr.Jansen and Anderson in Australia have described a non-surgical method in which the gametes are inserted into the fallopian tubes through the vagina and cervix under ultrasound guidance and therefore the procedure is called as vaginal GIFT. This technique requires a special set of catheters, which allow the doctor to reach the uterine ends of the fallopian tubes through the cervix. Once the catheter is accurately positioned (ultrasound can help in this), the gametes are injected into the tubes trans-vaginally (Vaginal GIFT). Since this technology does not involve surgery, the benefits to the patient are obvious. It becomes less expensive, requires no hospitalization and anesthesia, and there is no scar formation. Also the technique does require much more technical expertise than the conventional GIFT. However, the pregnancy rates with vaginal GIFT are less than with conventional laparoscopic GIFT.

Advantages and cost of GIFT technique: Pregnancy rates are higher for GIFT than for IVF, in fact, GIFT is about twice as successful as IVF. This higher pregnancy rate may be due to the type of patient accepted into GIFT programs or it may also be because for fertilization, *in* vivo, tubal environment is more "physiologic" for the gametes as well as the embryo than the *in vitro* environment. For GIFT technique, the fallopian tube acts as the laboratory and the embryo reach the uterus at a later stage in its development, as in the case of natural conception. Also, the endometrium is more receptive to the embryo in GIFT because of the greater time the embryo takes to reach the uterus. In addition, since conception (fertilization) occurs within the human body in GIFT, the procedure is considered morally acceptable to some religious groups that object to IVF. The cost of a GIFT treatment cycle varies from one program to another, falling within the basic range of Rs. 30,000 to Rs. 75,000 plus, which is typical for IVF.

Variations of GIFT have also been introduced recently with the names like ZIFT, PROST and TET or TEST, details of which are described below.

22.5 Zygote Intrafallopian Transfer (ZIFT)

A hybrid of IVF and GIFT has been developed as a newer technique in which both of these techniques have been combined. This is known as **zygote intrafallopian transfer** or **zygote intrafallopian tube transfer (ZIFT)**. A zygote is the cell formed by the union of a sperm and an egg. It represents the first or pronuclear stage in the life of an embryo. In contrast to GIFT, fertilization is done *in vitro* in ZIFT as in IVF and the zygotes (not the gametes as in GIFT) are transferred to the fallopian tube before cell division occurs. This technique also as with GIFT requires at least one good fallopian tube for transfer. Since the fertilized egg is transferred directly into the fallopian tubes in ZIFT, this procedure is also referred as **tubal embryo transfer (TET)**.

ZIFT is similar to *in vitro* fertilization and embryo transfer with the difference being that the fertilized embryos (zygotes) are transferred into the fallopian tube instead of the uterus. Both these techniques are favorable treatment for women who have severe infertility involving *in vitro* fertilization and in both techniques, the physician selects the best quality embryo for transfer into the female genital tract. As with IVF, in ZIFT procedure also eggs are stimulated and collected and then mixed with sperm in the laboratory dish. Fertilized eggs (zygotes) are then laparoscopically returned to the fallopian tubes in ZIFT from where they are carried into the uterus for implantation and development into a fetus. This procedure is more successful than GIFT because the physician has a greater chance of ensuring that the egg is fertilized.

22.6 Pronuclear Stage Tubal Transfer (PROST)

Pronuclear stage tubal transfer (also called pronuclear ovum stage transfer) is another ***in vitro*** fertilization procedure. It is absolutely similar to ZIFT but in PROST, transfer of the fertilized egg to the fallopian tubes is done at the pronuclear stage, that is a few hours earlier than is done in ZIFT. When a sperm penetrates an egg, the sperm introduces its nuclear material into the egg. Approximately 14 hours after penetration, two distinct pronuclei, one from the sperm and one from the egg are visible under the microscope. Pronuclei are taken as indicators that fertilization has occurred and the transfer to the fallopian tubes is done at this stage and therefore this technique is known as pronuclear stage tubal transfer. The fertilized egg before cell division begins is also called a "zygote" and in ZIFT, transfer of zygote to the fallopian tubes is done, that is a few hours later than pronuclear stage but before cell division begins.

22.7 Tubal Embryo Stage Transfer (TEST)

An extension of ZIFT is known as **tubal embryo stage transfer (TEST**). While zygote transfer is carried out as soon as fertilization is confirmed in ZIFT, embryos are not transferred for two or three days until cell division has begun in case of TEST technique. Thus, in tubal embryo stage transfer technique, a multi-cell-embryo of 2-cell, 4-cell, 8-cell stage is transferred to the fallopian tubes after ***in vitro*** fertilization.

Compared with IVF, these technologies such as GIFT, ZIFT, PROST and TEST has higher costs and risks related to laparoscopy. Also, there is lesser amount of diagnostic information about embryo development in GIFT technique. Therefore, these procedures are used only rarely. IVF is often the first port of call and its costs are usually less. If the ability of the sperm to fertilize the egg is proven but pregnancy does not result, GIFT/ZIFT may be attempted. The cost of ZIFT, PROST or TEST is usually greater than GIFT. Risks resulting from laparoscopy (which may be used to collect eggs) include pelvic infection, puncture of internal organs, and side effects from general anesthesia.

The assisted reproductive technologies, IVF, GIFT, ZIFT, PROST and TEST allow the reproductive tract time to recover from the mechanical manipulation before the gamete or zygote enters the uterus. . These techniques bypass the hazards of high acidity, unsuitable mucus, phagocytes and others (which might prevent fertilization), that sperm encounter in a female reproductive tract by bringing oocytes and sperm together in a laboratory dish in IVF and ZIFT, PROST and TEST or in woman's uterine tubes as in GIFT. In GIFT oocytes mixed with the partner's freshly ejaculated spermatozoa are inserted into the fallopian tubes, while in ZIFT, PROST and TEST oocytes freshly fertilized *in vitro* are inserted into the fallopian tubes. GIFT mimics the normal process of conception by uniting sperm and secondary oocytes in the prospective mother's uterine tubes, whereas ZIFT, PROST and TEST are more successful than GIFT because in these techniques, there are greater chances of ensuring that the egg is fertilized. However, for these techniques the patient must have at least one healthy tube for transfer of gamete or zygote. About 35 % of GIFT or ZIFT births are multiple births and a multiple pregnancy is at high-risk for both mother and fetus. Also, the success rate is limited, especially when only two or three oocytes are inserted. Some of the difficulties associated with these technologies may be related to abnormal endometrial preparation for implantation caused by the hormone treatments, or premature ovulation of incompletely prepared oocytes in addition to that of cost. Yet ZIFT, PROST, or TEST offers the best of both IVF and GIFT in terms of documentation of fertilization *in vitro* and higher pregnancy rates because of tubal transfer of fertilized eggs in various stages of further development.

22.8 Intracytoplasmic Sperm Injection (ICSI)

When infertility is due to impairments in sperm motility or due to the failure of spermatids to develop into spermatozoa, a newer technique called **intracytoplasmic sperm injection (ICSI)** is used. In this, an oocyte is fertilized ***in vitro*** by suctioning a sperm or even a spermatid obtained from the testis of an infertile man into a tiny pipette and then injecting it into the oocyte's cytoplasm. Once the zygote achieved by IVF reaches the 8-cell or 16-cell stage, it is introduced into the uterus using embryo transfer (ET) technology for implantation and subsequent growth.

22.9 Micro-injection fallopian transfer (MIF)

Microinjection fallopian transfer is the microscopic injection of a sperm into an ovum for *in vitro* fertilization followed by its transfer to fallopian tubes. This technique is useful for low sperm counts.

The assisted reproductive technologies are also useful in sex selection. The sex ratio defined as the ratio of males to females in most mammals at birth is near to one, but many prospective parents and cattle breeders would wish it otherwise. Selective infanticide has been extensively practiced in various human societies. Determination of fetal sex is possible by amniocentesis and chromosome analysis of the cells. Chromosome analysis technique involves the isolation of Y sperm from X sperm and, thus, sex ratio may be altered, in favor of male offspring whereby Y spermatozoa outdistance X spermatozoa. This is facilitated by the recent use of the dye quinacrine, which causes an intense fluorescence of Y-chromosomes, and consequently permits the ready identification of male cells. Prenatal sex selection of a fetus could then be followed by selective abortion of the fetuses of the undesired sex. Although, this approach might not be suitable for humans, yet it could prove to be of great value in stockbreeding. Sperm carrying an X-chromosome can be separated from those with a Y, the former being female and the latter male-determining factor. Using Sephadex gel filtration, a fraction rich in X-bearing sperm can be obtained. This technique and others may allow sex selection in artificial insemination and may be applied in cases of human hereditary diseases such as hemophilia to prevent genetic expression in the offspring. The process used to isolate Y sperm also selects out a fraction relatively free of cellular debris, dead spermatozoa, and morphologically and genetically abnormal spermatozoa. Genetic constitution of offspring may be controlled by selective marriages, that is, by discouraging some couples from marrying. Sex selection technique decreases the risk of transmitting the genetic defects to subsequent generations.

Summary

Several methods have been used to modify or stimulate the process of human and animal reproduction and also to treat severe cases of infertility in human male and female.

Assisted Reproductive Techniques (ART) are new techniques that have developed over several years to help infertile couples to have children and also in animal breeding to improve in farming and achieving better yielding and disease-resistant varieties.

Assisted reproductive technologies are artificial insemination (AI) with fresh or frozen semen, *in vitro* fertilization (IVF), embryo transfer (ET), gamete intrafallopian transfer (GIFT), zygote intrafallopian transfer (ZIFT), pronuclear stage transfer (PROST), tubal embryo stage transfer (TEST), intracytoplasmic sperm injection (ICSI) and micro-injection fallopian transfer (MIF).

Artificial insemination (AI) can be defined as the intra-vaginal or intra-cervical injection of spermatozoa to achieve fertilization. For artificial insemination, either husband's sperm or donor's sperm depending upon the degree of infertility in the male partner may be used and accordingly, it is known as AIH (artificial insemination using husband's semen) or AID (artificial insemination using donor's semen) respectively.

In vitro fertilization (IVF) is the "test tube baby" technology in which fertilization of egg and sperm is done in the glass receptacle in the laboratory and the embryo is transferred to the uterus. IVF is often used when a woman's fallopian tubes are blocked. First, medication is given to stimulate the ovaries to produce multiple eggs. Once mature, the eggs are suctioned from the ovaries and placed in a laboratory culture dish with the man's sperm for fertilization. The dish is then placed in an incubator. About two days later, three to five embryos are transferred to the woman's uterus. This is the embryo transfer technology (ET). If the woman does not become pregnant, it is tried again in the next cycle. Since most IVF programs super-ovulate patients to grow many eggs, there are often many embryos. These embryos are frozen and stored in liquid nitrogen and can be used later for the same patient so that she can have another embryo transfer cycle done without having to go through super-ovulation and egg harvest or may be donated or used for research work.

Gamete intrafallopian transfer or GIFT is similar to IVF, but is used when the woman has at least one normal fallopian tube. In addition, three to five eggs are placed in the fallopian tube along with the man's sperm for fertilization inside the woman's body.

Zygote intrafallopian transfer or ZIFT (also called tubal embryo transfer) is a hybrid of IVF and GIFT. In this technology, the retrieved eggs from the woman's ovaries are fertilized in the lab and the zygote (not the gamete) is replaced in the fallopian tubes rather than uterus.

Pronuclear stage tubal transfer or PROST (also called pronuclear ovum stage transfer) is another ***in vitro*** fertilization procedure. It is absolutely similar to ZIFT but transfers the fertilized egg to the fallopian tubes at the pronuclear stage.

An extension of ZIFT is known as tubal embryo stage transfer (TEST). While zygote transfer is carried out as soon as fertilization is confirmed in ZIFT, embryos are not transferred for two or three days until cell division (a multi-cell-embryo of 2-cell, 4-cell, 8-cell) has begun in case of TEST technique.

When infertility is due to impairments in sperm motility or due to the failure of spermatids to develop into spermatozoa, intracytoplasmic sperm injection (ICSI) technology is used. In this, an oocyte is fertilized ***in vitro*** by suctioning a sperm or even a spermatid obtained from the testis of an infertile man into a tiny pipette and then injecting it into the oocyte's cytoplasm. Once the zygote achieved by IVF reaches the 8-cell or 16-cell stage, it is introduced into the uterus using embryo transfer technology for implantation and subsequent growth.

Microinjection fallopian transfer (MIF) is the microscopic injection of a sperm into an ovum for *in vitro* fertilization followed by its transfer to fallopian tubes. This technique is useful for low sperm counts.

Questions

1. What are assisted reproductive technology? How are they beneficial to infertile couples?
2. Write notes on artificial insemination, in vitro fertilization, embryo transfer, intracytoplasmic sperm injection and pronuclear stage tubal transfer.
3. What are GIFT, ZIFT, PROST and TEST? How do they differ from each other and also from IVF?

Chapter 23

Family Planning

In the previous chapters we have learnt that several endocrine and neuroendocrine mechanisms regulate the physiologic mechanisms involved in the production, maturation, and transport of the sperm and egg, and in fertilization, implantation, and pregnancy. These mechanisms involve complex interactions amongst the external environment, the central nervous system, the hypothalamic hormones, and the pituitary hormones along with the gonadal functions and hormones. In addition to these interactions, in human, unlike most other mammalian species, coitus and ovulation are not synchronized. Also, the sexual receptivity of human female is not confined to the period of ovulation only and remarkable differences occur in reproductive ability of woman throughout the menstrual cycle. Therefore in humans, it becomes difficult to avoid unwanted births, and also to regulate the intervals between pregnancies. However, there are many possible sites at which reproductive processes in female as well as male can be altered to prevent fertilization, and/or implantation and as a result conception.

23.1 Contraception

The term **Contraception** literally means 'being able to block conception' (*contra* =against; *cept* =taking place). Contraception is usually understood to mean preventing fertilization, but reproductive physiologists also use it to mean the period of time from ovulation/fertilization lasting until implantation is completed. In simple terms contraceptive technologies mean fertility regulating methods, or fertility preventive methods, which help women/men to avoid unwanted pregnancies. The term's **birth control** and **family planning** also mean the same and refer to the voluntary regulation of the number of offspring produced by a couple. This regulation or control requires a method of contraception designed to avoid and prevent fertilization of an egg cell or implantation of a blastocyst and thus pregnancy following sexual intercourse. However, an expert committee of the WHO, in 1971 defined **family planning** in the following manner. It is " a way of thinking and living that is adopted voluntarily, upon the basis of knowledge, attitudes and responsible decisions by individuals and couples, in order to promote the health and welfare of the family group and thus, contribute effectively to the social development of a country".

Wide application of contraceptive technologies has resulted in increased delinking of human sexuality from reproduction. However, the key to birth control is the dependability of a couple on the contraceptive technique in use. Birth control techniques range from methods of preventing fertilization to the interruption of pregnancy at various stages. The contraceptive products currently available in the market have many sites of action for blocking pregnancy. They mainly interfere with one of the three physiological sites in reproductive process. These are sperm and ovum transport in the female reproductive tract (thus blocking fertilization), ovulation, and/or implantation of an egg. Table 23.1 gives various methods that interfere at different stages in reproduction to prevent the process of conception and pregnancy.

Table 23.1: Methods that interfere at different stages of reproduction in Human male and female to prevent the process of conception

Method of interference		Stage to prevent the process of conception
Male	Vasectomy	Transport of sperm down the male duct system
	Coitus interruptus, Condom	Deposition in the female vagina
Female	Birth Control Pill, Subcutaneous Progestin implants	Ovulation
	Tubal Ligation	Transport down of ovulated egg into uterine tube
	Spermicides Diaphragm Cervical Cap Vaginal Pouch	Movement of sperm through the female reproductive tract during sexual intercourse
	Morning after pill (MAP)	Union of sperm and egg after sexual intercourse
	Intra-uterine device (IUD) Progesterone mini-pill Depot-provera injection Morning after pill (MAP)	Implantation in properly prepared endometrium
	Medical termination of pregnancy through salting out, dilation and curettage (D and C), RU 486	Abortion of fetus, termination of pregnancy

23.2 Birth Control Methods

The contraceptive methods may broadly be grouped into two classes. These are the **Spacing methods** and the **Termination methods**. Further, the term **conventional contraceptives** are used to denote those methods, which require action at the time of sexual intercourse. All the contraceptive techniques used can be grouped in the following categories. These are **Natural methods, barrier methods, chemical methods, surgical methods,** and **miscellaneous methods**.

Natural methods of birth control are fertility awareness-based methods and require learning about the days in the menstrual cycle on which a woman can get pregnant. Barrier and surgical methods of contraception prevent meeting of male and female gametes and thus fertilization. On the other hand, chemical methods used for contraception may act by preventing ovulation and/or implantation.

Miscellaneous methods may include **Intra uterine devices (IUD), intra cervical devices (ICD)** or **vaginal rings, Lactational Amenorrhea (LAM)** and **Medical Termination of Pregnancy (MTP)**. An **Intra uterine device (IUD)** along with other devices is a kind of barrier method but shows different kind of action, and therefore, is described separately. Legal **abortion** and **medical termination of pregnancy** strictly speaking cannot be called a method of contraception. It is a technique performed to eliminate the products of conception or unwanted pregnancy, and therefore, is also described separately.

All the above-mentioned contraceptive methods are the spacing methods except the male and female sterilization in the surgical methods, which is used more as a terminal method of contraception. All these methods of contraception work by disrupting one of the three major steps in the reproductive processes. However, in spite of considerable progress that has occurred through evolutionary changes on most of the existing contraceptive technologies, yet no single method has evolved so far as an ideal method of birth control that can be considered as "**a perfect contraceptive**". Each method has its advantages and disadvantages even though today's spermicides, condoms, contraceptive pills, IUDs and surgical procedures are safer and more widely acceptable in comparison to their earlier prototypes.

The only method of preventing pregnancy that is 100 % reliable is the total avoidance of sexual intercourse.

23.3 Natural methods

Abstinence: The only method of birth control that is fully effective and safe is the complete avoidance of sexual intercourse. This is called **abstinence**. Theoretically, it sounds simple but it amounts to repression of a natural force. Also, it is liable to manifest itself in other directions such as temperamental changes and sometimes-even nervous breakdown. Therefore, it is not considered as a method of contraception, which can be advocated to the masses.

Coitus interruptus: In this method, the male partner withdraws the phallus (an externally protruding, tactile-sensitive male organ, usually refers to a penis) before ejaculation that is before climax is reached. Thus, in coitus interruptus ejaculate is deposited outside the vagina and because of this, it is also called a **male withdrawal** method. It is certainly the oldest method of reversible contraception and probably remains one of the most widely used on a global scale even today. During 18th and 19th centuries, coitus interruptus was widely practiced especially in Europe. However, this method requires high degree of motivation and perfect understanding between partners.
Advantages: It requires no supplies, specific preparation and also costs nothing.
Disadvantages: Even if successfully practiced, it is not an adequate safeguard against conception, because sperms may leak out before actual ejaculation occurs. It demands self-control of the male. It causes tension and strain, placing a heavy responsibility upon the male partner who feels guilty if he fails to withdraw in time. Also, it causes tension and fear in the female, since the male partner may fail to withdraw at the right time. Woman may not get orgasm and additional manual stimulation may be necessary for sexual satisfaction. Failure rate is quite high. This method offers no protection against transmission of sexually transmitted diseases (STDs).

Post-coital douche: Post-coital douche means washing of vagina after sexual intercourse. Washing with plain water, vinegar, and various other products have long been used for contraceptive purposes. It is intended to remove the sperm from the vagina after sexual intercourse. Also the chemicals used in post-coital douche have the ability to kill and/or immobilize the ejaculated sperms.
Advantages: It may be useful only as an emergency measure, e.g. if condom bursts.
Disadvantages: It is not a very effective method and the pregnancy rate is quite high. Sperms can reach the uterus within 90 seconds following ejaculation thus giving not much time for washing. Repeated use of strong solutions may cause damage to the vaginal wall. Also, this method is inconvenient and therefore, its use has declined drastically.

Prolonged lactation or Lactational amenorrhea method (LAM): Lactation is related to breastfeeding and amenorrhea means not having menstrual bleeding. In simple term, no menstrual bleeding means no reproductive cycle and no ovulation and thus no chance of conception.

For a long time women have known that they are less likely to become pregnant after a delivery if they breast feed their babies. This has led women to extend lactation deliberately with the intentions to delay or avoid pregnancy since ovulation is kept suppressed and amenorrhea is prolonged during the period of lactation. Not more than 5-10 % of women conceive during lactational amenorrhea. However, once menstruation returns continued lactation no longer offers any protection against pregnancy. Nearly 20-50 % women start menstruating by 6 months after childbirth. Giving baby "only" breast milk with little or no other food gives best protection from pregnancy. However, it is effective only for first 6 months after childbirth. Also, it does not provide protection against STIs or HIV/AIDS. Once the baby is 6 months or older, woman should use another method of family planning. Bleeding in first 8 weeks after childbirth does not count. However, LAM cannot be used if woman had two or straighter days of menstrual bleeding after eight weeks of childbirth.

Advantages: It costs nothing and requires no special preparation. Prolonged breast-feeding is practical in many developing countries, although it is not known how many practice it as a contraceptive measure.

Disadvantages: It cannot postpone pregnancy indefinitely, and pregnancy may sometimes occur even before the reappearance of menses after delivery. Prolonged breast-feeding may lead to, a) trauma to mother's nipple, and b) malnutrition of the child, if no supplementary food is given

Rhythm method (Safe period): The rhythm method is also called **timed coitus** or **natural family planning** and requires abstinence from sexual intercourse during a few days before and a few days after ovulation. Since complete abstinence, which is the only completely effective method of birth control, is unpopular for obvious reasons, many people practice periodic abstinence during the time of ovulation, when fertility is highest (that is why termed as rhythm method). Rhythm method is the only method approved by Roman Catholic Church. It was the first physiologically based contraceptive method developed in 1930s and was used in various cultures from South America to East Africa. This method takes advantage of the fact that a secondary oocyte is fertilizable only for 24 hours and is available for fertilization for 3 to 5 days in each reproductive cycle. This is because sperms can survive a maximum of 3 days in the female genital tract (survival time of two together, sperm and ovum becomes 3-5). Thus, the couple abstains from intercourse during this fertile period (3 days before ovulation, the day of ovulation, and 3 days after ovulation). However, the efficiency of this method in preventing pregnancy depends on the accuracy of predicting the time of ovulation.

Three methods are used to predict the time of ovulation in the menstrual cycle. The first involves monitoring of ovarian cycle and the length of menstruation for at least 6 months and avoiding intercourse on the days preceding and following ovulation (at mid-cycle). This method has a high failure rate because many women exhibit a large variation in length of monthly cycles. The second method involves daily monitoring of basal body temperature and avoiding intercourse on the days preceding and following ovulation, as the body temperature decreases during the period of ovulation (Figure 23.1). This method also has a high failure rate because the temperature shifts that occur during the ovarian cycle are small (usually less than one degree) and are difficult to be detected accurately. The third method of identifying the time of ovulation requires monitoring the consistency of cervical mucus. The cervical mucus becomes clear, thin, and stringy around the time of ovulation (Figure 23.2). Predicting ovulation on the basis of consistency of cervical mucus also has a high failure rate because of the difficulty of accurately identifying these changes.

In 1932, Ogino published his method of calculation for the fertile period and called it as **calendar rhythm method**. He assumed that ovulation occurs between 16th to 12th days before the onset of next menses (days 13-17 of the menstrual cycle). Counting 3 days as the maximum survival time of spermatozoa, he calculated that a woman is fertile from 19th to 12th days before next menstruation. Thus according to this schedule, a woman is fertile from day 10 to day 17 (both days inclusive) after onset of menstruation in a 28-day cycle. This is known as the '**unsafe period**' (fertile phase) during which coitus should be avoided. Rest of the days in a menstrual cycle is considered as the '**safe period**'. Statistically, day 14 is the most fertile day of the cycle.

Advantages: This is the only method approved by Roman Catholic Church. There are no side effects.

Disadvantages: Opportunity for sex act is reduced. The major problem with all the variations in the calendar rhythm method is that this method is based on a rough forecasting of a probable future event. Therefore, it is not suitable for use by woman with cycles less than 20 days or those with vary irregular cycles varying between 23 to 31 days. National Family Planning (NFP) includes temperature method and cervical mucus method but excludes calendar rhythm for using it as a contraceptive method. However, all these methods come under the category of '**periodic abstinence**' and rely primarily on signs and symptoms of fertile period of the cycle.

Basal Body Temperature (BBT) Method: A brief mention of this method has already been done in the rhythm method since change in body temperature is one of the symptoms considered in predicting the time of ovulation. In 1905 Van de Velde noticed that temperature of one of his patient dropped towards the middle of the cycle and this was followed by a rise to a plateau, which was maintained almost up to the next menstruation. He casually suggested that the low point of temperature reading might be related to ovulation. But it took almost 30 years to establish this character of ovarian cycle and use it as one of the natural contraceptive methods.

BBT or basal body temperature (at rest) is quickly influenced by a rise in plasma progesterone and in human the average mid cycle temperature shift is in the order of 0.2 ^{0}C or 0.6^{0}F (Figure 23.1). This technique aims to pinpoint actual day of ovulation more effectively than other symptoms. However, a combination of calendar method technique and BBT may be more effective to use in contraception. The effectiveness of the BBT method depends on: 1) great care in taking BBT daily with special BBT thermometers having expanded scales of 96-100 ^{0}F. It should be taken at the same time every morning before any physical activity. Although a woman can recognize the rise in temperature during each cycle, but illness or emotional tension can alter that. Also readings may be masked during periods of infection because the temperature changes are very small, only 0.2 - 0.4 ^{0}C (0.4 – 0.8^{0}F) and easy to misinterpret. In addition, sometimes the temperature rise coinciding with ovulation charts are non-interpretable.

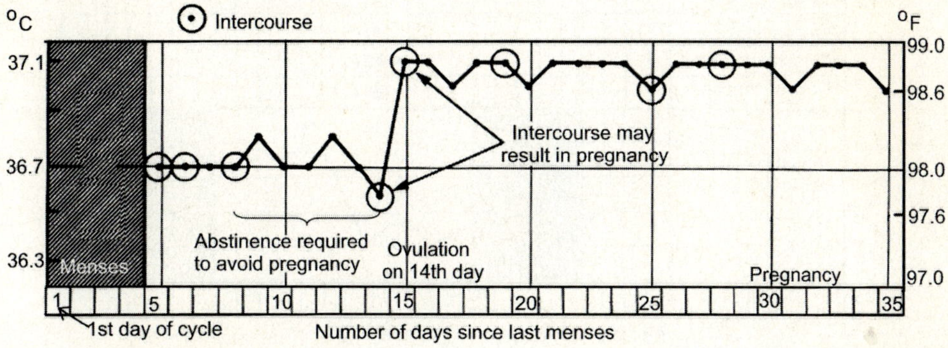

Figure 23.1: Basal body temperature method of birth control.

Advantage: It costs nothing and has no side effects.
Disadvantage: The major drawback of the BBT method is that abstinence is necessary for the entire pre-ovulatory period when no ovulation occurs as is common after menarche, during lactation, and around menopause. Thus, only a few couples use the temperature method alone as a means of contraception.

Cervical Mucus Method (Billings Method): Estrogen and progesterone regulate the secretory and physical-chemical properties of cervical mucus. In the pre-ovulatory phase, secretion of mucus by cervix increases under the stimulus of rising estrogen levels. After ovulation, under the influence of progesterone, mucus thickens and lessens in quantity.

According to Billings and his associates, the major features of vaginal mucus discharge are 1) menstrual bleeding is followed by a variable number of days when no loss of vaginal mucus is present. These are the infertile dry days. 2) Onset of mucus symptoms is characterized by appearance of increasing quantities of "cloudy" (sticky) secretion which is identified initially by a feeling of 'moistness' and then of 'sweatiness'. 3) Secretion of abundant, lubricating mucus identified by a feeling of wetness and having the physical characteristics of rawish of egg. Presence of such cervical mucus called "peak symptom", lasts for 1-2 days and its occurrence is an immediate forewarning of ovulation (Figure 23. 2). This mucus in female genital tract is most favorable for sperm transport. 4) After ovulation, mucus becomes thick, opaque and also diminishes in volume. The duration of this mucus symptom is variable and is followed by days when no vaginal mucus loss is observed. Sperm transport in this mucus is poor and is also 'hostile' to sperm. Abstinence should start on or day earlier to observation of clear cervical mucus after menses and must continue until 4th day after peak symptom. All subsequent days until menstruation begins again are considered infertile. Necessary precautions to be taken are 1) to avoid any confusion of cervical mucus with seminal fluid or vaginal secretions due to sexual stimulation. 2) Abstinence is recommended during entire first month of instruction. 3) During pre-ovulatory dry days, intercourse is not permitted on consecutive days, since new users can confuse seminal fluid with cervical mucus. Abstinence is necessary to ensure accurate observation of mucus.

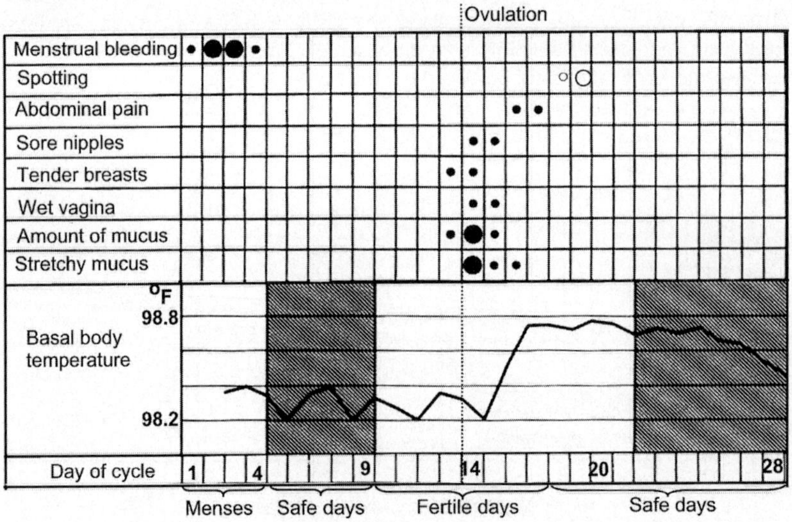

Figure 23.2: Sympto-thermal method of birth control.

Advantage: It costs nothing and has no side effects.
Disadvantage: Pregnancy may occur due to 1) when mucus flow begins too late, 2) because spermatozoa in the female reproductive tract are capable of fertilizing ova for 3 days, therefore, to provide adequate warning of fertile period, mucus flow must start more than 3 days before ovulation. 3) About 1/5th to ½ of the pregnancies due to method failure occur after intercourse on a pre-ovulatory 'dry day' especially the day before mucus is first noticed. 4) Sometimes peak symptoms occur too early that is, if it precedes ovulation by 3 days, not only would the ovum still be fertilizable but also the mucus could still permit sperm entry. 5) Many times mucus is not sensed or interpreted correctly; 7 to 25 % of women in various studies have reported difficulty in interpreting mucus patterns.

Sympto Thermal Method (STM): This method combines various techniques for identifying the fertile and infertile period of the ovulatory cycle. The signs of ovulation time in a cycle include increased basal body temperature; production of clear, stretchy cervical mucus; abundant cervical mucus; abdominal pain; inter-menstrual bleeding; self observed changes in position, texture and dilation of cervix; breast tenderness; edema and mood changes (Figure 23.2). World Health Organization (WHO) curriculum outline (1976-77) calls for abstinence from sex when calendar calculation indicates or when mucus is first noticed after menses whichever is earlier. If a couple abstains from sexual intercourse when the signs of ovulation are present and for 3 days afterwards, the chances of pregnancy are decreased. However, this method has its own difficulty. In some women, peak mucus symptoms and BBT rise do not coincide. Also, fertilization is quite likely if intercourse occurred up to 2 days before ovulation. Yet in contrast to temperature method, STM allows coitus before ovulation.

Advantage: It has advantages of all the natural methods with comparatively less failure rates and no side effects.

Disadvantage: Since the method is based on self-assessment of the ovulation time, failure rate may be high especially in cases of irregular menstrual cycles.

These natural methods do not work for all women. However, these may become more reliable and helpful with an "**ovulation predictor kit**" that detects the LH surge preceding ovulation. Further, two new variations on fertility awareness-based approaches have been introduced to help women track their fertile days. These are called the **Standard Days Method** and the **Two Day Method**. Couples can use the Standard Days Method to identify their likely fertile days and limit unprotected sex to days on which woman is not likely to be fertile. The Standard Days Method is based on the timings of the "fertile window" during the woman's menstrual cycle. A string of color-coded beads called Cycle Beads have been created to help women to keep track of their fertile days (Figure 23.3). The Cycle Beads represent a woman's menstrual cycle. To use Cycle Beads, a woman moves a rubber ring to the next bead each day to identify where she is in her cycle. The color-coded beads indicate whether she is on a fertile or infertile day. White bead signifies a fertile day and the couple must avoid unprotected sex at that time. A computer simulation have been used to develop this method, which took into account the variation in the timing of ovulation while minimizing the number of days that users must avoid unprotected sex. Their analyses concluded that the fertile period occurs most likely between days 8 and 19 of the menstrual cycle. This method works best for women whose menstrual cycles are between 26 and 32 days and is not effective for women having shorter or longer cycles than these. The Two Day Method on the other hand helps women determine whether they are fertile on any given day based on the presence or absence of cervical secretions. This method is based on the fact that a woman's cervical secretions are key to her fertility, and without secretions sperm have difficulty traveling to the egg. This method is appropriate for women with cycles of any length, regardless of regularity. To use this method, a woman must ask her two questions each day. These are i) "did I notice secretions today" and ii) "did I notice secretions yesterday". If she noticed secretions of any type either today or yesterday, she should consider herself to be in fertile phase of the cycle and must avoid unprotected sex. If the secretion is not noticed for two days consecutively, she is unlikely to get pregnant from sex taking place that day. However, couples that can use this method successfully are those who can avoid unprotected sex for about 10-15 days per cycle. But this method provides a simpler approach to identify the fertile days than either the Billings Ovulation Method or the Symptothermal Method, which also involve observations of cervical secretions.

Family planning methods based on fertility awareness, however, depend on commitment from and cooperation of both partners to avoid unprotected sex during the woman's fertile times. In addition, involvement of male partner is crucial to the effective use of these contraceptive methods. Also, these methods are impractical for those couples who cannot communicate about sex with each other and for women who lack the power to choose between when to have protected sex or not.

23.4 Barrier Methods

Barrier methods are the **mechanical** or "**occlusive**" methods that are designed in such a way as to prevent sperm from gaining access to the uterine cavity and uterine tubes. These methods are suitable for both men and women. Their popularity has increased recently because of contraceptive as well as non-contraceptive advantages. In addition to preventing pregnancy, barrier methods also provide some protection against sexually transmitted diseases (STDs) such as HIV infection, in contrast to other contraceptive methods and IUDs, which provide no such protection.

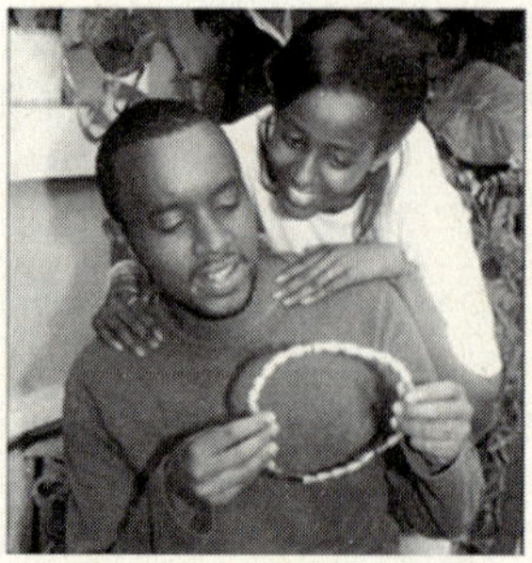

Figure 23.3: Standard days method, color-coded cycle beads help track the women's fertile days.

Barrier methods include condoms, caps, diaphragms, and contraceptive sponges. All these contraceptives prevent live sperm from entering the cervical canal by mechanical occlusions. However, these methods vary in effectiveness and to increase their contraceptive reliability, barrier methods are often used with chemical methods such as spermicidal creams, jellies and foams, which kill sperms.

Condoms: Condoms are penile sheaths for males (Figure 23.4). In India, it is better known by its trade name 'NIRODH' (a Sanskrit word meaning prevention). The prototype of the modern condom appeared in as early as the 16th Century as a sheath made of animal tissue. Condoms were the first modern family planning technology sold in pharmacies. The invention of vulcanization of rubber in mid 19th Century and the introduction of liquid latex in the 1920s made possible the production of cheap condoms, which were affordable by many. Condom is receiving new attention today as an effective, simple "spacing" method of contraception without any side effects. In addition to preventing pregnancy, condom protects both men and women from sexually transmitted diseases (STDs).

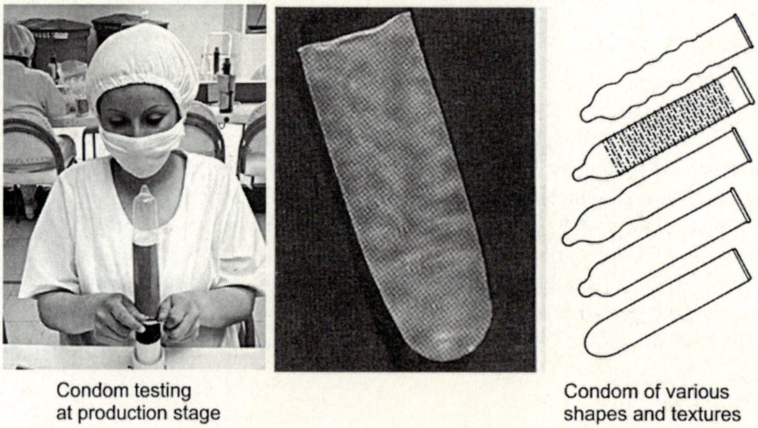

Figure 23.4: Condoms for Men.

Condoms are thin sheaths of latex (rubber) that is worn over the erected penis before intercourse thereby preventing sperm from entering the female reproductive tract. These are intended for single use only. To reduce the risk of bursting during use, it is important to leave half an inch or more at the teat end free and empty from air at the time of unrolling it on the erected male organ. Soon after the climax in male partner is over, the male organ gets smaller and the condom becomes loose. Therefore, it is very important that immediately after the climax, the male organ is carefully withdrawn holding the condom securely so as to prevent any leakage from the sides. Each condom is manufactured under strict quality control (Figure 23.4). Its dimensions are prescribed and is tested for tensile strength as well as for presence of minute holes by filling it with 300-ml water, suspending and wrapping it in absorbent paper. Strength rather than existence of holes are more important in ensuring its contraceptive reliability. If a condom bursts, the risk of pregnancy is much greater than a pinhole present in the condom. Today high-quality condoms are available in a range of sizes, thickness, shapes, textures, and colors to appeal to different customers (Figure 23.4). They include plain or reservoir-ended, straight-sided or shaped, smooth or textured, dry or lubricated, and an inexpensive or an expensive brand. Modern condoms are strong and durable with a shelf life of three to five years in temperate climates when stored properly. They deteriorate faster at higher temperatures and also when exposed to humidity, light, oxygen and certain chemicals. New designs of condoms are loose sheaths made of durable polyurethane plastic. Family Health International (FHI) is working with two lubricated models-one slips on the penis like a sock, and the other is rolled like the conventional latex condom. Compared with latex, plastic condom is stronger, longer lasting, less sensitive to heat and humidity, easier to manufacture, and is not damaged by oil-based lubricants.

In India, condom is manufactured mainly in two factories, Hindustan Latex (Trivandrum) and London Rubber Industries (Chennai). The Government has subsidized the cost of condom. It sells 3 brands of condoms-*Dry Nirodh*, *Deluxe Nirodh*, and *Super-Deluxe Nirodh*. Since the effectiveness of condom is increased if used along with some contraceptive cream or jelly, a recent addition to the range of condoms is the spermicidal condom. The lubricant contains the spermicide nonoxynol-9, commonly used in spermicidal foams, gels, suppositories, and sponges.

Advantage: It provides protection against pregnancy as well as sexually transmitted diseases (STD). Condoms prevent transmission of sexually transmitted diseases, including the infection that causes acquired immune deficiency syndrome (AIDS) and Venereal Diseases (VD). It is one of the most effective methods, and is widely used in all countries. It is simple to use, and can easily be used in all situations. It has no side effects. Finding intact condom after its use reassures the effectiveness of the contraception. Condoms are cheap and can easily be obtained from neighborhood outlets.

Disadvantage: Foreplay before the sexual act is interrupted. It may interfere with sex enjoyment in some couples.

Recently introduced **female condoms** are also becoming popular now a days (Figure 23.5). These are also called a **vaginal pouch** and resemble a small plastic bag. Vaginal pouch is made of two flexible rings connected by a polyurethane sheath. One ring is inserted to fit over the cervix, and the other ring remains outside the vagina and covers the female external genitalia. A woman inserts it into her vagina prior to intercourse. The device blocks sperm from reaching the cervix. The other brands of female condoms are **FC Female condom** and **Women's Choice Female Condom**. The FC female condom formerly called **Reality vaginal condom** is a polyurethane tube, 17 cm long, with flexible polyurethane rings at either end. The device is inserted like a diaphragm. The inner ring fits behind the pubic bone, and the outer ring covers the labia. The **vaginal sheath** known as the **Women's Choice Female Condom** is inserted like a tampon with a reusable plastic applicator. The Condom is shaped like a male condom but with a thickened inner tip that fits in the upper vagina and an outer ring that fits over the labia. Now a **latex panty** with a built-in "condom" is also available. A latex panty is with a built-in rolled pouch that fits over the opening of the vagina. Before intercourse, the woman pushes the pouch into the vagina. This device covers the entire perineum and outer genitalia, and provides maximum protection against all STDs also. However, female condom is six to eight times the average price of the male condom and like the latex male condoms, these are also not recommended for reuse.

Several newer female condoms which are made of less costly material include **FC2**, the **VA feminine condom** (also known as the **Reddy female condom**), and the **PATH Woman's Condom**. These are now in clinical trials. PATH Woman's Condom consists of a dissolving capsule intended to make insertion easier, a polyurethane condom pouch, and a soft outer ring, allowing for nearly universal fit. Once inserted, sections of urethane foam on the condom pouch allow the condom to cling lightly to the vaginal walls so that it does not move during use.

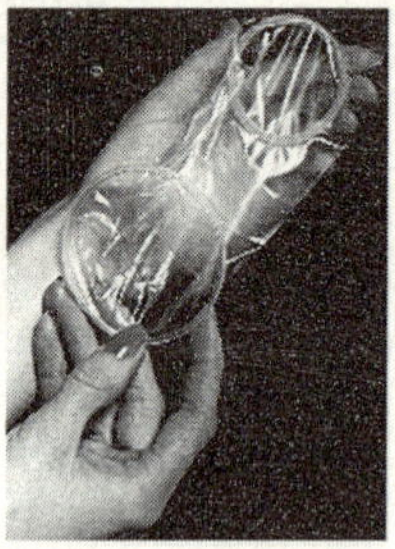

The Reality Vaginal Condom

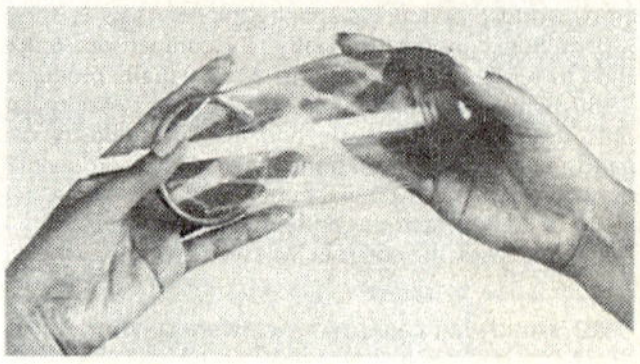

The Women's Choice
Female Condom with Applicator

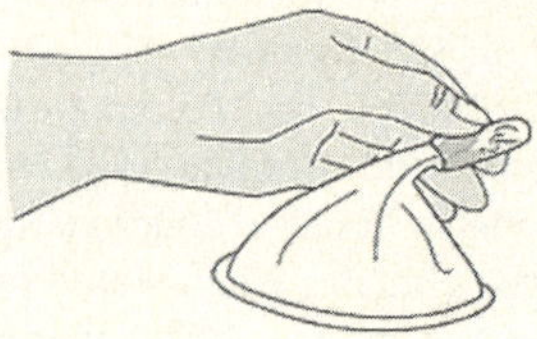

The Path- Female Condom

Figure 23.5: Condoms for Women.

Increasingly, companies are manufacturing male and female condoms in different materials to expand variety. New male condoms are being developed from non-latex materials and female condoms from latex. Manufacturing condoms from different materials will expand variety and also reduce cost, avoid allergic reactions that occur in some users and in turn will encourage their more use. Synthetic non-latex male condoms are made of polyurethane or styrene ethylene butylenes styrene (SEBS), a synthetic material commercially known as Tactylon. These have two advantages over latex condoms: I) they have a longer shelf life, and 2) can also be used with oil-based lubricants, which can damage latex condoms. In addition, some users feel that they have fewer odors, fit more comfortably, are less constricting, and transfer body heat better than latex condoms. Despite the greater breakage and slippage rates of these new condoms, most non-latex condoms are as effective as latex condoms in preventing pregnancies.

Caps: Caps, diaphragms, and sponges are vaginal barriers, and thus are for females. These are rubber or plastic devices that cover the entrance to the cervix and prevent sperm from entering the uterus. Such caps include vaginal diaphragms, cervical caps, vault caps, and vimule caps (Figure 23.6), made in various sizes and intended for repeated use along with spermicides. Diaphragm is a soft rubber vaginal cup with a metal spring reinforcing the rim. Cervical caps, which act similar to vaginal diaphragm, block the cervix only and can be worn for longer periods prior to their removal. These are held in place by suction but fitting a woman with a cap requires properly trained health personnel.

The Diaphragm: A German physician invented Diaphragm in 1882. That is why it is also known as "**Dutch cap**". Diaphragm is thin, hemispherical, rubber dome with a circular, rubber-covered metal spring reinforced rim (Figure 23.6). The external diameter of the rim is the size of the diaphragm and thus diaphragms are available in different sizes ranging from 50-105 mm (2-4 inches). Most women require diaphragms measuring 70-80 mm. Various types of diaphragms are available, such as, the flat spring type, the coil-spring type, and the arcing diaphragm (Figure 23.7). Both the flat-spring and coil-spring types fold on a single plane when compressed while the arcing diaphragm forms an arc and many women find it easier to insert. The diaphragm fits diagonally across the vagina covering the cervix (Figure 23.8 A, B and C). It is held in place by tension of the spring and by vaginal musculature. While the device acts as a barrier to most sperm, it does not fit tightly enough to entirely prevent the passage of all spermatozoa. Therefore, it is recommended to use diaphragm always with a spermicidal cream or jelly (Figure 23.8 D).

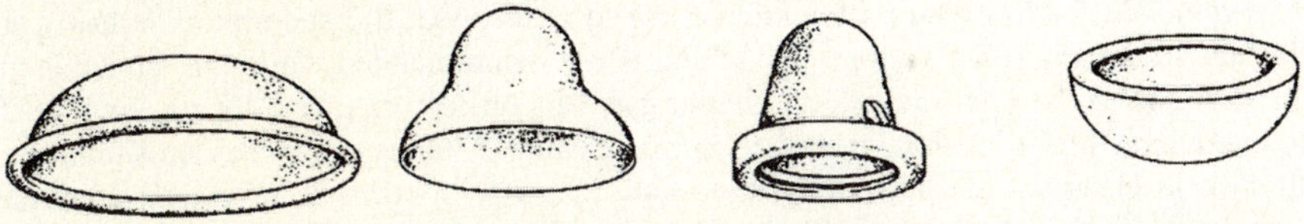

Figure 23.6: Intra-vaginal and Intra-cervical barriers for Women.

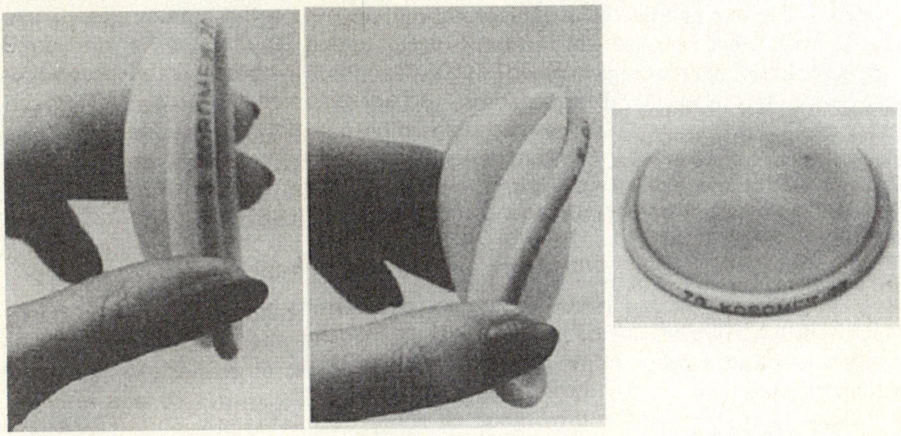

Figure 23.7: Three types of diaphragms for Women.

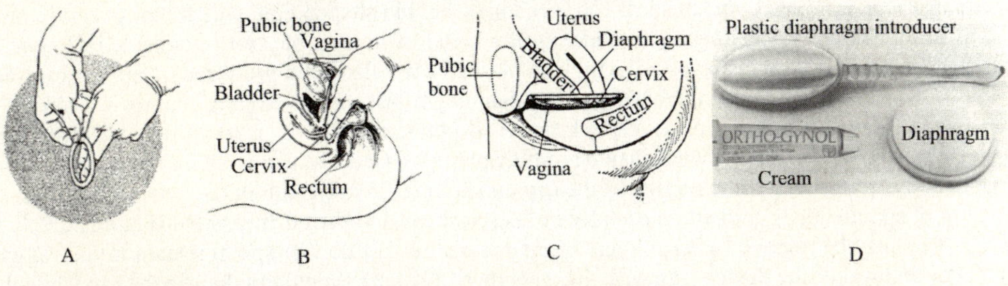

Figure 23.8: Steps in fitting of the diaphragm in Women, A- rim of the diaphragm is placed at the tip of the second finger, if diaphragm is of the correct size, the opposite rim will meet the place on the index finger marked by thumb, B- the index and second fingers are inserted deep into the vagina until tip of second finger touches the posterior vaginal wall, and the point on index finger is marked by thumb, C-correctly placed diaphragm in vagina and D-diaphragm with spermicidal cream and plastic introducer.

Proper use: Woman must learn to insert and remove the diaphragm correctly (Figure 23. 8 A, B and C). The diaphragm can be inserted with dome up or down. Most users insert with dome down to keep the spermicide (spermatocide) from falling out of the dome. Many women dislike inserting a diaphragm manually, they can use a plastic introducer for either coil-spring or flat-spring type diaphragms (Figure 23.8 D). The diaphragm can be inserted 6 hours or more before intercourse but when it is in place for more than 2 hours before coitus, application of additional spermicide is recommended. The device must not be removed for 6-8 hours after intercourse to ensure that the spermatocide has worked and that no live sperm remain in the vagina. Douching is not recommended while the device is in since it will dilute or remove the spermicide. A diaphragm can be left in place for as long as 24 hours following intercourse but if left longer, infection may result. After removal, device should be washed with mild soap in clean warm water, then dried and dusted with cornstarch or unscented talc. This protects the device from deterioration. It should be examined for damage before its use and must be replaced every year.

Advantages: It is highly effective if used properly. It is safe with no physiological or systemic effect in long term use. The user controls its use. It can be used only when needed. It can also be used during menstruation. It does not interfere with lactation. In developed countries, due to disillusionment with pill and IUD, many women are switching (or returning) to diaphragm.

Disadvantages: Its use requires high degree of motivation. It requires trained personnel to instruct the use of the device. It is relatively difficult to insert. It turns out to be expensive if used frequently, due to the cost of spermicide. In developing countries, with large rural population, diaphragm is not popular due to, a) lack of privacy for insertion and removal, b) lack of a ready source of water for cleaning it, c) lack of sufficient motivation among women to use it for every act of coitus, d) lack of clinical services for initial fitting of the device, and e) need for constant supply of spermicidal cream or jelly.

Nevertheless, the diaphragm still remains an excellent alternative for women who have conditions that contradict use of pill/ IUD or who do not wish to use these methods. It is especially suitable for women who are breast-feeding because it does not interfere with milk production. It is also a convenient method for women who engage in sexual intercourse infrequently because they do not need continuous protection.

Cervical Caps: Fredrick Adolph Wilde, a German gynecologist, first described the cervical cap in 1838. He called it as "cautchuk pessarium". It was a small rubber cap that was placed over the cervix and each cap was custom made, that is, a wax impression of the woman's cervix was used as a model or dye. The cap was introduced in England prior to diaphragm. Unlike diaphragm that blocks entire upper part of vaginal canal, the cervical cap is a small thimble-shaped cup, which blocks cervix only (Figure 23.6). Some cervical caps are made up of a metal or rubber, but most are made of Lucite, a clear rigid plastic. Flexible caps of polyethylene plastics have also been produced. Cervical caps are useful for those women who are unable to retain a diaphragm. Also in developing countries, 3 out of 10 women have uterine prolapsed or severe relaxation of pelvic muscles as a result of poor obstetrical care. These women can use cervical caps but not diaphragm. Cervical cap is held in place by suction rather than by spring tensions. The size of the cap varies from 22 to 31 mm in diameter. Before use, a 5cm strip of spermicide is applied on each side of cervical cap and then it is inserted (Figure 23.9 A, B and C). Cap may be removed after 6 hours of intercourse so that no live sperm remain in the vaginal canal after removal of the device. As with the diaphragm, the user should not douche the cap while the device is in its place in order to avoid dilution or removal of the spermicide. The cap is removed by tilting the rim away from the cervix thus breaking the suction (23.9 D).

Advantage: The cervical cap is nearly as effective as the diaphragm but has an additional advantage over the diaphragm. Because a properly fitted cap clings by suction deep in the vaginal canal, it is less likely than the diaphragm to be displaced during the intercourse. Cap can be left in place during entire inter-menstrual period and need to be removed only when menstruation is expected. However, this is generally not recommended due to collection of fluids inside emitting mal odor.

Disadvantage: Self-insertion and removal are somewhat more difficult because the cap must cover cervix, which is deep in the vaginal canal. Specially trained personnel must fit it initially.

During 1950 and 1960s, many manufacturers of diaphragms also produced cervical caps, but because of decline in the market, they discontinued making caps. The only company that still manufactures the cervical caps is Lamberts (Dalton) Limited in Britain with two brands of rubber cervical caps, Prencap and Prentif Cavity Rim.

Muang Sein, a New Delhi gynecologist in 1965 developed a flexible plastic (polyethylene) cervical cap (Figure 23.10) and found several advantages. Its advantages over those made of rubber are that it does not react with acidic vaginal fluids, does not deteriorate in hot climate, and is not damaged when used with spermicides that have an oil base.

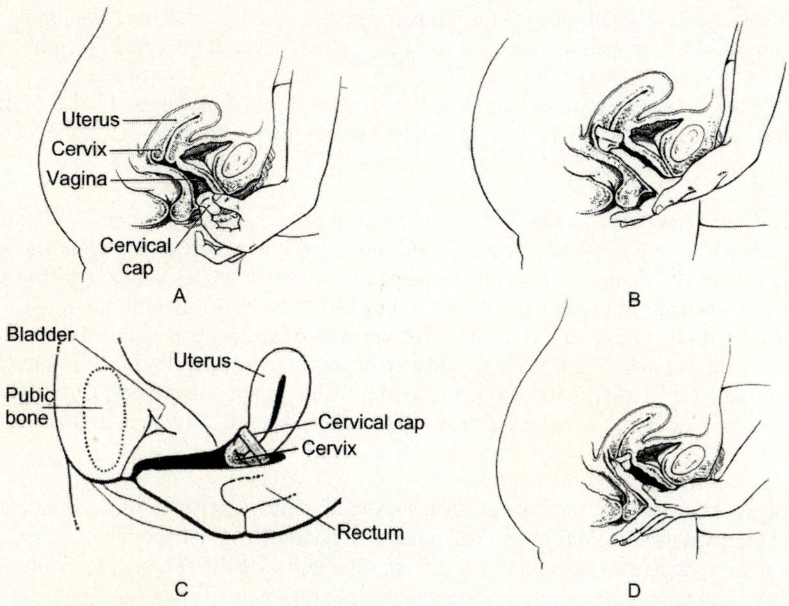

Figure 23.9: Steps in the insertion of a cervical cap in Women, A-a woman compresses the cap and pushes it into the vagina as far as possible, B-she checks its position over the cervix, C-it is held in place by suction, fits closely around the base of cervix and D-to remove, woman hooks her finger over the cap rim, dislodges it from the cervix, and pulls it out.

Two other intra-vaginal devices called the vault cap and the vimule cap (Figure 23.6) are often categorized as cervical caps. They combine the characteristics of both a diaphragm and the cervical cap, i.e. like the diaphragm, they cover an area beyond the cervix, and like the cervical cap, they cling to the vaginal roof by suction.

Vault (Dumas) Cap: Vault cap also called the Dumas cap, is made up of rubber or plastic and manufactured by Lamberts Limited. It is shaped like a circular bowl with a thick rim and thin center (Figure 23.6). It clings by suction to the vault or roof of vagina, following the contour of the cervix. Its size ranges from 50-75 mm and is used with a 5-cm strip of spermicide. It should be left in place for at least 6 hours after intercourse

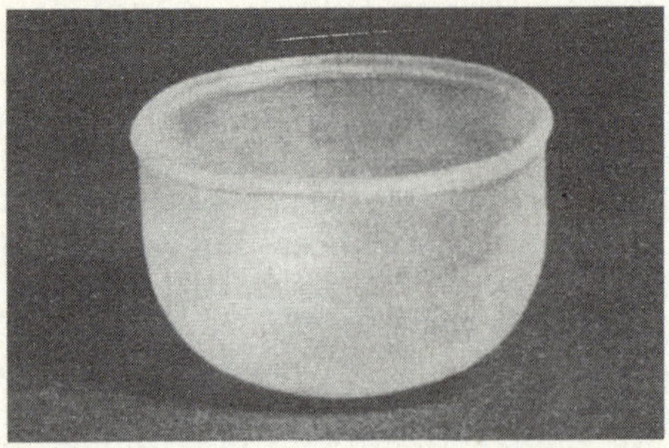

Figure 23.10:Cervical cap-flexible plastic type developed in India by Muang Sein.

Advantage: Vault cap is specially useful for women who are unable to retain a diaphragm because of poor muscle tone and for women who cannot use cervical cap because the cervix is either too short or has been torn.
Disadvantage: Like the diaphragm and cervical cap, a trained individual must fit the vault cap. One major criticism of the vault cap is that the male partner can sometimes feel the device during intercourse.

Vimule Cap: Vimule caps are also made of thick rubber or plastic. It is a combination of vault cap and cervical cap, having a dome-shaped portion to accommodate the cervix and a wide rim clinging by suction to vaginal vault (Figure 23.6). But unlike either, the vimule cap adheres with a very strong suction because a flanged rim permits the device to be pressed more firmly onto the roof of the vagina. Its size varies from 45 to 55 mm and is used with 5-cm strip of spermicide smeared to each side of the cap and over surface, but avoiding rim. It should also be left in place for 6 hours after intercourse.
Advantage: Vimule cap is useful for women who are unable to use diaphragm, cervical cap or vault cap due to poor muscle tone, a cytocele or a longer than average cervix. Lamberts Limited also manufactures it.

Vaginal Sponges: These are the natural sponges, soaked in, either vinegar or olive oil or an anti-sperm substance and are used as a vaginal plug. The modern version of vaginal sponge is a small disposable polyurethane foam sponge measuring 5 cm X 2.5 cm saturated with the spermicide, nonoxymol-9, and sold in India as '**Today**' (Figure 23.11). The contraceptive sponge 'Today' acts both, as **a chemical** and **a physical barrier**. The sponge when moistened with water releases the spermicide nonoxynol-9. The spermicide inactivates sperm while the sponge works to absorb them and block their passage into the cervix. As a contraceptive, the sponge has a failure rate of 15-30 %. It is as effective as the conventional diaphragm with spermicide among women who have never borne children, but is less effective among women with children.
Advantage: A major advantage of vaginal sponge is that it allows more spontaneity than other barrier methods since it can remain in place for up to 24 hours and also through more than one sexual act.

23.5 Chemical Methods

Chemical barrier contraceptives include **spermicides**, while the main chemical contraceptives for both males and females are hormonal preparations, and therefore are also known as **hormonal contraceptives.** Except for total abstinence or surgical sterilization, hormonal contraceptives when used properly are the most effective spacing methods of contraception.
Chemical Barrier Methods (**Spermicides** or **Spermatocides**): In 1960s, before the advent of IUDs and oral contraceptives, spermicides were widely used as vaginal chemical contraceptive. These are

creams, jellies and pastes that are squeezed from a tube (Figure 23.12), foams in the form of tablets and aerosols, suppositories and soluble films called C-film that are inserted manually. All of these contain sperm killing agent or spermatocides that make the vagina and cervix unfavorable for sperm survival. The commonly used spermicides are "surface-active agents" which attach themselves to spermatozoa, inhibit oxygen uptake by spermatozoa and kill them. The most widely used spermicide is nonoxynol-9, which kills sperm by disrupting the plasma membrane.

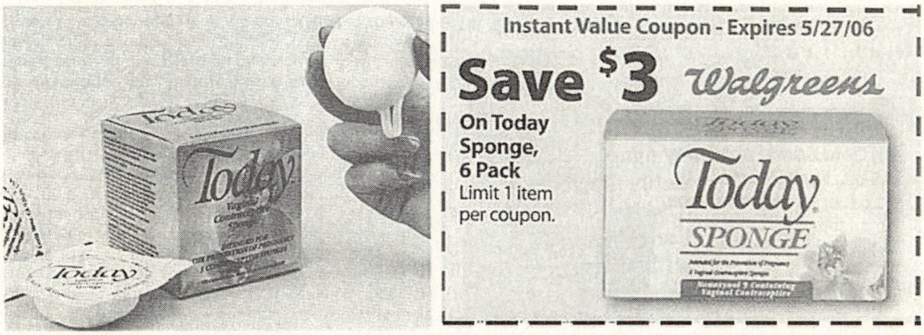

Figure 23.11: Contraceptive sponge 'Today' for Women.

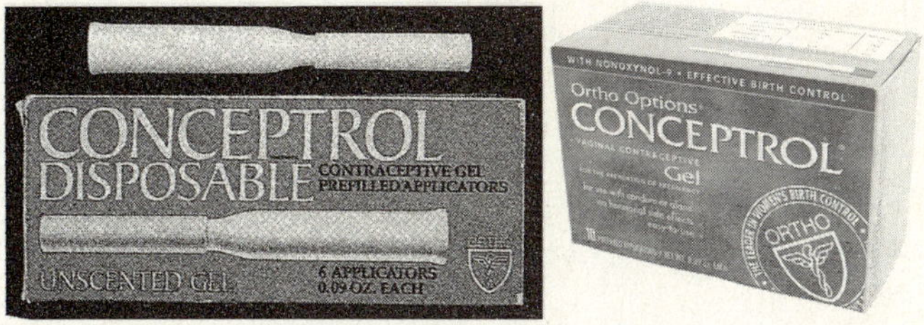

Figure 23.12: Spermicidal gel.

Spermicides were the second modern contraceptives widely available in pharmacies. W.J. Rendell (a pharmacist), who invented a soluble vaginal suppository made of cocoa butter and quinine, first marketed them in England in 1885. Common spermicides are usually a tablet and a suppository, but later are difficult to store because they melt in warm weather.

Advantage: These are available without prescription and are fairly easy to use. It also inactivates the AIDS virus and decreases the incidence of gonorrhea (bacterial infection of mouth and throat after oral-genital contact, in the vagina and penis after genital intercourse or in the rectum after recto-genital contact).

Disadvantage: Spermicides have a high failure rate when used alone. They are more effective when used together with a mechanical barrier device. They must be used almost immediately before intercourse and repeated before each sex act. Also, they must be introduced into those regions of the vagina where sperms are likely to be deposited. Sometimes, spermicides cause mild irritation or burning.

Chemical-Hormonal Contraceptives: Hormonal contraceptives if used properly are the most effective spacing methods of contraception. These can be **oral contraceptives** or **slow releasing (depot) formulations**. Oral contraceptives are in the form of **pills** and include i) **combined pill**, ii) **progesterone only pill** (**POP**), iii) **post-coital pill**, iv) **once-a-month** or long-acting pill and v) **male**

pill. Slow releasing hormonal contraceptive formulations include **injectables**, **subcutaneous implants** and **vaginal rings**.

Synthetic estrogens and **progestogens** are used in the hormonal contraceptives (Figure 23.13 A and B). Two commonly used synthetic estrogens are **ethinyl estradiol** and **mestranol** (Figure 23.13 A). The synthetic progestogens are classified into three groups. These are **pregnanes**, **estranes**, and **gonanes**. Pregnanes include **megestrol**, **chlormadinone**, and **medroxy progesterone acetate**, but pregnanes are now not recommended in oral contraceptives, as these seem to be involved in causing breast tumors. Estranes are also known as **19-nortestosterones** and are all metabolized to **19-norethisterone (norethindrone)** before becoming active. These include **norethisterone** and its acetate, **ethynodiol diacetate**, **lynestrenol** and **norethynodrel** (Figure 23.13 B). **Levonorgestrel** is the most favored gonane.

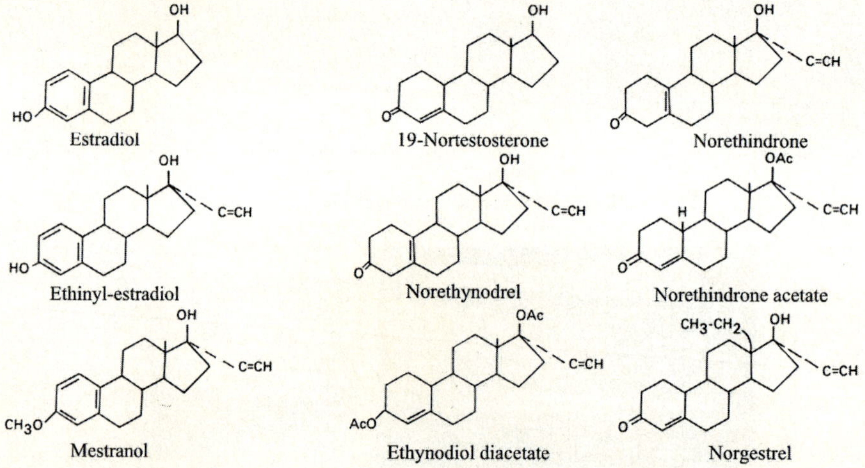

A B

Figure 23.13: Hormonal contraceptives, A-synthetic estrogens and B-progestogens.

Oral Contraceptives: Oral contraceptives are the most common and popular methods of contraception, usually referred as the **birth control pill**, or simply **"the pill"** (Figure 23.14). Currently available oral contraceptives consist of different combinations of synthetic steroids, an estrogen and a progestin (known as **combined** or **combination pills**), or a progestin alone (commonly called **progestin only pill** or **POP**).

The estrogen component in the pills consists of either 17 α-ethinyl estradiol-3-methyl ether (mestranol) or 17 α-ethinyl estradiol. All progestogens in the oral contraceptives are derivatives of testosterone minus a carbon atom at the 19 position known as 19-nortestosterone. All of these contain an ethinyl group at the 17 position. In addition to enhancing the activity of these compounds when taken orally, this structural modification prevents rapid hydroxylation and conjugation while passing through the portal circulation. Since the metabolism of the two estrogenic components is not similar and their biological activities are influenced by the particular progestin of the preparation, the estrogenic potency cannot be assessed by their weight alone. Furthermore, among the various progestins, there are differences not only in their progesterone activity but also in their androgenicity, anti-estrogenic activity, and their anabolic potency. Thus, the biologic activities of the combination type of the pills depend not only on the weight of the components but also on the synergistic effects of the two components and the intrinsic activities of the preparation.

Oral contraceptives are taken orally in the form of tablets. It is supplied in 28-tablet packets (Figure 23.14) and a popular one in India is **Mala D**. The first 21 identical tablets contain minute amounts of one of the two estrogens and one of the five progestins in the case of combined pills while the last seven tablets are hormone free. However, the progestogen only pills contain only small doses of the progestin without estrogen, but are used much less nowadays. The pill should be taken orally for 21 consecutive days beginning on the 5th day of the menstrual cycle, followed by 7 inert tablets during which menstruation occurs. The first day of menstruation is considered as the first day of the next cycle. The bleeding that occurs with the use of oral contraceptives is not like the normal menstruation, but it is an episode of uterine bleeding from an incompletely formed endometrium and it occurs due to the withdrawal of exogenous hormones. Therefore, it is called "**withdrawal bleeding**" instead of menstruation. The loss of blood in withdrawal bleeding is only about half of that which occurs in a normal menstruation. If bleeding does not occur, the woman is advised to start the second course one week after the preceding one. Normally, the woman menstruates after the second course of pills.

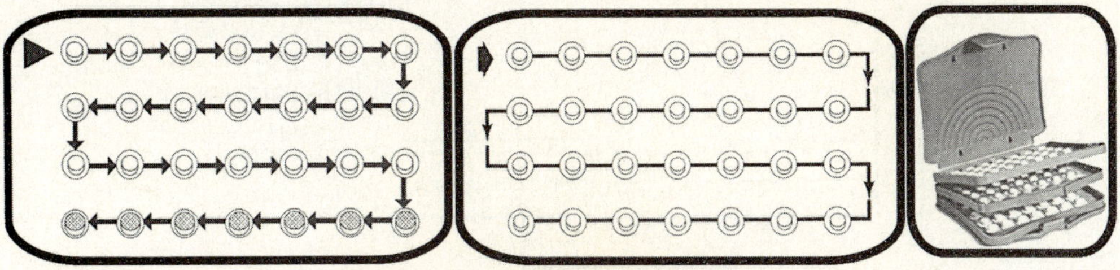

28 pills- 21 of one colour, 7 of another

Minipills- 28 or 35 pills of same colour

Seasonale- a new pill

Figure 23.14: Contraceptive pills for Women.

When taken under the combined regimen, the oral contraceptives are almost 100 % effective in preventing pregnancy. The omission of one or more tablets during any cycle significantly increases the risk of pregnancy.

Mode of action of pills: The action of the combined oral pill is to prevent pregnancy by blocking ovulation or implantation of a fertilized ovum in the uterus and also by preventing sperm transport (Figure 23.15). They act primarily by inhibiting ovulation through suppression of hypothalamic-releasing hormone, which in turn inhibit the release of follicle stimulating hormone (FSH) and luteinizing hormone (LH) from the pituitary gland (Figure 23.16). It is known that a rise in circulating levels of LH and FSH at the midpoint of the ovarian cycle stimulates maturation of the ovarian follicle, resulting in ovulation as seen in Figure 23.16 in the individuals who are not using oral contraceptives. Oral contraceptives suppress LH and FSH release and therefore, individuals who are on oral contraceptives show reduced levels of both FSH and LH. Therefore, follicular maturation does not occur, and ovulation is inhibited. Continuous use of oral contraceptives inhibits follicular maturation, ovulation, and onset of menstruation. Discontinuation of oral contraceptives for one week each month results in a drop in circulating levels of estrogen and progesterone, which stimulates the onset of menstruation and beginning of a new cycle. However, the contraceptive efficacy of birth control pills does not require monthly discontinuation of use.

Progesterone, contained in oral contraceptives, also interferes with conception in two additional ways. Firstly progesterone increases the viscosity of cervical mucus and therefore, blocks or restricts the entry of sperm into the uterus. Progesterone also inhibits tubal motility and delays the transport of the sperm and of the ovum to the uterine cavity. Secondly, progesterone interferes with implantation of the ovum in the uterus by inhibiting proliferation of the endometrial lining of the uterus, which is essential for implantation to take place (Figure 23.15).

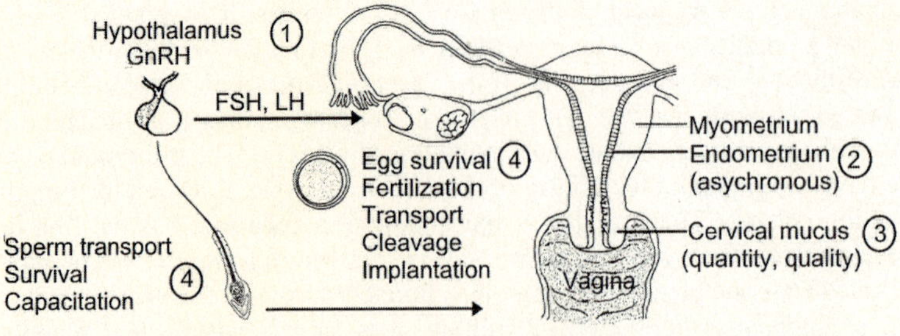

Figure 23.15: Mode of action of oral contraceptives.

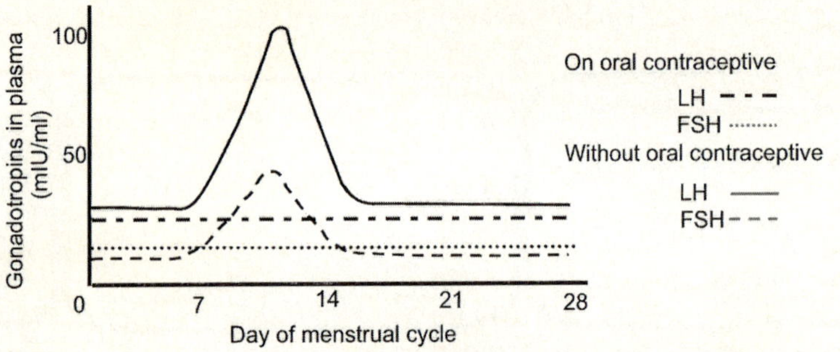

Figure 23.16: Plasma levels of gonadotropins during menstrual cycle in individuals not using oral contraceptive and of the ones those are on oral contraceptive.

The Department of Family Welfare, Ministry of Health and Family Welfare, Government of India has released three types of low dose oral pills under the brand names of MALA-N and MALA-D, each containing 0.3 mg Norgestrol and 0.03 mg Ethinil estradiol. Mala D is sold to the consumer under social marketing at a price of Rupees 2 per packet while Mala N is supplied free of cost through family welfare centers. It is a packet of 28 pills, 21 tablets containing contraceptive hormone and 7 iron tablets containing ferrous fumarate.

Advantage: Oral contraceptives, if used correctly, prevent pregnancy nearly 100 % of the time. They regularize the length of menstrual cycles and decrease menstrual flow and therefore decrease the risk of anemia. The pill also provides protection against endometrial and ovarian cancers and reduces the risk of endometriosis. Use of oral contraceptives virtually eliminates the chances of ectopic pregnancies. They also lower the rates of some pelvic infections. Oral contraceptives may also be used for **emergency contraception (EC),** the so-called **"morning after pill"**, when two pills are taken within 72 hours after unprotected intercourse and another two pills are taken 12 hours later, the chances of pregnancy is reduced by 75 %.

Disadvantage: Birth control pills can produce variety of side effects, including increased risk of nausea, constipation, elevations of blood pressure, skin rashes and salt retention with accompanying weight gain. Possible common side effects with pills are irregular bleeding, spotting or no monthly bleeding while headache, tender breasts and dizziness are less common side effects. The most serious side effect is increased risk of cardiovascular disease, which becomes significant in woman of over age 35 years who use both oral contraceptives and tobacco. Oral contraceptives increase the risk of benign liver tumors. They also decrease the quantity of breast milk among some lactating women.

Progestogen only pill (POP): In recent years, the **progestin-only oral contraceptives (POP)**, also called the '**minipills**' have become popular as these have less risk of cardiovascular diseases. Most women can safely use the minipill, but usually minipill is not recommended for the women who are breastfeeding a baby of 6 weeks or less or suffer with serious health conditions such as breast cancer, liver disease or jaundice, has blood clot in lungs or deep in legs. However, minipills do not suppress ovulation as effectively as combined oral contraceptives. Also, their other effects such as thickening of cervical mucus thus preventing implantation are not entirely reliable. Progestin only pill shows a 3-10 % failure rate and also a significant risk of ectopic pregnancy. Because progestin-only preparations do not seem to interfere with breast-feeding, minipills are best suited for lactating women who are partially protected against pregnancy by the suppression of fertility associated with breast-feeding.

Post-Coital Pill: Many combination birth control pills (marketed under various names including Ovral, Tetragynon, and Triphasil) are also used as **post-coital contraceptive**. These are commonly called as the **morning after pills (MAPs)**. **Mifepristone (RU486)**, so called **abortion pill**, developed in France is gaining lots of popularity as a MAP. It has proven to have a 96-98 % success rate with virtually no side effects. Mifepristone is an anti-hormone that, when taken during the first 7 weeks of pregnancy in conjunction with a tiny amount of prostaglandin to induce uterine contractions, induces miscarriage by blocking progesterone "quieting effect on the uterus".

Another type of morning after pill (post-coital pill) contains a very high level of estrogen. When this pill is taken shortly after unprotected intercourse, it promotes powerful contractions of smooth muscle in a woman's reproductive tract and may dislodge and expel a fertilized egg or blastocyst from the uterus. However, if the blastocyst has already implanted, intake of morning after pill may injure the blastocyst. In addition, the pill alters the endometrial lining of the uterus and prevent implantation of the fertilized ovum. However, high levels of estrogen contained in the morning-after-pill often induce severe nausea and vomiting, which have limited the use of this type of oral contraceptive.

Once-a-month Pill: **Once a month pill** is a **long acting contraceptive**. However, experiments using a long acting estrogen, **quinestrol** in combination with a short-acting progestogen in oral contraceptives have been disappointing. The failure rate is too high and bleeding tends to be irregular. Because of these reasons, this pill is not acceptable.

New drugs block periods and thus, menstruation becomes optional: A large section of reproductive health experts now a days are questioning the necessity for the monthly withdrawal bleed, which oral contraceptive users experience while taking the seven inactive pills or seven days without pills in each month's cycle. Women have long been manipulating hormonal contraceptives since almost the first pill arrived in 1960 to skip or block menstrual periods for events such as a wedding, sports competition or vacation. Two recent national surveys in United States found that approximately 1 in 5 women are using oral contraceptives to stop or skip their periods. Now new and upcoming contraceptive drugs are making things easier by blocking periods so that for young women with a world of choices, even the menstrual period becomes optional. Using the birth-control pills and other hormonal contraceptives, blocking of periods is becoming more popular, particularly among young women and those entering menopause.

New research has found that woman can safely and effectively use many **monophasic** (monophasic means that each active pill in the cycle contains the same amount of hormone) oral contraceptives continuously for a few cycles in a row, skipping the inactive pills. For example, **Seasonale**, a new continuous-use oral contraceptive launched in November 2003 by Barr Pharmaceuticals of Woodcliff Lake, N.J., U.S.A. limits periods to four a year. It contains 150 μg of the progestin levonorgestrel and 30 μg of the estrogen ethinyl estradiol and comes in a 3-month supply. Women take 1 active pill per day for 84 days and then take inactive pills for 7 days (Figure 23.14) for withdrawal bleeding. Continuous-use of oral contraceptives reduces the number of bleeding days (nearly four menstrual cycles annually) and related side effects. Many more such drugs will come soon in the market. **Seasonique** is a successor to Seasonale and is expected to reduce breakthrough bleeding and hormonal fluctuations even more. **Lybrel** is the first daily birth-control pill designed to be taken indefinitely. It is made by Wyeth of Madison, N.J., U.S.A. and is expected to come in U.S. market sometimes in 2006. Berlex of Wayne, N.J., U.S.A is developing its own birth-control pill for menstrual suppression. It has got approval for **Yaz**, a pill with only four days off hormones, reducing hormone fluctuations and premenstrual syndrome.

Drospirenone is the new progestin in the combined oral contraceptive **Yasmin** developed by Schering AG. Yasmin contains 3 mg of drospirenone and 30 μg of the estrogen ethinyl estradiol. Drospirenone-ethinyl estradiol pills are nearly as effective as other combined oral contraceptives but also provide other benefits in some such as reduction in acne and excess hair growth on body and less water retention. However, side effects are similar to those of the other combined oral contraceptives. **Desogestrel** is the progestin in the new pill **Cerazette** developed by Organon. Cerazette pill contains 75 μg of desogestrel and unlike other progestin-only pills that work mainly by making the cervical mucus thicker so that sperm cannot reach the egg, it works primarily by preventing ovulation. Also, desogestrel is unique among other POP in that a woman can take a pill as much as 12 hours late without reducing its effectiveness.

Male Pill: The quest for an efficient oral contraceptive for males has been disappointing. The challenge is to find substances that block production of functional sperm without causing erectile dysfunction, or interfere with their storage and maturation, prevent sperm transport in vas deferens or affect constituents of the seminal fluid.

Hormonal contraceptives for men have been in clinical stages of development for almost two decades and are now in phase III clinical trials in China. These studies are using testosterone or a combination of testosterone and a progestin to suppress sperm production.

Gossypol, a derivative of cottonseed oil was in news as male pill during the 1970s, but at present it is not in practice. It was thought to be useful for contraceptive purposes because gossypol is a chemical found in the seeds of cotton plants, which produce it in order to slow down the reproduction of the insects that eat cotton balls and seeds. This compound was also found to affect reproduction in mammals. Studies using gossypol for human involved over 8,000 men and it continued for over a decade. The researchers found that men taking daily a gossypol pill had reliable contraception and no complaints about change in libido. However, studies revealed two serious flows and these were disruption of potassium uptake and incomplete reversibility of infertility. Gossypol was found effective in producing azoospermia or severe oligospermia, but approximately 10 % men became permanently azoospermic after taking gossypol for 6 months. In addition, gossypol could be toxic too. Because of these reasons, gossypol was never used widely as a male contraceptive.

Depot or Slow Release Formulations: The term **depot** refers to a place of storing vehicles from where they are moved slowly. Similar type of approach has been utilized in contraceptive technologies to delay the rate of release of an active steroid for contraceptive effect from the site to prolong its biologic activity (that is why called depot). Techniques generally used to get prolonged effect of the chemical/steroid are, a) chemical modification of the steroid molecule by esterification and the use of ether derivatives, b) to render the steroid less soluble in form by altering the physiochemical characteristics of a compound (crystallization), and c) use of mechanical delivery systems (implants). **Depot steroid** is steroid hormone and synthetic analog conjugates that are slowly hydrolyzed to release the active components. They are used to achieve sustained effects when injected or implanted intramuscularly. Thus hormonal contraceptives besides being used as oral may also be categorized as injecatables and implants. As for the oral contraceptives, hormones used in contraceptive injectables and implants can be only progestins or a combination of both a progestin and an estrogen.

Mode of Action: The contraceptive action of hormone taken either through injection or implant (sustained-release systems), can be **central**, **peripheral** or **combined** (Figure 23.17). The most important factors involved in the mechanism of action are the type of drug (progesterone alone or combined estrogen-progesterone), the dose, mode of administration, (injection or implant), the formulation of the drug, and the duration of the therapy (Figure 23.18). The central effect of the contraceptive is inhibition of ovulation, which is achieved by the drug effect at the level of hypothalamus, pituitary and ovary resulting in depression of mid-cycle LH-surge, without greatly interfering with the tonic release of pituitary gonadotropins. Peripheral effects include suppression of endometrial growth (preparation for implantation) and secretion of hostile cervical mucus. The combined effects of two contraceptive hormones through injections or implants involve inhibition of ovulation and also suppression of endometrial growth. This results in prevention of implantation and also thickens cervical mucus.

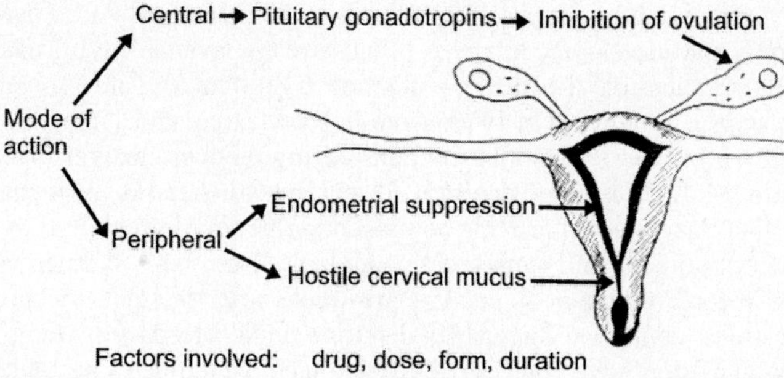

Figure 23.17: Mode of action of injectable contraceptives in Women.

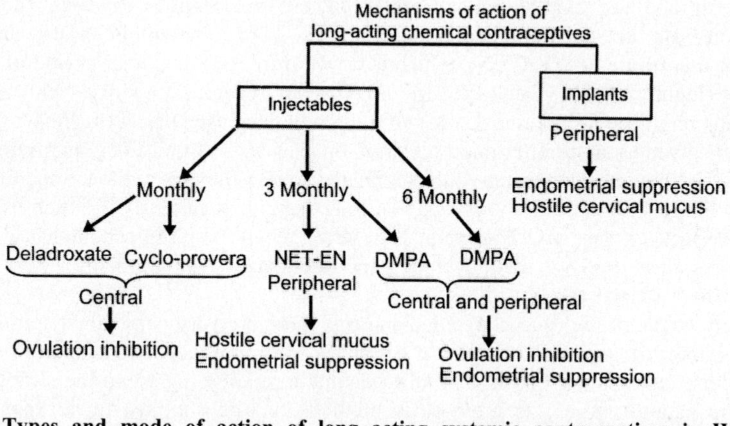

Figure 23.18: Types and mode of action of long acting systemic contraceptives in Women, DHPA-dihydroxyprogesterone acetate, EE-ethinyl estradiol, EC-estradiol cypionate, NET-EN-norethindrone enanthate and DMPA-depot-medroxyprogesterone acetate.

Injectable Contraceptives: The introduction of injectable contraceptives as long-acting pharmaceutical agents for fertility control fills a gap within the existing technology to suit a group of human society. The injectable contraceptives can be used once a month or once in two-three months or once in six months. Combined formulations are generally injected once a month compared with once every two or three month for progestin-only injectables such as norethindrone enanthate (NET-EN) and depot-medroxyprogesterone acetate (DMPA). Injectable contraceptives are highly effective, simple to administer, and are noninvasive. Acceptability of these contraceptives show an increasing demand for those women who have an intolerance for oral contraceptives, and for those in far rural areas where family planning services are difficult to reach. Also, the timing of injectable contraceptives is unrelated to coitus, and these are suitable for women who need continuous motivation for taking contraceptive or who are liable to forget or get confused about the proper use of oral contraceptives.

The progesterone component in injectable contraceptives is synthesized either from derivatives of progesterone or as esters of the 19-nor testosterone group. Almost all the forms used in monthly injectables are combined with a long-acting estradiol ester (such as valerate, enanthate, butyrate, cypionate, unducelate, and hexahydrobenzoate) to provide a reasonably acceptable cycle control. Trade name of combined injectables is **Cyclofem** (also known as **Cyclo-Provera**, **Lunelle**, **Novafem**, and **Feminena**) and **Mesigyna** (also known as **Norigynon**). Combined injectables have been studied since 1960s and several formulations have been used in some countries for the past two decades and even the newer combined injectables have been on the market now for years. These have become more widely known and used in recent years because of the availability of data on its safety and effectiveness. WHO accelerated the development of Cyclofem (Cyclo-Provera) for use in developing countries in response to requests in 1970s from India, Mexico, and some other countries for a safe and effective monthly injectable. Cyclofem contains **25-mg medroxyprogesterone acetate** and **5 mg estradiol cypionate** while Mesigyna contains **50-mg norethisterone enanthate** and **5 mg estradiol valerate**. Combined injectables provide contraception mainly by preventing ovulation and also by thickening the cervical mucus and suppressing endometrial growth. Women who stop using combined injectables can become pregnant as soon as six weeks after the last injection. Compared with progestin-only injectables, combined injectables disturb vaginal bleeding patterns to less extent and allow earlier return to ovulation once their use is discontinued. Combined injectables have gained greater attention after the approval of US Food and Drug Administration (FDA).

The three monthly injectables, on the other hand, are composed only of gestagens and two of these are popular and are available on market. These are **Depot- Provera (depot medroxy progesterone acetate or DMPA**) administered on a 3 or 6 monthly basis, and **Noristerat (norethisterone enanthate or NET-EN)**, which is active only for a maximal period of 12 weeks at a dose of 200 mg (Figure 23.18). Depo-Provera (DMPA) has been in use since 1960s and is accepted most widely with very little failure rate. Over two million women use Depo-Provera Worldwide. Depo-Provera, which is given as an intramuscular injection once every 3 months, contains a hormone similar to progesterone that prevents maturation of the ovum and causes changes in the uterine lining that make pregnancy less likely. Because Depo-Provera is long lasting, it takes 10-18 months after the last injection for its effects to wear off. Noristerat (NET-EN), a two-month injectable has also been in use as a contraceptive since 1966. It was developed and manufactured in Germany and is used by more than 200,000 women all over the World.

Advantage: Daily intake of the drug is avoided and it is therefore very convenient, and liked by many women. Furthermore, for women living great distances from contraceptive outlets or for women in overcrowded living quarters who wish or need to maintain privacy regarding their contraceptive use, injectables are a natural choice, as most other methods require supplies to be kept on hand and therefore, have high degree of acceptability. Injectable contraceptives are as effective as oral contraceptives and are more effective than IUDs. In rural areas, injectable contraceptives meet the demand of many patients. Use of these contraceptives has no relationship to coitus. The long-term effectiveness of injectables is a saving in patient's time and may be money too. These are well tolerated with very little side effects and show minimal incidence of non-menstrual complaints and absence of estrogen-linked annoying side effects, and the potentially serious estrogen complications. Depo-Provera and other progestin-only methods decrease the frequency and seriousness of sickle-cell crises and thus are the contraceptive of choice for women suffering from sickle-cell disease.

Disadvantage: Use of all injectables requires a doctor's care, because of potential side effects and risks. Once injected, the drug cannot be withdrawn to stop any side effects. Weight gain is a serious side effect, disliked by most women. Disruption of the menstrual cycle occurs. Uterine bleeding pattern becomes erratic, and most women experience irregular bleeding in the beginning followed by amenorrhoea. There is a delayed return of fertility on drug withdrawal. Personally, it is unsuitable for those women who dislike receiving injections. Women with a history of breast cancer, depression, asthma, kidney disease, high blood pressure, diabetes, migraine headaches, epilepsy, or strong family histories of these conditions should probably not use this method.

Mini injectable is a term introduced for the use of low dosage of DMPA or NET-EN (15 or 20 mg) as a monthly injectable. This progesterone-only, low dosage regimen has a contraceptive effect and overall incidence of side effects similar to those of minipills.

Contraceptive Implants: Other hormonal methods of contraception are **sub-dermal implants** of silastic capsules or rods containing different progestogen (Figure 23.19). Some of these are aimed to produce central inhibitory effects, but the majority of them acts via peripheral or combined inhibitory mechanisms (Figure 23.18). The most popular contraceptive implant is known as **Norplant** (Figure 23.19 A)**,** which contain the progestin levonorgestrel, also used in oral contraceptives. It consists of six slender hormone-filled capsules that are surgically implanted through a small incision one by one in a fan-shaped pattern under the skin of the arm or in the scapular region using local anesthesia. Another variant of contraceptive implant called **Norplant II** or **2** consists of two rods slightly longer than Norplant capsules and is easier to implant and to remove because there are fewer rods (Figure 23.19 B). Contraceptive implants slowly and continually release a progestin, which inhibits ovulation in much the same way, as do oral contraceptives, and also thickens the cervical mucus. Norplant is effective for a period of up to 5 years while Norplant II for at least 3 years. Removal of the device can reverse its contraceptive action. Unlike injectable contraceptives, this method is reversible at any time. However, removing the implants is usually more difficult than inserting them.

New research on contraceptive implants has focused on reducing the number of rods or capsules by using different progestins, minimizing side effects, particularly bleeding disturbances, and assuring that implants are safe for use while breastfeeding. The newer implants are similar to Norplant implants but offer several improvements. The new implants consist of one or two rods or capsules, and like Norplant implants, these are also inserted just under the skin of the upper arm to deliver progestins into the bloodstream. Most use rods rather than capsules. Rods differ from capsules in that they are filled with a mixture of steroid crystals and polymer. Capsules on the other hand, are hollow polymer tubes filled with free steroid crystals. New implant systems with fewer capsules or rods make insertion and removal much easier and produce fewer complications and less discomfort for users compared with Norplant's six capsules.

The new implants on the market are, **Jadelle** using only one rod as shown in Figure 23.19 C (formerly known as Norplant-2) releasing the progestin levonorgestrel and **Chinese No. 2** (also called **Sinoplant** or **Sino-implant**) that is nearly identical to Jadelle but contains 150 instead of 140-mg progestin. The **Etonogestrel implants (Implanon)**, a three-year contraceptive made by Organon USA of Roseland, N.J., is getting US approval in 2006. It is a single 30mm silastic rod with progestin etonogestrel implanted in the upper arm that stops menstruation in many women. The Population Council is developing contraceptive implant by the name **Nestorone (ST-1435)** with progestin levonorgestrel. It is a single rod implant made of a silicon rubber membrane that controls the release rate and is effective for two years. It is designed specifically for breast-feeding women. The Nestorone implant development program began in early 1980s and has completed phase II clinical trials. Lactating women have found the Nestorone implant acceptable but non-lactating women have complained of prolonged and irregular bleeding.

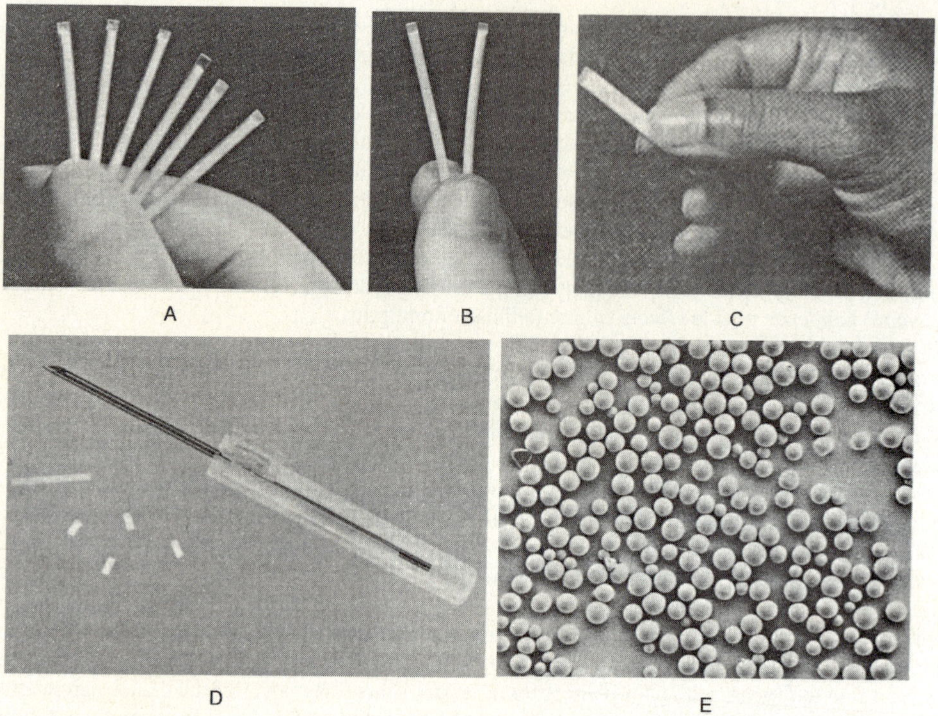

Figure 23.19: Contraceptive implants for Women, A-Norplant, B-Norplant II, C-Jadelle, D-Capronor, and E- norethindrone microspheres.

Currently biodegradable implants of polymer caprolactone (**Capronor 2**) or co-polymer caprolactone and trimethylene carbonate blend (**Capronor 3**) filled with 18 or 32 mg of levonorgestrel respectively are also used as contraceptives (Figure 23.19 D). The Capronor tubing is easier to insert and remove than Norplant's Silastic tubes in part because the caprolactone polymer has a slipperier surface and offers less resistance in body tissues. **Small pellet** made of 90% norethindrone (NET) and 10% pure cholesterol is another biodegradable implant (Figure 23.19 E). The hormone is released as the pellet gradually biodegrades over a 12-month period and then disappears completely within 24 months. During the first 12 months of implant, the period of contraceptive effectiveness, the pellet can be removed if desired.

Advantage: These are one time administration providing protection for a long period, and therefore, day-to-day vigilance is not necessary. It is as reliable as sterilization. Removal of contraceptive capsule quickly restores fertility.

Disadvantage: The side effects resemble those of progestin-only pills and injectables. Changes in bleeding pattern i.e. bleeding on more days per cycle, heavier bleeding, spotting between periods, infrequent or scanty bleeding, and amenorrhea (no bleeding at all) occur most commonly. Other side effects include headache, nervousness, nausea, dizziness, dermatitis, acne, change of appetite, hair loss, increase in facial or body hair, breast tenderness, and enlarged ovarian follicles. Ectopic pregnancy may occur.

Transdermal patch is a new hormonal contraceptive method for women that work by slowly releasing a combination of progestin and estrogen through the skin. Use of contraceptive patches is controlled by the user and requires attention just once a week. The trade name Ortho Evra or Evra today sells the only contraceptive patch on the market. It is a square patch 4.45 cms each side, resembling a light brown bandage (Figure 23.20 A). The patch contains three layers, an outer protective layer of polyester, a medicated adhesive middle layer, and a clear polyester release liner, which is removed just before application. The adhesive layer continuously delivers hormones through the skin into the bloodstream. The patch adheres well to the skin, allowing women to perform regular daily activities such as bathing, swimming, working etc. and can be placed on the buttocks, lower abdomen, upper outer arm or back etc, but not on the breast.

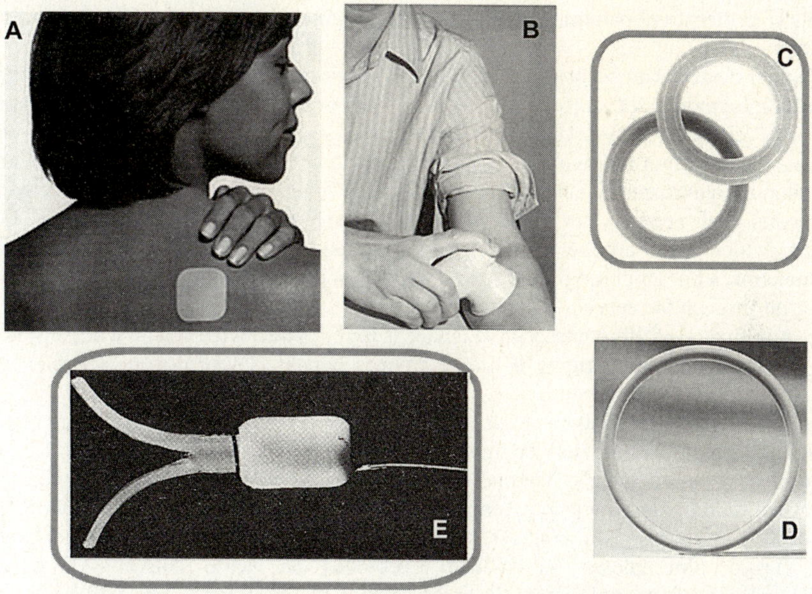

Figure 23.20: Contraceptives for Women, A-Woman with a transdermal patch, B- Spray-on contraceptive, C-vaginal ring, D- Nuva ring, and E-Intra-cervical Device.

The combined hormone formulation patch delivers 150 μg of the progestin norelgestromin and 20 μg of the estrogen ethinyl estradiol per day. A user wears the patch for one week, after which the patch must be replaced with a new one each week for a total of three weeks, followed by no patch for one week. The hormones released from the patch protect against pregnancy by preventing ovulation, thickening cervical mucus, and suppressing endometrial growth.

In addition, other transdermal contraceptives in different stages of development include **spray-on contraceptives** (Figure 23.20 B) and **gels**. The spray-on approach is a new technique for transferring a preset dose of fast-drying hormones onto the skin. The spray is absorbed almost instantaneously, so there is no risk of washing it off. The hormone in this technique gets collected as a reservoir within the skin, from which it then slowly diffuses into the bloodstream. In a clinical trial, 1.2 mg of Nestorone gel when applied to the skin daily for three months suppressed ovulation in 83% of participants.

The **vaginal rings** are a new way to deliver contraceptive hormones to the bloodstream. These are easy to use and the user can control their use. Vaginal rings can be used more correctly in comparison to the oral contraceptives. It is worn and positioned by the user herself in the vagina in a manner similar to an ordinary contraceptive diaphragm but need not be fitted or sized as precisely as a diaphragm since later work by blocking sperm entry into the cervix. It is worn for 3 weeks and removed for 1 week to allow menstruation to occur. Vaginal ring is a doughnut-shaped silicone rubber ring (Figure 23.20 C) that fits in the vagina and releases a constant dose of contraceptive steroids, either a progestin alone or a progestin and estrogen combined. Combined estrogen and progestin rings contain lower doses of hormones and cause fewer bleeding disturbances than combined oral contraceptives. Nuva Ring (Figure 23.20 D) is the first vaginal ring that is widely available. It releases a combined formula of a progestin and an estrogen. Because the steroids released by vaginal rings enter the circulatory system through the vaginal wall without first passing through the liver, lower doses are sufficient to produce the contraceptive effect. The technique has the potential advantages of little alteration in menstrual patterns, simplicity in use, high effectiveness, rapid reversibility and self-administration.

Vaginal devices can be grouped according to high or low release rate formulations. Vaginal devices with high amounts of steroids release them at dosages sufficient to inhibit ovulation. When these are used cyclically for 21 days of each menstrual cycle, endometrial development is sufficient to mimic normal menstruation following removal of the device. These devices also abolish the mid-cycle LH peak without significantly changing the normal FSH levels. Also, these can be left in place for longer intervals and need to be removed only when a bleeding episode begins. Low-dosage formulations, which need not be cyclically removed and replaced, allow normal ovulatory and menstrual function while inhibiting local reproductive processes such as cervical mucus production or sperm transport through the cervix.

Advantage: Acceptance of this contraceptive device is high. The device can be worn during all normal activities, and a woman can remove or insert devices herself. These do not interfere with sexual intercourse.

Disadvantage: Vaginal ring has a high expulsion rate. The contraceptive effectiveness and acceptability of such devices are now being studied further for improvements and also for the delivery of other hormones and chemicals. Vaginal devices are used for administration of prostaglandins to achieve cervical dilation and pregnancy termination and also for administration of spermicidal agents for contraceptive purposes. In contrast to these sustained-release preparations, a water-soluble polymeric plastic film known as "**C-film**" provides an acute delivery of a spermicide, nonylphenoxypolyethoxyethanol (Nonyl-9), to the vagina. The spermicide acts on the ejaculated sperm released during coitus to exert contraceptive effects.

Intra cervical devices (ICDs): These are small sized devices designed to remain in the cervix throughout the menstrual cycle for prolonged periods of time (Figure 23.20 E). In contrast to the placement of a vaginal device, medical personnel perform insertion and removal of the ICDs. Intra cervical devices are basically drug containing reservoirs, 10 mm long and 6 mm in diameter. Their size limits the selection of drugs to only highly potent compounds to be released from a cervical device. The ICDs with a surface area of 2.3 sq. cm contain enough norgestrel to maintain a release of 20-25 μg/day for four years. The daily release can be controlled downward relatively easily to as low as nearly 1 μg/day. This can be achieved by techniques such as reducing the reservoir drug concentration, by controlling surface area of the drug-containing portion of the reservoir to drug diffusion, or by a combination of these techniques. Intra cervical devices have been retained in place for periods up to 60 days without undesirable effects. However, acceptable retention, efficacy rates and long term safety remain to be established before these are made available for routine use.

The vaginal and the intra cervical devices may also be grouped and described under the miscellaneous methods of contraceptive technologies, since these are also devices just like the intra uterine device (IUD), which is inserted in the uterus for achieving contraception.

Currently, a lot of attention is being focused on new methods of **permanent contraception** for women that provide protection as good as achieved by surgical sterilization and are safer and easier to provide. Surgical female sterilization procedures involve tubal ligation, in which a woman's fallopian tubes are surgically cut or blocked by applying clips, rings, or heat. The most common surgical approaches are minilaparotomy and laparoscopy, described in details little later in this chapter in surgical methods. However, these approaches require skilled medical professionals and sterile conditions. In addition, minilaparotomy requires local anesthesia and laparoscopy requires general anesthesia. In contrast, these new contraceptive technologies do not involve surgery and increase an access to sterilization. The new developments focus mainly on **transcervical methods**. Some of the transcervical sterilization methods are already on the market and others are in clinical trials. These are fairly effective with only 0.2 to 2 pregnancies per 100 women in the first year of use. These are **nonsurgical methods** that reach the fallopian tubes through the vagina and uterus, and include use of **chemicals** such as **quinacrine**, and **plugs** (known as the **Adiana procedure**). **Quinacrine** is a chemical compound, which in the form of pellets. The pellets when inserted into the uterus, results in permanent sterilization by producing scarring (scar formation) to block the fallopian tubes. It can be provided by most trained health care providers, and does not require a physician. The **Adiana procedure** is also a transcervical sterilization method in which a clinician delivers a catheter through a hysteroscope into the fallopian tube and uses the catheter to apply low-level radiofrequency energy, creating a superficial lesion. The clinician then places a porous plastic implant, called a matrix, into the lesion. The matrix remains in the fallopian tube and the surrounding tissue and grows into it over the next 12 weeks. The ingrown tissue results in total closure of the fallopian tube. However, Adiana procedure requires use of an expensive hysteroscope. Therefore, it seems unlikely that this procedure is going to be introduced in the developing countries in the near future.

Micro coils, such as **Essure** (trade name, formerly named STOP) are already on the market. This is a spring-like device that a trained clinician using a hysteroscope inserts through the vagina into the uterus and then into each fallopian tube (Figure 23.21). Over three months following insertion, scar tissue grows into the device and permanently plugs the fallopian tubes so that sperm cannot pass through it to fertilize an egg. The procedure can be performed with a local anesthesia in less than an hour, and the woman quickly returns to her normal activities. Women need to use an additional temporary contraceptive method for first three months after insertion to allow time for scar tissue to form. After the scar tissue is formed, Essure is not reversible. Essure has been approved by regulatory agencies in Europe and in Australia, Canada, Singapore, Indonesia, Turkey and USA, but is unlikely to be introduced in developing countries in near future because of the high cost of the hysteroscope required for its insertion.

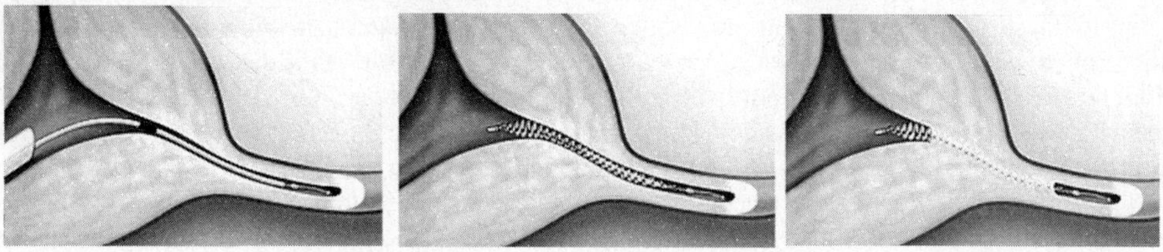

Figure 23.21: Microcoil Essure for Women.

Indian scientists at Delhi have developed **Intra Nasal Spray** of contraceptive steroids. The main advantage of such an approach is that extremely minute amounts of the hormone is administered and it reaches directly to the specialized area of the brain i.e. the hypothalamus and suppresses the central regulatory mechanisms that maintain cyclic reproductive activity in female. However, further studies on the spray are still in progress.

Birth control Vaccines: Most advanced research in contraceptive techniques involves several immunologic approaches for both men and women. Immunization with a vaccine prepared from beta subunits of human chorionic gonadotropin (HCG), a hormone produced in early pregnancy is being used in this technology. HCG immunization blocks continuation of the pregnancy. The antibodies appear in about 4 to 6 weeks and reach a maximum level after about 5 months, then slowly decline and reach zero levels after a period ranging from 6 to 11 months. Immunity can be boosted by a second injection. Two types of pregnancy vaccines employing variants of the beta subunit of HCG are now ready to go for clinical trials.

Similar type of injectable and steroid filled capsule as used for women has also been devised for **males** but they have not gained much popularity. Since Depo-Provera induces a marked depression in sperm count and motility in the male, it is not in practice.

Advances in male hormonal contraception have lagged behind advances in female hormonal contraception because of various reasons. One is that contraception has been seen as the woman's responsibility and the other is that caution has to be taken about the potential effects of hormone use on men's emotional and sexual well being. The potential side effects of female contraceptives appear minor in comparison with the large health benefits of avoiding unintended pregnancy and childbearing. In contrast, in case of men who do not face the risk of pregnancy and childbirth, the impacts of the side effects of contraceptive can appear relatively large.

Although several of new male contraceptives are close to market, none are currently available. Data from the United Nations Population Division World Contraceptive use 2003 on contraceptive use compiled primarily from surveys based on use of existing male contraceptives in developed region and in developing region shows clearly that family planning methods for females are more popular and are practiced more in comparison to those for males. Men should have access to contraceptives beyond condom and vasectomies. Researchers around the world are working toward male contraceptives that are potentially safer, more effective and more convenient than any contraceptives on the market today. These are heat methods, vas occlusion methods, hormonal methods, other pharmaceutical methods and new methods.

It is known that prolonged sitting in a hot tub can decrease a man's sperm count and men might be able to use this to their advantage as a source of inexpensive self-administered contraception. Researchers are trying to determine the reliability of the contraceptive effect of wet heat and suspensories. A man with sufficient determinations can undertake this method reliably for contraception.

Vas occlusion methods block the vas deferens while leaving the tube intact making reversal easier in comparison to vasectomy in which part of the vas deferens is removed. Injectable silicon plugs are being used by thousands of men in China for vas occlusion. Researchers in Canada and US are developing a pre-formed silicon plug called IVD that is implanted in the vas deferens. A new method of male contraception under development is **Reversible Inhibition of Sperm Under Guidance (RISUG)**. It is a clear polymer gel made of styrene maleic anhydride (SMA) mixed with dimethyl sulfoxide (DMSO). It was developed at the Indian Institute of Technology and the All India Institute of Medical Sciences in India. RISUG is injected into the vas deferens (the duct that carries sperm from the epididymis to the ejaculatory duct) and it results in long-term infertility by partially blocking the vas deferens and also by causing the membrane of the passing sperm to rupture, thereby disabling most sperm that do get through from fertilizing ovum. This contraceptive method for males has the potential advantage of being reversible. The side effects observed in the clinical trials are scrotal swelling in about one-third of participants. Toxicity and long-term follow-up studies of RISUG are being carried out. It is now in phase III clinical trials.

A number of hormones and other pharmaceutical compounds are being used to develop a "male pill" to suppress sperm production. **Anti-androgen, cyproterone acetate** (Figure 23.22) in low doses, when released from silastic capsules has shown to decrease sperm count and motility of spermatozoa. It also decreases the ability of spermatozoa to penetrate through the cervical mucus. However, the blood level of androgen also decreases with cyproterone acetate treatment and this is not desirable in case of men. A monthly or bimonthly injection or implant delivering testosterone only or a combination of testosterone and a progestin or gonadotropin-releasing hormone (GnRH) as a male hormonal contraceptive is now in phase II and III clinical trials. These prevent sperm production and provide men with a reversible and effective method of control of fertility. A new long-acting synthetic testosterone ester, 20 AET 1, now called **testosterone buciclate**, may be useful for maintaining libido and potency. After injection, this hormone forms a depot in the muscle and gradually releases testosterone over three months. **Analogues of luteinizing hormone releasing hormone, LHRH vaccines**, and some **herbal medicines** such as *Trippterigium wilfordii*, are also being studied as male contraceptives. Other drugs, such as an immuno-contraceptive or Dr. Joseph Hall's enzyme inhibitor pill are still in the conceptual stages of development. Also, two plant compounds, neem oil and papaya seed extract require further study.

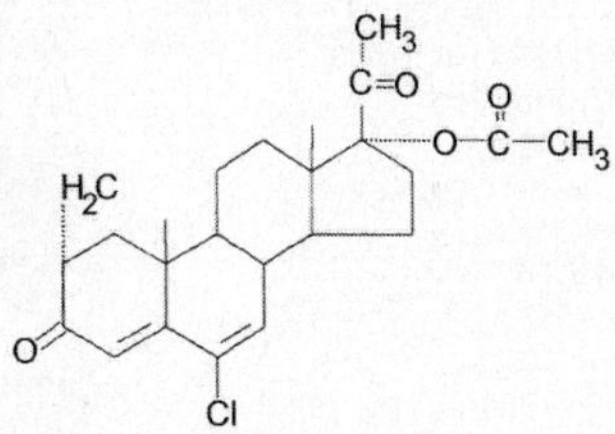

Figure 23.22: An antiandrogen- cyproterone acetate.

Gene-based approaches in contraception: With the recent advances in the discovery of genes and proteins functioning specifically in the reproductive tract, it may be possible to develop a contraceptive that target the genes controlling sperm and egg development or the proteins controlling the fusion of sperm and egg without causing side effects by affecting other body systems. However, these are at least a decade away from reaching the market.

In women, several novel approaches for contraception appear possible and one such is based on the molecules that are involved in the release of mature egg during ovulation. Identifying specific enzymes responsible for the release of an egg would allow for the development of a contraceptive that may prevent ovulation without disrupting the endocrine function. Further, scientists have discovered the zygote arrest I (ZARI) gene that plays a key role in the fusion of sperm and egg pronuclei. In female mice, pronuclei lacking this gene cannot fuse and thus show infertility. Therefore, it is believed that blocking ZARI I gene might produce contraceptive effect in human female.

In men too, discovery of gene and proteins are of great help in studying various processes such as maturation of spermatozoa, sperm penetration into an egg etc. Scientists have discovered a molecule in rats named Bin 1b that exists only in the epididymis, where sperm normally mature and gain motility. Bin 1b binds to the head of sperm and induce sperm motility. This action of Bin molecule could be blocked to achieve a contraceptive effect by preventing sperm penetration into egg. Further, a set of genes, known as Catsper, that encode a series of calcium ion exchange channels specific to the male reproductive tract have been discovered. Study of these genes would help to develop a contraceptive drug that could act as calcium channel blocker.

23.6 Surgical Methods

The most effective form of birth control, with the exception of abstinence, is **surgical sterilization** (Figure 23.23). Sterilization is a procedure that renders an individual incapable of reproduction. That is why these methods are also referred to as **terminal methods**. It includes **vasectomy** in the male and **tubectomy** or **tubal ligation** in the female. Sterilization has enjoyed a recent increase in popularity because it is safe, effective and permanent. Currently, female sterilization accounts for nearly 85 % of all the sterilization's in India and male sterilization for 10 to 15 %.

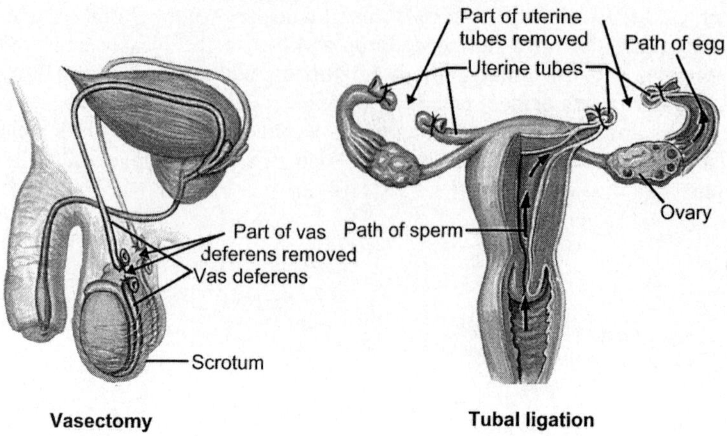

Figure 23.23: Surgical methods- vasectomy in Human male and tubal ligation in Human female.

Vasectomy in Male: Vasectomy is a voluntary male sterilization (Figure 23.23). It is a simple surgical procedure that is performed within 10 to 15 minutes under local anesthesia. As illustrated in Figure 23.24, vasectomy consists of a small surgical incision on each side of the scrotum to expose a small section of the vas deferens. The vas deferentia are severed, and the ends are tied, clamped, or cauterized to prevent sperm transport through the vas deferens. Vasectomy does not interfere with sperm production. Following vasectomy, sperm accumulates in the epididymis, where they are engulfed and destroyed by phagocytosis.

A refined and improved technique of vasectomy is known as **no-scalpel vasectomy**. It substitutes a small puncture for one or two small incisions in the scrotum (Figure 23.25). Details of the procedure are illustrated and described in the figure itself. No-scalpel technique reduces pain, complications, and operating time, in addition to minimizing bleeding and tissue trauma.

Now a days **vas occlusion methods** are also being tried to block the vas deferens. These methods involve **injections** or **devices** inserted directly through the skin and into the vas deferens without pulling the vas deferens out of the scrotum. Injections of polyurethane or silicone given directly into the vas deferens eliminate surgery entirely. The injected liquid polyurethane or silicone hardens within 10 minutes into solid plug that blocks passage of sperm. The vas occlusive devices are contraceptive plugs, which are surgically inserted in the vas to block the passage of sperm. Vasocclude is a new instrument used for applying clips to the vas deferens. Compared with conventional occlusion methods, these new techniques may cause less tissue damage and may be more easily reversible.

The **Intra Vas Device** (**IVD**-originally called the **Shug**) is a device that is implanted into the vas deferens. The new intra vas device uses two plugs in each vas deferens, so that any sperm passing by one plug will be stopped by the second. In animal studies, the technology proved effective and reversible. Placing and removing the IVD does not require special surgical training. It could be provided as a contraceptive choice in cases where no-scalpel vasectomy can be provided. In a pilot study, IVD drastically reduced number of sperm in the ejaculate of all the 30 men participants. Phase II clinical trials will assess the IVDs safety, ability to block the vas deferens and overall contraceptive effectiveness

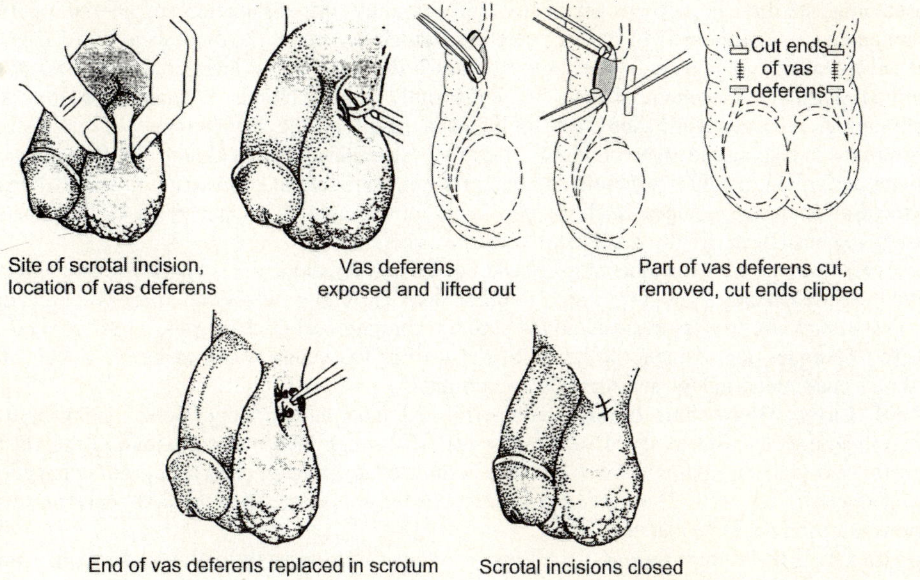

Figure 23.24: Steps involved in vasectomy in Men.

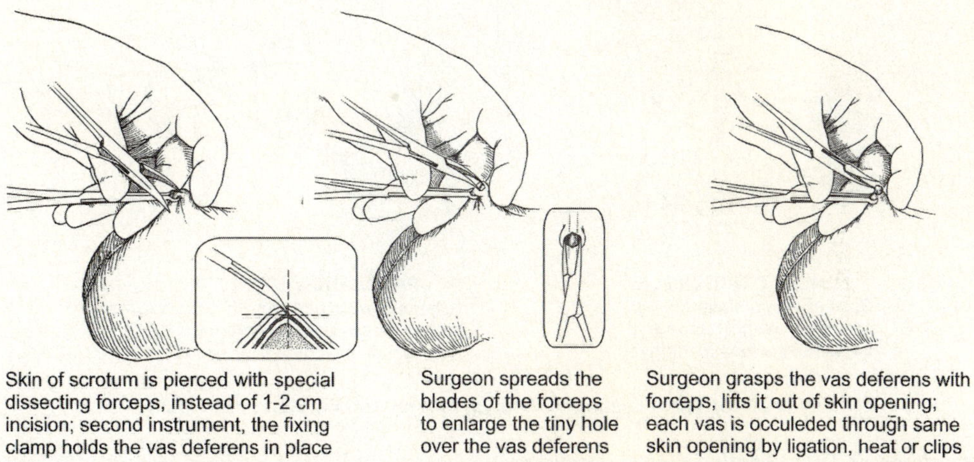

Figure 23.25: Steps involved in no-scalpel vasectomy in Men.

Advantage: Vasectomy does not interfere with the synthesis or release of testosterone from the testes. It does not affect erection, ejaculation, or orgasm in any way. Vasectomy is economic, safe and a very effective method of contraception, with failure rates below 0.15 %. Post-surgical complications, which can include bleeding, infection, and swelling of scrotal tissue due to sperm leakage, are rare. No long-range health risks appear to be associated with vasectomy. It is potentially reversible. Vasectomy does not seem to exert long-term harmful psychological or behavioral effects.

Disadvantage: Men regard genital operation as a form of castration. They also do not accept the fact that they are permanently infertile since ability to father a child is a sign of masculinity for them. Post-vasectomy sterility is not instantaneous and requires the dissipation of stored spermatozoa. Spontaneous re-anastomosis of the vas deferens, which occurs in 1% of vasectomized men, may be caused by sperm granuloma. Vasectomy causes a decrease in the levels of dihydrotestosterone in seminal plasma but without altering it significantly in the blood. Some men may show an immunologic reaction following vasectomy, as a result of the development of circulating auto-agglutinins in response to obstructive azoospermia. Electrocautery and chemically induced vasectomy can be performed rapidly but these techniques are not reversible in comparison to surgical vasectomy. Extravasal occlusive devices, such as clips and intraluminal occlusive plugs or threads used for vasectomy must be surgically removed to restore vas potency.

Vasovasostomy: Post-vasectomy sterility can be restored by surgical anastomosis of the vas deferens, called vasovasostomy. The two most common and currently successful operative procedures for vasovasostomy are two-layer, intraluminal suture technique, and double layer, microscopic technique. These techniques approximate the layers of the wall of vas deferens and make the lumen of the vas deferens continuous and the anastomosis "watertight".

Double-Layer, Microscopic Technique is performed under an operating microscope using 9-0 nylon sutures throughout. Six to seven sutures are placed through the mucosa, including the elastic layer directly next to the mucosa and when lineup is completed, a watertight and leak proof connection of the vas deferens is achieved. The outer muscularis and the serosa are then sutured separately using 9-0 nylon sutures in the same manner.

Two Layer, Intraluminal Suture Technique employs two to three through-and-through, intraluminal muscularis-serosal sutures, called as "anastomosing sutures".

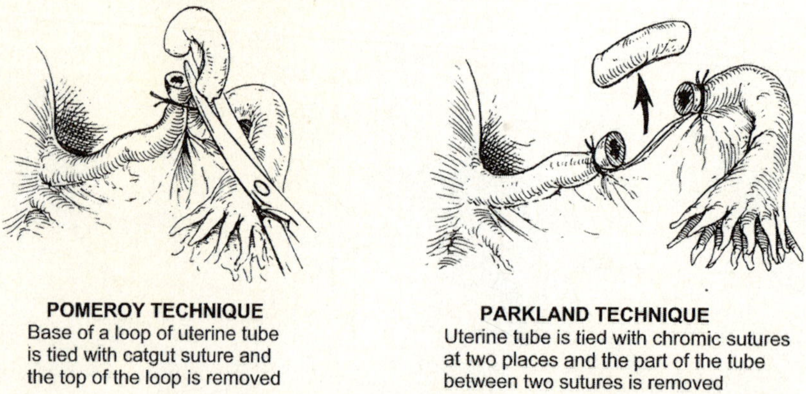

Figure 23.26: Tubal ligation in Women, Pomery and Parkland techniques.

Tubectomy or Tubal ligation: Female sterilization involves blocking of the Fallopian tubes that carry eggs from the ovaries to the uterus (Figure 23.23). There are two ways to reach the tubes. **Laparoscopy** method consists of an abdominal incision to permit insertion of an instrument called a **laparoscope**. Laparoscope is a fiber-optic instrument that can be inserted through the abdomen to view the internal organs. The surgeon sees the fallopian tubes through this thin tubular instrument and applies rings, clips or cautery (heat), to block the tubes for both ovum transport to the uterus and sperm transport to the fallopian tubes. **Minilaparotomy** method consists of making a small incision in the abdomen, moving each tube to the incision, ligating (tying) each tube, and removing a segment of the tube from tubes of both sides. The tubes are ligated or tied by two common techniques. These are **Pomeroy technique** and **Parkland technique** (Figure 23.26). Both these methods are very effective and very safe. When performed after childbirth, tubal ligation often consists of placing two ligatures around the mid-section of each fallopian tube and removing the intervening segment. Reversal surgery is major abdominal surgery that involves removal of damaged tube parts, aligning the remaining segments and suturing them together to create a secure connection. Reconnecting the tubes is quite difficult because they are small and slippery. Women who undergo reversal surgery are at an increased risk of ectopic pregnancy.

Advantage: Voluntary female sterilization is number one method of family planning in the world. Tubal ligation is a very effective method of preventing pregnancy. Post-surgical complications, which can include bleeding and infection, are rare. As with vasectomy, no long-range health risks appear to be associated with tubal ligation.

Disadvantage: The reversal surgery may not be successful in some cases as per the needs. Sometimes reconnection of the severed ends of the fallopian tube (**anastomosis**) after sterilization occurs spontaneously, allowing pregnancy to take place. Emotional reactions may occur in a few cases. Autoimmunization can also cause problems.

23.7 Intra Uterine Devices (IUD)

Another type of contraceptive method is the intrauterine device (IUD), which can be worn by the females in the uterus for extended periods of time (Figure 23.27). It works mainly by stopping sperm and egg from meeting. Most women can use IUDs including women who have never been pregnant.

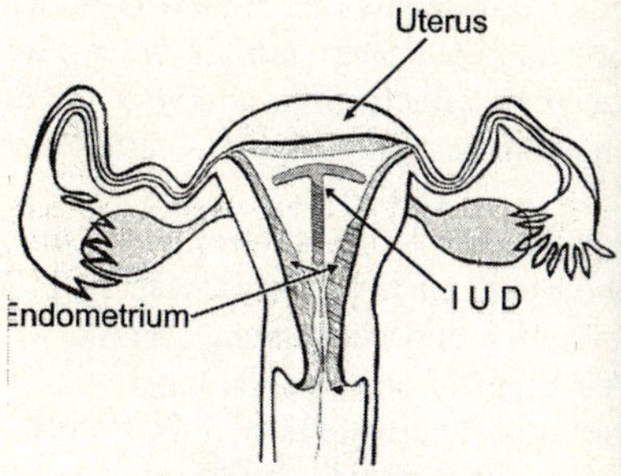

T-shaped framed IUD

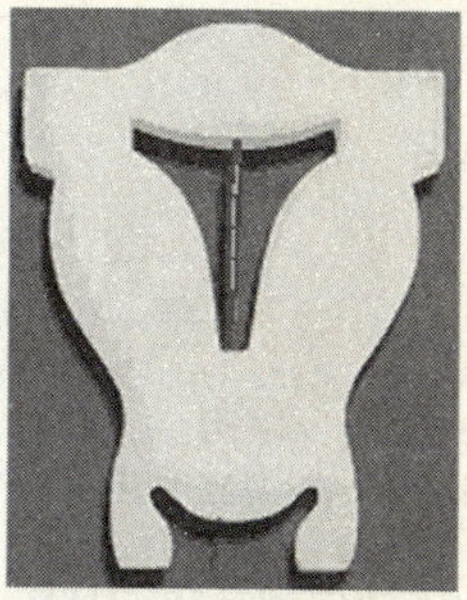

Frameless IUD Gyne Fix

Figure 23.27: Intrauterine device for Women.

The control of conception by introducing a foreign body into the uterus was known to the Arabs in the Middle East from ages. They were controlling conception in camels by introducing a small round stone into each uterine horn of a female camel. Based on this knowledge a device was made and first used in 1909. This original device was made of silkworm gut. In 1929, Grafenbergh, a German gynecologist opened a new chapter in the history of intra-uterine devices (IUD) for contraception by an IUD made of silver in preventing conception. He achieved a failure rate of only 1.6 %. In 1934, Ota made a new device in Japan called Ota ring, which is still in use today. In 1959, Japanese were the first to utilize plastic material in the manufacture of IUDs. This led to a huge interest in intrauterine contraception and resulted in the development of modern IUDs.

The IUD is made of either plastic or metal (copper, or stainless steel) and is inserted by a physician into the uterus through the vagina and cervix (Figure 23.28). Using IUD is many times safer and more effective in preventing pregnancy than oral contraceptives, condoms, spermicides, any barrier method, or Natural Family Planning method. IUD does not leave the womb but move around inside the body without coming in the way during intercourse, although sometimes the man may feel the strings. It does not rust inside the body, even after many years. IUD is very effective contraceptive with little to remember and women can soon become pregnant when IUD is taken out. For older woman, IUD should be removed one year after her last menstrual period (i.e. menopause).

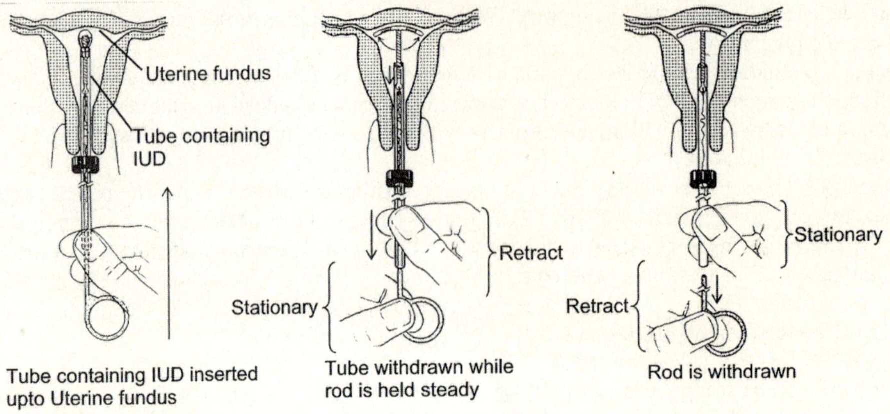

Figure 23.28: Steps involved in insertion of copper Ts, Multiloads, Nova T, and Progestasert in Women.

Types of IUD: IUDs can be classified as either **non-medicated (inert) type** or **medicated type**. Of the eight types of IUDs widely used, two are non-medicated and six are medicated. The medicated IUDs were developed to increase their contraceptive effectiveness and also to reduce their side effects. However, they are more expensive and also need to be changed after a certain period to maintain their effectiveness.

The first modern IUDs appeared in the early 1960s and were in use throughout the world for more than three decades. These were non-medicated, made of polyethylene, a biologically inert plastic and millions of women found them safe, effective and convenient. These were the **Lippes Loop** (Figure 23.29) and the **Margulies Spiral**. The Lippes Loop was the most widely used non-medicated IUD outside China. This IUD is no longer used internationally. The other major types of non-medicated IUDs are flexible stainless steel rings, either round or in the shape of the uterine cavity and made with a single or double coil (Figure 23.28). These rings have been widely used in China only.

However, in the late 1960s, researchers discovered that adding copper to a plastic IUD frame increased its effectiveness, thus allowing use of devices of sizes smaller than the all-plastic devices. Thus, medicated IUDs were introduced which had copper or hormones added to a plastic frame. The non-medicated IUDs are often referred to as the **'first generation IUDs'**. In the medicated IUD types, the **copper** IUDs comprise the **'second generation'** and the **hormone releasing** IUDs as the **'third generation'** of IUDs. The copper IUDs included the **Cu-7**, the **Tcu-200**, and the **Multiload-250** (MLCu-250) (Figure 23.28). These IUDs carried copper wire with a surface area of 200-250 mm^2. Following this, 'second generation' copper IUDs were introduced with several innovations such as more copper wire, copper sleeves, and/or a silver core to the copper wire, denoted by Ag in the IUD name. These changes increased the effectiveness and also extended the effective life span of the device. The second generation IUDs includes **TCu-380A, TCu-220C, Multiload-375** (MLCu-375) and **Nova T** (Figure 23.29). **Hormone-releasing medicated IUDs** constantly release small amounts of steroid hormone into the uterus to further prevent pregnancy. For example, **Progestasert** (Figure 23.28) contain 38 mg progesterone released at a rate of 65 μg/day for one year, and a longer lasting **LNG-20** IUD contains 52 mg of levonorgestrel released at a rate of 20 μg/day and lasts for at least five years. Various types of IUDs are shown in the Figure 23.29.

Researchers continued to develop new IUDs to reduce expulsion rates and side effects. Among these is T-shaped copper IUD, the Cu-SAFE 300, which is smaller, lightweight, and flexible and can be inserted without a plunger. It is designed to move towards the uterine fundus when the uterus contracts. In yet another device, a copper bearing IUD with a T-shaped frame called Sof-T, the tip of each end of its arm consists of a soft ball designed to prevent uterine perforation and to block the opening to the fallopian tubes in order to prevent sperm from entering. Frameless IUD has also been designed, called the FlexiGard 330, GyneFix™, or CuFix PP330. The frame-less IUD is made without the plastic T-shaped frame common to most other types of IUDs. It consists of six copper sleeves (copper cylinders) tied together on a surgical nylon thread (string) and is anchored one centimeter deep into the fundus or top of the uterus. The thread is knotted at one end, which is anchored in the muscle of the fundus.

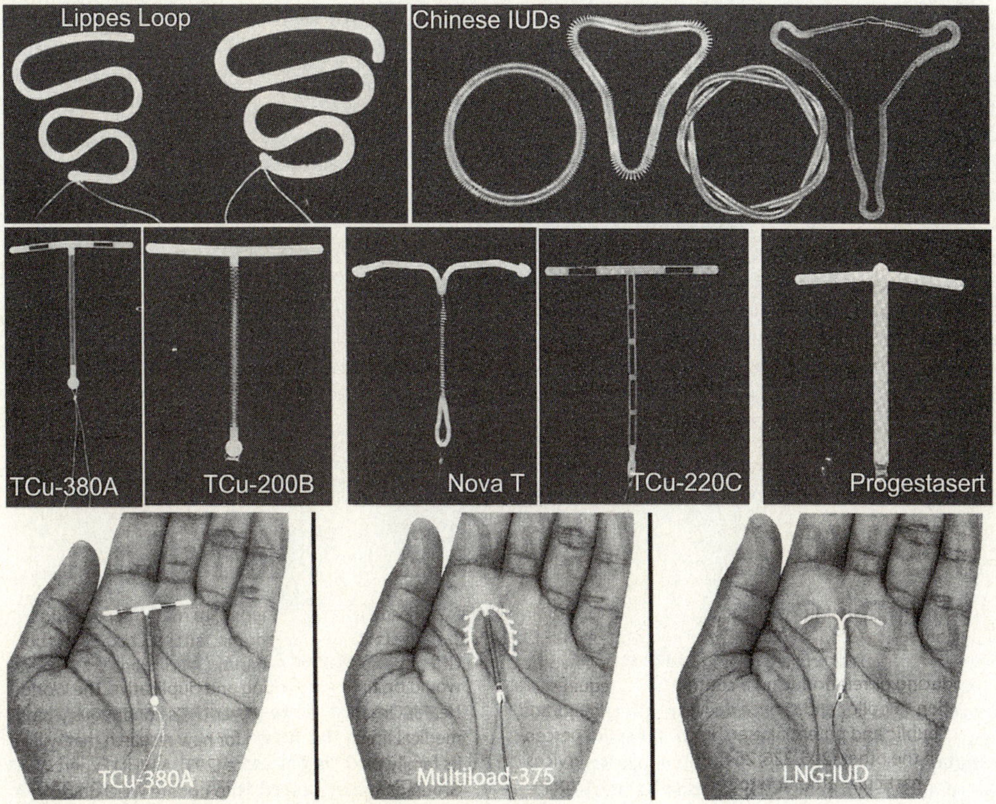

Figure 23.29: Various types of non-medicated and medicated IUDs.

Many of the early IUDs were named after their inventors, for example, the Lippes Loop after Jack Lippes of the US. However, with recently developed IUDs, manufacturers have conducted market research to come up with product name that suggests effectiveness, reliability, and other positive images. For example, GynoPharma, the company that market the Tcu-380A in the US, used focus-group discussions and surveys to decide on the name ParaGard for the Tcu-380A as this name suggests a modern and effective IUD.

Mechanism of Action of IUDs: IUDs prevent sperm from fertilizing ova, and not as believed earlier by inducing a local inflammatory reaction in the endometrium of the uterus, which prevents implantation of the ovum. Medicated IUDs produce other local effects that may contribute further to their contraceptive action. Copper IUDs alter the function or survival of sperm or ova before they can meet. Copper seems to enhance the cellular response in the endometrium and also affects the enzymes in the uterus, thus affecting the motility, capacitation and survival of sperm. The hormone releasing IUDs, such as LNG-20 IUD has primarily a hormonal mode of action. These IUDs work by thickening cervical mucus so that sperm cannot pass through it, thus preventing fertilization of ova. Also, they maintain high levels of progesterone in the endometrium, and thus relatively low levels of estrogen, thereby sustaining an endometrium unfavorable to implantation.

Effectiveness of IUDs: Among various types of IUDs known, the Copper T 380A (Tcu-380A) is now the most widely available and used IUD, and is approved for up to 10 years of use. In addition to Tcu-380A, the Tu-220C, the Multiload-375, the Nova T, and the LNG-20 are other IUDs currently available and are in practice. All these are more effective than oral contraceptives and at par with injectables, implants and voluntary sterilization. The hormone-releasing LNG-20 IUD may be the most effective of all IUDs, with just 0.3 pregnancies per 100 women. Because modern IUDs prevent pregnancy very effectively, they avert many maternal deaths, and thus rank among the best family planning methods for protecting women's lives. Proper IUD insertion (Figure 23.30) reduces the risks of pregnancy and all major side effects such as expulsion, bleeding, and pain, perforation, and infection. IUDs can be inserted safely at any time during the menstrual cycle as long as pregnancy is ruled out. Postpartum insertion also is safe and is convenient. IUDs can safely be inserted after spontaneous or induced abortion except in women with pelvic infections. The IUD is an ideal contraceptive method for lactating women because it has no effect on the quantity or composition of breast milk. Like insertion, IUD removal is usually a routine and uncomplicated procedure and can be done at any time of the menstrual cycle. Most women who discontinue IUD use to become pregnant, conceive as rapidly as nonusers of IUDs.

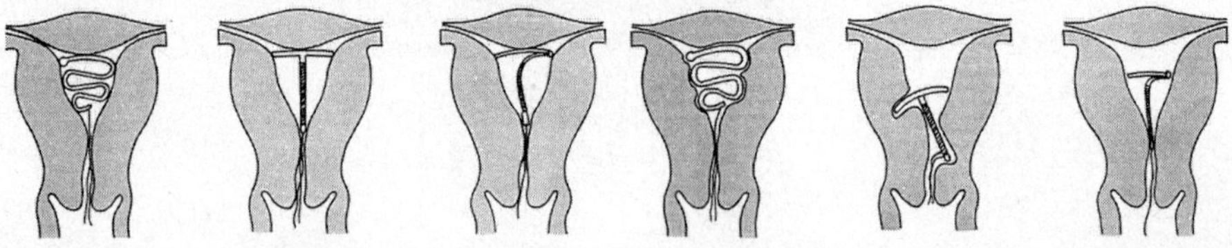

Figure 23.30: Proper and improper insertion of IUDs in Women, first three-properly positioned Lippes Loop, T Cu-200 and Cu-7 and next three-a Lippes Loop too large for the uterus and is pressing into and irritating the endometrium, Tu-200 is perforating the cervix, and Cu-7 is too small for the uterus and has slipped or been forced out of position by uterine contractions; improperly placed IUDs produce higher rates of pregnancy, expulsion and removal for bleeding or pain.

Advantage: IUD remains a generally safe, effective, and useful form of birth control. . It has long-term effectiveness, which is comparable to that of tubal ligation. Failure rate is very low. It needs one time decision and action. It is not associated with sex act. It is economical. Hormone-releasing IUDs, by reducing menstrual bleeding, may actually protect against anemia. It is suitable for a large-scale family planning program.

Disadvantage: Side effects of IUD include uterine bleeding, spasm and cramping of uterine muscles, pelvic infection, and perforation of the uterine wall, however, second generation medicated IUDs are much more effective and have fewer side effects than unmedicated IUDs. Because of side effects, some women discontinue use of IUDs unless properly educated and reassured. IUDs do not prevent

AIDS. IUD use does increase the risk of developing pelvic inflammatory disease (PID) and sometimes this leads to tubal infertility.

New IUDs now on the market make their insertion and removal easier and reduce rate of expulsion, pain, and bleeding. These advances could lead to a greater acceptance and use of the IUD. New IUDs include the progestin-releasing intrauterine system (IUS), and IUDs without the conventional T-shaped frame. Progestin releasing IUD is marketed under the name Mirena. It gradually releases levonorgestrel, which makes menstruation lighter and less painful. The frame-less IUD is marketed as GyneFix. It is anchored into the uterine wall, and this design cause less pain and bleeding than framed devices.

The Ideal IUD Candidate: The Planned Parenthood Federation of America (PPFA) has described the ideal IUD candidate with the following characteristics. A woman i) who has borne at least one child, ii) has normal menstrual period, iii) has no history of pelvic disease, iv) is willing to check the IUD tail, v) is in a monogamous relationship, and vi) has access to follow up and treatment of potential problems.

It has been found that IUD is not a method of first choice for nulliparous women (who have not been pregnant earlier). They show problems of expulsion, abdominal pain, and pelvic infection. Smaller IUDs, such as copper T are better suited to the small uterus of the nulliparous women in case they cannot use or accept alternative methods of contraception. The American College of Obstetricians and Gynecologists, in 1985 stated that IUDs are "not recommended for women who have not had children or who have multiple partners, because of the risk of PID leading to possible infertility". Also, it cannot be used for woman who shows unusual recent vaginal bleeding or infection/problem in female organs or the one who is at high risk for STIs.

Timing of IUD Insertion: The IUD can be inserted at anytime during a woman's reproductive years, except during pregnancy. The most suitable time for insertion of IUD is during menstruation or within ten days of the beginning of menstruation. This is because the diameter of the cervical canal is greater at this time than during the secretory phase. Also, the uterus is relaxed and the myometrial contractions, which might tend to cause expulsion, are at a minimum. Insertion of IUD can also be done during the first week after delivery, known as **postpartum insertion**. However, special care is required for insertion at this time because of greater risk of perforation during this time, as well as high expulsion rate. Insertion after 6 to 8 weeks of delivery is called **post-puerperal insertion**, and this has many advantages over post-partum insertion. It can be easily combined with the follow-up examination of the woman and her child. Some side effects observed after insertion are some cramps for several days and some spotting for a few weeks. But these are not the signs of illness. The other common side effects are longer and heavier periods, bleeding or spotting between periods and more cramps or pain during periods. These may get less after a few months.

Change of IUD: An IUD cannot be used indefinitely. It must be changed after the prescribed period of use. Inert IUDs such as Lippes Loop may be left in place if there are no side effects for as long as required. However, copper devices cannot be used for too long because copper corrodes and mineral deposits build up on the copper affecting the release of copper ions. These IUDs have to be replaced periodically at intervals of 2-4 years or as per recommendations. It is also true for the hormone-releasing intrauterine devices. Fertility is not impaired after removal of a device provided there has been no episode of pelvic inflammatory disease (PID) when the device was in the uterus. In addition, there is no evidence of increased risk of cancer and teratogenesis associated with use of IUDs.

23.8 Abortion and Medical Termination of Pregnancy

The word abortion has a Latin root (*Ab* = abnormal and *oriri* = to born). It refers to the premature expulsion of the products of conception or fetus from the uterus, living or dead, but of recognizable size. In case of human, it usually occurs before the 20th week of pregnancy. Generally the aborted fetuses are non-viable. In medical terms, the **abortion** is defined, as the **medical termination of a pregnancy (MTP)** before the fetus is capable of extra-uterine life. The condition, in which fertilized eggs and embryos are lost before the recognizable size is reached, is known as **early embryonic death.**

Causes and types of Abortion: There can be various **causes** of abortion such as **physical** like trauma or accidental injuries; **toxic** due to chemicals or drugs; **psychological**; **hormonal**; **nutritional**; **infectious diseases** like viral, protozoan or fungal; **hereditary** and **miscellaneous**. Abortion is of two types:

- **Spontaneous Abortion**-It is a naturally occurring abortion, also called a **miscarriage**. All abortions not induced are spontaneous even if an external cause such as trauma or disease is involved.
- **Induced Abortion**-Ii refers to deliberate interference with a pregnancy with the intention of terminating it and this is referred to as **medical termination of pregnancy** or **MTP** in short.

Abortion to some extent can be performed intentionally by the pregnant woman herself or by another person, may be medical or non-medical. When birth control methods are not in use or fail to prevent a pregnancy, an induced abortion is performed. The incidence of abortion is increasing as more women try to avoid unwanted births and like to keep their families small. Between 30 and 60 million abortions are induced worldwide every year, making abortion one of the most prevalent means of preventing childbirth and a method of family planning today. Inserting a twig or other object into the cervix can mechanically induce abortion. This may however lead to uterine and intestinal perforation and subsequent peritonitis. Other non-medical methods of inducing abortion include eating or drinking quinine, laundry bluing, or many other chemicals. These can lead to poisoning, renal failure, or intense vomiting causing dehydration, and eventual death unless proper care therapy is instituted. The most common method of illegal abortion worldwide is insertion of a foreign object, like a urinary catheter, or *sonda*, into the vagina and cervix.

A major cause of death among women of reproductive age in developing countries is illegally induced abortion. Four different approaches can reduce mortality from illegal abortion. These are, encouraging the use of contraceptive method instead of abortion, legalizing abortion, allowing medically trained practitioners to perform abortions for health reasons, and improving clinical management of abortion complications. Abortion, when performed by a trained provider in aseptic conditions is relatively safe, but when performed by inexperienced people or under unhygienic conditions, as is generally the case with illegal abortion, then mortality, morbidity, and long-term complications become much greater. Four major factors determine the mortality and morbidity from both legal and illegal abortion. These are: the method used to induce abortion, the skill of the provider, the duration of pregnancy and the accessibility and quality of medical facilities to treat complications of abortion. In India facilities available during induced abortion and its clinical management has improved since the time abortion has been legalized.

Some terms, which are commonly used in abortion research, are incomplete abortion, septic abortion, abortifacient etc. Abortion that is followed by infection is the **septic abortion** while the **incomplete abortion** is the presence of retained products of conception in the uterus after a spontaneous or induced abortion. A drug or other substance used to cause a pregnant woman to abort is called an **abortifacient**. Abortion is usually measured by **rates**, which relate numbers of abortions to population, or by **ratio**, which relate the number of abortions to the number of events such as live births, deliveries, or pregnancies.

Methods of Abortion: W.E. Brenner classifies midtrimester abortion methods into four categories. These are **surgical evacuation** (for example, hystertomy, hysterectomy, dilation and curettage, vacuum aspiration), **intrauterine injection of solutions** (for example, hypertonic saline, prostaglandins, urea, glucose), **intrauterine insertion of devices** (for example bougie, metreurynter), **extra-uterine** (oral, intravenous, intramuscular, intravaginal), **administration of drugs such** as oxytocin, prostaglandins. A single method or several in combination may be used to induce abortion. However, five general types of techniques are now followed in current clinical practice to induce legal abortion. These are, i) **Curettage procedures**, ii) **Intrauterine mechanical devices**, iii) **Intrauterine instillation of abortifacient agents**, iv) **Extra-uterine administration of abortifacient agents**, and v) **Hysterotomy and Hysterectomy**. As shown in the Figure 23.31, any of these procedures of abortion can be performed depending on the number of weeks of pregnancy. All these procedures are described below in details.

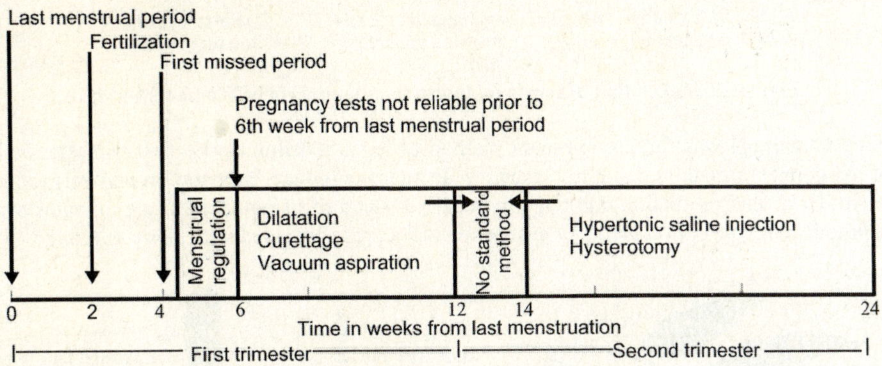

Figure 23.31: Methods of pregnancy termination selected by number of weeks of pregnancy in Women.

1. Curettage Procedures: The word curette means a surgical instrument used for scraping tissue from a body cavity. Thus, curettage procedures are those, which are employed surgically to evacuate the contents of the uterus containing the products of conception. These methods are simple, efficient and safe and are subdivided into four types.

- **Menstrual regulation or endometrial aspiration or menstrual extraction** is relatively new means of suction curettage designed for use within a few weeks after the first missed menses. A cannula of appropriate size is connected to the source of the suction then inserted into the uterus. The uterine contents are aspirated with rotatory motion of the cannula.
- **Suction Curettage or vacuum aspiration** with rigid cannulas is the principal type of abortion procedure used in many countries. Suction curettage has two parts, the first is the dilation of the cervix, and second is the evacuation of the products of conception by suction. Either para-cervical or general anesthesia may be used for the abortion. The cervix is gradually dilated by introducing a series of progressively larger tapered cylinders known as **dilators** over a period of several minutes. The cervix can also be dilated more slowly by means of **laminaria tents,** which must be properly inserted into cervix (Figure 23.32). These are hygroscopic sticks of sterile dried stems of marine plant commonly called Commelina plant (Figure 23.33) which when exposed to moisture in cervix, expand to several times their original diameters. Most expansion occurs over the first 4-6 hours after insertion. After adequate dilation has been accomplished, a suction cannula with a diameter in millimeters of approximate gestational age is inserted. The cannula, connected to an

electrically powered vacuum pump by clear flexible tubing, is rotated gently to aspirate the products of conception.

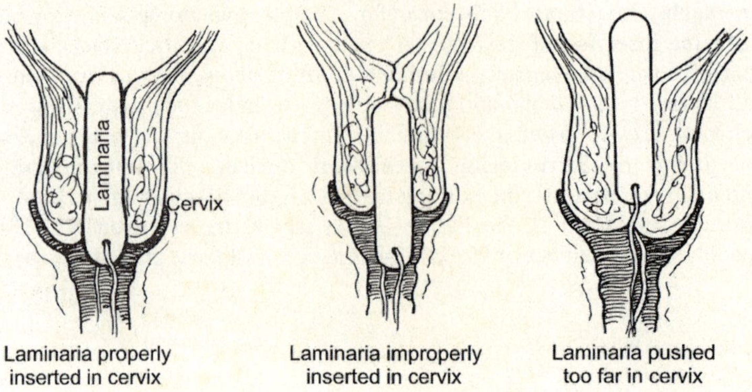

Figure 23.32: Dilation of cervix by insertion of laminaria in Women's cervix.

- **Sharp Curettage** was the predominant method of legal abortion in the first trimester before the suction curettage method came into practice. In sharp curettage, preparation and cervical dilation are similar to that of suction curettage, however, instead of using suction, the operator evacuates the products of conception using sponge or ovum forceps combined with sharp curettage.

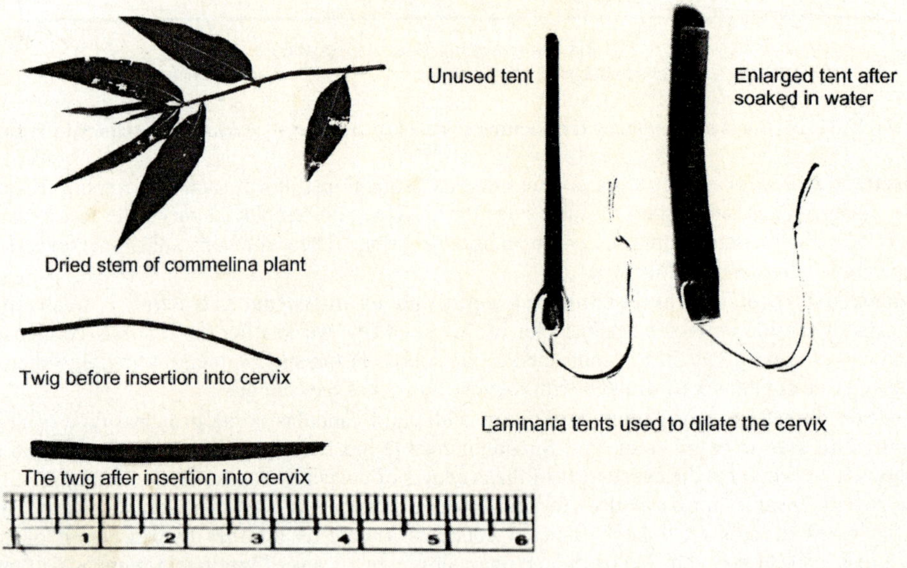

Figure 23.33: Laminaria tents-unused and enlarge, and dried stem of Commelina plant, used as cervical dilators in Ghana, twigs shown are before and after insertion into the cervix of Women.

- **Midtrimester Dilation and Evacuation (D and E)** involves cervical dilation followed by evacuation under para-cervical or general anesthesia with a total operation time of usually less than 30 minutes. Because the cervix must be dilated to larger diameters in order to empty larger uteri, some operators rely on overnight placement of multiple intra-cervical laminaria, while others accomplish more rapid dilation with large caliber dilators. The uterus is then emptied using sponge forceps, heavier crushing forceps, suction curettage, sharp curettage, or a combination of these.

2. Intrauterine Mechanical Devices: One of the oldest methods of abortion has been insertion of a foreign body into the uterus. Devices used to induce abortion have been **catheters**, **bougies** (large, slender and soft rubber catheters), **laminaria**, **balsa**, and **metreurynters** (a rubber bag or an intrauterine balloon similar to a 30 ml Foley catheter). These devices are used primarily in Japan. They cause uterine irritation or inflammation, which results in uterine contractions and fetal expulsion. Common disadvantage with all the foreign body methods was introduction of high rates of infection and also long abortion times in comparison to alternative abortion methods. In addition, hospitalization and continuous medical care is required during the prolonged period of confinement. Also, there is a high incidence of live births associated with these methods. Therefore, this method is least desirable and is not considered a primary method of abortion, although laminaria or metreurynters may be used to augment other techniques when medically indicated.

3. Intrauterine Instillation of Abortifacient Agents: The instillation (slow injection) techniques are the most common and widely used of all methods of abortion in the mid-trimester of pregnancy. The intrauterine infusion of hypertonic solutions, such as saline, glucose, or urea, or of uterotonic agents like prostaglandins $F_{2\alpha}$($PGF_{2\alpha}$), induces uterine contractions, resulting in expulsion of the products of conception. The abortifacient agents can be injected into either the intra-amniotic space (within the amniotic sac) or the extra-ovular space that is outside the fetal membranes (Figure 23.34). Extra-ovular instillation of saline is generally less effective than intra-amniotic instillation. Natural prostaglandins and their analogues are effective in inducing abortion at any stage of gestation. Prostaglandin $F_{2\alpha}$ stimulates uterine contractions directly and produces faster abortions than hypertonic solutions, which act indirectly and has higher success rates in first 48 hours. However, because $PGF_2\alpha$ is rapidly metabolized, a second dose is frequently used to hasten abortion in about 30 % 0f patients. Intravenous oxytocin infusions have been used to augment $PGF_2\alpha$. Also the combined effects of laminaria insertion permit the use of smaller doses of $PGF_2\alpha$. Although transient gastrointestinal side effects, such as nausea, vomiting, and diarrhea are often associated with the administration of prostaglandins, serious complications are rare.

4. Extra-uterine Administration Of Abortifacient Agents: Various routes have administered a number of different abortifacient agents, however Food and Drug Administration have approved only prostaglandin E2 vaginal suppositories. These may be used for abortion of approximately 13 weeks gestation and in cases of fetal death *in-utero* through 28 weeks.

5. Hysterotomy and Hysterectomy: Prior to the development of safer techniques for mid-trimester abortions, major abdominal or vaginal operations were the important methods of abortion. Hysterotomy is the incision of the uterus. It is similar to a cesarean section and the abdominal approach is used exclusively as it is simpler and allows concurrent tubal sterilization. In this procedure, after making a laparotomy incision, the operator incises the uterus, evacuates the products of conception either manually or by curettage and then closes the wound as per any standard surgical operation. Hysterectomy on the other hand is the surgical removal of uterus, partially or completely. Since the morbidity and mortality rates of hysterotomy and hysterectomy were high, these operations are not used as a method of abortion these days. Hysterectomy performed to remove a pregnant uterus, as a method of abortion should be restricted to pre-existing gynecologic pathological cases or to unique circumstances only.

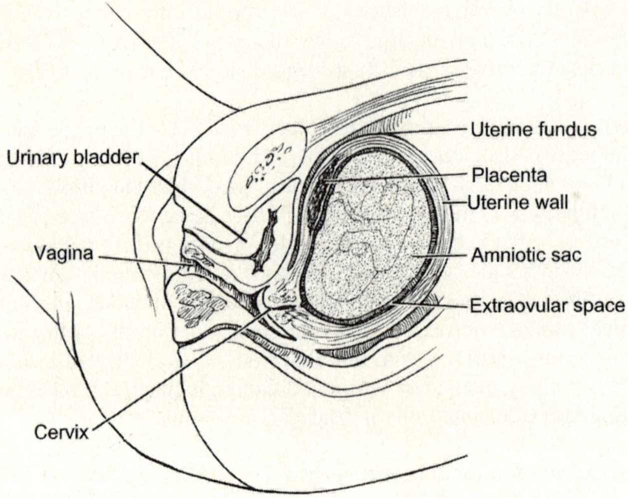

Figure 23.34: Female reproductive organs during midtrimester pregnancy, showing 'amniotic sac' and 'extra ovular Space' in Women's uterus.

Although abortion is a safe surgical procedure now yet, two predominant factors influence the morbidity of abortion. These are i) the gestational age and ii) the abortion technique. The risk of abortion morbidity increases with advancing gestational age. The lowest complication rate for induced abortion occurs at 7-8 weeks of gestation and it is 0.3 per 100 abortions. It increases progressively to a maximum of 2.26 per 100 abortions at 21-24 weeks of gestation (Table 23.2). Although abortion technique is related to gestational age, yet curettage technique used for inducing abortions are the safest with suction curettage having the lowest major complication rate (0.4%), followed by sharp curettage (0.9%), instillation techniques (1.9%), hystertomy (14.9%), and hysterectomy (16.1%) as indicated in Table 23.3.

Table 23.2: Relationship of gestational age with complication rate in women

Gestational Age (Weeks from last Menstrual Period)	Complication Rate (Complication/100 Abortions)
6	0.36
7-8	0.27
9-10	0.45
11-12	0.77
13-14	1.37
15-16	1.91
17-20	2.16
21-24	2.26

Certain drugs, most notably RU 486, can induce a so-called non-surgical abortion. **RU 486 (mifepristone)** is a steroid, structurally similar to progesterone (Figure 23.35). It crosses the cell membrane and binds to the progesterone receptor in the cytoplasm of target cells, forming an inactive complex and thus blocking the action of progesterone. Administration of RU 486 causes shedding of the endometrial lining either before implantation occurs or after it (within the first 49 days after conception). It is a contra-gestin and thus counteracts the uterine conditions necessary for gestation.

In practice, RU 486 is given in a single dose. A form of prostaglandin E (misoprostol), which stimulates uterine contractions, is given later (36-48 hours after RU 486) to aid in expulsion of the endometrium. The success rate of RU 486 is more than 95 percent and in most cases, embryo along with all the endometrial fragments are expelled within 24 hours. RU 486 can be taken up to 5 weeks after conception

Table 23.3: Relationship of complication rate and type of abortion procedure used in Women

Abortion Procedure	Complication Rate As Per 100 Abortions
Suction Curettage	0.4
Sharp Curettage	0.9
Instillation of Abortion Tent	1.9
Hysterotomy	14.9
Hysterectomy	16.1

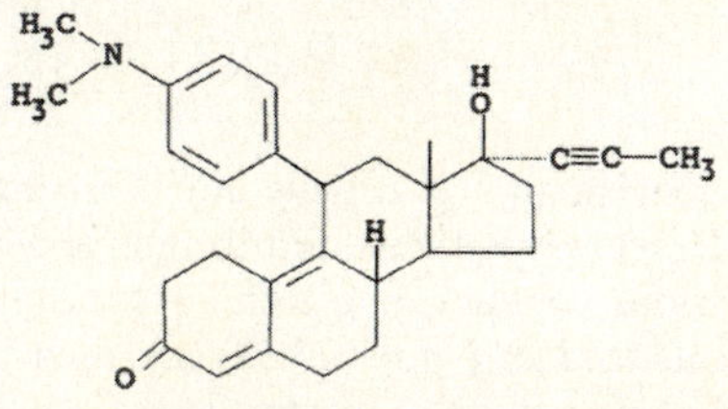

Figure 23.35: Structure of RU 486 (mifepristone).

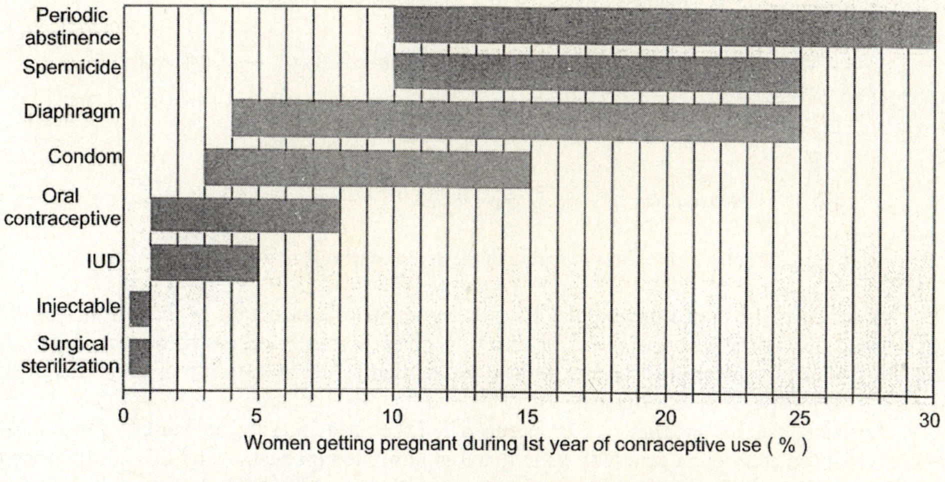

Figure 23.36: Failure rates of various contraceptives used Worldwide.

Heavy bleeding may follow any abortion procedure. Therefore, it must be performed with medical facilities where women can be monitored and treated if necessary. Since India liberalized its abortion laws in 1972, the number of legal abortions has increased every year, but substantial number of illegal abortions still takes place. The main reason for illegal abortion to be more dangerous than legal abortion is that illegal abortions are often performed by unskilled, untrained providers, traditional practitioners or midwives or attempted by the woman herself in unhygienic conditions using crude instruments or toxic agents. Generally, doctors working in clean surroundings using modern techniques and sterile equipment perform legal abortions only. Not only higher death rates but also more complications occur with illegal abortions. However, because it is not possible to get correct data on illegal abortions, it is difficult to determine which factors contribute most to the higher health risks involved with illegal abortions.

All the methods described above are used worldwide as the need for contraception varies with age, health, marital status, pregnancy interval, sexual behavior, emotional and socioeconomic factors, moral and hazards of pregnancy. No single method is universally recommended and all of them show some failure rates (Figure 23.36). The most effective method is the one that a couple will apply correctly and use consistently without omissions and errors. Clinical effectiveness of a contraceptive technology refers to the protection from unwanted pregnancy achieved by actual users including the effects of carelessness and other human manifestations. The combined use of two contraceptive methods provides a higher degree of effectiveness than either method used alone.

Summary

Contraception means to block conception. It usually refers to the technologies that can prevent transport of sperm or ova in the female genital tract, fertilization and/or implantation and thus, prevent pregnancy. To achieve this, various contraceptive techniques using different sites in reproductive physiological processes (as summarized in Figure 23.37) are used to prevent unwanted pregnancy. Various methods of birth control along with their mechanism of action, advantages and disadvantages and their failure rates are summarized in Table 23.4.

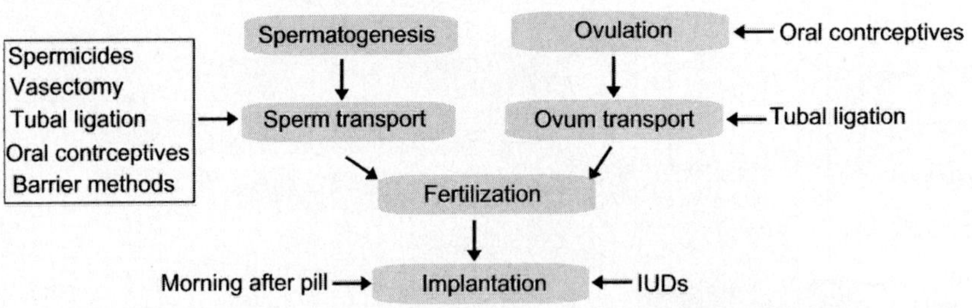

Figure 23.37: Sites of action of different contraceptive methods.

Abortion is the premature expulsion of the products of conception or fetus from the uterus, living or dead, but of recognizable size. In case of human, it usually occurs before the 20th week of pregnancy. In medical terms, **abortion** is defined as the **medical termination of a pregnancy (MTP)** before the fetus is capable of extra-uterine life.

Abortion can be spontaneous or induced. There can be several causes of spontaneous abortions. Induced abortion is generally done to avoid unwanted pregnancy and this is called medical termination of pregnancy or MTP. There are several procedures for MTP and these are performed according to the weeks of pregnancy

Table 23.4: Summary of various methods of birth control used for Human male and female

Contraceptive Method	Mechanism Of Action	Advantages	Disadvantages	Failure Rate(%)
None				85
Natural				
Rhythm method	No intercourse during fertile period		Hard to predict ovulation time	9-20
Coitus interruptus	Removal of penis from vagina before ejaculation	No cost and side effects	Difficult	4-18
Sympto thermal	Various methods combined to predict onset of fertile period		Not suitable for irregular cycles	2-20
Barrier				
Condom	Worn over erect penis, or within vagina, keeps sperm out of vagina		Can break and reduces excitement in male	2-12
Condom and spermicide	Keeps sperm out of vagina, kills sperm that escapes	Protects against STD	Disrupts spontaneity and reduces sensation in male	2-5
Vaginal pouch	Inserted into vagina prior to intercourse and it blocks sperm from reaching cervix		Decreases sensitivity	5-21
Diaphragm and spermicide	Kills sperm and blocks uterus	In-expensive	Disrupt spontaneity, messy, needs to be fitted by doctor	6-18
Cervical cap and spermicide		Cheap, can remain for 24 hrs.	May slip out of place, messy, needs to be fitted by doctor	6-18
Spermicidal foam and jelly	Kills sperm and blocks vagina	In-expensive	Messy	3-21
Spermicidal suppository		Easy to use and carry	Irritates some users	3-15
Surgical				
Vasectomy	Sperm cells never reach penis	Permanent, Does not interrupt spontaneity	Require minor surgery	0.15
Tubal ligation	Egg cells never reach uterus	Permanent, Does not interrupt spontaneity	Requires surgery, entails some risk of infection	0.4
Hormonal				
Oral contraceptive	Prevents ovulation, and implantation, thickens cervical mucus	No effect on sex act, lower cancer risk, menstrual flow	Raises risk of cardio-vascular disease, causes weight gain, and breast tenderness	3
Depo-Provera	Prevents ovulation, alters uterine lining	Easy to use	Menstrual change and weight gain	0.3
Progesterone implant (Norplant)	Prevents ovulation, thickens cervical mucus		Menstrual changes	0.3
Other				
Intrauterine device (IUD)	Prevents implantation	Does not interrupt spontaneity	Severe menstrual cramps, increases risk of infection	3

Questions

1. Why is coitus interruptus unreliable?
2. What is rhythm method and what factors make it less reliable than some other methods of contraception?
3. Describe the natural methods of birth control.
4. Describe two methods of contraception that use mechanical barriers.
5. Describe the chemical methods of contraception.
6. What substances are contained in oral contraceptives?
7. How do an oral contraceptive, an injectable contraceptive and a contraceptive implant prevent pregnancy? Discuss their advantages and disadvantages.
8. How does an IUD prevent pregnancy?
9. Describe the surgical methods of contraception for a male and for a female.
10. Compare the various kinds of birth control methods and their effectiveness.
11. Why do some methods of birth control protect against sexually transmitted diseases, whereas others do not?
12. Define abortion. Discuss various methods, which can be adopted to terminate a pregnancy.

Chapter 24

Demography

Community health, medicine, and reproduction are all vitally concerned with population. This is because health in a group depends upon the dynamic relationship between the number of people in a community, the space that they occupy, their reproductive age and the acquired knowledge, which they utilize to fulfill their daily needs.

24.1 Demography

Demography is defined as the scientific study of human population. It basically deals with the changes in population size, its composition and distribution in space through five "demographic processes". These five processes are fertility, mortality, marriage, migration, and social mobility. The main source of demographic statistics in India is population censuses, National Sample Surveys, registration of vital events and adhoc demographic studies. Attitude surveys have shown that awareness of family planning is widespread and in general people are found to be in favor of family planning, yet rate of contraceptive use by a couple in developing countries is low. Studies have shown that only 6 percent population in Pakistan, 27 percent in Bangladesh and 43.5 percent in India use family planning methods to control population increase. This is because of common myths and beliefs, which persists amongst mass of people. These myths can be, children are the gifts of God, every Hindu must have a son in a family and many more like this. Low adoption of family planning methods by a mass of people is essentially due to lack of awareness and education regarding health and welfare of a family and requires a socio-economic change in a community through education to improve standards of living by adopting a small family norm. A number of terminologies are used in studying population dynamics in relation to family planning and these are described below.

24.2 Demographic Cycle

The history of world population suggests that there is a **demographic cycle** of **five stages** through which a nation passes. The **first stage** is **high stationary** and is characterized by a high birth rate and a high death rate, which cancel each other, thus keeping the population stationary. India was in this stage till 1920. The **second stage** is **early expanding** and in this, the population expands as the death rate begins to decline while the birth rate remains unchanged. Many countries in South Africa and Asia are in this phase. The **third stage** is the **late expanding** stage and in this, the death rate declines further, and birth rate also tends to fall as a result, the population continues to grow because births exceed deaths. India has entered this phase. The **fourth stage** is **low stationary** and is characterized by a low birth as well as death rate so that the population becomes stationary. Most of the industrialized countries fall in this category. In the **fifth stage**, which is the **declining** stage, the population begins to decline since the birth rate becomes lower than the death rate. Some East European countries such as Hungary and Germany fall in this category. Table 24.1 indicates reduction in the crude birth and death rates in some selected countries. Key factors in fertility decline include changes in Government attitudes towards growth, spread of education, increased awareness and services offered through family planning programs etc. Improved health conditions have also decreased the death rate.

Table 24.1: Crude birth rate and death rate in some countries during 1960 to 1999

Country	Crude Birth Rate			Crude Death Rate		
	1960	1985	1999	1960	1985	1999
Bangladesh	51	40	28	25	15	9
China	36	18	16	15	7	7
India	43	32	25	21	11	9
Nepal	46	43	34	29	18	10
Singapore	38	17	14	8	5	5
Sri Lanka	36	25	18	9	6	6
Thailand	46	26	16	17	8	7

24.3 Growth Rates

Growth rate is the net residual obtained after subtracting crude death rate from the crude birth rate. The growth rate is not uniform in the world. In many European countries, growth rate is less than 0.5 % per year while in developing countries it is much more. For example, growth rate is around 2.8 % in Africa and 1.9 % in Asia. At present India's population is second to that of China, and according to UN projections, India's population will reach 1.52 billion by the year 2050 and will be highest in the world. Table 24.2 gives the population of India since 1901 to 2001. **Density of population** is defined as the number of persons living per square kilometer. The trend of density of population in India is given in Table 24.2

Table 24.2: Population density and sex ratio of India from 1901 to 2001

Year	Total Population in million	Density/ Sq. Km	Females/ 1000 Males
1901	238.4	77	972
1911	252.1	82	964
1921	251.3	81	955
1931	279.0	90	950
1941	318.7	103	945
1951	361.1	117	946
1961	439.2	142	941
1971	548.2	177	930
1981	683.3	216	934
1991	843.9	267	927
2001	1027.0	324	933

Survival of human societies depends on **fertility**. There are two extremes of the fertility scale, infertility on the lower end and excessive fertility on the other. Various parameters used as determinants to measure fertility in context of different patterns of population change are given here to familiarize with various techniques used in demography.

Population education: Population education is defined as "an educational program designed for the study of the population in the community, nation and world with the purpose of developing rational and responsible attitudes in the young ones and also positive behavior toward the situation". The population education program is influenced by the specific national situation as well as by political and educational goals. In Indian context, it is designed at the school and university level to bring home and discuss the consequences of uncontrolled population growth, benefits of a small family, the economic and statistics of population growth, its distribution and relation to the standards of living.

General Fertility Rate: General fertility rate is the number of live births in a calendar year per thousand women who are in the reproductive age, that is between 15 to 45 or 49 years. General fertility rate may exceed 100, especially in high fertility areas since the denominator is smaller than the figure for general population.

Child-Woman Ratio: When accurate figures on births are not available, this rough index of fertility is used. Child/Woman ratio is the number of children below 5 years of age per thousand women who are in reproductive age.

Pregnancy Rate: Pregnancy rate is the ratio of number of pregnancies in a year to married women in the ages from 15 to 44 or 49 years. It includes all pregnancies such as live births, stillbirths or abortions or pregnancies that had not yet terminated.

Abortion Rate: Abortion rate is the number of all types of abortions per 1000 women of child- bearing age.

Abortion Ratio: Abortion ratio is the number of abortions performed during a particular time period divided by the number of live births over the same period.

Marriage Rate: Marriage rate is the number of marriages in the year per 1000 population.

$$\text{Crude Marriage Rate} = \frac{\text{Number of marriages in the year}}{\text{Mid-Year population}} \times 1000$$

However, demographers consider general marriage rate a more sensitive rate, as it is more accurate when computed for women than for men because more men marry than women do at the older ages.

$$\text{General Marriage Rate} = \frac{\text{Number of marriages within one year}}{\text{Number of unmarried persons age 15-49 years}} \times 1000$$

Sex Ratio: Sex composition is one of the basic demographic characteristics of the population. Sex ratio is defined as the number of females per 1000 males. Table 4.2 gives the trends of sex ratio in India from 1901 to 2001.

Family Size: Family size refers to the total number of persons in a family. In demography, it is the total number of children a woman has borne at a point in time.

Fertility: Fertility is the actual bearing of children. However, some demographers use the term **natality** in place of fertility. Fertility depends upon several factors such as, age at marriage, duration of married life, spacing of children, economic status, cast and religion, education, nutrition, family planning, social and cultural factors etc. It can be measured by a number of indicators.

Age-Specific Fertility Rat: Age-specific fertility rate is the number of live children in a fixed period of time born to women in a specific age group. It can be represented as the "number of live births in a year to thousand women in any specified age group". It is a more sensitive indicator of fertility but is usually not available for all communities and countries.

Age-Specific Marital Fertility Rate: Age-specific marital fertility rate is the number of live births in a year to thousand married women in any specified age group.

General Fertility Rate (GFR): General fertility rate is the "number of live births per thousand women in the reproductive age group (15 to 44 or 49 years) in a given year". It is a better measure of fertility than crude birth rate as the denominator is restricted to the number of women in the childbearing age, instead of whole population.

$$GFR = \frac{\text{Number of live births in an area during the year}}{\text{Midyear female population age in the same area in same year}} \times 1000$$

Cumulative or Completed Fertility: Cumulative fertility rate is the total number of children ever born per thousand women in a cohort who have completed their childbearing period.

General Marital Fertility Rate (GMFR): General marital fertility rate is the number of live births per thousand married women in the reproductive age group, i.e. 15 to 44 or 49, in a given year.

Total Fertility Rate (TFR): Total fertility rate is obtained when the age-specific fertility rates are summed and multiplied by 5, since 5-year age grouping is commonly used in demography. It also refers to an approximate magnitude of completed family size. Total fertility rate is the average number of children cohort of thousand women aged 15-49 would have during their childbearing period if exposed to a current set of age-specific fertility rates and survive until menopause. A total fertility rate of two means, that two children replace each couple. Thus, TFR gives the approximate magnitude of completed family size.

Total Marital Fertility Rate: Total marital fertility rate is the average number of children that would be born to a married woman if she experiences the current fertility pattern throughout her reproductive span.

Crude Birth Rate: Crude birth rate is the most common measurement of fertility for national and international comparisons. It is the number of live births in a calendar year per thousand midyear (counted as of July 1) populations. It can be represented by the formula:

$$\text{Birth Rate} = \frac{\text{Number of live births during the year}}{\text{Estimated mid-year population}} \times 1000$$

However, the measure does not reflect early changes in fertility or account for differences in the age and sex composition of populations as it considers the total population rather than only woman in reproductive ages. Therefore, the crude birth rate must be standardized for comparative purposes.

Gross Reproduction Rate (GRR): Gross reproduction rate is a measure of replacement of mothers by daughters who are potential mothers. It indicates how many female babies would be born to thousand women during the childbearing years if the age-specific fertility rates remain constant and if every woman entering the childbearing years survives, assuming no mortality until menopause. Summing the age-specific fertility rates, multiplying the total by 5 and multiplying the product gives the gross reproduction rate. In other words, multiplying the total fertility rate by the proportion of births that are female (usually 49 %) is the gross reproduction rate. Since the measure is calculated for each woman, thousand divides the final product. Though theoretical, yet this rate is preferred by demographers. Gross reproduction rate, higher than 2 indicates high fertility in a population.

Net Reproduction Rate (NRR): The gross reproduction rate may be refined to net reproduction rate by taking into account deaths occurring during the reproductive years of women or the age-specific mortality rates. It not only requires age-specific fertility and mortality rate, but also female life tables. Therefore, NRR is a demographic indicator. The level of NRR in India was 1.5 in 1990. NRR less than 1 indicate reproductive performance below replacement level, whereas value 1 is equivalent to attaining approximately the 2-child norm.

24.4 Family Planning

WHO defined family planning as "a way of thinking and living that is adapted voluntarily upon the basis of knowledge, attitudes and responsible decisions by individuals and couples, in order to promote the health and welfare of the family group and thus contribute effectively to the social development of a country".

24.5 Family Welfare Program

Family welfare programs aims to improve the quality of life of the people. This term is used to replace the family planning as people associate family planning in their minds either with sterilization or they equate it with birth control. In India, the objective of the Family Welfare Program is to stabilize the country's population through "small family norm". This program initially adopted the model of 3-child family and symbolized it by the inverted red triangle. However, in 1980s after realizing the seriousness of the increasing population, it started stressing on 2-child norm. A significant achievement of this Family Welfare Program in India is seen in terms of a drop in fertility rate from 6.4 in 1950s to 3.1 in the year 2000. At present all efforts are being made at the national level through such programs as to reach a Net Reproduction Rate of 1 by the year 2006. This is equivalent to attaining approximately the 2-child norm.

Eligible couples: An "eligible couple" refers to a currently married couple where the wife is in the reproductive age (between the ages of 15 and 45). In India, there are approximately 150 to 180 such couples per 1000 population, and on an average 2.5 million couples are joining the reproductive group every year. These couples need family planning services. The "Eligible Couple Register" is a basic document for organizing the family planning programs and is regularly updated by its each functionary for the area falling within his jurisdiction.

Target couple: The term target couples has been coined to pinpoint the couples that are a priority group within the "eligible couples" and this term is applied to a couple that has had 2-3 living children. The family planning program is largely directed to such couples. Now this term has been broadened to include even families with one child or even newly married couples with a view of accepting the idea of family planning.

Couple protection rate (CPR): Couple protection rate is defined as the percent of eligible couples that are effectively protected against childbirth by one or the other approved methods of family planning (e.g. sterilization, IUDs, oral pills, condom etc.). It is an indicator of the prevalence of contraceptive practice in the community and the demographers are of the view that the demographic goal of NRR = 1 can be achieved only if the CPR exceeds 60 %. This means that CPR is a dominant factor in the reduction of net reproduction rate.

Fertility trends: The level of fertility in India is beginning to decline. This is evident by the following figures. The crude birth rate was about 49 per thousand population during 1901 to 1911, 31.3 per thousand population in 1991, and 26.1 per thousand populations in 1999. The fertility trends show inter-state variations too and this is clear form the following statistics. At least ten states or union territories (UT) have achieved net replacement levels (Kerala, Tamil Nadu, Goa, Chandigarh, Delhi, Mizoram etc.), while twelve states or UT have a total fertility rate of 2.1 to less than 3.0 (Karnatka, Andhra Pradesh, Maharashtra, Gujrat, Punjab, West Bengal, Himachal Pradesh etc), and eleven states/UT (Orissa, Bihar, Uttar Pradesh, Madhya Pradesh, Assam, Haryana, Rajasthan etc.) have a total fertility rate of over 3.0.

Fecundity and Childlessness: Fecundity is the reproductive potential or ability to conceive in a person. It refers to the probability of conception in a fixed period of time, usually a year. Fecundity term is many times used to refer to the numbers (and sometimes the quality) of gametes produced. It is same as fertility, which is defined as the ability to produce or production of offspring. Childlessness, if not voluntary, is the result of the inability to conceive indicating infertility, inability to bring a pregnancy to term due to fetal loss, or death of an infant, that is child loss.

24.6 National Population Policy 2000

Population policy generally refers to policies intended to decrease the birth rate or growth rate. India formed its first "National Population Policy" (NPP) in April 1976 calling for an increase in the legal minimum age of marriage from 15 to 18 for females and from 18 to 21 years for males. The policy was modified in 1977, and the new policy statement reiterated the importance of the small family norm without compulsion and changed the program title to "family welfare program". "National Population Policy 2000" is the latest in this series, and it reaffirms the commitment of the government towards target free approach in administering family planning services. It gives informed choice to the people to voluntarily avail the reproductive health care services. The new NPP 2000 deals with women education, empowering women for improved health and nutrition, child survival and health, the unmet needs for family welfare services, health care for the under served population groups, adolescent's health and education, increased participation of men in planned parenthood, and collaboration with NGOs. The main objective of NPP 2000 is to bring the total fertility rate (TFR) to replacement levels by 2010 and the long-term objective is to achieve requirements of suitable economic growth, social development and environment protection. It is anticipated that National Population Policy 2000 if fully implemented will bring down the population to 1107 million in the year 2010 instead of 1162 million as projected by the Technical Group of Population Projections. The planning commission has observed that the achievements are lagging behind the proposed goals for the year 2002 with the present demographic situation in the country. Therefore, the end of the Ninth Five-Year Plan has formulated fresh targets to achieve the earlier goals.

24.7 Pearl's Index

Pearl's index is defined as pregnancies per hundred woman-years of exposure (HWY). It is a mathematical formula for determining the relative efficacy of contraceptive methods, irrespective of the number of women using the method and length of time considered. Raymond Pearl of Baltimore, in 1932 introduced this formula for calculating contraceptive efficiency, and hence named as Pearl Index. It is expressed as a pregnancy rate among users of the method measured in terms of pregnancies per hundred woman-years, by multiplying the number of pregnancies by 1200 (the number of months in 100 years) and dividing by the number of months of use. The "number of pregnancies" includes all pregnancies, whether this had terminated as live births, stillbirths or abortions or had not yet terminated. Pearl's Index can be represented as

$$\textit{Pregnancy rate per 100 woman-years (HWY)} = \frac{\textit{Number of pregnancies}}{\textit{Number of months of use}} \times 1200$$

For example, 300 women used a method for 2 years, i.e., 300 x 24 months, with 6 pregnancies reported during that time. The Pearl Index as per calculations given below comes to 1 pregnancy per 100 women years.

$$\textit{Pregnancy per 100 women years} = \frac{6}{300 \times 24} \times 1200 = 1$$

With this index, one may compare the relative efficiency of two methods, even though the number of women using each method and the lengths of time for which they use the method differ. Pearl Index, though a somewhat crude indicator is useful for obtaining estimates. A modification of the Pearl Index is a measure of contraceptive effectiveness or the failure rate per 100 woman-years of contraceptive use. These indices have been superseded by a life-table method, which computes the risk of pregnancy more precisely.

24.8 National Family Welfare Program

India was the first country to launch a nation wide family planning program in 1952. Family planning was declared as "the very center of planned development" during the Third Five Year Plan (1961-66), with the emphasis on education for motivating people for acceptance of the "small family norm". Introduction of Lippes Loop in 1965 brought structural reorganization of the program resulting in the creation of a separate Department of Family Planning in the Ministry of Health in 1966. Government of India in the Fourth Five-Year Plan (1969-74) gave it a top priority. In 1972, the Medical Termination of Pregnancy (MTP) was introduced. Major changes occurred in the Fifth Five-Year Plan (1975-80). The country framed its first "National Population Policy" in April 1976. Forced sterilization in 1976 led to the defeat of Congress in 1977 and Janata Government came into the power. This Government formulated a new population policy and the Ministry of Family Planning was renamed as "Family Welfare". The program moved in healthier directions and from January 1977, the 42nd amendment of the constitution made "Population control and Family Planning" a concurrent subject in its program. The family planning program is now accepted purely on voluntary basis. Greater goals were achieved with the launching of the Rural Health Scheme in 1977 as it involved local people. In 1983, the National Health Policy approved by Parliament laid down the long-term demographic goal of net reproduction rate (NRR) equal to 1 by the year 2000, implying a 2-child family norm. The Sixth and Seventh FiveYear Plans were set to achieve these goals. The Universal Immunization Program was started in 1985 to reduce mortality and morbidity among infants and young children. Various other programs were also implemented to take care of Maternal and Child Health (MCH) during the Seventh FiveYear Plan. During 1992, these tasks were grouped under Child Survival and Safe Motherhood (CSSM) program. In 1994, International Conference on Population and Development in Cairo recommended implementation of United Reproductive and Child Health Program (RCH). The Government of India has evolved National Population Policy 2000 to promote family welfare. It must be stated here that from a small amount of 0.65 crores during the First Five

Year Plan, the investment has reached to Rs 14170 crores during the Ninth Five Year Plan period to promote family welfare policies.

Evaluation of Family Planning Program: Evaluation is a process of making judgements about selected objectives and events by comparing them with specified value standards for the purpose of deciding alternative course of action. Evaluation is done to improve the design and delivery of family planning services. It is a technical activity and thus requires trained personnel, statistical facilities and adequate information and data. WHO Expert Committee in 1975 has suggested five types of evaluations for the assessment of family planning in health services. These are:

- Evaluation of need in terms of health, demographic and socioeconomic requirement for family planning,
- Evaluation of plans in terms of assessment of family planning program,
- Evaluation of performance in terms of services, responses, cost analysis and other activities in implementing the family planning programs,
- Evaluation of effects of the program in terms of changes in knowledge, attitude, behavior and motivation and
- Evaluation of impact of the programs in terms of family size, birth interval, age of mother at birth of first and last child, number of abortions etc. The Family Welfare Program in India are doing well with the objective of birth control and these programs also aim now to improve the quality of life of the people.

Unmet need for family planning program: This concept was first explored in 1960s, when data from surveys of contraceptive knowledge attitude and practices (KAP) showed a gap between some women's reproductive intention and their contraceptive behavior. This group was then described by the term "KAP-gap" and one of the first published use of the term "unmet need" appeared in 1977. In 1978, Charles Westoff based on World Fertility Survey data from five Asian countries published first comparative estimates of unmet need for limiting births. The concept of "unmet need" for family planning is applied to married women, who are sexually active and are not using any method of contraception, including their partners, and prefer to avoid becoming pregnant. The unmet need for spacing the births is the same as the unmet need for limiting the births.

Unmet need is a powerful concept for family planning and is defined on the basis of women's response to survey questions. It posses a challenge to family planning program, to reach and serve millions of women whose reproductive attitude resembles those of contraceptive user, but due to some reasons are not using contraceptives. The most common reason for unmet need are the unsatisfactory services, lack of information, fear of side effects associated with contraceptives, and opposition from husband. According to the National Family Health Survey-2 (1998-1999), approximately 16 % of currently married women in India have an unmet need for family planning. It is highest (27%) among women below 20 years of age and is mainly for spacing the births rather than for limiting the births. It is also high (24 %) for women of 20 to 24 years with nearly 75 % of the need for spacing the births, but is mainly for limiting the births in women aged 30years or more. Further, unmet need for family planning is higher in rural areas than in urban areas. It also varies with religion and women's education.

Sociology of Family Planning: The problem of family planning is essentially a problem of social change. The contraceptive technology is not a short cut to this problem. Therefore, implementation of the social changes, which can affect fertility, is very important. In this regard, mass education and communication play a key role so that people understand the benefits of a small family. This can be achieved by raising the age of marriage, increasing the status of people, education and employment opportunities of women, old age security, compulsory education of children, accelerating economic changes designed to increase the per capita income etc.

Voluntary Organizations: Voluntary organizations play an important role in population control programs. Some of the well known voluntary agencies in India are the Family Planning Foundation and the Population Council of India, the Family Planning Association of India, the Indian Red Cross, the Indian Medical Association, Rotary Clubs, Lions Clubs, Citizens Forum, and Christian Missionary and Private Hospitals.

The International Planned Parenthood Federation (IPPF) is the world's largest private voluntary organization at the international level with headquarters in London. It supports family planning services in developing countries. Some of the other organizations are the United Nations Fund or Population Activities (UNFPA), the US Agency for International Development (USAID), the Population Council, Ford Foundation, the Pathfinder Fund and World Bank besides WHO and UNICEF. All these agency help in funding family planning research , services, training and information program designed to reduce family size.

Summary

Demography is the scientific study of human population. There is a demographic cycle of five stages through which a nation passes. The first stage is high stationary, the second is early expanding, third is late expanding, fourth is low stationary while fifth is declining stage of the population cycle.

Growth rate of a population is the net residual obtained after subtracting crude death rate from the crude birth rate. It can be controlled by using a family planning method by a couple voluntarily in order to promote the health and welfare of the family and in turn to contribute effectively to the social development of a country.

Family Welfare Programs improve the quality of life of the people.

National Population Policy 2000 was developed to educate women, empower women to take care of health and nutrition of children and also to take part in national health improvement programs.

Pearl's Index represents a way of evaluation of contraceptive method. It is expressed as a pregnancy rate among users of the contraceptive method measured in pregnancies per hundred woman-years by multiplying the number of pregnancies by 1200 and dividing by the number of months of use. India was the first country to launch a nation wide family planning program in 1952.

Evaluation of family planning is done to improve the design and delivery of family planning services.

Voluntary organizations play an important role in population control programs. Such organizations in India are the Family Planning Foundation and the Population Council of India, the Family Planning Association of India, the Indian Red Cross, the Indian Medical Association, Rotary Clubs, Lions Clubs, Citizens Forum, and Christian Missionary and Private Hospitals. Such organizations at international levels are the International Planned Parenthood Federation (IPPF), United Nations Fund or Population Activities (UNFPA), the US Agency for International Development (USAID), the Population Council, Ford Foundation, the Pathfinder Fund and World Bank besides WHO and UNICEF.

Questions

1. What is demography? Why demography is useful in family planning?
2. Write notes on Pearl Index, fertility rate, pregnancy rate, abortion rate, sex ratio, marriage rate, child woman ratio, marriage rate, fertility, reproduction rate, and couple protection rate.

Part IV
Animal Husbandry

- Breeding in Cattle
- Nutrition and Reproduction
- Poultry

Chapter 25

Breeding in Cattle

The term fertility means to produce abundantly. But in breeding in farm animals, it has a limited sense since reproduction is limited by the normal physiology of each species beyond which it cannot normally reproduce. The sexual maturity in males is attained comparatively later than in the females yet the reproductive span is longer in males than in females. Propagation rate in any species is dependent on several factors. These can be length of breeding season, duration of gestation, average number of young ones produced in each litter, the suckling period and the reproductive span in an individual animal. In addition, reproduction is also dependent on genetic and environmental factors. Therefore, in measuring optimum levels of fertility in an animal, one has to consider the genetic makeup as well as the environmental conditions such as climate, plans of nutrition, water, hygiene, soil management etc. For example, Sindhi and Gir cows reared under climatic conditions of the Decan Plateau in India showed reduced fertility when transferred and reared in heavy rainfall area in Konkan districts as compared to the local cattle. Similarly Dangi cattle thrives well in heavy rainfall areas while Khillar cattle though considered stronger and faster do not adapt well in heavy rainfall areas with regard to rate of fertility, but shows good fertility in their home tract. In 1951, Lagerlof postulated that fertility of an animal is largely dependent on its endocrine constitution, and the inherent capacity of reproduction in an animal is predetermined by its hereditary influences while Laing (1954) mentioned that even if a female is very fertile, its fertility is dependent on the viable and briskly moving spermatozoa in the reproductive tract, reaching the site of fertilization at a proper time to fertilize the ovum. A delay or obstruction reduces the fertility even if both partners are very fertile.

In the economics of livestock industry, main object in the field of animal husbandry is to prolong the useful productive life of a high yielding animal. This is entirely dependent on high levels of fertility during the reproductive span in the life of an animal. During recent years, attention has been focused on the selection of animals of special breed showing high fertility. Such stock is reared on the farm under controlled environmental conditions with proper nutrition and is used for further propagation using various methods to improve their reproductive efficiency. These methods can be **artificial insemination (AI), induction and synchronization of ovulation, embryo transfer** and **pregnancy diagnosis**. However, work with large animals necessitates adequate housing and handling facilities for each species used. It is essential to have sorting pens and chutes for separating animals for treatments, surgery, and pregnancy diagnosis. These facilities are important but can be varied to meet the needs of a specific program. A spacious and clean area is essential for surgery and the embryological laboratory should be located adjacent to the surgery room but completely separate.

25.1 Artificial Insemination Technique

Artificial Insemination (AI) is defined as artificial deposition of semen in the female genital tract. The first documented report of successful use of artificial insemination was by Italian physiologist L.

Spallangini in 1780 when he impregnated a bitch. In India, Samoath Kumaran used artificial insemination for the first time in 1939 at Palace Dairy Farm in Mysore.

Artificial insemination is the most important technique ever devised for the genetic improvement of animals. This is possible because a few highly selected males produce enough spermatozoa to inseminate thousands of females per year whereas only relatively few progeny per selected female can be produced per year by embryo transfer. Artificial insemination has been demonstrated successfully in cattle, sheep, goats, horse, dog, cat, and poultry and in a variety of laboratory animals and insects. AI facilitates cross breeding and requires maintenance of only one breed on the farm.

Semen and AI Technique: Semen is the complete discharge of the male during normal ejaculation. It has two major components, the spermatozoa or cellular elements and the seminal plasma or liquid portion. Semen is creamy or milky in appearance with yellowish to gray color. The consistency of semen varies from a relatively low viscosity in the dog and rabbit to a high viscosity in cats, and to actual gel formation in most rodents and primates. The number of sperm and the volume of seminal plasma ejaculated depend on the species. Variations in the volume of semen ejaculated are due largely to the amount of secretion from the accessory glands. However, many factors such as frequency of ejaculation, season of the year, age, environment, nutritional state, and general health of the animal play important roles in semen production.

The technique of artificial insemination requires the following main steps:
i) Collection of semen from male, ii) Evaluation of semen quality, iii) Semen dilution/extension, and iv) Deposition of semen in the female reproductive tract.

i) Collection of Semen: Collection of semen requires the following.

Management of Males: Production of high quality semen depends upon males that have been kept under good conditions. Well fed young males at an approximate age of 12 months in bulls, 7-8 months in rams, goats and boars and 24 months in case of stallions can be used for semen collection.

Physical condition of Males: Production of good quality semen depends on the physical health of the male to a great extent. Exercise is important for the general health of the animal, and bull studs frequently put bulls on mechanical exercisers. However, this does not seem to affect fertility. Feeding has a profound effect on the rate of sexual development in all farm animals. Testis size in males is also important as it is highly correlated with the sperm producing potential of the animal.

Housing of males that are used for semen collection should be convenient and comfortable for the animals and safe for the handlers.

Preparation of Bull: Pre-collection stimulation of a bull is important to get increased ejaculate volume and percentage of motile spermatozoa. Sexual preparation of bulls prior to semen collection increases the number of spermatozoa in the semen. Stimuli that are effective in increasing the sexual response in bulls are changing the teaser, changing the location of teaser, bringing a new bull into the collection area and also on false mounting. Various combinations of these may be tried for semen collection in case of sluggish males.

Time for collection: Semen collections are made during early morning before feeding, as bulls are alert and fresh during morning hours.

Frequency of semen collection must be compatible with satisfactory conception rate. The usual practice is to collect semen from a bull once a week. However, two or even three successive collections may be obtained from the same bull. From young bulls, collections may be obtained twice in a week. Increasing the frequency of semen collection decreases the number of sperm per collection, but it increases the sperm number obtained per unit of time. Therefore, frequent ejaculation of superior sires provides more spermatozoa to inseminate more females.

Methods of Semen collection: Collection of semen using a correct technique is the most important task of any AI program. A number of methods have been used to collect semen but natural ejaculation using a teaser is the most successful one.

- **Electro-ejaculation Method:** This method was devised by Gunn (1936) for ram and later modified by Laplaud and Cassou (1948) for its use in bull. In this method weak alternating current is provided to the sacral and pelvic nerves through electrodes placed in rectum by hand or on probe for ejaculation of semen. The penis usually erects and the semen is collected without the possibility of contamination in the prepuce. Secretion from the accessory sex glands takes place at lower voltage and ejaculation at higher voltages. Semen samples obtained by this method are usually of large volume containing lower concentration of sperm. But the fertility and the number of spermatozoa in the semen obtained are equivalent to the samples obtained by using artificial vagina method. Electro-ejaculation method is preferred only when males cannot be trained for artificial collection of semen or when they refuse to serve the artificial vagina. However, it is rarely used in normal routine as it causes discomfort to the animal and also results in variable reactions.

- **Massage Method**: Massaging by way of the rectum of the vesicular glands and ampullae of the vas deferens can induce semen flow. This method can be used successfully in bulls for collection of semen when an electro-ejaculator is not available. But semen collected by this method is likely to get contaminated with urine or it gets imbalanced in its composition in comparison to the one collected using artificial vagina. Also, the semen so collected contains lower concentration of sperm than that obtained in ejaculates collected by using artificial vagina. Thus, it is considered as an outdated method.

- **Collection on dummy cow or Manikin**: A dummy cow is prepared of strong, heavy, steel frame and covered properly with hard numda and leather to give appearance of a normal cow. An artificial vagina prepared in the usual manner is fixed at suitable height in the rear of the dummy at the time of collection of semen. Dummies have an advantage over live mounts in providing stability and over teaser females in permitting disease control. However, majority of bulls do not show interest in such dummy cows.

- **Live Mounts and Teasing Procedures:** Live mounts using a teaser female are the most successful techniques for routine semen collection. Males in this procedure should be restrained to minimize lateral as well as forward movement and still provide easy access for semen collection. In this procedure selection of a teaser is also important and an estrogen-treated female may provide added incentive during the training period.

Selection of a Teaser Cow: It is essential to have a teaser cow on which the bulls are expected to mount during artificial collection of semen. The cow as far as possible should be of the same breed and color. Teaser should be of medium height as bulls are either reluctant to mount or find difficulty in mounting in extreme cases. In addition, the teaser cow must be physically strong and docile so as to bear the weight of the bull easily during mounting, and also does not get irritated in case she has to stand for a long time in the service crate for collection of semen from bull. It is better to select a cow, which has done 2-3 calving. A pregnant cow and a cow in heat should not be used as teaser. Also, a recent calve must not be used as a teaser until about a month or so by which time there is cessation of the lochial discharge. An ovariectomized cow is recommended for use as a teaser. Teaser cow must be cleaned before she is brought to the service crate and it is better to tie her tail with a rope on one side so that swinging of the tail does not cause any obstruction while directing the penis into an artificial vagina.

Preparation of an Artificial Receptacle for Collection of Semen: Artificial vagina (AV) made out of a hollow rubber serves best for the purpose. It consists of an outer cylinder measuring 20-40 cm in length. The outer edges of the cylinder are ruptured to have firm grip by the inner sleeve. A value is fixed at about 5 cm from one end on the outer cylinder to allow water and air to enter in artificial vagina. A thin soft rubber sleeve with a diameter of 7.2 cm is rolled over on both ends of outer cylinder and is tightly held by thick rubber bands. A 20 cm long rubber cone is fixed at valve end with a sterilized graduated 10 ml glass tube to receive the semen (Figure 25.1). Proper temperature, lubrication and pressure are important in the preparation of artificial vagina to elicit thrust and ejaculatory reflex. The artificial vagina is pre-warmed with hot water and refilled to bring the inner temperature of 40-46 ^{0}C when ready for use. Half to two third capacity of the artificial vagina must be filled with warm water. Sterilized, neutral white Vaseline is used to lubricate artificial vagina, as it is nontoxic to sperms. Insulation bag may be fixed on the graduated glass tube, especially in cold season to avoid temperature shock on the semen.

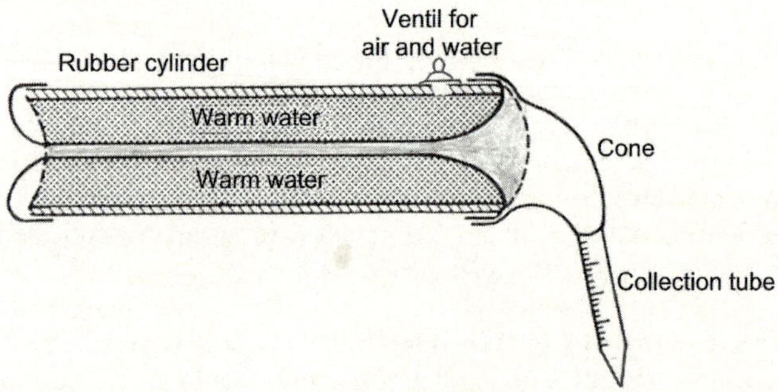

Figure 25.1: Artificial vagina used for collection of semen in Bull.

Semen Collection Room: A quiet place must be selected for semen collection. The attendant and veterinarian must not use too bright color clothing as it distracts attention of the bull. The bull must be allowed to mount when there is proper erection of the penis, and this time, the penis is deflected and directed into artificial vagina by grasping the prepuce. After the thrust reflex, artificial vagina should be withdrawn.

Factors Affecting Semen Production: After sexual maturity, maximum semen production and reproductive capacity are usually reached by 4-7 years of age in cattle and then it declines. Generally full spermatogenesis is reached at about 9 months of age. Testes show a relative decrease in weight after about 2 years of age and a gradual decrease after 5 years of age. Bulls up to 6 months of age secrete more androgens per gram testes than older bulls. The continental breeds reach sexual maturity at an early age of about one and a half year whereas, in indigenous breeds of cattle in India, the average sexual maturity in bulls occurs between 2 to 3 years of age. Long distance transportation of breeding bulls shows a transitory effect on the average semen volume. Seasonal effects on spermatogenesis are also observed in some bulls. Day light hours, ambient temperature, disease, nutrition quality and genetic inheritance affect the semen quality. Therefore, to overcome all these factors, semen from best quality proven bulls may be collected, preserved and used whenever required.

ii) Evaluation of Semen Quality is necessary for assessing the potential fertility of semen sample. Properly protected semen from cold shock during semen collection and kept at temperature slightly below body in a labeled test tube identifying the source of semen is evaluated for its quality. The semen is examined for color, volume, consistency or density, mass activity, motility of spermatozoa and sperm concentration. Semen having uniform opaque appearance indicates high sperm concentration while translucent samples contain few sperm. On the other hand, semen with a curdy appearance indicates infection of the reproductive tract and therefore, should not be used. Proper care must be taken in handling the semen. Volume of the semen can be determined from the calibrated collection tube and the percentage of progressively motile sperm can be estimated using a microscope. The proportion of live to dead sperm is estimated with the help of nigrosin-eosin stain. The **density of spermatozoa** (number of spermatozoa per milliliter of semen) is accurately determined as to find out the number of females that can be inseminated with the optimal number of spermatozoa from that sample.

iii) Preservation of Semen: It is generally known that ejaculated spermatozoa do not survive for long periods and a sudden drop in temperature affect spermatozoa of all species. High temperature storage (39 ^{0}C) is also destructive to spermatozoa. Therefore, proper preservation of semen is very important.

Semen dilution/extension: Fertilizing capacity of the spermatozoa in the semen must be preserved with the help of diluting agent for a long period so as to increase its services to a number of females. It is estimated that 500-1000 cows can conveniently be inseminated with preserved semen from a single ejaculate.

A number of diluents have been used to **preserve the quality of semen**. The basic idea of dilution of semen is to preserve fertilizing capacity of spermatozoa for a long period. The prerequisites of a satisfactory diluent should be to maintain the following: I) the osmotic pressure isotonic with bull blood and capable of maintaining it during preservation, 2) a proper balance of mineral elements essential for a live sperm cell, 3) the nutrients for both aerobic and anaerobic metabolic processes for survival of sperm cells, 4) lipoproteins and lecithin to protect against cold shock and agitation, 5) provision of chemical means for buffering toxic end products of sperm cell metabolism and to prevent harmful shifts in pH as lactic acid is formed, 6) a source of reducing substances to protect the sulphydryl containing cellular enzymes, 7) inhibits bacterial growth and 8) increase volume of the semen so that it can be used for multiple inseminations.

A variety of buffers may be used to maintain an approximate neutral pH and an osmotic pressure of nearly 300 milliosmoles that is equivalent to that of semen, blood plasma and milk. Lardy and Phillips (1939) were the first to report the protective action of egg yolk against cold shock to spermatozoa, and also to describe the yolk phosphate dilutor for preserving cattle semen which consisted of one part of fresh yolk from hen's egg and one part of phosphate buffer. Salisbury *et al* (1948) found better bull-sperm viability and good fertility results with the use of sodium citrate in place of phosphate buffer. Addition of carbohydrates such as glucose and/or fructose as a source of energy in diluents results in an increase in motility and survival of spermatozoa but showed no effect on increase in conception rate.

Semen ejaculates, which are completely bacteria free, cannot be collected in routine collection from bulls. Therefore, it is highly advisable to use antibiotics such as streptomycin, penicillin, polymyxin B etc. in the semen extenders to guard against bacterial contaminants as a routine practice.

Minimum number of spermatozoa required per insemination to obtain an optimum fertility rate, is 5-10 million motile cells from bulls of known fertility.

Cooling of semen is done to prolong the viability and fertilizing capacity of spermatozoa by reducing the metabolic activity to a minimum. Rapid cooling adversely affects the motility of spermatozoa. Therefore, for preservation, semen is diluted wholly or partially prior to cooling. Then the diluted semen vials are wrapped with cotton wool, placed in a beaker containing water and these beakers are transferred to the refrigerator for further cooling to 5 ^{0}C.

Deep-Freezing of Semen: The only practical method in long-term preservation of semen is deep-freezing as it arrests the metabolic processes of spermatozoa. This is called **cryopreservation**.

For many years the emphasis in artificial insemination programs was on the use of unfrozen semen. This was because of the loss of some viable cells during freezing. Still the first insemination using deep-frozen semen was performed by Stewart (1951) in co-operation with Polge and Rowson and out of 5 inseminated cows, one became pregnant. Now most cattle are inseminated with frozen semen as it offers the user a wide variety of choice of semen. Also, deep freezing permits the semen samples to be collected at one time and place for the use at other places and even after long periods of storage.

Ampoule freezing method, pellet freezing method and straw freezing method are different methods of cryopreservation. However, Ampoule method and Pellet freezing method are now outdated. The general principle for deep-freezing of semen requires the semen diluents to contain **glycerol**. Glycerol usually protects sperm against the lethal effects of freezing and thus acts as a cryoprotectant. After equilibration, the suspension is frozen according to special rules and thereafter stored either by using dry ice (-79 ^{0}C) or liquid nitrogen (-196 ^{0}C) as the cooling medium. Resistance of sperm to deep freezing varies with different species of animals. Ice crystal formation damages the sperm cells. Bull spermatozoa are very sensitive to thermal shock. Thus, the freezing rate is an important factor even in the presence of glycerol. Use of glycerol in diluents enables freezing to be carried out slow enough to avoid thermal shock to spermatozoa in semen.

For preservation, fresh semen is selected on the basis of estimation of sperm concentration in the ejaculate and also on the rate of mass activity and motility shown by the sperm. Deep-freezing for preserving the semen can be done by two methods. One is **slow freezing** using ampoule and the other is **instant freezing** using pellet and straw. Slow freezing in ampoule method is carried out in alcohol – CO_2 ice bath or can be transferred to liquid nitrogen container for long preservation. However, this method is now outdated. Pellet freezing is used by Japanese using sugar solutions containing 5-5.5 % glycerol with equilibration of 5-10 hours. The semen is placed in small drops of 0.5-0.2 ml using micro syringe for 10 minutes on dry ice, then it is transferred into the containers and stored in liquid nitrogen. In the straw-vapor freezing, the equilibrated straws after drying in cold cabinet are arranged on freezing ramps with the help of straw spreader. The freezing rate varies with the depth of vapor in the tank, liquid nitrogen level in relation to the straws and number of straws frozen at a time, volume of semen and type of diluents. Approximately 600 mini-tubes or 300 medium straws can be frozen at a time on a grill in 250-liter container. Once the straws are frozen, they are placed in goblet, which are then immersed in liquid nitrogen.

The basic principle of any cold storage is that the cold chain must not be broken. Frozen semen is stored at -79 ^{0}C by using solid CO_2 (dry ice) and alcohol, -190 ^{0}C by using liquid air, -196 ^{0}C by using liquid nitrogen, and –296 ^{0}C by using liquid helium. Storage of frozen semen in liquid nitrogen is the most convenient and accepted method all over the world. The semen must be stored for one month in the container in which it is frozen, and then it should be transferred to another long-term storage container to safeguard against the spread of Foot and Mouth disease of bull. After freezing, the semen can be stored in big insulated thermos flasks or in special storage chambers. However, it is cheaper and genetically advantageous to use semen from outstanding sires promptly, rather than to store it for long periods. With semen kept at –70 ^{0}C, it has been possible to obtain good fertility even after storage for more than five years but in general the fertilizing capacity of deep frozen semen drops progressively with time. Once preserved, semen can be transported to long distances by road, sea or air.

Deep-frozen semen in liquid nitrogen storage container is supplied to service places for insemination. Thawing of frozen semen is essential immediately before use. Two factors are important for thawing the frozen semen. The first one is that the melting of frozen semen must go as quickly as possible to prevent re-crystallization of water into bigger crystals, and this can be done by thawing frozen semen in straws at + 34 ^{0}C for 15 seconds in water kept in a thermos flask. The second factor is that after thawing, the straws must be quickly fitted to the inseminating gun previously warmed to avoid cold shock. Insemination from the frozen semen is done in the following manner: The straw is removed from the goblet with the help of forceps, and is shaken vigorously once or twice to remove liquid nitrogen from the cotton plug. Then the straw is placed in warm water at + 34 ^{0}C in the thermos flask. Rubbing it vigorously warms the chamber of the insemination gun. The straw is dried with tissue paper, held vertically with the cotton plug or ball downwards, and is cut at right angles through the air space to remove the powder plug or sealed plug (take the sheath from the container and fix it over the straw to ensure the firm union between the straw and sheath), and is quickly fitted to the inseminating gun previously warmed to avoid cold shock. The semen is inseminated in the cervix of cow as shown in the Figure 25.2.

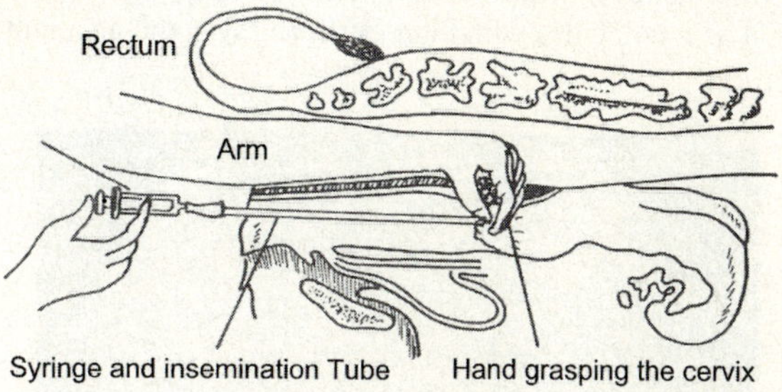

Figure 25.2: Artificial insemination technique in Cow (Recto-Vaginal).

iv) Deposition of semen (Insemination) in the Female Reproductive Tract in Cattle: Insemination technique involves deposition of the semen in the cervix of a cow at appropriate time of the estrous cycle. It is performed during the later part of the heat period in cattle in order to give best chance for the viable spermatozoa to meet the ovum for successful fertilization. The dairy cow is usually inseminated while standing in a stanchion/stall. Stress should be avoided during insemination. High fertility using AI program can be achieved by using the following: 1) high quality semen, 2) proper technique of thawing and of insemination, 3) healthy females in sound breeding condition must be used for insemination, and 4) insemination must be done at the proper time of the estrous cycle.

Actual insemination is done with a 2 ml plastic or glass syringe having outside diameter of 6 mm and inside diameter of 1mm. Sufficient numbers of inseminating pipettes are sterilized, dried, individually wrapped with paper and are once again sterilized in hot air oven. These pipettes are then packed in stainless steel containers. Similarly syringes and rubber connections are also sterilized and stocked. Diluted semen, 0.8-1.2 ml is sucked into the pipette. The vulva area of the cow to be inseminated is cleaned with dry cotton. The lips are dilated and the pipette with semen is inserted into the vagina. The semen is lead to the mid-cervix and then pipette is slowly withdrawn. To obtain high conception rate, viable sperm must be in the vicinity of the egg and capacitated shortly after ovulation. Since it is difficult to detect ovulation, insemination must be timed relative to estrus.

The two main methods of AI generally followed in different species are i) **Speculum method for small animals** such as sheep, goat etc., and ii) **Recto-vaginal method for the large animals** such as cow, buffalo, mare etc.

With the **Speculum method**, it is possible to dilate the vagina, locate the cervix and introduce the pipette into the cervix for deposition of semen. But now days, **recto-vaginal** or **cervical fixation** method is more widely used all over the world as by this method, it is possible to perform intra-uterine inseminations (Figure 25.2) which is not possible by the speculum method. Mid-cervix is considered to be the most ideal site for deposition of semen as it activates and motivates the spermatozoa and increases the capacitation of spermatozoa, which is necessary for fertilization. Also, cervical insemination gives higher conception rates than deposition of semen in other parts of the genital tract. This may be due to the fact that cervical mucus arrests the possibility of ascending infection.

For successful AI, detection of heat in cattle is very important. The time of insemination and proper detection of estrus is possible with the help of crystallization pattern of cervical mucus. During estrus, there is copious secretion of mucus from cervical glands and it can be observed hanging from the cow's vulva. A uniform smear can be prepared on a clean glass slide from this mucus, air dried, and observed under the low power of microscope. It appears like the leaves of fern tree (Figure 25.3). Thus, it is possible to judge the period of estrus and time of insemination from the appearance of crystallization pattern which takes the form of long leaves with long venation and sub-venation with clear minute crystals on it as it coincides with high estrogen level and also indicates that ovulation is to follow soon.

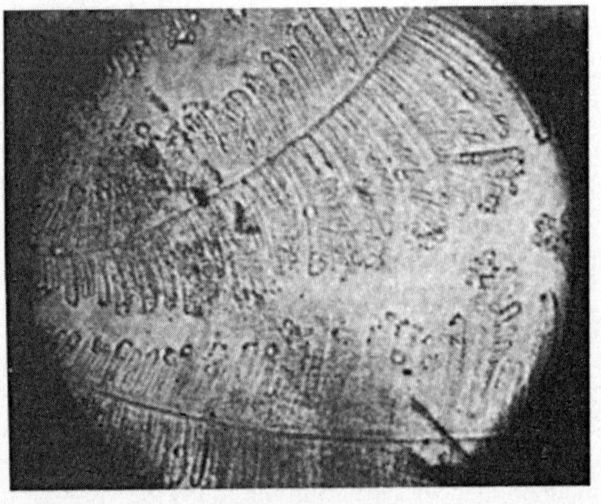

Figure 25.3: 'Fern patterns" of cervical mucus at estrus stage of the cycle in Cow.

Following the onset of heat, the optimum period during which a satisfactory conception rate can be obtained is of considerable importance in the economics of livestock production. There is a wide range in the heat period of cows from 3-28 hours, average being 18 hours, depending on genetic factors, environmental conditions and nutrition. Proximity of bull is also important for the duration of estrus. Insemination should not be done after parturition until the uterus involutes fully and the female starts cycling normally. Also, cows should not be inseminated before 50 days after calving for best conception rates.

The bull spermatozoa can remain viable in the intra-uterine tract for about 30 hours, the stallion spermatozoa in the mare for 48-72 hours, the ram spermatozoa in the ewe for 22-42 hours, and the boar spermatozoa in the sow for about 24 hours. The average life of an unfertilized ovum is 12-24 hours. In cows maximum fertility is claimed if insemination is done during the last 8 hours of heat (Table 25.1). Cows detected in heat during morning hours must be inseminated during afternoon hours on the same day, while those coming in heat during afternoon or the evening hours, must be inseminated next morning to get fairly good conception rate.

Table 25.1: Relation of insemination time and conception rate in Cows

Insemination Time	Conception Rate (%)
Beginning of heat	44
Middle of heat	82.5
End of heat	75
Six hours after heat	62.5
Twelve hours after heat	28
Twenty four hours after heat	12
Thirty six hours after heat	8
Forty eight hours after heat	Nil

Higher fertility rates are obtained with insemination done about 24 hours before the end of the estrus in mare, during the latter half of the estrus period in ewe, before the middle of estrus in sow, during early part of estrus in bitch, and between 6th to 8th day after the onset of estrus in cats. The cows must be handled very carefully during insemination. Any excitement at that time leads to the release of adrenalin that may inhibit sperm travel within the genital tract. Lower conception rates are obtained in cows that are either completely quiet or highly nervous.

Systemic recording of the field's record and data is essential in AI organizations. There must be detailed records of bull, semen quality, insemination details etc. in the form of separate registers.

Advantages and Constraints of Artificial Insemination (AI) :

Advantages of AI: The main advantages of artificial insemination are: i) It increases the use of superior sires. ii) It allows evaluation of young sires for progeny testing program. iii) Small quantity of semen obtained in service center can be extended with suitable dilutors to inseminate large number of animals. iv) AI helps in disease prevention control. v) It is beneficial to small farmers who cannot keep breeding bull for fertility purpose. vi) The farmer can have services at his doors, thus avoiding catching of infection during transport of semen etc. Such semen can easily be transported to any part of the country. vii) More number of cows or buffaloes coming in heat on one/same/successive day can be served by this method. viii) It is possible to preserve semen by refrigeration or cryopreservation for long duration and future use. ix) AI allows maintenance of satisfactory fertility records. x) It is a golden tool for rapid improvement and upgrading of livestock for economic traits. In natural mating method certain breeds of bull may not mate with certain other breeds of cow due to physical disparity. In AI method, the semen of any breed can be introduced into the cow for conception. Normally a bull can give good and healthy service only for 6-8 years. Old and injured sires that may not be able to inseminate cows in routine way can be made use of by collecting their semen artificially for AI programs.

Constraints of AI: There are few limitations of AI and these are i) A team of trained veterinarians and technicians is a pre-requisite at a work place. ii) There is inherent danger of contamination of semen at a number of stages. Therefore, it requires a very careful handling during the complete process, i.e. from collection of semen to insemination. iii) Cost is little high for establishing AI laboratory, equipment and deep-freezing facilities. Also high cost is involved in transportation of technicians, liquid nitrogen containers and preserving the semen samples at the site of insemination.

However, the advantages of AI over natural breeding are too many and distinct, and therefore, AI is used now very commonly as a method of breeding in livestock, especially in cattle and buffaloes.

25.2 Embryo Transfer Technology (ETT)

Embryo Transfer (ET) is a technique in which embryo is produced from highly genetically superior females called donors and is transferred to recipients to act as foster mothers for the growth and development of the fetus. Walter Heape in Cambridge carried out the first successful embryo transfer in 1890 in species of rabbits. Potentialities of the technique, however, both as a research tool, and as a practical aid in animal husbandry were not realized until twentieth century.

Embryo Transfer Technique and its Importance: In farm animals, number of times a female can become pregnant is severely limited due to the extended duration of gestation. But with embryo transfer technique, number of offspring that a female can produce in her lifetime can be greatly increased by repeatedly allowing her to become temporarily pregnant. The embryos are recovered from such females in early pregnancy and transferred to the reproductive tracts of other females to complete gestation. These females are then used again after sometime to produce another set of embryos (Figure 25.4). Depending on the species, embryo transfer involves the use of gonadotropins to induce the donor female to super ovulate, and then synchronizing it with the recipient to show estrus and ovulation. Various steps involved in ETT are as follows.

- Selection and management of donor animals,
- Selection and management of recipient animals,
- Synchronization of estrus both in donor and recipient,
- Superovulation of donor animal,
- Breeding of donor animals by AI or natural service,
- Collection or recovery of embryos,
- Examination, evaluation, selection and isolation of embryos,
- Embryo transfers in recipients for implantation and further development,
- Pregnancy diagnosis and proof of parentage of the offspring, and
- Cryopreservation of surplus embryos.

All these steps are essential for the overall success of embryo transfer technique and require attention to all the points to a greater or lesser degree. However, transfer preparations necessarily vary somewhat with different species of animals.

Herd Management: Herd management must be considered the first priority for any embryo transfer program to be successful, since many times the best animals may yield poor results if attention is not given to the welfare, health and nutrition of both donor and recipients.

25.3 Induction and synchronization of ovulation and pregnancy diagnosis

The mammalian ovary contains enough oocytes to produce many times the normal number of eggs. For example, bovine ovaries contain nearly 133,000 primordial follicles but all of them do not mature to form functional gametes. In animal husbandry, artificial insemination has been an important method for the widespread distribution of desirable genes by way of the spermatozoa. Similar genetic improvement through the use of egg is greatly limited in domestic farm animals due to small number of offspring and also due to the inability to utilize the potent ova. However, this has become possible due to the recent developments in assisted reproductive technologies. Donor cows of good breed are used for collection of ova in embryo transfer technology (Figure 25.5).

Induction of ovulation: In order to induce ovulation in anestrous or acyclic females, a single follicle or group of follicles is stimulated to develop to a state of maturity so that luteinizing hormone (LH) or a hormone with LH-like properties such as human chorionic gonadotropin (hCG) could induce ovulation.

Many studies are now directed to the methods for super ovulating various animals, fertilizing the eggs *in vitro*, recovering the fertilized eggs from Petri dish or tubes, and finally transferring them to the recipient females.

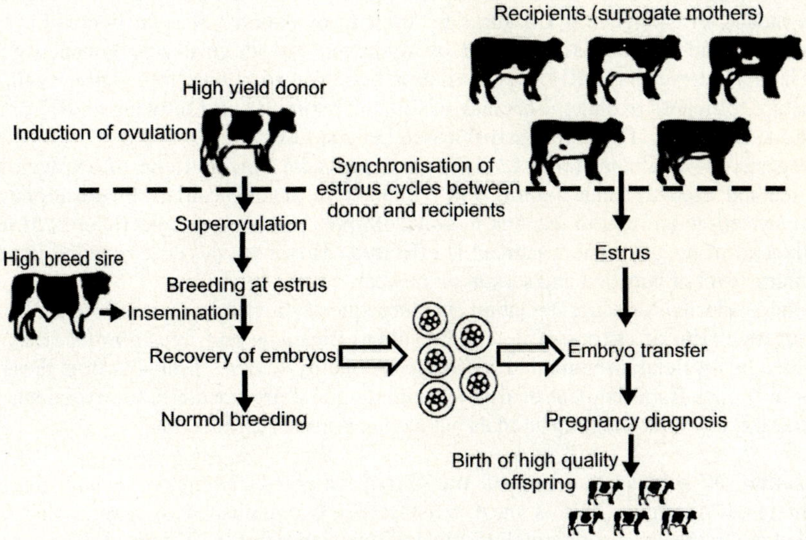

Figure 25.4: Various steps involved in embryo transfer technology in Cattle.

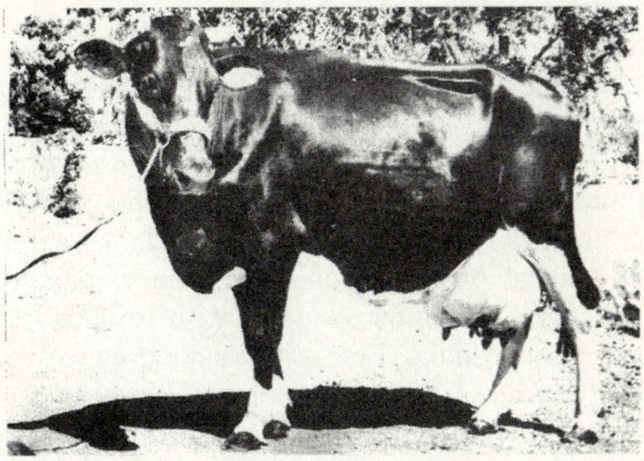

Figure 25.5: Donor Cow for embryo transfer technology.

Super ovulation: It is the stimulation of ovaries to produce more than the normal number of ovulatory follicles so to release more ova than normal. It is practiced in animal husbandry to harvest a larger crop of fertilized ova (about five folds).

Studies on super ovulation provide basic information about ovarian functions such as the process and physiology of maturation of follicular oocytes. Further, super ovulation is used to increase the litter size in monotocous species such as cattle and sheep. The successful use of embryo transfer is a most significant development in cattle improvement programs.

Treating the animals with gonadotropins induces super ovulation. Two types of gonadotropins commonly used to super ovulate cows, buffaloes, sheep, and goats are pregnant mare serum gonadotropins (PMSG) and follicle stimulating hormone (FSH). These are administered during the mid-luteal phase of estrous cycle. Once follicle growth has been stimulated with either FSH or PMSG, it is necessary to administer LH or HCG about 48 to 96 hours later in order to induce ovulation. In some cases, administration of LH/HCG is not required because developing follicles secrete enough estrogen to induce an endogenous LH surge to result in ovulation. Also, it is possible to stimulate endogenous FSH and LH release followed by ovulation by administering gonadotropin-releasing hormone (GnRH). However, GnRH does not normally induce additional follicular growth, although it causes a mature follicle to ovulate. This lack of follicular stimulation following GnRH administration is related to short half-life of endogenously released LH and FSH.

Progesterone treatment for 7-12 days combined with gonadotropin or estrogen is the most successful method used to induce estrus and ovulation in acyclic cattle. Progesterone primes the reproductive system to allow it to respond to gonadotropins and a single injection of PMSG in such a regime at the end of progesterone treatment is effective. However, the dose required depends on the breed of animal, level of nutrition and season of the year.

Donors selected for super ovulation and subsequently for embryo transfer must be genetically superior with regularity of estrous cycle and breeding efficiency, and free from diseases. Generally donors are bred by artificial insemination with superior quality semen. Embryos from these donors are collected on 6-8 days from the date of first insemination and are transferred to recipients, which are generally inferior, low milk-yielding animals but having normal reproduction.

Synchronization of estrus: Survival of transferred embryos requires a hospitable intrauterine environment in all species. This is most satisfactorily accomplished by transferring embryos to recipients that are in the same endocrinological condition as the donor. This is achieved in practice by use of recipients that are naturally or artificially synchronized at estrus with the donor female. There are a number of ways to achieve estrus synchronization, all of which can yield a high degree of synchronization without producing fertility problems.

Mainly the secretion of progesterone from corpus luteum controls the time of estrus and ovulation in cyclic domestic animals presumably through a negative feedback effect on gonadotropin secretion. Thus, the regulation of the cycle in domestic animals really means controlling the life span of the corpus luteum. The life span of corpus luteum can be regulated by several procedures. These are: I) long-term progesterone administration, and 2) use of progesterone combined with luteolytic agent. Various factors affect the life span of corpus luteum of domestic animals. These are injections of oxytocin during the early luteal phase, estrogen treatments, administration of LH antibodies, presence of foreign bodies in uterus, irritation of uterus with irritants like iodine solution or benzyl alcohol, and administration of prostaglandin. Few of these are used to synchronize estrus. In cattle, a luteolytic dose of prostaglandin $F_{2\alpha}$ causes regression of corpus luteum and a precipitous fall in progesterone leading to follicular growth, estrus and ovulation within two to four days.

The importance of synchrony was first clearly demonstrated by experiments involving surgical transfer of embryos from a donor female at one stage of pregnancy to the uterus of a recipient female at a different stage. Embryo transfer give a higher success rate if donor and recipient female are at the same stage of development, or better still (since transfer may slightly retard embryonic development) if the donor is somewhat more advanced in development than the recipient. Synchronization has been shown to be necessary in rabbits, mice, rats, sheep and cows. Embryonic mortality that occurs sometimes in natural pregnancies around the time of implantation is probably due to faulty synchronization.

Estrus Detection: In embryo transfer technologies, whenever natural or artificial synchronization of estrus is used, detection of estrus is a crucial step for it to be successful. In cattle, the strongest criterion for detecting behavioral estrus is standing rigidly of the concerned cow for mounting by other cattle that could be male or female.

Insemination: Whether donors are bred naturally or artificially, several inseminations at 12-hour intervals, beginning nearly 12 hours prior to expected ovulation and continuing until at least 12 hours after ovulation, are highly recommended for obtaining best results.

Embryo Collection: Embryos can be collected from the oviducts or uteri either by slaughtering or by excision of the reproductive tract or from the intact animals. Generally, it is done in intact animals either by **non-surgical method** or by **surgical method** (Figure 25.6). Ova representing 40-80 % of the corpora lutea can easily be recovered from superovulated intact animals. However, recovery rates are slightly higher in the cases of excised tracts.

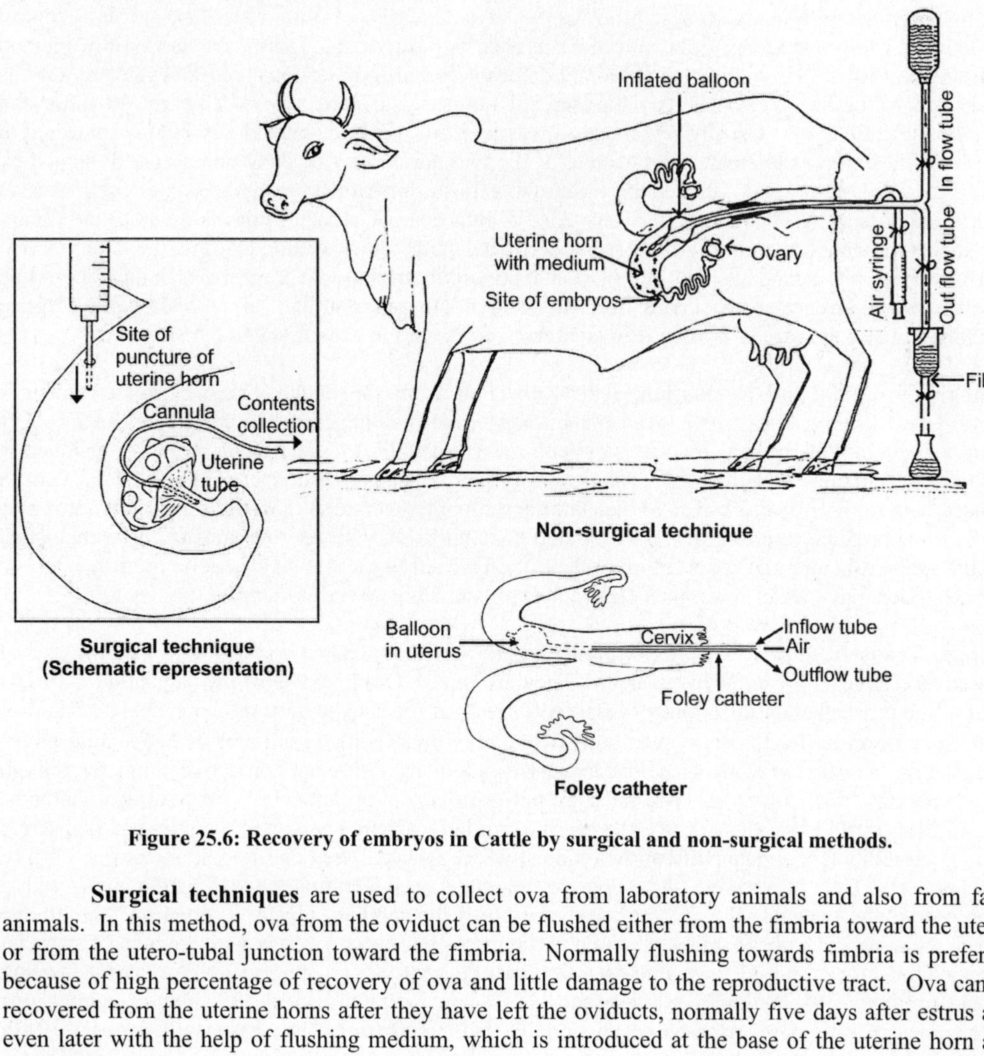

Figure 25.6: Recovery of embryos in Cattle by surgical and non-surgical methods.

Surgical techniques are used to collect ova from laboratory animals and also from farm animals. In this method, ova from the oviduct can be flushed either from the fimbria toward the uterus or from the utero-tubal junction toward the fimbria. Normally flushing towards fimbria is preferred because of high percentage of recovery of ova and little damage to the reproductive tract. Ova can be recovered from the uterine horns after they have left the oviducts, normally five days after estrus and even later with the help of flushing medium, which is introduced at the base of the uterine horn and flushed towards the tubes. The flushed medium containing ova is collected through a blunt syringe needle or a small glass tube inserted into the lumen through a puncture wound in the uterine wall (Figure 25.6). Two to twenty milliliter of the medium is used to flush the oviducts, whereas ten to hundred milliliter of the medium is used to flush the uterus depending on its size.

In cattle, buffalo and horses, **non-surgical** approaches developed by T. Sugie are commonly used to collect embryos. The advantage of non-surgical method is that it does not cause damage and adhesions to the reproductive tract. Also, it can be repeated for a number of times. The cervix of the animal is often dilated with an expander to facilitate the insertion of the collection device (Figure 25.6). In cows, embryos usually enter the uterus on day 4 after estrus. Embryos are collected non-surgically 6-8 days from the date of first insemination. Prior to day 5, embryos are in the oviduct and after day 8, it may be difficult to visualize them as they might have escaped from zona pellucida. The embryos are collected either by i) **continuous flow, closed circuit system**, or ii) **interrupted syringe method**. A combination of these two systems may be used, as both are equally effective when done properly. Continuous flow, closed circuit system offers the advantage of cleanliness, sterility and fluid control but requires additional tubing and connections as seen in figure 25.6. The interrupted syringe method is faster and allows embryo searching before the flush is completed. Various types of catheters, such as Rush catheter or Foley catheter may be used for non-surgical collection of embryos in cattle and buffaloes (Figure 25.6). Usually seven days after the estrus, superovulated donor cow is subjected to "flushing" to retrieve the embryos. Flushing of the two horns must be done one by one followed by filling of the donor's card. Immediately following flush, antibiotics are infused into the uterus to reduce the possibility of uterine infection. Also a high dose of prostaglandin is given to the donor. This helps the donor to return to the normal hormonal status quickly and also kills the embryos that may have been left behind and thus eliminates the possibility of multiple pregnancies in the donor. It is possible to make repeated recoveries from the same donor with the help of successful non-surgical methods and also, ova are now often recovered from cows without superovulation.

Embryo Isolation and Evaluation: After collection from the donor, ova are isolated under a microscope. Embryos must be kept viable in the nutrient medium for the period between recovery from the donor and transfer to the recipient. The medium should be buffered to maintain a physiological pH of 7.2 to 7.6. It is better to keep embryos at room temperature (15-25 ^{0}C) than to subject them to the repeated cycles of incubator and room temperature. Paraffin oil is used frequently to cover the medium to prevent evaporation and contamination with microorganisms. Ova that show normal gross structure and are from one-cell to the hatched blastocyst stage can be used for embryo transfer. Generally ova of fewer than eight-cells are transferred to the oviducts.

Embryo Transfer: Genetically inferior but having normal reproduction and low milk yielding animal is used as recipients for **embryo transfer**. They are injected with 25 mg of prostaglandin, 24 hours prior to the prostaglandin injections of respective donor in order to achieve proper synchronization of their estrous cycles. Recipients synchronous with that of donor with a limit of $\pm$ 24 hours are used for ET. Embryo transfer to recipients is done by surgical methods or through non-surgical transfer, though in case of cattle, the embryo survival rates are not nearly equal to that achieved by surgical methods. For surgical transfer into the oviduct, the tip of a capillary pipette containing the embryos is inserted into the infundibulum and ampulla of the oviduct, where embryos are deposited in one or two drop of medium. Also embryo transfer can be done in the uterus by puncturing the wall of the uterus with a blunt needle and expelling the embryos from the tip of the capillary pipette inserted into the uterine lumen. Non-sugical embryo transfer is done in the uterus through the cervix with the help of artificial insemination straw gun 6-12 days after estrus. Extra embryos are cryopreserved. Successful freezing of cattle embryos by Wilonut and Rowson, 1973 and Willadson *et al*, 1978 and simultaneous development of microprocessor based on portable embryo freezers have hastened progress in **'On**

Farm Embryo Freezing'. Figure 25.7 represents diagrammatically a simple apparatus used for cooling samples. It is developed by Leibo *et al* in 1970. It consists of an inner, double-walled glass vessel that has been evacuated and contains 95 % or 100 % ethanol (any other organic solvent with a freezing point of –90 ^{0}C can be substituted) as a coolant. A variable speed stirrer is placed to mix the ethanol to prevent the establishment of thermal gradients. Sample tubes, which have been prechilled to approximately the bath temperature, are placed into the ethanol. Use of dry ice should be avoided and instead, for cooling this entire assembly, liquid nitrogen should be used contained in a standard 4-litr wide mouth Dewar flask. This apparatus requires little attention except to maintain the level of liquid nitrogen in the outer flask. Temperature of the samples and bath can be monitored continuously with the help of thermocouple attached to temperature recorder. Survival of frozen embryos using this apparatus is unaffected by the length of storage.

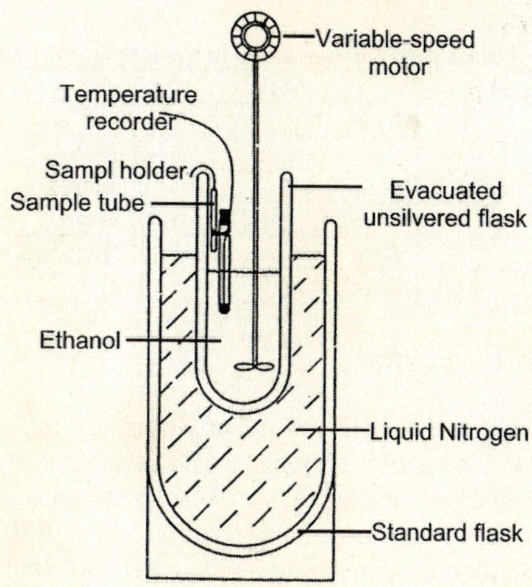

Figure 25.7: Diagrammatic representation of the apparatus used to preserve Mammalian embryos by freezing.

25.4 Pregnancy Diagnosis

It is normally desirable to know the success of the embryo transfer as soon as possible after transplantation. Cattle can be diagnosed pregnant by rectal palpatation of the uterus and ovaries at 35-40 days after breeding. Success rates vary considerably even within the same organization and same species, but the embryo survival rate after transfer in some cases can reach to 80% or more.

Proof of Parentage: Proper records must be maintained for proof of parentage so as to be aware of the breeding or insemination status of each donor and each recipient.

Advantages and Limitations of Embryo Transfer Technology:

Advantages of ETT: i) The most important advantage of ET is the production of calves from genetically superior females and their faster multiplication. ii) It results in the production of calves of the desired sex. iii) It helps to preserve endangered breeds. iv) It allows export and import of embryos rather than of live animals. v) With the import of frozen embryos, risk of introducing contagious diseases is minimized. vi) ET produces identical calves for research purposes and provides a real alternative for the production of twins as well as clones and chimeras. vii) ETT allows getting of calves from infertile animals. viii) ETT helps to develop pathogen free herds. ix) ET helps in building up a seed stock of a superior germ plasm. x) And the principal advantage of ET is the increased reproduction capacity and it decreases the generation interval.

Limitations of ETT: Few limitations of ET are high initial capital investment, and requirement of highly qualified personnel. In embryo transfer technique, donor and recipient animals must be critically selected.

Table 25.2 gives the terms of two sexes (male and female) of various mammals used as livestock in animal husbandry. The terms **bovine** and **ovine** are used to represent characteristics of cattle and sheep (and related animals) respectively.

Table 25.2: Terms used for two sexes in various mammals used as livestock

Animal	Male	Female
Bull	Black Bull	Buffalo
Goat	Bucks	Does
Horse	Stallion	Mare
Ox	White ox (Bull)	Cow
Pig	Boar	Swine (Sow)
Sheep	Ram	Ewe

25.5 Induction of Early Puberty in Cattle

In cattle, age does not determine the onset of puberty, instead relative growth and body weight influences the onset of puberty. The period of puberty also varies in different breeds. The average age at puberty in exotic (Bos taurus) cows ranges between 8 to 18 months, 24 to 30 months in Indian cows of well-defined breeds and 36 to 48 months in non-descript cows. Buffaloes under Indian conditions reach puberty between 24 to 48 months, depending on the breed and environmental conditions.

Onset of puberty in cattle depends on the following factors:

- **Breed**: In general, it is observed that the breeds with smaller individuals gain puberty much earlier than those, which are taller.
- **Climate**: Tropical climate or Temperate Zone helps in early induction of puberty than the other climatic areas.
- **Season of Birth**: It is a surprising phenomenon that season of the birth of the individual determines its onset of puberty. For example, individuals born in January tend to attain puberty at an earlier age than those born in April.
- **Sex**: It is observed that the females attain sexual maturity earlier than males in case of cattle.
- **Environment**: It is observed that the individuals bred in a group or those females which had presence of a male member near them attain sexual maturity or puberty much faster compared to individuals that are bred alone.
- **Genetic**: Age of puberty varies between species, breeds and strains. Cross breeding minimizes the pubertal age, whereas indiscriminate breeding delays the onset of puberty.
- **Nutrition**: Nutrition has a profound influence on the onset of puberty. Usually well-fed heifers reach puberty at an earlier age than those poorly fed. Underfeeding has adverse effect on pubertal age and the delay is variable depending upon the type of nutrition. Mineral and trace element deficiencies also greatly influence the onset of puberty.

  Therefore, these factors must be kept in mind in inducing early puberty in cattle.

Need for Induction of Early Puberty in Cattle: Early puberty brings early lactation in the cattle, which is a feature required for prolonged lactation for high milk yield. Puberty can be induced early in cattle by giving certain hormones

- **Progestin Method**: By giving progesterone, changes can be induced in the cattle, which get mature earlier and start estrous cycles. Progesterone can be mixed in their drinking water or mixed in their feed such as hay etc. It is done for 14 days. After its removal or withdrawal, estrous begins in the cattle within 2-3 days.
- **Prostaglandin Method**: By injecting prostaglandin for 10-11 days, puberty can be induced early in cattle.
- **Prostaglandin plus Progestin Method**: This method reduces the time period of induction of puberty in cattle. In this method, both prostaglandin and progesterone are given to induce early puberty in cattle. Prostaglandin is given orally as one dose on 6th day during the treatment followed by progesterone for next 7 days. The induction of puberty occurs faster this way.

In addition, proper diet and nutrition with better husbandry and other sanitation conditions should be maintained for onset of early puberty in cattle. Puberty is attained when a certain weight or body mass has reached at a particular age. Also, puberty is genetically determined.

25.6 Increasing Milk Yield in Cattle

Milk collection and use of milk by man started from very ancient time. With the advent of time, man started domesticating cattle because cow, goat, sheep and buffalo produce milk in quantities that is far in excess of the needs of their young, and this is harvested by man for his own and his children's nurture. Therefore, he began rearing good breeds of cow in order to obtain more milk. World statistics show that in 1955, there were about 877 million cattle in the world and out of these, nearly 278 millions were in Asia. India had the largest number of cattle, nearly 178 millions. Since milk forms an important part of food, there was always a need to improve milk yield of cows. To achieve this, artificial (supplementary) feeds and nutrient foods were manufactured. In the latter half of the 19th century, dairying technology made striking advancements in this direction and India has now high milk yielding breeds of cattle.

Dairying is the production and marketing of milk, usually of cow and buffalo (cattle) and its products. Dairying technology includes the care of cattle, their breeding, feeding, management and milking. Breeding techniques and application of science of genetics in stock improvement programs of cattle tremendously increased the production of new breeds with high milking capacities.

NDDB (National Dairy Development Board) brought 'operation flood' in India, which made it the second largest milk producing country in the world. This is called the 'white revolution'.

Breeds of Cattle: India has 26 breeds of cattle belonging to two distinct species classified as *Bos indicus* (ox) and *Bos bulbalis* (buffalo), the former is the more domesticated form. Cattle are classified in three groups depending on the purpose they serve to man. These are draft breeds, dairy breeds and dual-purpose breeds. Draft breeds are for pulling carts, ploughing fields' etc and are well built with cows having poor milk yield. Examples of Indian draft breeds are Malvi, Nagore, Amrithamahal, Hallikar, and Kangayam. Dairy cattle are high milk yield breeds with extended lactation periods, and bullocks are of poor draft qualities. Examples of dairy breeds are Gir, Sindhi, Sahiwal and Deoni. Dual-purpose breed is meant for both, draft works as well as milk yield. Therefore, the bullocks are useful in draft works, while cows are good in milk yields. Examples of dual-purpose breeds are Haryana, Krishna Valley breed, Ongole and Tharparkar. In addition, many milk yielding breeds of cattle are imported and reared in India and are classified as exotic breeds. These are Holstein-Friesian,

Jersey, Ayrshires, Brown Swiss and Guernsey. Breeding farms are now established in many parts of India to raise crossbreeds and improve the milk yielding capacity of the indigenous cows.

Milk Production: The onset of lactation in general occurs around parturition but in some high yielding cows, it may be necessary to begin the regular withdrawal of milk before parturition to relieve the pressure that develops in the udder. Initial secretion of milk is thick and yellowish in color and is called **colostrums**. It is high in fat, protein and immunoglobulins and low in lactose. In cattle, composition of this secretion changes from that of colostrums to the normal milk over the first four days of lactation. This milk yield increases steadily to reach a peak at eight to nine weeks and then steadily declines over the remainder of the lactation period. As long as the animal remains non-pregnant, reduced levels of milk production can be maintained for long periods with sufficient diet.

Lactation days are an important trait among dairy breed cattle. Extended lactation with steady yield per day is a desirable trait. The period between lactation and calving during which cow does not milk are called **dry days**. Cows are usually mated at the first or second estrus period after parturition, that is, 8-9 weeks after parturition. If pregnancy occurs, cow produces very little milk around 28th week of pregnancy or around 40 weeks after the previous parturition and remains dry until next parturition. This dry period is essential in cattle if high yields are to be obtained in the next lactation. A desirable good breed gives around 20-40 kg milk with 10-11 months of lactation and a short dry period. Factors that limit the increase in daily milk yield to a peak at eight to nine weeks are genetic capabilities, diseases, poor husbandry conditions or accidents. Table 25.3 gives the lactation days of few important breeds of cattle.

Table 25.3: Lactation days of some important breeds of Cattle

Breed	Lactation days
Ayrshire	305
Gir	320
Holstein	365
Holstein-Haryana cross	360
Jersey	365
Jersey-Haryana cross	340
Sahiwal	310
Sindhi	298

The number of time a cow is milked in a day also tells upon its trait and in India more than 90% of the herds are milked twice a day. The number of times a cow is milked per day, the more is the milk yield. The milk yield initially increases with age and number of calving, but later on it decreases. Most of the traits of milk yielding in cattle is influenced by environmental and nutritional factors rather than purely genetic. Therefore, milk yield in cattle can be improved by paying proper attention to the environmental and nutritional factors along with proper management and disease control.

Breeding of cattle: Reproduction and milk yield is closely related in cattle as lactation represents the final phase of the reproductive cycle and the physiological state of the mammary gland is limited to the reproductive state of the animal. Breeding is resorted for raising good milk yielding varieties or dairy breeds, in addition to for other purposes. Earlier selective breeding was attempted based on conventional knowledge, but now cattle keeping and stock improvement is done in a very scientific manner. Dairyman maintains a record of pedigree information, breed type, reproductive efficiency, and milk production with lactation days. Crossbreeding of dairy cattle is carried out with the help of improved programs in order to increase the milk yielding capacity of the herd. Crossbreeding is the mating of animals belonging to two different breeds. Improved breeding techniques include artificial insemination and embryo transfer technologies with the help of which high milk yielding breeds can be achieved

Proper Management of herd: Milk yield in dairy animals depends upon besides genetic, many other factors such as nutrition, proper care and management, housing conditions, exposure to hot climate for varying period's and disease control. Exposure to hot climate affects the dairy animals directly. This is in contrast to the indirect effects of climate imposed via the fodder and pests. Direct climatic conditions evoke short and long-term reactions in dairy animals to show changes in the efficiency of their production as well as in reproduction. The summer season has a cumulative effect on animals in the form of heat stress, shortage of fodder and poor quality of fodder. It has been noticed that milk production reduces drastically during summer in all types, i.e. in high-grade crossbreeds, low-grade crossbreeds and buffaloes. As a homoeothermic measure, the animals cut down heat production in the body by reducing feed intake and utilization or try to get rid of excess heat or it may bring into operation both of these. Such a strain on the part of buffalo is against the interest of the farmers since he is interested in more milk production.

Hence, there is a need to take special efforts on the part of farmers or managers so that animals are protected well against the effects of summer season and produce more milk or at least the same quantity as produced during other part of the year. There are several factors responsible for day-to-day fluctuation in milk yield. For example, to obtain good milk yield, the cow should be milked as soon as possible after milk ejection has occurred and is important to maintain a regular routine in preparation for milking. The milk ejection reflex, like other reflexes can be inhibited under conditions of stress. This inhibition is effected through a block of the release of oxytocin. If these factors are controlled well or are taken care properly, milk yield will not be affected drastically.

The major component of milk is water in which the solid constituents are suspended. The solid constituents are proteins, fats and lactose. All these constituents are formed within the alveolar cell and the cell content of milk is used as an index of health of mammary gland. In milk, proteins are in the form of casein, fat contents in the form of triglycerides and carbohydrates occur as lactose. The lactose content of milk is largely responsible for the osmotic pressure exerted by milk and therefore, its concentration in milk determine the amount of water secreted or resorbed by the epithelial cells. A number of **factors are responsible for day-to-day fluctuations in milk yield**. These are:

- **Physiological Factors**: These include the physical state of the animal. A healthy, physiologically fit animal will be affected less by factors such as stress, heat, water deprivation etc. Lactation can be maintained for long periods at a reduced level as long as the animal remains non-pregnant, stays healthy, receives sufficient food and is milked regularly.
- **Environmental Factors**: These include season of calving and climate; feeding methods and nutritional status; frequency of milking; holding time; stage of lactation; feeding and milking time.
- **Other Factors** include temperament, weaning, udder stimulation, disease and use of drugs. Factors that limit the increase in daily yield to a peak at eight to nine weeks, such as genetic capabilities, poor husbandry conditions, disease or accidents, will affect the daily yield adversely for the remainder of that lactation period.

Following Efforts and Practices may be taken to Increase Milk Yield and to Reduce Summer Stress:

1. Protection against thermal stress

- Preventing incidence of direct as well as indirect solar radiation on animals by providing, a) green covers, i.e. trees, landscaping, and b) proper sheltering or housing. The shelter should be simple under which animals can retire when it is hot and humid. It should be good loafing area, with minimum of walls to allow free flow of air. It must have temporary barriers for exceptionally bad weather. There must be feeding facilities round the clock especially at night in the summer.

- The existing sheds may be improved by the following steps to reduce the thermal stress: i) The surface of the floor in the shed should be made even by leveling off ridges and filling up pits. The surface can be paved with bricks or at least made hard by good ramming. ii) The farmer's cattle sheds may be having a roof made of straw or mud or GI sheets or asbestos sheets. Straw and mud roof may be leaky and may harbor insects and pests. In rainy season they may leak. Therefore, if money permits, it is better to replace such roofs with better materials. iii) Farmer's traditional cattle sheds are made very close to or in between living quarters and the roof is made too low. This makes the shed dark inside and the air movement is also poor. To make it better, the roof should be raised to proper height, which is six feet at the eaves. iv) Overcrowding is another problem in traditional sheds. Farmers should take care to provide at least 40 Sq. feet area per cow and 45 Sq. feet per buffalo in the sheds. This makes the animals more comfortable.

2. Reducing Body Temperature by

- Washing/Wallowing/ Sprinkling/ showering water on animals during the hot part of summer days.
- Providing cooled drinking water.
- Providing cooling devices such as fans, wet curtains/ khas-khas panels etc.

3. Improve Feed Consumption by

- Feeding green fodder throughout the year and silage/hay during scarcity of green fodder.
- Provision for night feeding during summer (DF).
- Grazing only if green pastures/grass lands are available early in the morning and late in the afternoon.
- Supplementation of mineral mixture.
- Avoid abrupt change in the composition of ration, for example R & C ratio and G & DF ratio. If change is necessary, do it gradually.
- Feed energy balance ration to high yielding animals in early stage of lactation.
- Feeding time should not be changed frequently. Feeding 2-3 hours before milking is ideal.
- Avoid feeding unpalatable feeds to high yielding animals.

4. Improving Reproductive Efficiency through

- Protection of lactating animals, breeding bulls and teaser bull against thermal stress.
- Heat detection with young teaser bull.
- Use marker on the belly of teaser bull in summer.
- Keep close observation of all open cows.
- Scheduling of heat detection and AI during cooler part of the day.
- Insemination at optimal time with good quality semen.

5. Milking Parlor and Milking Management

- Milking parlor should provide proper environment. It should be comfortable in all seasons.
- Hygienic conditions should be maintained in the parlor.
- It should be free from flies, unusual noise, and fright. All these will result in incomplete milk ejection.
- Since milk ejection reflex can be inhibited under conditions of stress, a disturbance free environment must be maintained in the milking parlor.
- Factors influencing let down of milk of the animal should be followed in a definite sequence, may be conditioned or natural, and should not be changed.

- Milking intervals should be uniform. Twelve hours is ideal.
- Correct method of milking should be used, either machine or hand milking.
- Milkier should be trained and do not change him frequently.
- Milking should be done quickly in 5-6 minutes.
- On an average a milkier should milk 10-12 animals in one time.

6. Protection from Cold Winds in Winter

- Provide proper bedding to sick animals and calves.
- Protect against cold winds by making gunny bags curtains.
- Grooming of animals.
- Increase source of energy in severe cold.

Once all these points are taken care properly in housing and managing the cows and buffaloes, milk production will not be affected much due to severe changes in the environment or season. Balanced and nutritious feed, enough drinking water, comfortable temperature and hygienic housing etc. work synergistically in increasing the milk yield in cattle.

Summary

Various methods are used to improve reproductive efficiency in farm animals. These are artificial insemination (AI) and embryo transfer technology (ETT).

Artificial insemination technique involves semen collection, its evaluation and preservation and finally its deposition in the cervix of a cow at appropriate time during the later part of the heat period.

The main advantage of AI is increased use of superior sires for raising progeny. It also helps in preventing and controlling the spread of diseases. It is beneficial to small farmers who cannot keep breeding bulls.

Embryo transfer technology (ETT) is a technique in which embryo is produced from highly genetically superior females (donors) and transferred to recipients to act as foster mothers.

The essential steps in ETT are selection and management of herd for donors as well as recipients, synchronization of estrus both in donors and recipients, superovulation of donor animal, breeding of donor animals by AI or natural service, collection of embryos, selection and evaluation of embryos followed by embryo transfer in recipients, cryopreservaton of surplus embryos, and pregnancy diagnosis. Main advantages of embryo transfer technology are production of calves from genetically superior females and their faster multiplication, production of calves of desired sex, export and import of embryos rather than live animals, and getting calves from infertile animals. It also helps to preserve endangered breeds.

In cattle, age does not determine the onset of puberty; rather it depends on breed, climate, season of birth, environment and management of the animal in dairy farm. Early puberty brings early lactation, so it is desirable to induce early puberty in cattle. Giving certain hormones can induce early puberty.

High milk yielding varieties can be obtained through AI and ETT. But these breeds must be managed properly during extreme summer and winter, with proper nutrition and hygiene conditions. In addition, there are other factors responsible for day-to-day fluctuation in milk yield. All these factors must be taken care properly to improve milk yield in farm animals such as cattle.

Questions

1. Discuss various techniques of improving reproductive efficiency in farm animals.
2. How can puberty be induced early in cattle?
3. Discuss various mechanisms by which milk yield may be improved in cattle.

Chapter 26

Nutrition and Reproduction

Role of nutritional factors and body composition in determining the onset of puberty has been of great interest among scientists from many years. The age of menarche in United States and in many western countries has decreased by about four months for each decade between 1850 and 1950 due to upliftment of socio-economic status of the society. Nutrition plays an important role in the onset of puberty; and malnutrition has been found to delay menarche. For optimal performance in livestock and cattle, efficiency in the metabolic processes of production as well as reproduction is an essential pre-requisite. Reduction in the age of puberty increases the economic efficiency of calf production in cattle etc.

Recent advances in nutrition clearly indicate that all dietary nutrients are required in proper quantity and in proper proportion not only for somatic cell functions but also for gonadal cell functions. All nutrients whether in micro or macro requirements function synergistically in the development and maintenance of the reproductive system in both male and female. Inanition is inadequate intake of one or more nutrients in the diet. Most of the effects of nutrition on reproductive performance are reflected through the anterior pituitary hormones, which in general, affects the hormonal metabolism of the gonads. This means that normal development of the reproductive organs and their proper functioning in adults are dependent not only on the endocrine glands composing the hypothalamo-hypophyseal-gonadal axis but also on other factors as well such as nutrition. Common nutritional factors that are important in maintaining reproduction in mammals include caloric, protein, vitamin, and mineral deficiencies.

Variation in food availability also acts as a proximate regulator and an ultimate cause of seasonal reproduction. A continuous excess of food characterizes no wild habitat. Food availability shows great variations from season to season and year to year and in most habitats some individuals experience undernourishment either routinely or periodically. If severe enough, this affects their reproduction regardless of other environmental concerns.

26.1 Effect of Diet on Male Reproductive System

The two basic functions of the male gonads are to produce gametes and secrete steroids. Spermatogenic activity can be estimated from testis morphology and examination of semen samples while androgen secretion can be estimated from urinary steroid levels, accessory gland weight, and from analysis of accessory sex gland secretions, i.e. fructose and citric acid. Androgen secretion precedes spermatogenesis.

The reproductive organs of the adult are more resistant to changes imposed by diet than are those of the immature animal. In addition, nutrition affects the endocrine rather than the spermatogenic function of the testis. Thus, 28 weeks of underfeeding produced little change in sperm density and motility in mature animals, although seminal vesicle function was reduced. In the male rat, partial or complete starvation, results in testis hypofunction but there is no reduction in testicular nitrogen. Loss of Leydig cell function results in cessation of spermatogenesis and this is evident by the atrophy of the accessory sexual organs and by an alteration in accessory gland secretion. Severe dietary restriction is associated with the absence of spermatozoa in the seminiferous tubules as well as in the epididymis. The human male suffering from chronic malnutrition exhibits hypogonadism. The testes atrophy and size of the seminiferous tubule decreases with thickening of basement membrane and small Leydig cells. These individuals excrete significantly subnormal amounts of 17-ketosteroids. Acute starvation may also decrease urinary 17-ketosteroid and androgen levels to as much as 50 %, with recovery evident on feeding. Figure 26.1 represents influence of food restrictions on hormonal pathways that maintain reproduction in a male mammal.

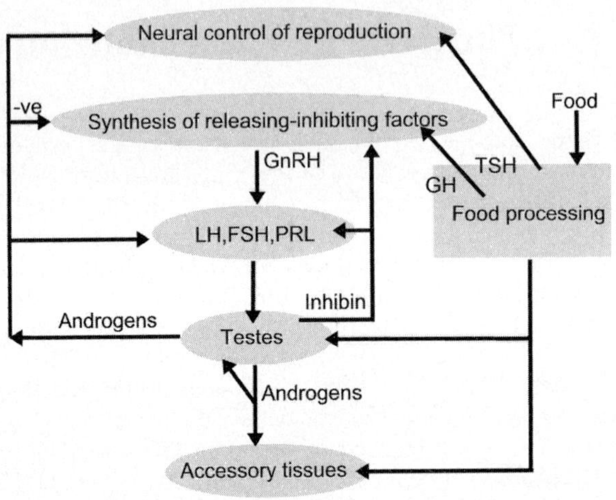

Figure 26.1: Schematic hormonal pathways to show influence of food restriction on maintenance of reproduction in a male Mammal.

Underfeeding young male causes retarded sexual development and delayed puberty. This is due to the suppression of endocrine activity of the testes. It is seen that well-fed young bulls come into semen production 2-3 months sooner than poorly fed animals. Motile spermatozoa appear in Holstein bull calves as early as 37-43 weeks of age with high plan of nutrition and in these, sperm concentration is twice as much as that seen at 80 weeks of age. Both of these traits are affected by under nutrition or with food containing less protein diet. Undernutrition or low protein diet affects the sperm concentration and motility, semen volume, and sex libido (sex desire/drive). In some cases, even gonads do not develop fully and androgenic functions are not normal. Reduced protein intake may decrease the weight of seminal vesicles and there may be even cellular desquamation of tubular spaces. Fructose and citric acid levels may decrease in semen leading to poor quality of semen. Underfeeding is equally bad to rams as it affects sperm density and motility, semen volume per ejaculate but may not affect libido. With increase in dietary protein, sperm density improves in rams. Underfeeding cause thirty days delay in first appearance of spermatozoa as compared to control in boars. The effects of under nutrition may be corrected in mature animals by feeding them large amounts of food whereas it is less successful in young animals because malnutrition causes permanent damage to the germinal epithelium of the testis. Quality of protein is also important for the normal physiological events in the testicles.

Food deprivation depresses a male rat's reproductive capacity in complex ways. In the laboratory, restriction depends on actual amount of food given each day, length of time for which food restriction is imposed, and the developmental stage of life cycle. In general, steroidogenesis is more sensitive to food restriction than is spermatogenesis. Food restriction imposed during early in life, before spermatogenesis begins, greatly delays the onset of this process. But once spermatogenesis begins, food restriction only if severe and prolonged, inhibits it. On the other hand, sensitivity of steroidogenesis to food restriction persists throughout lifetime. Spermatogenesis as well as steroidogenesis is adaptively susceptible to chronic food restriction in some adult deer mice.

Complete starvation prevents maturation of immature animals. Furthermore, marked undernutrion in 700 boys, 7-16 years of age, was associated with genital infantilism in 37 % and cryptorchidism in 27 %. Restriction of food intake to one-half of the normal in maturing bull calves had a marked delaying effect on the onset of secretions from seminal vesicles but a lesser delaying effect on spermatogenesis. Limiting the food intake to one third of the normal did not prevent the immature rat testis from forming spermatozoa at the same time as their controls. When testis maturation was prevented by inanition, a raid growth and maturation occurred on refeeding but full body size is not attained.

Food restriction has a potent effect on LH secretion but less on FSH secretion, thus indicating the relative insensitivity of spermatogenesis and great sensitivity of steroidogenesis to food restriction. LH pulsing seems to be completely blocked by restricting food intake in a young male rat to a level that allows only maintenance of body weight but not the growth (Figure 26.2). A return to *ad lib* (unlimited) feeding initiates the pulsatile release of LH. In the rhesus monkey, chronic food restriction depresses the frequency of LH pulses in castrated males and this treatment has little effect on FSH secretion. However, in humans, FSH secretion seems to be more sensitive to food restriction. Food restriction profoundly depresses the secretion of growth hormone (GH), thyroid stimulating hormone (TSH) and prolactin in addition to LH. This suggests that initiation of secretion of GH and TSH could lead to a depression of general metabolic processes which in turn result in an insensitivity of the testes and accessory tissues to LH and testosterone respectively.

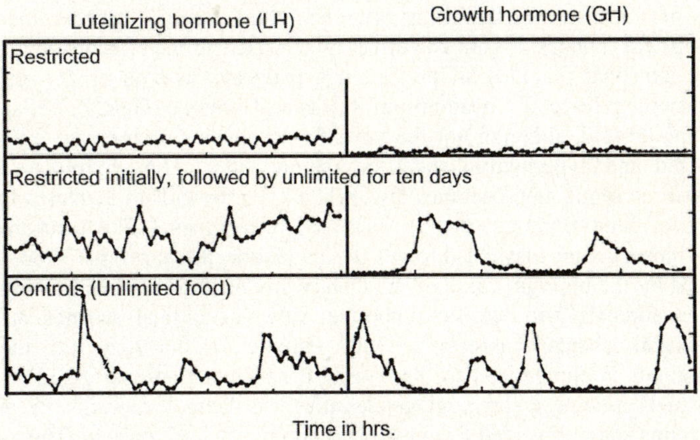

Figure 26.2: Patterns of circulating levels of luteinizing hormone (LH) and growth hormone (GH) in three 60-day-old male Rats, maintained at 60 % expected body weight by food restriction, treated similarly, followed by *ad lib* food for 10 days, or allowed to grow normally (controls).

Androgen secretion can be assessed by measuring the levels of fructose and citric acid in the ejaculate as these are secreted by the seminal vesicles under the influence of testosterone. Luteinizing hormone (LH) treatment enhances the testicular activity before puberty and such bull calves when fed on a high plan of nutrition shows a pronounced increase in fructose and citric acid levels in the ejaculate and these calves reach puberty at about 7 months of age (Figure 26.3). In contrast, when LH treated bull calves are fed on a low plan of nutrition, they show a poor response in terms of these constituents in ejaculate and also show delayed puberty.

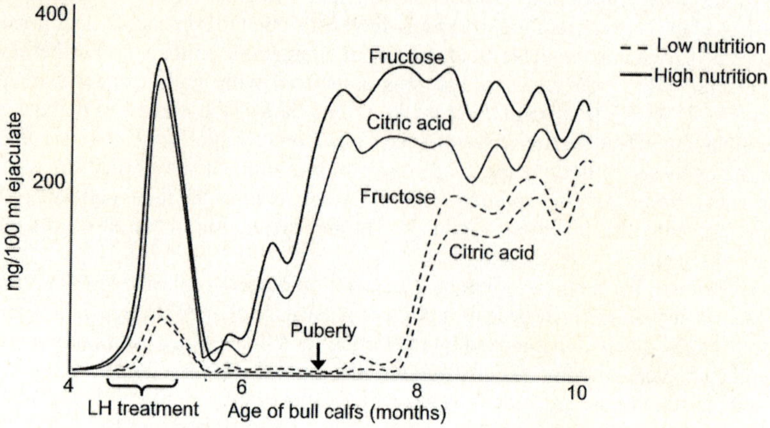

Figure 26.3: Effect of LH treatment on the testicular activity of identical Bull Calves before puberty kept on high nutrition and on low nutrition, the former showed a pronounced increase in the amount of fructose and citric acid in the ejaculate in response to LH treatment and showed normal puberty at about seven months of age, while the later animal showed a poor response to the same dose of LH as indicated by decreased levels of fructose and citric acid in the ejaculate and delayed puberty by about three months.

Influences of nutrition on the testis are direct and are not entirely mediated through hypophyseal gonadotropin changes. Figure 26.1 gives an overview of the effect of food restriction on a male's reproductive axis that includes all presumptive pathways as well as the steroid-dependent depression of the pulsatile release of Gonadotropin Releasing Hormone (GnRH), LH and testosterone. The importance of the thyroid, although not the same for all species, is apparent from the effects of prolonged hypothyroid and hyperthyroid states on reproduction. Hypothyroidism affects steroid metabolism (androsterone production becomes low) while hyperthyroidism increases the appetite and enhances absorption of food from gut due to increased metabolism. The mechanism of thyroid hormone action on reproduction may be through the regulation of nutritional processes as thyroid function is influenced by the biologic value of the dietary protein and the specific amino acids fed to the individual. The adrenals also play an important role via cortical steroids on nutrition and reproduction. Gonadal changes associated with chronic malnutrition are more severe in adrenalectomized animals in comparison to the ones that had intact adrenal glands. Adrenal gland influences metabolism of proteins, and hypoglycemia influences the male reproductive organs.

Immature animals are prevented from maturing when diets lack protein. The minimal amount of dietary protein, which support reproduction, lactation, and growth, is 16.7 %. Feeding of protein-free diet for 15-30 days after weaning to immature rats, prevented maturation of testes and accessory sex organs. Supplements of 5 % liver to the casein-free diet had no effect, but a diet containing 6 % or more casein permitted the formation of spermatozoa in the testis and also showed an increase in the testes weight (Table 26.1). When 6 % casein diet was fed to immature animals for 30 days, 50 % of the rats exhibited some spermatozoa with little increase in testis weight but the seminal vesicle weight doubled. It was found that the gain in testis weight and the biochemical composition of the immature rat testis are both influenced by the nutritive value of the protein fed to the animal.

The testis of normal immature rats contains 85 % water, 10.5 % proteins, 4.5 % lipid, and detectable glycogen. Proteins of lower nutritive value (wheat, gluten, peanut flour, gelatin) permit some increase in the testis weight, but testis protein concentration decrease, percentage of water increases, and lipid and glycogen remain unchanged (Table 26.2). The enzyme β-glucuronidase, frequently associated with growth processes exhibited no change in concentration as the testis matured or prevented from maturing by a protein-free diet. Feeding protein of varied biological value not only influences the weight and composition of the testis, but also the release of androgen, which is more profoundly altered. When a 22-day old male rat is fed a 20 % casein diet for 30 days, the seminal vesicles and ventral prostate weights increases 9-10 fold in comparison with initial control weight. Seminal vesicle weight as related to body weight does not increase in animals fed 20 % wheat gluten.

Table 26.1:Effect of protein diet on testes of immature Rats

Diet (Casein)	Testis Weight (mg)	Sperm %
Initial Control	329	0
65 % for 30 days	1747	100
20 % for 30 days	1694	100
6 % for 30 days	824	50
3 % for 30 days	380	0
0 % for 30 days	140	0
0 % plus 5 % liver	112	0
0 % plus 5 % yeast	119	0

Table 26.2: Effect of nutrition on testis composition in immature Rats

Diet	Final Body Weight (gm)	Testis Weight in gm and constituents in %			
		Weight	Protein	Fat	Glycogen
Initial Control	61	273	72.7	30.1	0.19
20 % Casein	128	1468	72.3	30.4	0.11
5 % Casein	61	684	62.4	29.2	0.26
20 % Wheat gluten	82	1017	64.6	34.0	0.18
20 % Peanut flour	81	1257	66.1	28.8	0.11
20 % Gelatin	53	210	-	-	0.10
Fox chow	115	1515	70.3	30.3	0.15

Withholding of dietary protein from an immature rat for 30 days does not impose a permanent damage. Refeeding of protein permits rapid recovery of testis weight and also the appearance of spermatozoa. 70 % of all animals recovers in 30 days when fully fed, whereas only 25 % recovers when 6 % casein is fed. Recovery of androgen secretion is somewhat slower than that of the tubules as estimated by seminal vesicle weight. If the diet is varied so that calorie intake per gram is reduced to half while retaining the dietary casein level at 20 %, immature rat testis growth is prevented.

Variations in protein quality are a reflection of amino acid deficiencies, and it interferes with testis maturation. Protein metabolic levels are higher in the tissue of young growing animals and the body is more dependent on dietary protein level and quality for maintenance of the metabolic nitrogen pool than in adult animals. On the other hand, body protein reserves in adult animals permit internal shifts of nitrogen to the metabolic pool and the tissues when dietary sources are reduced or endocrine imbalances are imposed. Thus, when low protein diet is fed to adult male rats for 60-90 days before the sperm disappeared, the animals do not mate. Amount of semen and sperm production by sheep is related to the dietary protein level. Removal of protein from the diet for 30 days show little effect on the adult rat testis weight, spermatogenesis, or nitrogen content. However, seminal vesicle weight reduced to 50 %. Prolonged protein depletion is required before the testis exhibited a loss in protein and a reduction in size. A loss of spermatozoa is not observed consistently, although some testes become completely atrophic. Decreased weights of accessory organs of reproduction in these animals reflect the disappearance of androgens from circulation. Interstitial cell atrophy is also noted in rats that are fed a low vegetable protein diet. Sterility may or may not be induced with diets containing 65 % protein but a 15 –18 % dietary level of a poor protein such as maize or gelatin decreases sperm motility and increases the number of abnormal sperm.

Adequate dietary protein cannot maintain reproductive function if the diet is calorie deficient. Thus a decrease in seminal vesicle weight is related to a decrease in dietary calories when protein levels are kept constant. However, increasing the dietary protein slows the weight loss of the accessory sex glands imposed by calorie restriction. Alterations in testis function occurred due to inadequate protein diet is corrected by feeding normal levels of protein diet.

Linoleic, linolenic, and arachidonic acids are designated as essential fatty acids but the physiologic role of these substances is not clearly understood. Nevertheless, dietary essential fatty acid levels influence the male reproductive organs. Adequate level of fat in diet is essential for boars to show normal testes weights. High fat diets may enhance testicular weight, whereas removal of fat from the diet resulted in a degeneration of the seminiferous tubule as evidenced by intracellular vacuolation and a reduction in the number of spermatids and spermatozoa. After feeding a fat free diet for five months, the rat testis becomes devoid of sperm. Testis degeneration occurs despite dietary supplements of vitamin A and E.

Vitamins are also important constituents of nutrition. A lack of vitamin has little effect on testes weight, but such diet influences the Leydig cells and prevents the growth of the accessory sex organs. Testicular dysfunction as judged by failure of sperm formation or atrophy of the secondary sex organs has been observed in deprivation of thiamin, riboflavin, pyridoxine, calcium pantothenate, biotin and vitamin A and E. Vitamin E deficiency in the rat results in a specific and irreversible damage to the testis. Tubular damage may proceed to the point where only Sertoli cells remain but the interstitial cells are not influenced. Similar changes occur following vitamin E deficiency in the guinea pig, hamster and bird; however, a little or no effect of an absence of vitamin E is noted in the rabbit and mouse or in livestock or man, although vitamin E is present in human testis. Dietary vitamin A or carotene deficiency leads to testicular degeneration in farm animals. Testis damage induced by vitamin A deficiency can be reversed, but vitamin A therapy in man for oligospermia which is not due to lack of vitamin shows no effects.

Other vitamin deficiencies also influence the testis. A chronic lacks of ascorbic acid cause a degeneration of both Leydig cells and seminiferous tubules. Serious anatomic and functional impairments of testes are noted in pantothenic acid deficiency. Development of the rat testis and seminal vesicles is retarded by a biotin deficiency, but the animals do not exhibit marked alterations in other endocrine organs. Testosterone hastened the development occurred due to vitamin deficiency and enhanced the severity of biotin deficiency in both sexes, thereby suggesting a hormone-vitamin relationship in male reproduction. Gonadotropins failed to promote spermatogenesis in vitamin A or vitamin E deficient rats, but the atrophic accessory sex organs of vitamin A depleted rats are stimulated by gonadotropin treatments. Lack of vitamin A favored an enhanced response to pregnant mare serum gonadotropin (PMSG) when the ratios of seminal vesicle weight to body weight are computed. The failure of gonadotropins to stimulate testis tubules suggests a special effect of avitaminosis A and E on the responsiveness of the germinal epithelium of seminiferous tubules. Vitamin deficiencies do not prevent the seminal vesicles from responding to androgens. Restricting the calorie intake of vitamin A deficient rats retarded the curative effects of vitamin A deficient animals.

Little information is available concerning the effects of trace mineral deficiencies upon male reproductive functions. Iodine deficiency may result in poor libido and low semen characteristics in bulls while supplementary feeding of copper, cobalt, zinc and manganese results in improvement in sperm production. Plant estrogens exert adverse effects on male accessory organs. Many chemicals and ionizing radiations interfere with spermatogenesis

Overfeeding and obesity induce libido and enhances sexual activity in males. This has been observed in boars, rams and bulls particularly during hot weather.

26.2 Effect of Diet on Female Reproductive System

Mammalian species generally exhibit a delay in sexual maturation when food intake is subnormal before puberty. If inanition is imposed on adults, ovarian atrophy with associated changes in cycles is observed. War famine induced a decrease in fertility and a greater incidence of menstrual irregularities in human beings. Chronic undernutrition involves ovarian atrophy with associated amenorrhea and sterility. The ovarian morphologic changes are similar to those occurring due to aging. Urinary estrogens become subnormal exhibiting amenorrhea when assessed with limited food intake.

The nutritional requirements of primates other than man have been studied in female baboons. The intake of vitamins and other essential nutrients is found to be of the same order as that recommended for man. Calorie intake varied with the menstrual cycle, being least during the follicular phase and maximal during the 2-7 days preceding menstruation. Various diets are studied to assess their importance in maintaining the normal menstrual rhythm. The feeding of maize alone, assorted vegetables and fruits or maize, skimmed milk and fat lead to menstrual irregularities or to amenorrhea. The mechanism regulating ovulation is the first to be deranged. The addition of various vitamins or of animal protein does not correct the menstrual disorders. However, inclusion of ox liver in the diet does maintain the menstrual rhythmicity.

In cows and buffaloes, the level of nutrition markedly influences the puberty and in general, the higher growth rate, the earlier it will reach sexual maturity. Underfeeding in terms of less protein or energy or both affect the rate of growth thereby delay in sexual maturity because puberty is a function of live weight rather than age. In crossbred cows undernutrition causes long anestrous periods. Plasma progesterone peak delays significantly. This may be partly due to increase in estrous cycle length.

In lower mammals inanition hinder vaginal opening and delay puberty and also the maturation and functioning of ovary. In females, it appears that onset of puberty is coupled to growth in terms of body weight, rate of growth, fat content, fat-to-lean ratio, and food intake. There is specific regulation of gonadotropin secretion by some yet unknown mechanisms, more universally constant facet of the body's energy or nutrient processing systems, according to which, the female's prepuberal increase in gonadotropin secretion could occur only when both internal and external energetic conditions predict success for lactation.

Chronic food restriction as in male profoundly depresses GnRH secretion and hence LH and the gonadal steroid secretion in the female, but have less effect on FSH secretion. Also, as in the male, accessory organ responsiveness to exogenous steroids is depressed by chronic food restriction, indirectly via either prolactin insufficiency or metabolic depression. Although, there is minimal effect of food restriction on FSH secretion but folliculogenesis *per se* is little impaired. Food restriction seems to delay follicle atresia, at least in the adult. On the other hand, ovulation occurs less frequently in response to exogenous gonadotropin in starved mice.

LH secretion can be manipulated in the female rat by varying food availability and can be best seen in relation to puberty. Figure 26.4 illustrates that young females maintained for several weeks at 50 % of expected adult body weight by restricting their food intake showed suppressed episodic release of LH. After several weeks of such treatment, these rats were returned to *ad lib* feeding. This resulted in rapid body growth, LH pulsing, and ovulation. The repetitive LH pulse was initiated in some rats within 12 hours, most within 24 hours and most ovulated during the 3rd or 4th dark period. Administration of this hormone in a pulsatile manner to food-restricted females' yields a normal sequence of endocrine and ovarian changes that culminates in normal pubertal development and ovulation despite a total lack of body growth. Food restriction depresses GnRH secretion in the young female rat both directly and by enhancing negative feedback sensitivity to estradiol.

In the adult female rat, we know little about the relative sensitivity of the various stages of the estrous cycle to acute food restriction. It is noticed that food restriction by total deprivation for one day on the day of estrus, just before ovulation preceded and followed by *ad lib* food, resulted in modest prolongation of the following ovulatory cycle. If food deprivation is imposed for 2 days on a female mouse during diestrus, the next ovulation delayed by one full week. Total food deprivation blocks the estrous cycle of the Syrian hamster, and interestingly this block is overcome by giving the hamster unlimited access to drinking water containing glucose, without access to any protein or fat.

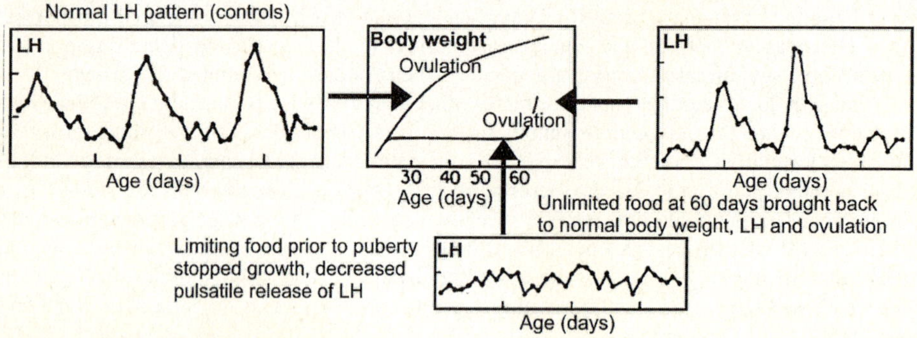

Figure 26.4: Patterns of changes in blood levels of LH in individual female Rats in relation to body growth, which is manipulated by varying food availability.

Chronic food restriction has potent effect on the estrous cycle in livestock in relation to puberty and sometimes also in relation to the onset of seasonal breeding. However, in comparison to rats and mice, these large animals with their much larger energy reserves are much less susceptible to short-term food deprivation, but chronic underfeeding apparently suppresses ovulation in much the same way as it does in rodents. Underfeeding may disturb the reproductive system by altering the secretory pattern of sex hormones, such as progesterone or even LH.

Submaintenance levels of food also affect reproduction in ewes. There is lengthening of estrous cycle, increase in the incidence of silent heat and decrease in estrous intensity. On high plan nutrition, embryo mortality rate becomes less. In swine also, underfeeding of gilts delays the puberty weight and high energy diet is beneficial to attain early puberty weight. If gilts are given maize as a single ingredient, they never show estrous as a result of multiple deficiencies. High protein diet is advantageous to show better ovulation rates. However, protein quality is also important and approximately 25 % of animal protein in diet is required, otherwise puberty gets delayed. Gilts given feed rich in energy and protein show higher ovulation rates and pituitary weights. Riboflavin in adequate quantity ensures good viability of litters in pigs.

Vitamins and minerals are also important for growth and reproduction. Marginal deficiencies affect selectively the function of one particular organ or tissue or even all organs of reproduction. For example, importance of zinc, copper, cobalt, and manganese and vitamins such as A and E has been recognized in the process of reproduction in both sexes in achieving higher sexual activity and fertility. Calcium deficiency at parturition leads to feeble uterine contractions and this may result in difficult parturition. Phosphorus deficiency leads to poor follicular development resulting in infertility. Inadequate phosphorus causes reduced voluntary feed intake, slower growth and impaired reproduction. A severe deficiency of phosphorus can lead to delay in the onset of puberty and post-partum estrus because of inactive ovaries whereas its moderate deficiency may be associated with repeat breeding. The calves of phosphorus deficient dams may be born still or weak. Supplementing phosphorus in feed improves calving and increases percentage of animals coming in heat. Copper deficiency in rats results in reproductive failure with death and resorption of fetuses. In cows, copper deficiency causes suppression of estrus and estrous cycles associated with atonic condition of uterus. Inactive ovaries, delayed or depressed estrous and retained placenta is also attributed to copper deficiency in dairy cattle. Sodium has to be supplemented regularly in food, as it is not stored in any tissue and is liable to be excreted quickly through the excretory channels if not replenished. Sodium deficiency leads to low sodium and potassium ratio in blood and tissues, and this result in poor reproductive performance. Manganese is an activator of a number of enzymes in both somatic cells and gonads. Its deficiency affects reproductive system. Zinc is closely associated with vitamin A function, therefore, deficiency in any of these delays sexual maturity. Pituitary gland shows cystic conditions as a result of vitamin A deficiency. Iodine is required for its incorporation into thyroxin, hormone of the thyroid gland. Its deficiency leads to goiter, which in turn disturbs the whole metabolism of the body and affects reproduction. In cattle, iodine deficiency can impair ovarian activity and fertility.

26.3 Effect of Diet in Females on Pregnancy and Lactation

The human male once attains adulthood is presented with the problem of maintaining the body tissues built up during growth period. However, in addition to this, human female has to take care of replacement of menstrual losses after every menstrual cycle, and also the female (and in all viviparous species) is presented with even more formidable demands in the event of pregnancy. Therefore, nutrition plays more important role in the life of females in comparison to that of males.

The role of nutrition in pregnancy and lactation has always received considerable attention. However, the effects of long term food restriction on pregnancy and lactation has proved difficult since these stages of the female reproductive cycle obviously do not occur in such situations and hence cannot be studied if food restriction is severe enough to block ovulation. Therefore, to study the effect of food on pregnancy and lactation, the amount of food available must be insufficient for these stages but must be sufficient for ovulation to occur.

A limitation of nutritional needs during pregnancy can lead to loss of the embryo or fetus. During the first 15 days of pregnancy, a rat may gain 50 gm of weight and most of it is maternal, associated with an increase in food intake. The increased food intake in early pregnancy provides a reserve for late pregnancy when fetal growth is rapid. Placental secretions are also associated with the active anabolic state of second half of pregnancy. Protein is the most important component of nutrition during pregnancy. Complete removal of protein from the diet beginning at the time of mating does not prevent implantation but does induce almost complete embryonic loss. Also, a successful pregnancy requires proteins of good nutritional quality, and the caloric intake must be adequate. However, protein deprivation during later part of pregnancy decreases maternal weight without showing an ill effect on fetal or placental weight.

Essential fatty acid deficiency during the initial stages of pregnancy does not interfere with the development of the fetuses or parturition in rat but pups may be born dead. Vitamin deficiencies influence the course of a pregnancy. For example, moderate deficiency of vitamin A damage the fetuses without interrupting pregnancy. Vitamin A access also proves detrimental to pregnancy. Deficiency in vitamin E leads to resorption of fetuses. Lack of choline, riboflavin and B_{12} induce fetal abnormalities and interrupt gestation. Choline deficiency is detrimental to placenta while riboflavin lack may impair carbohydrate use and/or induce electrolyte disturbances, and B_{12} is concerned with the synthesis of nucleic acids. Deficiency of thiamine, pyridoxine, pantothenic acid and folic acid individually can interrupt a pregnancy. It seems that the basic physiologic alteration resulting from all these deficiencies is a deprivation of ovarian hormones.

In general, demand for food in females' increases greatly during late lactation in comparison to pregnancy and early lactation. Therefore, effects of food deprivation initiated on day 2 of pregnancy in rat for 24 or 48 hours shows little effect on the number of young born. Food deprivation in mice later in lactation after having invested a great deal of effort in their young shows that mothers often die before consuming any of their young and this is inspite of their depleted fat reserves and their greatly increased need for food. However, in early lactation period, female mice consume some of their young ones when confronted with an absence of food, keeping some alive if possible. Deermouse females employ a different strategy. Whenever their energy constraints become too large during early or late lactation, they simply consume their entire litter and reinitiate an estrous cycle.

Food availability undoubtedly acts as the most important cause for seasonal reproduction in many wild populations of mammals. Even domesticated livestock often require food supplements during winter in order to maximize their reproductive performance. Thus, supplementing food to natural habitats containing wild mice as studied in Australia increased the percentage of pregnant and lactating mice during late winter (Figure 26.5). The number of eggs ovulated and ultimately the number of lambs born can be increased in ewes kept on poor pasture by giving them supplement food for a few weeks prior to mating.

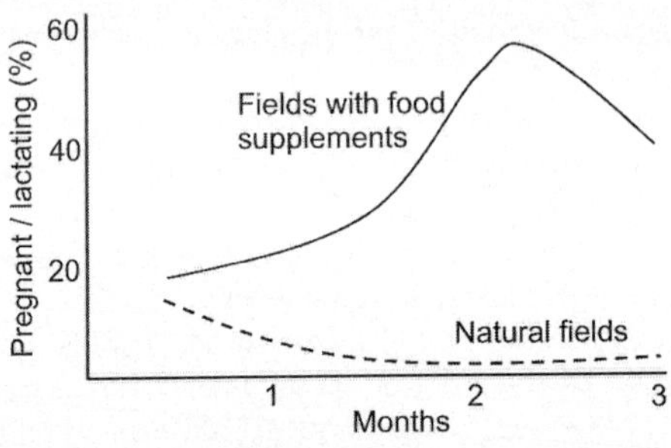

Figure 26.5: Effect of adding supplement food to natural habitats containing wild Mice in Australia in late winter.

The nutritional status of mother appears to influence the quantity of prolactin (PRL) secretion during lactation. An improvement of maternal diet causes a significant reduction of PRL release in all stages of lactation. The persistently higher PRL levels found in undernourished mothers appear to ensure milk synthesis by preferentially channeling nutrients to the breast. However, the lower PRL levels associated with improved maternal nutrition shortens the period of postpartum infertility despite prolonged breast-feeding.

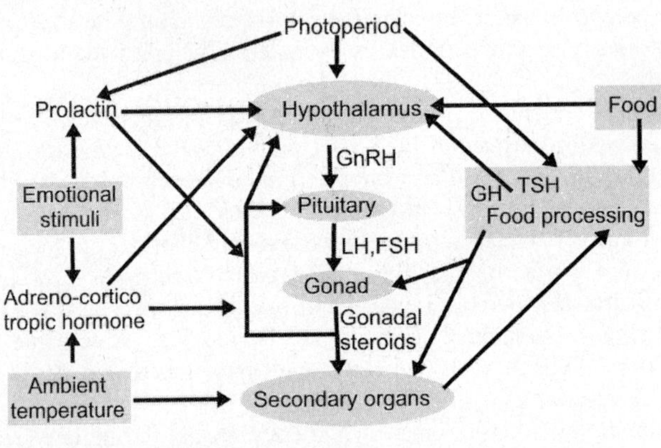

Figure 26.6: Schematic representation of influence of food availability and other environmental factors via endocrine pathways on reproduction in Mammals.

Figure 26.6 summarizes the effect of food availability along with other environmental factors on various endocrine pathways to influence reproduction in mammals.

Summary

Of the many environmental factors that can influence reproduction in mammals, availability of food plays a very important role. It can act as a proximate regulator of reproductive performance in many individuals. Effects of underfeeding or malnutrition in both sexes are more severe in immature than in mature animals and can be corrected to some extent by *ad lib* supply of food.

Food restriction suppresses the pulsatile release of GnRH directly and also indirectly by enhancing negative feedback sensitivity to the gonadal steroids.

LH secretion is affected more by food restriction than FSH in both male and female. Thus, steroidogenesis is affected more than gametogenesis at least in the adult by food restriction.

Food deprivation early in the life of a male seriously affects spermatogenesis. However, oogenesis in females is less affected by food restriction.

Food deprivation decreases reproductive performance indirectly by inhibiting the secretion of GH, TSH, and prolactin.

Food restriction that allows ovulation have little effect on pregnancy but have most potent effects on lactating female when the demands for calories and nutrients are highest and is partly due to decrease in prolactin secretion.

Vitamins and minerals are also important for growth and reproduction. Marginal deficiencies affect selectively the function of one particular organ or tissue or even the organs or reproduction. Importance of zinc, copper, cobalt, and manganese and vitamins such as A and E has been recognized for the presence of reproduction in both sexes to achieve higher sexual activity and fertility.

Questions

1. Discuss the role of diet on male reproductive system.
2. Discuss the effects of diet on female reproductive system.
3. Discuss the role of nutrition on pregnancy and lactation.

Chapter 27

Poultry

The term 'poultry' includes fowls, domestic ducks, turkeys, guinea fowls and geese. However, in day-to-day references poultry deals mainly with chicken and fowls.

Domestication of fowls originated in India. It was initially for cock fighting but later the main objective of poultry diverted to egg and meat production. Poultry and poultry farming forms a substantial source of food protein for the human population and practically in all country poultry farming is carried out to some extent for this purpose. In India, poultry has gained considerable importance in the last few decades with the introduction of exotic breeds of fowls. Thousands of farms exist at present where a large number of fowls are bred and reared for egg and meat production. In India number of egg laying hens increased during 1961 to 1980 from 35 to nearly 100 millions and egg production from nearly 2500 to 12500 millions.

27.1 Selection of Breed

Specific poultry stocks are available for egg and broiler production. The present day fowls reared for egg or meat purposes are crossbreeds of Leghorns and Rhode Islands with indigenous breeds. For egg production, breeders in poultry farming try to raise efficient egg-laying strains. Success in raising chickens for egg production depends largely on good quality stock and efficient management. Good stock for breeding is secured by selection and others of undesired traits are removed from the stock. This is called **Culling**. Following characters are considered during selection of good breeds.

- **Pedigree information**-Breeds with good ancestry records such as the rate of egg laying, size of eggs produced etc. is selected for breeding. A breed with an average record of laying annually 250-280 eggs is preferred.
- **Appearance**-Good health and vigor are required characteristics for a good laying hen. Many features in appearance of a bird indicate it's laying capacity and condition. Therefore, following characters must be taken into consideration during selection of a good breed (Table 27.1).

Table 27.1: Comparison of characters of an egg-laying and non-laying Hen

Character	Egg-Laying Hen	Non-Laying Hen
Abdomen	Large and triangular in outline.	Small, and not triangular.
Beak	Short, and even mandibles.	Mandibles uneven, and overlapping.
Comb	Full, soft, and bright red.	Dry, hard and dull colored.
Ear	Proportionate and bright.	Small and dull.
Head	Clear-cut and alert.	Coarse and masculine.
Pubic bones	Wide apart by 2/3 fingers thickness.	Closely placed with very little space in between.
Vent	Moist, wide and expanded.	Coarse and masculine.

- **Moulting** or **Molting**-Molting is the process by which old feathers are shed by the hen to replace with new ones. Molting and egg laying capacity of a hen are inter-related. Good layers molt late, quickly and begin production of eggs while poor layers molt late, slowly and take a long time to complete their molt and then begin production of eggs
- **Pigmentation**-Pigmentation of skin is related to the formation of eggs in the ovary. By observing the depth of pigmentation, one can judge the egg laying condition of the hen. The disappearance

of yellow pigment from the skin begins from the vent and then extends to the eye rings, ear lobes, beak and shank. The approximate period for which the hen has been laying eggs can be determined by the order of disappearance of pigment from the body.

- **Sexual maturity**-Early maturing fowls lay more number of eggs than late maturing ones. Sexual maturity is influenced by food, length of the day, climate and season. Chicks hatched during January to March usually mature earlier and the breeders must select early maturing breeds of fowl to obtain good results.
- **Egg cycle**-It is the persistency or continuity of egg laying during a period. A good breed lay one egg every day for a long period, pause for a day or two and then resume laying.
- **Broodiness**-It is the tendency of a laying hen to sit over the eggs to hatch. Prolonged broodiness lowers the production capacity of eggs by the hen. Therefore, non-broodiness hens are selected for breeding.
- **Trap nest record**-Trap nesting is observing a hen for 3-4 days a week for determining the egg production of a hen. It is also useful to study the nature of the egg.

27.2 Reproductive Physiology and Endocrinology of Hen

Birds are **"Uni"-polytocous** animals in which many eggs are matured, but **ovulated singly**, and laid in clutches, in contrast with some **"multi"-polytocous** mammals, such as rats, in which many eggs are ovulated simultaneously.

Genetic selection has made the domestic hen one of the most remarkable and potentially most prolific reproductive organisms among the higher vertebrates. The reproductive pattern of hen differs from that of mammals in many important aspects, and the first one is that hens do not show a cyclic pattern of reproduction as seen in mammals, although avian reproduction is characteristically cyclical, usually seasonal. Gonadal development occurs in response to stimulatory environmental cues and in turn promotes courtship and mating behavior. Reproductive organs control whole reproductive phases in hen, and the follicular and oviduct functions continue at the same time. Most hens lay eggs in clutches. A clutch consists of one or more eggs, followed by a day of rest, which is succeeded, by another egg or series of eggs, depending on the genotype of the hen. A prolific hen lays five or more eggs in a clutch. Clutches of 50-100 eggs are common and they are separated by not more than one day of rest. Many hens lay 365 eggs in one year.

Compared with mammals, avian endocrinology is poorly understood and is even less known in males than in females. The most obvious external characters that distinguish male from female are comb growth, spur development, calls, behavior, fat deposition, feather shape & pigmentation and the width of the pelvic bones. These characters are under the influence of steroids. They are more directly involved in reproduction by affecting the growth of the oviduct, the breakdown of the occluding plate, protein synthesis within the oviduct and the movement of the egg down the oviduct. About nine hormones are directly involved in the reproductive physiology of birds.

Reproduction in female can be divided endocrinologically into two distinct phases, the one in which physiologic mechanism leads to sexual maturation and the other in which the processes result in development of single egg. Difficulties in ovarian endocrinology arise because similar hormone is active in each phase and one phase is superimposed on the other. Left ovary produces steroids during early embryogenesis and the estrogen present may be responsible for the suppression of the right ovary and at the same time without the presence of right ovary, the right oviduct fails to develop further.

The functional morphology of the ovary is basically similar to that of mammals. But, in contrast to mammals, the bird has no well-defined estrous cycle. Instead, reproductive activity of the ovary is continuous during the part of the breeding season devoted to egg laying. In the domestic fowl, it may be extended almost indefinitely by the provision of suitable environmental conditions. Follicle maturation is sequential. Each day, with few exceptions, a new follicle reaches maturity and only this follicle ovulates in response to LH-stimuli although all follicles are subjected to some LH stimulation as LH is present in general circulation.

As the birds reach sexual maturity, they become photosensitive and it is this change, which is responsible to future sexual development. In response to changing day length, the hypothalamus alters the output of gonadotropin releasing factor. There has been much speculation about the specific trigger for LH release. Estrogen, progesterone and androgen all seem to be involved. Increase in plasma LH occurs approximately at the same time when an increase in estrogen, androgen, and progesterone occurs in the plasma. Light may affect reproductive activity through at least three pathways: i) eyes, ii) pineal glands, and iii) through its direct effect on hypothalamus.

A characteristic feature of avian reproduction is that a successive egg of a sequence is laid later called "lag" during the day. This is brought about by LH release occurring later during the dark period and not by the length of the time the egg spends in the oviduct. It seems that LH release occurs only during dark period. If there is no LH release, there will be no ovulation. After the paused day (twenty-four hours later) the following sequence is initiated by the next onset of darkness and the cycle is repeated. Estrogen and progesterone play an important role in production of egg.

Estrogens have many functions. They bring about the breakdown of the oviducal plate and increase the uptake of calcium from the gut. It acts on liver to produce the yolk protein, increase deposition of body fat, causes changes in vascular system, stimulates growth of the oviduct, brings about the pubic bones to "spread". Estrogens directly control lipoprotein synthesis in the liver. Estrogen plays an important role in deposition of calcium in the bones and helps to bring about the typical "female" behavior.

Progesterone is involved in calcium metabolism, growth and functioning of oviduct, and feedback effect on gonadotropin production. Progesterone plays a regulating role in luteinizing hormone (LH) release and ovulation. Calcium metabolism in the gut and in the bone is also under the influence of steroid hormones.

Androgens play part in oviduct growth, differentiation and development of secondary sex characteristics.

The control of the hypothalamo-pituitary-gonadal axis in birds may also be modified by the actions of other hormones, particularly by prolactin, thyroid hormones, and adrenal corticoids. The adrenal hormones may be involved in the entrainment of rhythmical hormone secretion while reproductive function is strongly influenced by thyroid hormones, the circulating concentrations of which reflect changes in environmental conditions such as food availability, temperature, and photoperiod. Somatic growth in the bird interacts with environmental factors and results in puberty, sexual maturation, and reproductive activity.

The reproductive systems of the adult male and female birds are acquired after a period of somatic growth, since the bird must be sufficiently well grown to take parental responsibilities and to lay eggs large enough to produce hardy nestlings. Once somatic maturity has been achieved, many photoreceptive species such as chickens, ducks etc. then attain sexual maturity, even when exposed to nonstimulatory environmental conditions, for example, short days or constant darkness. The onset of sexual maturity is, however, usually triggered by environmental conditions that stimulate the hypothalamo-pituitary-gonadal axis, provided this axis is fully developed and is responsive to these stimuli. The development of the hypothalamo-pituitary-gonadal axis in turn depends on the maturation of the neuroendocrine pathway's control of GnRH release. This is in response to day length or steroid feedback. In photoperiodic species the increase in day length during spring increases testicular size and androgen secretion in parallel with increased gonadotropin release. Unlike mammalian species the onset of puberty appears to be age-rather than size-related and is triggered by a suppression of the negative feedback pathway controlling gonadotropin release, facilitating increased FSH and LH release in response to environmental stimuli, such as light. The onset of sexual behavior normally occurs before the attainment of adult circulating gonadal steroid levels.

As birds approach the completion of their reproductive span, aging results in the laying of fewer and less fertile eggs by the females, and in the males in suppression of mating frequency and sperm production. This decline in reproductive function probably results from a loss of gonadal steroid receptors at target sites and because of an increase in the threshold required for the induction of hormone action. A decrease in the 5α-reductase pathway is probably also casually involved in the suppression of reproductive activity in aging males.

Egg formation involves the transport of large quantities of materials across biological membranes and formation of many new substances particularly specific proteins and lipids. Liver also plays an important role in egg formation. Size of egg and its composition are affected by many factors, such as genetic, environmental, and physiological.

27.3 Role of ovary and ducts in egg formation

Avian Ovaries: In majority of Aves, only left ovary is functional. The right ovary though present in embryos, persists only for a few days after hatching, and becomes vestigial in adult females. This is due to early production of steroid hormones by the left ovary. The right ovary becomes functional only when the left functional ovary is either removed surgically or destroyed but this development depends on the age at which the functional ovary has been removed. If the ovary is removed from the chickens, which are less than twenty days old, the rudiment hypertrophies into a structure resembling a testis that is capable of spermatogenesis. Since, the Wolffian duct system does not develop in the genetic females, there is no duct connection between the testis and the copulatory organs. If the ovary is removed at a higher age, the rudiment develops into functional ovary that is capable of ovulation. However, such females do not have an oviduct on the side of the rudiment gonad, and there is no way to conduct the ovulated eggs to the outside. Operations at intermediate ages cause the rudiment to form an ovotestis having germ cells of both sexes in an undifferentiated condition. In cases of development of testis or ovotestis after the loss of the functional ovary, the genetic female develops all sex characteristics of the male, including a large red comb, male plumage, crowing, and male copulatory behavior toward the normal female.

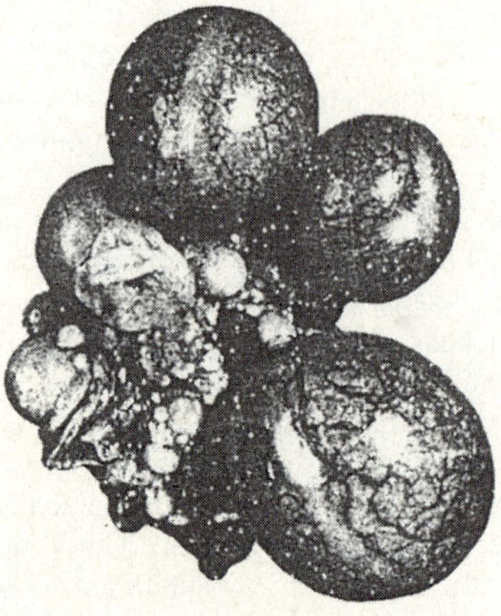

Figure 27.1: Ovary of a Hen.

Morphologically, avian ovary differs from the mammalian ovary. It is relatively enormous structure because of the huge amount of yolk deposited in the individual eggs (Figure 27.1). The ovary contains two major lobes and within each lobe, large numbers of follicles are carried on follicular stalks (Figure 27.2). The developing avian ovum fills the follicle and contains a large amount of yolk compared to which the germinal portion of the egg is negligible in size. There is no antrum and follicular fluid in the follicle. The wall of the mature follicle is composed of several cell layers. Granulosa cells, which are involved in both hormone production and yolk deposition line the avian follicle and the arrangement of theca interna (steroid producing) and externa (connective tissue) is however, similar to that found in mammals. Within the granulosa layer is the vitelline membrane surrounding the ovum.

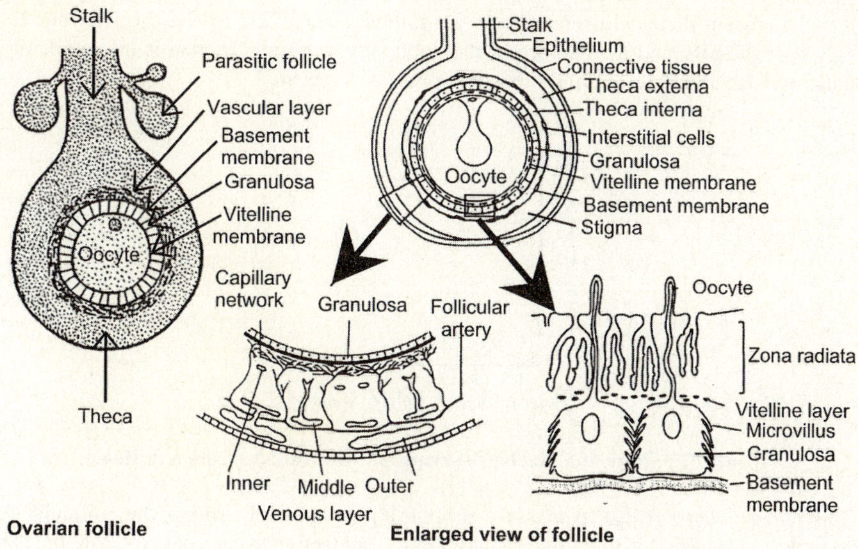

Figure 27.2: Histology of ovarian follicle and follicle wall in Chick.

In the left or functional ovary, there are several clearly recognizable groups of follicles though each merge into the other in order of increasing size. The largest group consists of numerous microscopic follicles consisting of an oocyte covered by the first stages of a granulosa and a theca. The next group consists of follicles of about 1-3 mm diameter, within which primordial yolk is formed. These are also numerous. Larger follicles of 4-8 mm diameter with a more yellowish color and 6-25 in numbers are present. The most obvious group consists of 5-7, yellow colored follicles, which reach a size of nearly 35-mm diameter at ovulation. This group of follicles is graded into a hierarchy consistent with daily ovulatory sequence and for convenience they are often designated as F_1, F_2...with the largest being identified as F_1. Each gap in the hierarchy usually coincides with a predicted future **pause-day** (break between one sequence and the next). Position of gap depends on the bird's laying record and may occur at any position in the hierarchy. The development of the hierarchy of follicles is rigidly controlled, so that there is an orderly progression with in the chicken and one is ready to ovulate each day. How this hierarchy of development is maintained is not fully understood. One of the factors in this may be the supply of oxygen, nutrients, and hormones via the blood supply, which is regulated by both adrenergic and cholinergic innervations.

The final stage of follicular growth is linear (Figure 27.3). Avian follicles are the fastest growing structures found in higher vertebrates. It starts with a diameter of less than a millimeter and weight less than 100 milligrams, and in nine days it grows to a mature size weighing 18-20 grams. It accomplishes this with the help of complex circulatory system. The main feature of the circulatory system is an enormous development of the venous supply, which is arranged in three concentric layers around the follicle, and terminates, in an extremely fine venous capillary network enveloping the growing ovum (Figure 27.2). In contrast, the arterial supply to the follicle is poorly developed. The system depends on getting the blood into the venous network, where it stays long enough to permit the transfer of the yolk antecedents to the ovum. The intricate follicular circulator system serves primarily one of the larger follicles, but is also utilized by smaller follicles, which grow in large numbers on the same follicular stalk on which the large follicle is growing. When the largest follicle ovulates, spiral arteries in its wall become constricted, thus reducing the blood flow to the empty follicular sac. In spite of the reduced blood flow to the ovulated follicle sac, vascularization remains sufficient to permit rapid growth of the smaller follicles clustered along the follicle stalk. One of these is destined to enlarge more rapidly than the rest, and as it enlarges, its blood system rapidly increases in complexity until it reaches ovulatory size and ruptures, and the whole process is repeated.

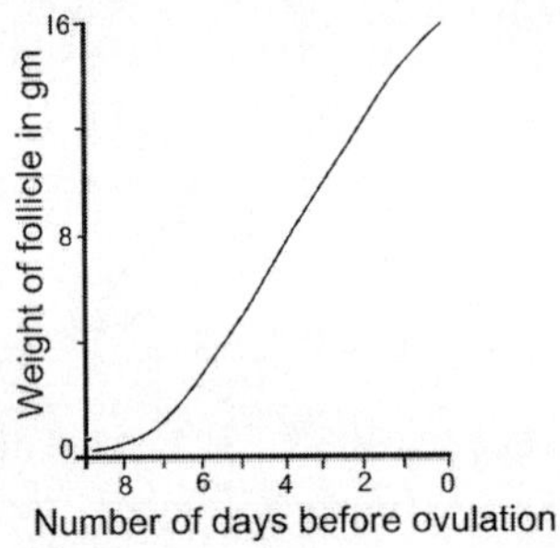

Figure 27.3: Rate of follicular development with yolk deposition in Hen.

The avian oocyte grows to massive proportions, completely filling the follicular covering, unlike that in the mammals. Also, the follicle has a thick connective tissue coat covering the theca. The theca differentiates into a theca interna and externa but the general cells of the interna are not steroidogenic. Instead, interstitial cells are present which have the characteristics of steroid producing cells.

The ovarian follicles accumulate only yolk. The outer follicular membrane is called stigma. Ovulation occurs through the rupture of stigma due to LH release. Once ovulation occurs, an empty follicle shrinks but remains visible for a considerable time. No structure comparable to the mammalian corpus luteum is formed in birds, but empty follicle seems to play a role in the reproductive cycle of chickens.

Ovarian Steroid Hormones: In comparison to mammals, steroidogenesis within the ovary of the birds is still poorly understood. Figure 27.4 shows the hormonal patterns in the blood plasma of laying hens during a 24-hour cycle. In the laying hen, the interstitial cells of the ovary, including the follicular theca, and the granulosa cells of the 5-6 large yolk-filled follicles have the capability of synthesizing and secreting sex steroid hormones. Androgen as well as estrogen stimulate ovarian development and do not inhibit pituitary gonadotropins. The granulosa cells of a particular follicle are only enzymatically competent to produce hormones in the last 6-7 days of its lifetime that is after it reached a size greater than 5 mm. During this time, the activity of the penultimate enzyme in the steroid biosynthetic chain called 3β-HSD (Δ^5-3β-hydroxysteroid dehydrogenase) in the granulosa increases linearly along with follicle weight. The granulosa cell produces only progesterone in response to LH. The interstitial cells of the follicular theca metabolize progesterone to androstenedione and testosterone, which is aromatized to estrone and 17β-estradiol respectively. There are marked qualitative and quantitative differences in enzymatic activities of the thecal cells of the follicular hierarchy. During the day, the concentration of LH and the steroid sex hormones are small. At the onset of dark or slightly later, there is a small rise in the concentration of LH with minor concomitant changes in the concentrations of progesterone and androgens. About 4-11 hours later or approximately 6 to 8 hours before ovulation, concentration of LH increases. This result in a LH peak of 2-3 fold greater concentrations than the basal values observed during the day. The LH increase is accompanied by increased concentrations of progesterone, testosterone, estrone and 17β-estradiol (Figure 27.4). Though pregnancy is absent from birds, yet, the ovarian hormones are needed for the production of a yolky egg surrounded by a layer of egg white, membranes, and shell (Figure 27.5). Synthesis of the yolk precursors by the liver is initiated and maintained by ovarian steroids, which are also responsible for the production of egg white proteins and the massive growth and differentiation of the oviduct. The later is an essential prerequisite for synthesis of egg albumin. Alone, neither progesterone nor the androgens have a major effect on reproductive physiology of birds, but they act synergistically with estrogens to affect oviduct development and egg white production. Furthermore, some hormone actions must occur in sequence. For example, progesterone can only stimulate avidin (egg white) production after estrogens have stimulated oviduct development. Estrogens and androgens together play a major role in calcium homeostasis in laying birds. The postovulatory follicle does not contribute significantly to the sex hormone pattern observed in the plasma of the laying hen during ovulatory cycle.

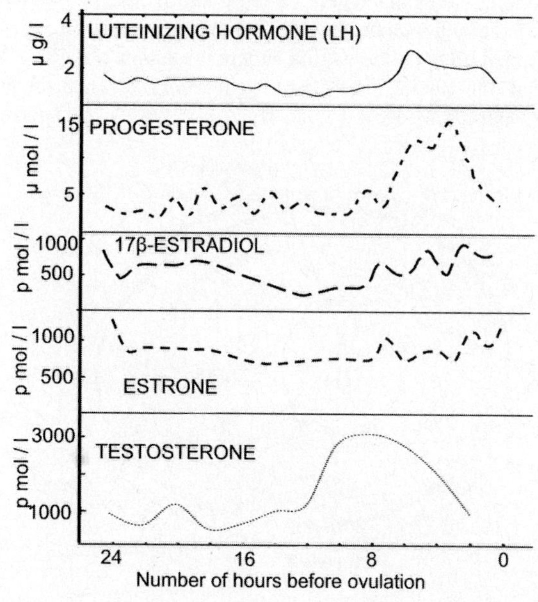

Figure 27.4: Hormonal patterns during a 24-hours cycle in blood plasma of laying Hen.

Avian Oviduct: The avian duct system is a tube of almost uniform diameter with a single unilateral distention near the cloaca. In most of the birds, only the left half of the Mullerian duct system persists and the right half degenerates completely or persists only in the rudimentary form. It is the source of yolk protein and phospholipids.

On the basis of anatomical features, it is possible to distinguish the following parts: **infundibulum**, **magnum**, **isthmus**, **shell gland**, and **vagina** (Figure 27.6). Infundibulum consists of funnel, or fimbria, that actively engulfs the shed ovum. It is the chalaziferous region, in which the chalazae-two coiled, spring-like cords that extend from the yolk to the poles of the egg are formed. Magnum, also called the albumen-secreting region, is the longest portion of the oviduct. It has thick walls, and its lining is thrown into folds in which secretory cells unlike yolk proteins not formed in the ovary are present. Most of the proteins and albumen are found in the oviducal tissues. White of the egg is deposited around the yolk as it passes through this region. Avidin is found in the epithelial goblet cells and tubular glands of the oviduct produce ovalbumen and lysozymes and estrogen is involved in their production. Progesterone may be involved in the formation of only one protein i.e. avidin. Release of the formed proteins occurs as developing egg passes down the magnum. Next region of the oviduct is called isthmus and there is a distinct, externally visible line of demarcation that girdles the whole duct, known as the magnum-isthmus junction. The egg acquires the soft-shell membrane in this part of the oviduct. From the isthmus, the egg passes into the caudal expanded portion of the duct called the "shell gland" or uterus. It is joined to the isthmus by a short neck. This region is called so as the egg acquires the hard calcareous shell here. The egg remains in the shell gland for nearly 20 hours. During the first 6 hours, clear, watery fluid produced from the neck region passes on to the egg, this process is called plumping and it results in the two-fold increase in the mass of egg white. Plumping may continue throughout the time egg stays in shell gland. Calcification of egg starts during its stay in the shell gland. The oviduct does not store calcium and about 20 % of the calcium come from the blood, when egg passes through the shell gland. Rotation of egg around the polar axis leads to the completion of formation of chalazae (which were secreted in the infundibulum) and stratification of the albumen takes place here. Shell gland is responsible for the formation of thick cuticle and pigmentation of the egg. Once the egg formation is completed in the shell gland, egg is expelled through short s-shaped tube, called vagina, where it remains only for a short time and becomes coated with mucus to seal the shell pores, and to prevent bacterial invasion. Vagina helps in fertilization of the egg, as sperms are stored in it, since it contains the sperm storage glands that is typical of birds.

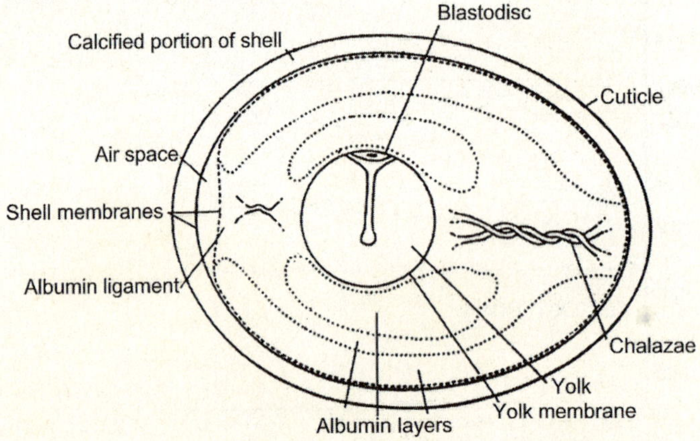

Figure 27.5: Structure of egg of Hen.

The chick oviduct is complex. In about twenty-six hours, it transports the egg to the vagina and outside and secretes about 40 grams of material, consisting of 10 grams of solids and 30 grams of water. The time spent by the egg in different parts of avian duct are summarized in Table 27.2. One may note that the egg spends maximum time in shell gland, where secretion is least by weight but 98 % of these are solids and calcium carbonate and traces of other minerals are deposited at the rate of 0.3 gram per hour.

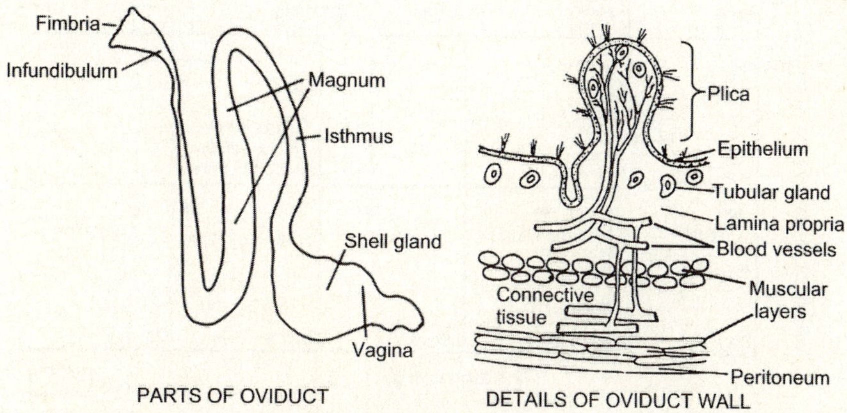

Figure 27.6: Structure of the oviduct and its wall in adult Hen.

Table 27.2: Time spent by egg in different parts of Avian oviduct

Region of Oviduct	Average length (cm)	Contribution by each region of the duct			Time spent by egg (Hours)
		Kind	Amount (gms)	Percent solids	
Infundibulum	11.0	Chalaza	.....	.....	0.25
Magnum	33.6	Albumen	32.9	12.2	3
Isthmus	10.6	Shell membrane	0.3	80.0	1.25
Shell gland	10.1	Calciferous shell	6.1	98.4	18-22
Vagina	6.9	Mucus	0.1	......	1/60

Histologically, oviduct consists of external peritoneum coat or serosa, middle muscular layer, with outer longitudinal and inner circular, the connective tissue layer carrying the blood vessels and nerves, and the innermost mucosa layer (Figure 27.6). In the young chick, the mucosa is a simple, unfolded lining but as sexual maturity approaches, the oviduct begins to be stimulated by estrogen and progesterone, so that the mucosa becomes intricately grooved and folded into primary, secondary, and tertiary folds to form glands. Numerous glands are found throughout the length of oviduct. The cells in these glands vary in type from simple, tall, columnar to transitional, columnar at the height of secretory activity, and secrete substances characteristic of that region. Most of these cells are ciliated.

Transport of egg through oviduct and oviposition: The transport of egg in oviduct is same in all domestic poultry or birds. Ovulation in the majority of hens under ordinary daylight conditions occurs in the morning hours, never after 3.00 P.M. The ovulated egg spends about 3 ½ hours acquiring the albumin coat in the magnum part of the oviduct, 1-¼ hours in the isthmus part for the formation of the soft shell membranes, and then 21 hours for the formation of the calciferous shell in the uterus, or shell gland. Thus, egg formation requires 25-26 hours in total. Ovulation of the next egg in the clutch occurs 30-60 minutes after oviposition of the previous egg. Therefore, the hen normally runs behind schedule, ovulating later each successive day and eventually it will be as late as 2.00 or 3.00 P.M. before the next ovulation should take place. When that point is reached, ovulation is held in abeyance (as it does not occur after 3.00 pm), and laying is interrupted for one or sometimes several days before a new clutch is started for ovulation occurring very early in the morning (Figure 27.7). Based on these regulated timings, it is easy to time oviposition and predict next ovulation time once the clutch length of a hen has been determined by observation. It is not known, how the oviposition is initiated, but both hormonal and neural factors are involved in egg laying.

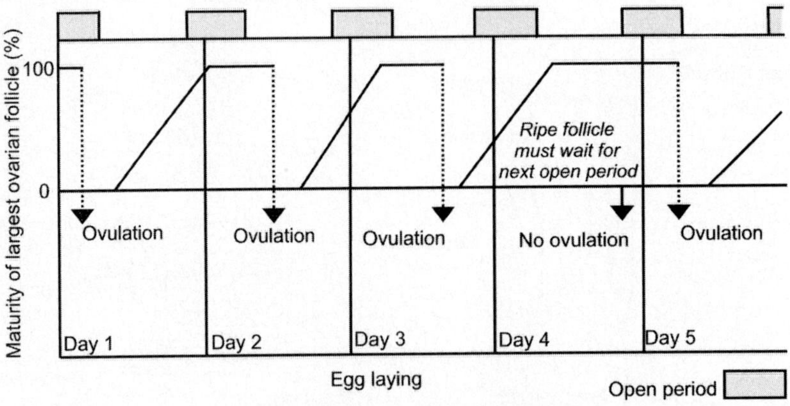

Figure 27.7: Sequential pattern of egg laying in Hen.

The length of the clutch determines the productivity of a hen. It depends on the interval between oviposition and the following ovulation. The larger that interval, fewer eggs will be produced in one clutch. Hens laying twenty, thirty, or more eggs in one clutch accomplish this by two means, one is by shortening the interval between oviposition and ovulation to a few minutes, and second by shortening the time the egg spends in the shell gland to as little as eighteen hours.

Clutch length is governed by the amount of gonadotropin produced by the pituitary gland. However, in hen, the rate of FSH secretion is not controlled, as in the mammalian females, by the flow of follicular estrogen. Further, the pituitary of the hen has been found to be very resistant to estrogenic inhibition because of the almost continuous and the cyclic maturation and ovulation of eggs in chickens. And also, in the normally laying hen there is a steady and continuous flow of FSH and of some LH from the pituitary. In the hen with the short clutch the valve is set for a low but steady flow of FSH and in the hen with the long clutch the valve is opened wider for a more rapid but still steady outpouring of FSH.

The ovum is picked up after ovulation by the fimbria of the oviduct and conducted into the magnum where it acquires the albumen layers. Two hormones control albumen secretion in the magnum; one is estrogen, and the other is androgen or progesterone, either of which acts on estrogen developed magnum and cause formation of albumen granules and their release into the lumen. Following this, actual secretion of albumen from the glands into the lumen is elicited by the presence of any foreign body in the magnum, be it an ovum or anything else. Having acquired albumen during the two and a half or three hours in the magnum, the egg moves on to the isthmus, where the shell membranes are secreted. This part of the oviduct is histologically distinguishable from the magnum, but is controlled by the same hormones in the same manner and sequence as they do on the magnum. The egg spends one and half-hours in the isthmus, and once it acquires the soft-shell membranes and some water, it moves on to the shell gland or the uterus. Here the egg spends about twenty- two hours and acquires the calcareous shell around it. The endocrine control of the shell gland differs from that of the upper regions of the oviduct in that estrogen alone causes the shell gland's growth and development as well as the mobilization and secretion of the calcium salts needed for the formation of the shell. Estrogen is known to mobilize calcium from bones, leading to hypercalcemia, which is typical of laying hens and can be induced in the non-laying hens and males by injection of estrogen. Estrogen also encourages osteoblastic activity in the bone and hence deposition of calcium. However, how estrogen accomplishes simultaneously these opposite effects is not clear, but it does so with the cooperation of parathyroid hormone. The egg moves through the various segments of the reproductive tract at different rates and the secretions of the hypothalamus control this.

During copulation, spermatozoa are deposited into the vagina, where they are stored for up to 2 weeks, in specialized areas known as sperm "glands" or sperm host glands. Following oviposition, spermatozoa are released and transported up the oviduct to the infundibulum where the ovum from the next ovulation is fertilized.

27.4 Photoperiodism

Photoperiodism is the onset of reproductive activity in response to increasing day length in an organism. There is no doubt that light plays an important role in determining the reproductive periodicity in animals. However, in some, it governs only macro-periodicity as in sheep by determining the onset of the breeding season (but does not play a major role in governing estrous cycles within the breeding season) and in others such as birds (chickens), light governs micro-periodicity as well for not only the breeding season itself but also the laying of eggs within clutches is controlled by light. The development of photo refractoriness and subsequent photosensitivity following short-day exposure suggests that some birds can distinguish between long and short days and hence measure the passage of time of dark and lighted periods. Two hypothetical models have been described which may be involved in the measurement of day length. The first is based on the "hourglass" principle and involves some chemical that is synthesized during the day and broken down during the night and when the photoperiod is long enough, the chemical accumulates and triggers the hormonal induction of reproduction. The alternative hypothesis is based on the interactions of the light/dark cycle with an internal daily rhythm or clock, linked to either an external or internal coincidence model. The external coincidence model possibly involves pineal gland, the suprachiasmatic nucleus of the hypothalamus and the retina of the eye in an interlocking system (Figure 27.8). The daily cycle of light and dark entrains the circadian rhythm to exactly 24-hour and the daily rhythm is of sensitivity to light (photosensitivity) during a critical period of a few hours each day. When light is coincident with the sensitive phase, reproductive development occurs. The internal coincidence model involves two circadian rhythms-one is entrained by dawn and the second by dusk. As the day length changes, the two rhythms change in position relative to each other. When the correct alignment is achieved, the system is activated and causes the cascade release of GnRH, LH and FSH, and also of the gonadal steroids. Experimental evidence demonstrates the existence of "external coincidence model". However, it seems that different species may differ in the photoperiodic mechanisms involved in reproduction.

Photoperiodism in Hen: Reproductive potential of any animal depends on its genetic makeup and it is possible to alter it now by selective breeding (see chapter 25). However, in birds/poultry, the most important factor in attaining sexual maturity is an increasing day length (photoperiod) and is regulated by hypothalamus-pituitary axis. The strength of light above a very low level and the wavelength of light are not important in this regard. Photoperiodism or the 'effective length of light' in hen has a direct and major role to play in the,

- Attainment of sexual maturity in terms of age, and
- Ovulation

Sexual Maturity: It has been observed that around puberty, the hen become photosensitive. Light brings about the development of gonads in both the male and female sexes. The length of daylight must not be less than 16 hours and it should not exceed more than 17 hours. Fluctuation in the light – dark periods brings about ovulation in mature hen.

Ovulation: Hens lay eggs "in clutches". A clutch consist of a number of eggs which are laid daily (one egg/day) in wild hen until all the eggs of a clutch are laid and this brings a '**Pause Day**' when no eggs are laid and the next day beginning of next clutch starts. This phenomenon occurs continuously in a hen during ovulation:

Mechanism of Photoperiodism: Two distinct types of environmental influences determine seasonal breeding in birds and other animals. These are ultimate and proximate factors. The ultimate factors such as food, weather, reproductive readiness determines the optimal breeding season, while proximate factors trigger the development of gonads and secondary reproductive organs, to anticipate the breeding season.

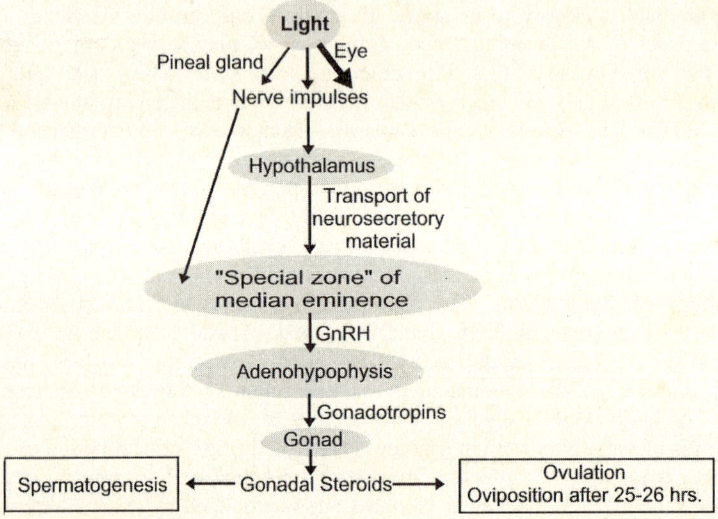

Figure 27.8: Schematic representation of the mechanism of photoperiodic stimulation of hormones resulting in spermatogenesis in Hen and ovulation in domestic Fowl.

In case of birds, day length is the prime proximate factor, and its increase in winter/spring promotes reproductive development in many avian species. Once the photoperiod has exceeded a critical number of hours, light rapidly (within 24 hours) exerts a stimulatory effect on both FSH and LH secretion as a result of increased hypothalamic drive and release of GnRH (Figure 27.8). The rate of gonadotropin secretion is proportional to both the intensity and length of the photoperiod up to a species-specific maximum. Gonadal growth and steroidogenesis are induced and facilitated by expression of positive gonadal steroid feedback and by the suppression of the negative feedback mechanism controlling gonadotropin release.

Soon after the first egg of a clutch is laid, LH brings about ovulation. It is stimulated by some neuroendocrine reflex, which in turn is stimulated by length of light period. This happens 60-90 minutes after the oviposition of one egg. This egg takes 24-26 hours in the shell-gland before it is laid the next day, after a 'lag' of about 2 hours than the previous day. The next ovulation starts around 60-90 minutes later and the process is continued until the LH surge happens to occur in light and therefore, due to some unknown phenomenon, the ovulation does not take place, this brings about the 'pause day' (Figure 27.7). Next ovulation occurs on next onset of dark. This is how the phenomenon of photoperiodism is explained by ovulation mechanism in hen.

27.5 Methods to Increase Egg-Production in Poultry

Total egg production depends on the length of the day period but rate of laying of egg is also important and this depends on the length of the sequence. For example, a fowl laying three-egg sequences can attain a maximum of 75 % egg production while the one having twenty four-egg sequences can reach to 96 %. Yet, there are a number of ways by which egg production can be increased in poultry farms. Proper care and management of poultry birds is one of the important factors in this. Care and management of birds in poultry farms is called **rearing** and this is carried out in large scale in commercial farms to help in increasing the egg production. The following does this:

- **Housing**: The housing of poultry must be clean, spacious and noise free,
- **Sanitation**: Proper sanitation conditions must be maintained to prevent diseases, healthy stock of hen must be used for better quality of eggs.
- **Watering**: Water must be provided at an approachable place and precautions should betaken to avoid spilling of water or leakage,
- **Lighting**: A proper lighting of 16 hours period must be provided to the hen, and care must be taken that light period should not exceed 17 hours,
- **Overcrowding**: Overcrowding must be avoided at all costs as it leads to poor egg quality and quantity in hen,
- **Feed**: A nutritious high protein, high calorie feed must be provided as ovulation and oviposition requires expenditure of a lot of energy. Nutritional deficiencies affect egg production and simultaneously, excessive amounts of certain substances may have deleterious effects on egg production. Feeding artifactual foodstuffs, such as drugs may be beneficial in certain cases. However, a balance must be maintained between therapeutic and toxic effects,
- **Calcium**: Calcium is involved not only in shell formation but also in regulating total egg production. Birds on a calcium-deficient diet produce eggs if given gonadotropin (as control of production of oocytes is through pituitary gonadotropin), but die due to severe skeletal defects.
- **Culling**: Proper culling and selection should be done and infected/ hostile animals must be removed from the stock as soon as possible to maintain health of other animals,
- **Debeaking**: Debeaking must be done properly to avoid breakage of eggs by the bird,
- **Routine Check-up**: The animals should be checked time to time for any communicable /non-communicable diseases,
- **Vaccination**: Animals should be vaccinated against any sort of communicable diseases as disease results in decreased egg production and increase in defective eggs,
- **Records**: A complete record of egg production, diseases and vaccination must be maintained,
- **TLC** or **Tender Loving Care**: The stock must be handled with love and care.

Eggs meant for hatching and rearing must be selected very carefully since the performance of the chicks produced depends on the quality of eggs. Incubation of eggs can be done by natural or artificial means to get best results followed by brooding or proper care of the new borne. Following features increase the frequency of egg laying in birds: These are, Early sexual maturity, Late molt, Persistency, Removal of eggs from nest, Increased light, Non-broodiness, and Short-winter-pause.

Rate of Egg Laying: Normally a hen lays one egg a day for several successive days before missing a day and this is called a **clutch**. The number of eggs laid in a clutch is heritable. Hens laying more eggs in a clutch produce more eggs than hens laying fewer eggs per clutch. Hens, which lay throughout the year are called **persistent layers** while the ones, which lay during a particular time of the year are the **seasonal layers**. Some birds enter a short non-laying period called **winter pause** consisting of 2-10 or 6-10 days. Good layers have high persistency and a very short winter pause. **Removal of eggs** from the nest increases the rate of egg laying. **Presence of eggs** in the nest switches off the pituitary secretion and stimulates the secretion of **prolactin**, which is responsible for the maternal instinct in hen. This leads to stoppage of egg laying and hen becomes **broody**.

Summary

Domestication of fowls and other birds for egg and meat production is termed as poultry. India had 114.4 million poultry birds which produced nearly 2120 million eggs during 1961-62, and by 1971, the number increased to about 139 million birds producing 6040 million eggs. Among different states in India, Andhra Pradesh produced the largest number of eggs followed by the West Bengal and Tamil Nadu.

Birds are Uni-polytocous animals in which many eggs are matured, but ovulated singly and laid in clutches.

Gonadal differentiation and oogenesis is completed before hatching. The reproductive system of the adult male and female birds are acquired after a period of somatic growth. Unlike mammalian species, the onset of puberty appears to be age-rather than size-related.

The onset of sexual maturity is usually triggered by the environmental stimuli, such as day length, light, temperature, food, social status, interactions etc. Photoperiod is a potent stimulator of sexual maturation.

Light may affect reproductive activity through at least three pathways. These are eyes, the pineal gland and through its direct effect on the hypothalamus. Relative importance of these three pathways is not known, but main one appears to be eye.

The reproductive activity is controlled by the brain in response to the neural information received about the external stimuli. This is reflected in gonadal steroid activity, which is indirectly controlled through the output of gonadotropin-releasing factor (GnRH) from the hypothalamus. GnRH regulates the synthesis and release of pituitary gonadotropins, FSH and LH, which in turn stimulate gonadal growth and steroidogenesis and LH results in ovulation.

The onset of sexual behavior normally occurs before attaining the adult levels of circulating gonadal steroids.

In adult bird, ovary is a large organ containing the developing yolk-filled follicles. This comprises a mass of very small follicle, a hierarchy of large developing ones, and those regressing after ovulation.

The wall of mature follicle is composed of several cell layers, involved in both hormone production and yolk deposition.

The timing of ovulation is strictly controlled and it normally occurs in the domestic fowl approximately 30 minutes following oviposition of the previous egg. Ovulation occurs every day in a sequence at progressively later times until a clutch of eggs is laid. Then there is a missed day, followed by another sequence of ovulation, starting at a similar time to the previous initial ovulation.

Oviposition is the process by which the egg is moved from the uterus through the vagina and hence to the exterior. The timing of oviposition is precisely controlled in the chicken, approximately 26 hour following ovulation and 30 minutes prior to the ovulation of the next ovum in the sequence. This control is very precise.

In addition to photoperiods, proper care and management is also very important in increasing egg production in poultry.

Questions

1. Discuss the ways by which egg production may be increased in poultry.
2. Discuss the role of photoperiods in egg production.

Acronym

A (A^0)	Angstrom unit(s) (10^{-10}m.0.1nm)
ABP	Androgen binding protein
ACh	Acetylcholine
ACTH	Adrenocorticotropic hormone
ADH	Antidiuretic hormone (vasopressin)
AH	Assisted Hatching
AI	Artificial Insemination
AID	Artificial Insemination by Donor
AIH	Artificial Insemination with Husband's sperm
ANF	Atrial natriuretic factor
AMH	Anti-Mullerian hormone (Mullerian duct inhibitor)
cAMP	3',5'-Cyclic adenosine monophosphate/Cyclic AMP
ARE	Androgen response element
ASF	Acrosome stabilizing Factor
A-Z test,	Aschheim-Zondek test ("mouse test"), a pregnancy test
CBG	Corticosteroid-binding globulin
CG	Chorionic gonadotropin
CT	Cytoplasmic Transfer
cGMP	3',5'-Guanonosine monophosphate/Cyclic GMP
CLIP	Corticotropin-like intermediate lobe peptide
CRH	Corticotropin-releasing hormone
CS	Chorionic somatomammotropin; Placental lactogen
DES	Diethylstilbesterol
DHEA	Dehydroepiandrosterone
DHT	Dihydrotestosterone
DIFI	Direct Intrafollicular Insemination
DIPI	Direct Intraperitoneal Insemination
DOT	Direct Oocyte Transfer
E_1	Estrone
E_2	Estradiol
E_3	Estriol
EBPS	Estrogen binding proteins
EGF	Epidermal growth factor
EIPs	Estrogen induced proteins
EPF	Early pregnancy factor
ER	Estrogen receptor
EREs	Estrogen response elements
ERT	Estrogen replacement therapy
ET	Embryo Transfer
FDA	Food & Drug Administration
FET	Frozen Embryo Transfer
FGF	Fibroblast growth factor

FSP	Fallopian Tube Sperm Perfusion
FSH	Follicle-stimulating hormone
FSHRH	Follicle-stimulating hormone-releasing hormone
GAP	GnRH-associated peptide
GH	Growth hormone
GHRH/GRH	Growth hormone-releasing hormone
GHRIH	Growth hormone release-inhibiting hormone; Somatostatin
GIFT	Gamete Intrafallopian Transfer
GnRH/ LRH	Gonadotropin-releasing hormone, Gonadoliberin
GUT	Gamete Uterine Transfer
HCG/hCG	Human chorioic gonadotropin
HCS/hCS	Human chorionic somatomammotropin
hGH	Human growth hormone
HMG	Human menopausal gonadotropin
hPL	Human placental lactogen
hCS	Human chorionic sommatomamotropin
HPA	Hypothalamic-pituitary-adrenal
hPRL	Human prolactin
hPUTH	Human placental uterotropic hormone
HRE	Hormone regulatory element
ICI	Intracervical Insemination
ICSI	Intracytoplasmic Sperm Injection
IFI	Intrafallopian Insemination
IGF	Insulin-like growth factor
IPI	Intraperitoneal Insemination
IUGR	Intauterine growth retardation
IUI	Intrauterine Insemination
IVF/ET	*In Vitro* Fertilization/Embryo Transfer
IZF	Intrazonal Fertilization
LH	Luteinizing hormone
LHRH	Luteinizing hormone-releasing hormone
LPH	Lipotropin
LRH	Luteotropin-releasing hormone
LTH	Luteotropic hormone
MEN	Mutiple endocrine neoplasia
MESA	Microsurgical epididymal sperm aspiration
MIF	Mullerian inhibiting factor
MMTV	Murine mammary tumor virus
MOET	Multiple Ovulation and Embryo Transfer
MRF	Melanocyte-releasing factor
MRH	Melanocyte release-inhibiting hormone
MRI	Magnetic resonance imaging
MRIH	Melanocyte-releasing factor
MSA	Multiplicatio-stimulating activity
MSH	Melanocyte-stimulating hormone
NGF	Nerve growth factor
3ß-OHSD	3ß-Hydroxysteroid dehydrogenase
17ß-OHSD	17ß- Hydroxysteroid dehydrogenase
PCR	Polymerase chain reaction

PG	Prostaglandin
PgR	Progesterone receptor
PMSG	Pregnant Mare Serum Gonadotropin
PL	Placental lactogen
POST	Peritoneal Oocyte and Sperm Transfer
PRH	Prolactin releasing hormone
PRIH/PIH	Prolactin release-inhibiting hormone
PRL	Prolactin
PROST	Pronuclear Stage Tubal Transfer
PSA	Prostate-specific antigen
PTH	Parathyroid hormone
PZD	Partial Zona Dissection
QCT	Quantitative computer-assisted tomography
ROSNI or ROSI	Microinjection of round spermatid nuclei injection into oocytes
SCNT	Somatic Cell Nuclear Transfer (reproductive cloning)
SHBG	Sex hormone-binding globulin
SIFT	Sperm Intrafallopian Transfer (Transvaginal)
SRIH	Somatostatin/Somatotropin release-inhibiting hormone
SRY	Sex-determining region on the Y chromosome
STD	Sexually Tansmitted Diseases
SUZI or SZI	Subzonal Sperm Injection
T_3	Triiodothyronine
T_4	Thyroxine; Tetraiodothyronine
TBG	Thyroid-binding globulin
TDF	Testis-determinig factor
TDI	Therapeutic Donor Insemination
TEBG	Testosterone-estrogen-binding globulin
TESA	Testicular Sperm Aspiration
TESE	Testicular Sperm Extraction
TEST	Tubal Embryo Stage Transfer
TET	Tubal Embryo Transfer
Tfm	Testicular feminization
TFNA	Testicular Fine Needle Aspiration
TIFT	Transcervical Intrafallopian Transfer
TRH	Thyrotropin-releasing hormone
TSH	Thyroid-stimulating hormone; Thyrotropin
TUFT	Transuterine Fallopian Transfer
TV-TEST	Trans-Vaginal Intratubal Embryo Stage Transfer
VIP	Vasoactive intestinal polypeptide
ZIFT	Zygote Intrafallopian Transfer
ZP	Zona Pellucida
ZPG	Zero Population Growth

Glossary

Abortifacient	Any agent that involves expulsion of an embryo or immature fetus.
Abortion	Spontaneous or artificially induced expulsion of an embryo or immature fetus.
Acromegaly	Endocrine disorders caused by excessive secretion of growth hormone.
Acrosome	The apical portion of male sperm, it permits penetration of the ovum.
Acrosome reaction	Chemical and morphological changes in the head of a capacitated spermatozoon, with release of enzymes, that precedes and is essential for fertilization.
Addison's disease	Severe adrenocortical hormone deficiency.
Adrenalectomy	Surgical removal of the adrenal glands.
Anestrus	Absence of estrus cycles.
Agonist	Any compound, such as a drug that can activate a receptor.
Androgens	The male sex steroid hormones, principally testosterone.
Anti-androgens	Agents that oppose the effects of male type gonadal steroid hormones.
Antidiuretic hormone	A hormone released from the posterior pituitary that controls water permeability in the kidneys.
Anti-estrogens	Agents that block estrogen action.
Arachidonic acid	A phospholipid whose synthesis is activated by many hormones and neurotransmitters.
Azoospermia	Inability or failure to produce spermatozoa.
Blastocyst	A hollow sphere of cells in the early stages of embryogenesis.
Capacitation	In reproduction, the ability of sperm to fertilize an ovum.
Castration	Gonadectomy, removal of testes.
Chimera	An individual with some cells of one genetic type and some of another.
Climacteric	In women, the symptoms and the endocrine events associated with cessation of ovarian cycles and continues through completion of menopause
Climax	Peak, the highest point of sexual excitement.
Clitoris	The female homologue of a part of the penis.
Clomiphene	2-chloro-1, 2-diphenylvinyl phenoxy triethylamine, a non-steroidal anti-estrogenic agent.
Clone	Genetically identical progeny of a single parent cell.
Colostrum	The yellowish, watery secretion, low in lipid content and devoid of lactose, produced by eutherian mammary glands shortly before and for 1-2 days after parturition.
Corpus albicans	A white body, usually scar-like that is formed after copus luteum degenerates.
Corpus luteum	A yellowish body, usually formed from emptied ovarian follicle after ovulation.
Cortical reaction	A process that occurs in an oocyte soon after fertilization and zona reaction, as an initial response to sperm penetration.
Cretinism	A condition caused by thyroid hormone deficiency that begins during infancy.
Cryopreservation	Cooling embryos, gametes, or other organisms to maintain them in dormant state from which they can be returned to normal functions when rewarmed.

Cryoprotectant	Glycerol, dimethylsulfoxide (DMSO), and other substances used to prevent the formation of ice crystals when organisms, chemical, or specimens for microscopy are frozen.
Cryptorchidism	Retention of testes within the abdominal cavities in humans and other species.
Cushing's disease	Disorders in which excessive production of glucocorticoids is stimulated by adrenocorticotropic hormone.
Decidua	The endometrial tissue that borders the uterine lumen.
Defeminization	Masculinization, loss of an "inherent" tendency to acquire or display feminine characteristics.
Depo-Provera	A trade name for medroxyprogesterone, a hormonal contraceptive.
Down-regulation	A decrease in receptor density caused by the binding of a hormone, neurotransmitter, or neuromodulator to a cell
Dwarfism	Stunted growth caused by a deficiency of growth hormone.
Dysmenorrhea	Painful menstruation.
Dyspareunia	Persistent genital pain in women, during and following coitus.
Ectopic pregnancy	Pregnancy in which implantation occurs at a site other than the uterus.
Ejaculation	Rapid discharge, usually of semen.
Embryo	An organism in early stages of development.
Endometriosis	An inflamatory condition in which endometrial tissue occurs and grows atypically in the pelvic cavity.
Embryo transfer	Artificial insertion of one or more young embryos into the oviduct or uterus.
Epididymis	The male reproductive tract between the sites of sperm production and the vas deferens.
Erection	Swelling of the penis caused by its engorgement with blood.
Estrogen	Naturally occurring 18-carbon steroid hormones with aromatic rings and synthetic agents that invokes similar response.
Estrous cycles	Ovarian cycles of subprimates.
Estrus	The phase of estrous cycle (heat period).
Exocrine	Secretion in the direction of free surface.
Fecundation	To make fertile, artificial fecundation is artificial insemination.
Fecundity	Reproductive potential, numbers of gametes produced.
Feedback control	Regulation of one component of a reaction system by another of the same system.
Ferning	Formation of leaf-like patterns in uterine cervix mucus collected during the estrogen-dominated perifollicular phase of a menstrual cycle, dried on a glass slide or cover slip, and viewed under a light microscope, used as an indicator of the timing of ovarian cycle phases.
Fertilization	Syngamy, union of two gametes to form a zygote.
Fertilization cone	A pointed projection from an oocyte surface that forms at the site of entry of a spermatozoon.
Fertilization potential	The change in the electrical properties of an oocyte plasma membrane that occurs almost immediately after fertilization, it confers protection against polyspermy.
Fertilization site	Place where the sperm and oocyte unite.
Fetation	Intrauterine fetal growth and development.
Feticide	Killing or destruction of a fetus usually by artificial means.
Fetoplacental unit	A complex formed from placental and fetal components across which nutrients, respiratory gases, metabolites, and regulators are exchanged.

Fetus	A conceptus that has acquired the morphological features characteristic of its species.
Follicle	In the ovaries, the structure containing the ovum, granulosa cells, follicular cells, and theca cells.
Follicular phase	The phase of the menstrual cycle that precedes ovulation.
Freemartin	A virilized or hermaphroditic calf with female type (XX) chromosomes, whose abnormal development is attributed to Mullerian duct inhibitor, testis determining antigen, and/or other factors released prenatally by a normal male twin fetus that shares the same placental circulation. In most freemartins, the gonads are ovotestes.
Freeze drying	Lyophilization, technique for preserving hormones, vaccines and other biological materials.
Galli-Mainini test	"Frog" test for pregnancy.
Gelding	A castrated horse.
Genital hypoplasia	It is the incomplete development of the genital organs.
Genitalia	Genitals, usually the externally visible reproductive organs.
Germ cells	Gametes, spermatozoa and ova.
Gestagens	Progestins.
Gestation period	The time normally required to complete prenatal development.
Gigantism	An abnormal increase in body size caused by excess growth hormone.
Gilt	A young female swine, especially one that has not produced a litter.
Gonad	Any organ specialized for the production of gametes.
Gonadectomy	Surgical removal of the gonads, it can be orchidectomy or ovariectomy.
Gonarche	Initiation of spermatogenesis, or of ovarian cycles at puberty.
Gonadotropic hormone	A generic term that includes the anterior pituitary hormones FSH and LH.
Gonadotropin releasing hormone (GnRH)	The hypothalamic releasing factor that controls the secretion of FSH and LH from the anterior pituitary.
Granulosa cells	Cells in the ovary that nurture the ovum.
Gravida	A pregnant woman.
Growth hormone	An anterior pituitary hormone that has widespread effects on growth, development, and organic metabolism.
Gynecomastia	Breast enlargement in males.
Gynecology	Specialized branch of medicine that deals with the diagnosis and treatment of female reproductive system disorders.
Gynogenesis	A type of sexual reproduction, in which spermatozoa activate oocytes, but do not contribute genetic components to the embryo (Parthenogenesis).
Hemicastration	Removal of one testicle or ovary.
Hermaphrodite	An individual with gonads that produce both male and female type gametes.
Hermaphroditism	It is often termed as intersex and is a combination of both sex characters, i.e. the genitalia may resemble to certain degree to male type and also to female type.
Hirsutism	Excessive growth of hair, especially in women.
Hormones	A term initially applied to specialized organic molecule endocrine glands and transported via the bloodstream to distantly located target organs.
HCG	Human chorionic gonadotropin, a placental hormone that maintains the corpus luteum during pregnancy
Hydatid mole	Developmental abnormality of the placenta.
Hyperplasia	Increased growth of a tissue or organ by proliferation of the cell types normally present in that location.

Hypertrophy	Excessive growth via enlargement, but not proliferation of the cells of an organ or tissue.
Hypophysectomy	Surgical removal of the pituitary gland.
Hypothalamus	The region of the brain that controls the release of hormones from the pituitary.
Hysterectomy	Surgical removal of the uterus.
Implantation	Blastocyst penetration into and interaction with endometrial cells (Nidation).
Impotence	Inability to achieve penile erection and ejaculation.
Impregnation	The act of making pregnant.
Inanition	Inadequate intake of one or more nutrients.
Insemination	Delivery of spermatozoa to female reproductive tracts.
Intersex	An individual of a bisexual species that has characteristics intermediate between those of a female and a male.
Kallman's syndrome	Delayed puberty due to gonadotropin deficiency as a result of GnRH deficiency.
Labor	Parturition.
Lactation	Milk synthesis and release.
Lactogenesis	Milk synthesis.
Lactogens	Agents that stimulate mammary gland stimulation and/or milk production.
Lactoglandin	A neurophysin-like protein made in mammary glands.
Laparoscopy	Examination of the abdomino-pelvic cavity with a laparoscope.
Laparotomy	Surgical incision through the abdomen, usually to gain access to the peritoneal cavity and its components.
Lee-Boot effect	Suppression or prolongation of ovarian cycles of mice and some other rodent species when females are housed in groups and isolated from males.
Leydig cells	Cells in the male reproductive system that secrete testosterone.
Legal sex	The gender officially assigned to an individual usually at the time of birth, and usually on the basis of phenotype.
LH surge	The rapid, massive release of luteinizing hormone (LH) that precedes, and is essential for ovulation, mediated primarily by a rapid rise in luteinizing hormone releasing hormone levels in most species with estrous cycles.
Libido	Sexual interest or desires or drive.
Lordosis	The characteristic posture assumed by females in response to vulval stimulation during receptive phase of estrous cycles.
Lordosis quotient	Mount ratio, within a specified tie period, the number of lordosis responses to stimulation, divided by number of mounts by a nonspecific males.
Luteal phase	In the menstrual cycle, the phase immediately after ovulation and before menstruation.
Lutectomy	Removal of one or more corpora lutea.
Luteinization	Morphological changes associated with conversion of an emptied Graafian follicle to a corpus luteum and/or the biochemical changes associated with acquisition of the ability to secrete large amounts of progesterone.
Luteolysins	Physiological or pharmacological agents that promote corpus luteum degeneration.
Luteolysis	Corpus luteum demise.
Luteomas	Tumors comprising hyperplastic luteal cells.
Luteotropin	Luteinizing hormone.
Mammary glands	Epithelium-derived glands of mammals that produce milk when prepared by sufficient amounts of hormones presented in the right sequences, and others that sustain the function.

Mammogenesis	Mammary gland development.
Menarche	The onset of menstruation.
Menopause	Cessation of ovarian and menstrual cycles.
Menorrhagia	Excessive blood loss during menstruation.
Menorrhea	The blood loss associated with normal menstrual cycles.
Menstrual cycle	A monthly cycle of ovulation and menstruation in the female.
Menstruation	The monthly shedding of the uterine lining.
Mestranol	17α-ethinylestradiol 3-methyl ether, an orally effective estrogen receptor agonist.
Metafemale	Superfemale.
Minipills	Oral contraceptive preparations that contain progestins but no estrogens.
Mittelschmerz	Slight to severe back pains halfway through the cycle, indicating ovulation.
Monogamy	The reproductive pattern in which one male and one female form an exclusive, stable mating pair.
Monospermy	Fertilization by a single spermatozoon.
Morning after contraceptives	Agents taken postcoitally to avoid pregnancy.
Mullerian duct	The structure in the embryonic gonad that gives rise to the fallopian tubes, uterus, and proximal vagina in the female.
Neuroendocrine	A term referring to the control of pituitary hormone release by the central nervous system.
Neuromodulator	A substance that acts to alter the effect of a neurotransmitter.
Neurotransmitter	A chemical released by a neuron that activates specific receptors on a second neuron, muscle cell, or gland.
Nonsteroidal estrogens	Substances other than steroids that bind to estrogen receptors and mimic the effects of the hormones, e.g. diethylstilbesterol.
Nurse cells	Cells that support the survival, differentiation, and/or functions of other cells, e.g. Sertoli cells.
Oocyesis	Ovarian pregnancy
Ootid	A mature ovum.
Oophorectomy	Ovariectomy, surgical removal of the ovary.
Orchitis	Inflammation of the testes.
Oschea	Scrotum.
Ovarian aplasia	It is the absence of ovary.
Ovarian dysgenesis	Faulty or incomplete ovarian development.
Ovarian hypoplasia	Incomplete development of ovary.
Ovariectomy	Oophorectomy, surgical removal of ovaries.
Ovary	The female gonad.
Ovulation	The release of a mature ovum from its follicle.
Oxytocin	A posterior pituitary hormone that causes uterine contractions and milk let-down.
Pampiniform plexus	A tendril-like arrangement of blood vessels.
Panhypopituitarism	Deficiency of all adenohypophysial or of all pituitary gland hormones.
Parabiosis	Surgical joining of two animals.
Parathyroid glands	Glands near the thyroid that secrete parathyroid hormone.
Parathyroidectomy	Surgical removal of the parathyroid glands.
Persistent estrus (PE)	Constant estrus.
Photoperiodism	Regularly recurring responses of living organisms to cyclical changes in the wavelengths, intensities, and/or duration of environmental light.

Pituitary gland	An endocrine gland located below the hypothalamus.
Placenta	The organ that develops from maternal and fetal tissue and serves as an interface between the maternal and fetal circulation.
Placental lactogens	Somatomammotropins.
Polyandry	Reproductive strategies in which females mate with more than one male.
Polycystic ovary (PCO)	Several disorders in which the ovarian stroma hypertrophies and produces excessive amounts of androgens.
Polyestrous	Having more than one estrous cycle per season.
Polygamy	Polyandry or polygyny, mating with more than one partner.
Polygalactia	Excessive milk production.
Polymastia	Presence of more than the usual number of mammary glands.
Polymenorrhea	Too frequent menstrual cycles, metrorrhagia.
Polyspermy	Fertilization of an oocyte by more than one spermatozoon.
Polythelic	Having more than the usual number of breast nipples.
Polytocous	Giving birth to multiple young following a single pregnancy.
Polythelia	It means extra teats, and these extra teats may be located in between the normal teats when they are called as intercalary.
Post-coital contraceptives	Agents that promote extrusion of newly formed conceptuses and/or block implantation.
Post coitum	After mating.
Posterior pituitary	The region of the pituitary gland that secretes ADH and oxytocin.
Precocious puberty	Sexual maturation at an earlier age than is characteristic for the species.
Pregnancy	The condition of a mother from the time of conception or implantation to parturition.
Premenstrual syndrome	PMS, severe distress that recurs regularly in some women during the late luteal phases of their menstrual cycles.
Priming	In endocrinology, stimulation of synthesis of the receptor by one hormone for another.
Progesterone	A female sex steroid, secreted by the corpus luteum, and placenta and affects uterine development.
Prolactin	One of the anterior pituitary hormones, it stimulates milk secretion by the mammary glands.
Proliferative phase	In the menstrual cycle, the phase before ovulation during which the endometrium of the uterus is increasing in thickness.
PROST	Pronuclear ovum stage transfer, an *in vitro* fertilization procedure.
Prostaglandins	A group of modified fatty acids that act as chemical messengers.
Prostate	A gland in the male that secretes fluid in the urethra.
Prostatein	A steroid binding prostate gland protein.
Protogyny	A form of sequential hermaphroditism.
Pseudohermaphroditism	More common in man with testes in abdominal cavity or beneath the skin in scrotal region, external genitalia resembles female with enlarged clitoris, vulval configuration and urination in dorsal arc.
Pseudopregnancy	Condition in which symptoms associated with pregnancy occur in females that are not carrying conceptuses.
Pubarche	The first menstruation of sexual maturation.
Puberty	Attainment of the ability to produce mature gametes.
Raphe	A visible site where bilateral structures have joined.
Salpingectomy	Removal of fallopian tubes.
Salpingitis	Inflammation of the uterine tubes.

Secretory phase	In the menstrual cycle, the period between ovulation and menstruation during which the uterine lining develops a secretory characteristics.
Segmental aplasia	It is a complete or partial absence of one or both Wolffian ducts.
Seminal plasmin	A 5.4K enzyme in seminal fluid that contacts sperm at the time of ejaculation, inhibits sperm motility and acrosome reactions, and can also block RNA synthesis.
Seminal vesicles	Glands that secrete fluid into the vas deferens in males.
Seminiferous growth Factor (SGF)	A 15.7K acidic peptide made in large amounts by prepubertal Sertoli cells.
Seminiferous tubules	It is the sites of sperm production in the males.
Sertoli cells	In the male, the cells that line the seminiferous tubules and "nurture" sperm maturation.
Sertoli cell factor (SCF)	Factors controlling Sertoli cell functions, e.g. inhibins, SGF.
Sex determination	Mechanisms whereby an individual acquires the gonad type characteristic of one gender of the species.
Sex differentiation	Changes in cells of indifferent gonads that lead to formation of embryonic testes or fetal ovaries.
Sex factor	Fertility factor also called F factor.
Sex ratio	The relative numbers of males and females in a population.
Sex reversal	A change to gonadal sex function of the opposite gender.
Sex steroids	Steroids produced by gonads, e.g estrogens, progesterone, testosterone.
Sex steroid binding globulin (SSBG)	Plasma proteins that bind steroids with high affinity but differ from hormone receptors, also called Sex hormone binding globulin (SHBG), Testosterone-estrogen binding globulin (TeBP).
Sex vesicle	Germinal vesicle.
Somatomammotropes	Placental lactogens.
Sperm	A single spermatozoon or sperm cell.
Spermacrasia	Abnormally low numbers of sperm in ejaculates.
Spermateliosis	Spermatid maturation to spermatozoa, also called Spermiogenesis.
Spermatid	One or two small, round, haploid cells formed when a secondary spermatocyte completes meiosis.
Spermatogenesis	It is a process that converts diploid sperm cell to an immature spermatozoon.
Spermatocides	Spermicides, agents that kill spermatozoa.
Spermatocoele	A cyst in the scrotum that contains spermatozoa, formed when seminiferous tubules are partially obstructed.
Spermatocytogenesis	Differentiation of primary spermatocytes from spermatogonia.
Spermatolysins	Spermolysins, agents that destroy sperm plasma membranes.
Sperm capacitation	The final stage in the preparation of spermatozoa for acrosome reactions. It usually proceeds in the uterus or oviduct, and involves changes in the cell surfaces and the release of enzymes.
Spermiation	Extrusion of fully formed spermatozoa from Sertoli cells, along with some testicular fluid.
Spermiogenesis	Spermatid maturation to spermatozoa.
Spinnbarkeit	The tendency for uterine cervical mucus to form threads when stretched between two glass slides or coverslips.
Spontaneous ovulators	Animals in which ovarian cycles are endogenously controlled, and mating stimuli are not required for ovulation.
Sterilization	Surgical removal or destruction of organs required for reproduction, such as gonadectomy, vasectomy, or salpingectomy.
Steroid hormones	Hormones with steroid-type structure.

Steroidogenesis	Biosynthesis of steroid hormones.
Stratified	In layers, as in stratified epithelium.
Streak gonads	Ovaries or testes that have never completed development.
Suckling reflex	Responses initiated in the mother when a suckling infant stimulates nerve endings in the nipple region that communicate with hypothalamic neurons.
Superfecundation	Fertilization, after a single ovulation, of more than the usual numbers of oocytes
Superfemale	A female mammal with more than two X (but no Y) chromosomes.
Superfetation	Formation of large numbers of fetuses than can be accomplished by the uterus and carried through the gestation period or fertilization of a second oocyte released when a fetus is undergoing prenatal development.
Symphysis pubis	Joint between the pubic bones.
Symptothermal methods	Modifications of rhythm method for contraception to detect ovulation time.
Syndrome	The signs, symptoms and other characteristics of a disease.
Syngamy	Union of gametes.
Testibumin	A Sertoli cell protein chemically related to albumin and α-fetoprotein, induced by follicle stimulating hormone (FSH) and testosterone.
Testicular feminization	A sex differentiation disorder caused by androgen receptor defects that block the ability to respond to testosterone and dihydrotestosterone.
Testicular hypoplasia	Underdevelopment of seminal epithelium, resulting in markedly smaller, freely movable and palpable testis in the scrotal sac.
Testins	Two related proteins made by Sertoli cells of testes that contain germinalcells.
Testes	The male gonads.
Testis determining antigens/genes/factor (TDA)	DNA segment on Y chromosomes that initiate masculinization of mammalian embryos.
Testosterone	The main male sex hormone secreted by the testes.
Thecal cells	A type of cell found in the ovaries.
Thymectomy	Surgical removal of the thymus gland.
Thyroid gland	A gland in the neck that secretes thyroid hormone.
Thyroidectomy	Surgical removal of the thyroid gland.
Trimester	A three month period; for some purposes, human pregnancy is divided into first, second and third trimesters.
Tropic	Going toward, can be used as a suffix as in gonadotropic.
-Tropin	A suffix for agents that go toward a structure as in thyrotropin.
Tuber cinereum	A mass of grey matter that forms part of the floor of the third ventricle of the brain and is continuous with the infundibular stalk.
Turner's syndrome	Sex differentiation disorder associated with X chromosome defects.
Ultrasonography	Use of sound waves of with frequencies above the range detectable by human ears. It is a noninvasive technique that uses sound waves to visualize the position and size of the fetus and placenta.
Umbilicus	The structure that marks the former placenta attachment site.
Up-regulation	An increase in receptor density caused by the presence of a hormone.
Urethra	The tube that connects the bladder with the exterior.
Urogenital sinus	An embryonic structure that give rise to most of the vagina in females and to prostate glands in males.
Urogenital swellings	Embryonic structures that fuse to form the scrotum in males and give rise to labia majora in females.
Uterine	Derived from or characteristic of the uterus.

Uterine cervix	Distal end of uterus that projects into the vagina through which spermatozoa enter and neonates are expelled.
Uterine "milk"	Fluids secreted by endometrial cells during pregnancy in some mammals to provide nutrients for and prolong the survival of preimplantation blastocysts.
Uterine tubes	Fallopian tubes or oviducts.
Uterotropic	Going toward, or stimulatory to the uterus.
Uterus	Hollow female reproductive organs specialized in mammals for implantation, nurturing of conceptuses and parturition.
Vagina	The muscular canal connecting the female uterus with the exterior of the abdomen.
Varicocele	Abnormally dilated spermatic cord veins, usually painful, and associated with oligospermia.
Vas deferens	Muscular tube on each side of the body in the male reproductive system between the epididymis and the urethra.
Vasectomy	Ligation or insertion of plugs or valves into vasa deferentia to block sperm delivery to the ejaculate.
Vasovasostomy	Surgical anastomosis of the vas deferens following post-vasectomy.
Viable	Capable of survival, term applied to fetuses sufficiently mature to survive outside the uterus
Viability test	Determination of the numbers of surviving organisms of a species or cell type relative to others, under specified conditions
Viviparous	Live-bearing, females giving birth to living young ones that can survive without protective coats and stored nutrients.
Vulva	Region that includes labia majora, labia minora, vaginal vestibule and vaginal orifice of the female mammal external genitalia.
Wether	A gonadectomized lamb.
White heifer disease	It is due to arrested development of the Mullerian duct system, the uterus and the vagina are incompletely developed but the ovaries and the vulva are always normal.
Whitten effect	Induction of regular ovarian cycles in female mice and some other rodents whose cycles have become lengthened, irregular, or arrested following confinement in group cages in the absence of males, by introduction of an adult male of the species.
Witch's milk	A milk-like fluid released by the mammary glands of neonates.
Wolffian duct	Part of the embryonic gonad that develops into the male reproductive ducts, and disappears in the female.
XO	Turner's syndrome, second X chromosome is usually lost by nondisjunction during gametogenesis.
XX	Normal sex chromosome pattern for females.
XXX	Superfemales.
XXXY/XXXYY	Abnormal sex chromosome pattern.
XXY	Abnormal sex chromosome pattern associated with Klinefelter's disease.
Yellow body	Corpus luteum, the term is appropriate for women and many other vertebrates, but the structures are not yellow in all species.
ZIFT	Zygote intrafallopian tube transfer, a technique used for couples with fertility problems.
Zinc fingers	Components of many proteins, composed of two pairs of cysteinyl moieties that chelate zinc, the group includes receptors for steroid hormones.

Zinc fingers	Components of many proteins, composed of two pairs of cysteinyl moieties that chelate zinc, the group includes receptors for steroid hormones.
Zona pellucida (ZP)	A clear non-cellular layer on the surface of an oocyte, zygote or blastocyst secreted by stratum granulose cells.
Zona pellucida proteins	Species specific glycoproteins that contribute to fertilization and the events that soon follow, ZP1, ZP2, and ZP3 are present in relative amounts.
Zona reaction	Changes in the surface of a fertilized secondary oocyte initiated by the cortical reaction.
Zoogonous	Viviparous.
Zoosperm	Spermatozoan
Zuclomiphene	The cis form of clomiphene, a mixed estrogen receptor agonist or antagonist.
Zygote	The diploid cell that forms soon after an oocyte is fertilized.

Index